Imaging of the Airways
Functional and Radiologic Correlations

Imaging of the Airways Functional and Radiologic Correlations

EDITORS

DAVID P. NAIDICH, MD
Professor of Radiology
Department of Radiology
NYU Medical Center
New York, New York

W. RICHARD WEBB, MD
Professor of Radiology
Chief, Thoracic Imaging
University of California, San Francisco
San Francisco, California

PHILIPPE A. GRENIER, MD
Professor of Radiology
Chairman of the Department of Radiology
Pitié-Salpêtrière Hospital
Université Pierre et Marie Curie
Paris, France

TIMOTHY J. HARKIN, MD
Assistant Professor of Medicine
Division of Pulmonary and Critical Care Medicine
Director of Bronchoscopy
Department of Medicine
NYU Medical Center
New York, New York

WARREN B. GEFTER, MD
Professor of Radiology
Chief, Thoracic Imaging Section
Associate Chair, Department of Radiology
Hospital of the University of Pennsylvania
Philadelphia, Pennsylvania

LIPPINCOTT WILLIAMS & WILKINS
A **Wolters Kluwer** Company
Philadelphia • Baltimore • New York • London
Buenos Aires • Hong Kong • Sydney • Tokyo

Acquisitions Editor: Lisa McAllister
Managing Editor: Kerry Barrett
Developmental Editor: Luzselenia Loeb
Project Manager: Fran Gunning
Manufacturing Manager: Ben Rivera
Marketing Manager: Angela Panetta
Production Services: Nesbitt Graphics, Inc.
Printer: Quebecor World Kingsport

530 Walnut Street
Philadelphia, PA 19106 USA
LWW.com

Printed in the USA

Cover image of lung, courtesy of Ewald R. Weibel, MD, DSc. Used with permission.

Library of Congress Cataloging-in-Publication Data
Imaging of the airways : functional and radiologic correlations / David P. Naidich ... [et al.].
p. ; cm.
Includes bibliographical references and index.
ISBN 0-7817-5768-1
1. Airway (Medicine)—Imaging. I. Naidich, David P. [DNLM: 1. Diagnostic Techniques, Respiratory System. 2. Diagnostic Imaging. 3. Respiratory Tract Diseases—diagnosis. WF 141 I31 2005]
RC734.I43I46 2005
616.2'004754—dc22

2005002295

10 9 8 7 6 5 4 3 2 1

Dedication

To Our Wives:

Jocelyn, Teresa, Harmony, Dominique, and Marlene

Contents

Preface

During the past decade an ever-accelerating revolution has been taking place in imaging technology. Most important, this includes the introduction and now widespread availability of both multidetector CT scanners that use 4, 8, 16, and now even 64 detectors, as well as positron emission tomography (PET), including combined PET–CT scanners. Opening new vistas in evaluating thoracic disease, their use now constitutes an essential aspect of routine clinical care. In addition, a host of new imaging techniques are being developed, including the exciting prospect of employing agents such as hyperpolarized helium to noninvasively evaluate airway physiology using magnetic resonance imaging.

In this same period, equally important advances have been made in both diagnostic and especially therapeutic bronchoscopy. Interventional techniques for the relief of airway obstruction caused by endobronchial lesions, in particular, have rapidly evolved and multiplied. This includes, among others, the use of photodynamic therapy, cryotherapy, electrocautery, balloon dilatation, and argon plasma coagulation. Additionally, the science of airway stenting has continued to evolve, enhancing the ability to maintain airway patency once the obstruction has been relieved. Along with surgery, radiation therapy, and chemotherapy, interventional bronchoscopy now legitimately is one of the mainstays for treating endobronchial malignancy. In addition to these techniques, parallel advances in airway visualization have also taken place, including the introduction of ultrathin bronchoscopes, autofluorescence bronchoscopy, and the evolving field of endobronchial sonography.

Given these developments a text specifically dedicated to evaluating airway disease is clearly needed and, in particular, a text that takes a global approach by emphasizing the relative contributions of all currently available technologies to the evaluation and treatment of patients with airway abnormalities. It is our contention that only by assessing the relative merits of these techniques in relation to each other can we hope to optimize patient care. To this end we have combined the talents of experts in the complementary fields of radiology and bronchoscopy to write this volume.

Chapter 1 is devoted to the basic principles of imaging, including a detailed review of bronchial anatomy. Chapter 2 includes a detailed assessment of the relationship between CT and bronchoscopic visualization of airway lesions and is followed by individual chapters devoted to specific anatomic portions of the bronchial tree. Chapter 3 includes an in-depth review of lesions involving the trachea and mainstem bronchi, and Chapter 4 is a thorough review of the role of imaging for assessing bronchiectasis. Chapter 5 is devoted to the evaluation of small airway disease. This is especially appropriate given the huge impact that high-resolution CT has made in recent years to the diagnosis of this remarkably varied entity. Finally, Chapter 6 is dedicated to the rapidly emerging field of physiologic airway imaging. Although still in their infancy, it is not overoptimistic to envision these novel techniques as someday becoming indispensable in routine clinical care.

We hope that this volume will serve both as an introduction to those first approaching imaging and as a thorough review for more knowledgeable readers. The continued rapid evolution in our understanding of imaging technologies is a great challenge to us as authors and clinicians, made all the more pressing by the need to address these clinical issues on a daily basis. We hope that this volume will ultimately make this task easier for all.

Acknowledgments

We wish to acknowledge all those in our many institutions—especially our Residents and Fellows—who so generously gave of their time and energy to contribute to the completion of this text.

We would also like to extend special recognition to the following individuals.

From New York University Medical Center, New York

We wish to thank Drs. Doreen Addrizzo-Harris, Ioannis Vlahos, Jane Ko, Ami Rubinowitz, Barry Leitman, and Georgeann McGuinness for their assistance in developing this text. A special thanks is also extended to Dr. Ed Lubat at the Hackensack Hospital, New Jersey, for his generous contributions to this text. We also extend our most sincere thanks to the many CT technologists so instrumental in insuring the highest possible image quality, including: Emilio Vega, Bernhard Assadourian, Alba Cardona, Tania Yeargin, Nelly Patino, Melanie Moccaldi, John Sebellico, and Phil Fontana. Finally, it cannot be overemphasized that this work could not have been completed without the invaluable assistance of the members of our photoradiology department, Martha Helmers and Tony Jalandoni, who so willingly spent their time and energy to insure that this project could be completed.

From Pitié-Salpêtrière Hospital, Paris

We warmly thank Catherine Beigelman-Aubrey, MD, and Michel Brauner, MD, from the Department of Radiology, and Frédérique Capron, MD, from the Department of Pathology, for their considerable contribution to the preparation of figures in Chapter 5.

Imaging of the Airways
Functional and Radiologic Correlations

Introduction to Imaging Methodology and Airway Anatomy

1

With the introduction and widespread availability of multidetector computed tomography (CT) scanners capable of providing continuous and/or overlapping high-resolution, near-isotropic thin sections throughout the lungs in a single breath hold, virtually all the lobar, segmental, and subsegmental bronchi can now be routinely identified in nearly all cases. In combination with advanced image processing techniques, including multiplanar reconstructions (MPRs), 3D surface renderings, and virtual endoscopic views, CT is now well established as the noninvasive imaging procedure of choice to evaluate virtually the entire gamut of diseases affecting the airways (1). Clinically, this includes evaluating patients presenting with chronic cough, dyspnea, chest pain, and hemoptysis (2–4). To date, CT has proved especially valuable in identification of occult airway pathology, including in patients with suspected airway malignancy with normal or nonlocalizing chest radiographs (5); evaluation of airway patency in patients in whom either partial or complete airway obstruction from a variety of causes is suspected (6,7); and identification of inflammatory airway disease, especially the diagnosis of bronchiectasis (8–10). In addition to these indications, CT has also become an invaluable tool for diagnosing diseases involving the small airways (11–17). As discussed in greater detail in Chapter 2, CT has also become an indispensable tool for assessing potential interventional techniques including, among others, the selection of appropriate patients for transbronchial needle aspirations (18) as well as patients with airway obstruction requiring stents (19).

IMAGING TECHNIQUES

The introduction of multidetector CT scanners capable of both prospectively and retrospectively providing high-resolution near-isotropic images throughout the entire thorax in a single breath hold has vastly simplified the task of imaging the airways. This is because it is now possible to use a single "generic" acquisition protocol for essentially all cases, including those specifically referred for evaluation of potential airway pathology. Although technical parameters vary depending on the type of scanner used, a few basic principles apply to nearly all current multidetector scanners. These include use of the thinnest possible collimators (typically 0.75 to 1.5 mm) and the shortest available scan times (i.e., subsecond image acquisition to minimize respiratory motion), with z-axis coverage to include the entire thorax in a single breath-hold period (typically a pitch of between 1 and 2). These parameters allow routine prospective reconstruction of both contiguous 5-mm sections (imaged with appropriate mediastinal and lung reconstruction algorithms, respectively) and high-resolution 1- to 1.5-mm sections reconstructed every 10 mm using an appropriate edge-enhancing algorithm. In effect, current-generation multidetector CT scanners maximize imaging flexibility by turning every study into both a routine and a high-resolution examination. Depending on the individual case, additional retrospective thin sections can then be reconstructed through appropriate regions of interest to clarify potential endobronchial abnormalities. In those cases for which MPRs or virtual bronchoscopic images are desired, contiguous and/or overlapping high-resolution 0.75- to 1.5-mm images also can be prospectively and/or retrospectively reconstructed. These techniques represent a considerable improvement over conventional CT in the era before multidetector CT in which the sensitivity and specificity of CT for detecting obstructive lesions of the respiratory tract, for example, were reported to be as low as 60%, leading some investigators to consider CT inadequate, for example, as a method for initial evaluation of the airways in patients with suspected lung cancer or hemoptysis, (20,21).

In addition to the imaging parameters mentioned previously, other considerations include dose as well as the use of contrast enhancement. In patients for whom the primary indication is visualization of the central airways, in particular, low-dose (40 to 80 mA) technique should be used to minimize radiation exposure (22). Boiselle et al. (23) conducted a combined phantom and clinical study of the effect of radiation dose on multiplanar and 3D image quality using both single-detector and multidetector CT scanners. They found that, although image quality was consistently superior with multidetector CT, no distinguishable differences in image quality could be identified comparing images obtained at 40, 120, and 240 mA, respectively. Similar considerations apply when the primary indication for performing CT is to visualize the peripheral airways and lungs. Low-dose techniques should also be standard for evaluating airway pathology in pediatric patients as well as younger individuals, especially women of child-bearing age (24).

Although there are no definitive guidelines regarding intravenous contrast administration, use of iodinated contrast media allows improved visualization of peribronchial and parenchymal abnormalities. It should be routinely used, in particular in patients in whom there is suspicion of mediastinal or hilar disease or radiographic evidence of parenchymal consolidation or collapse

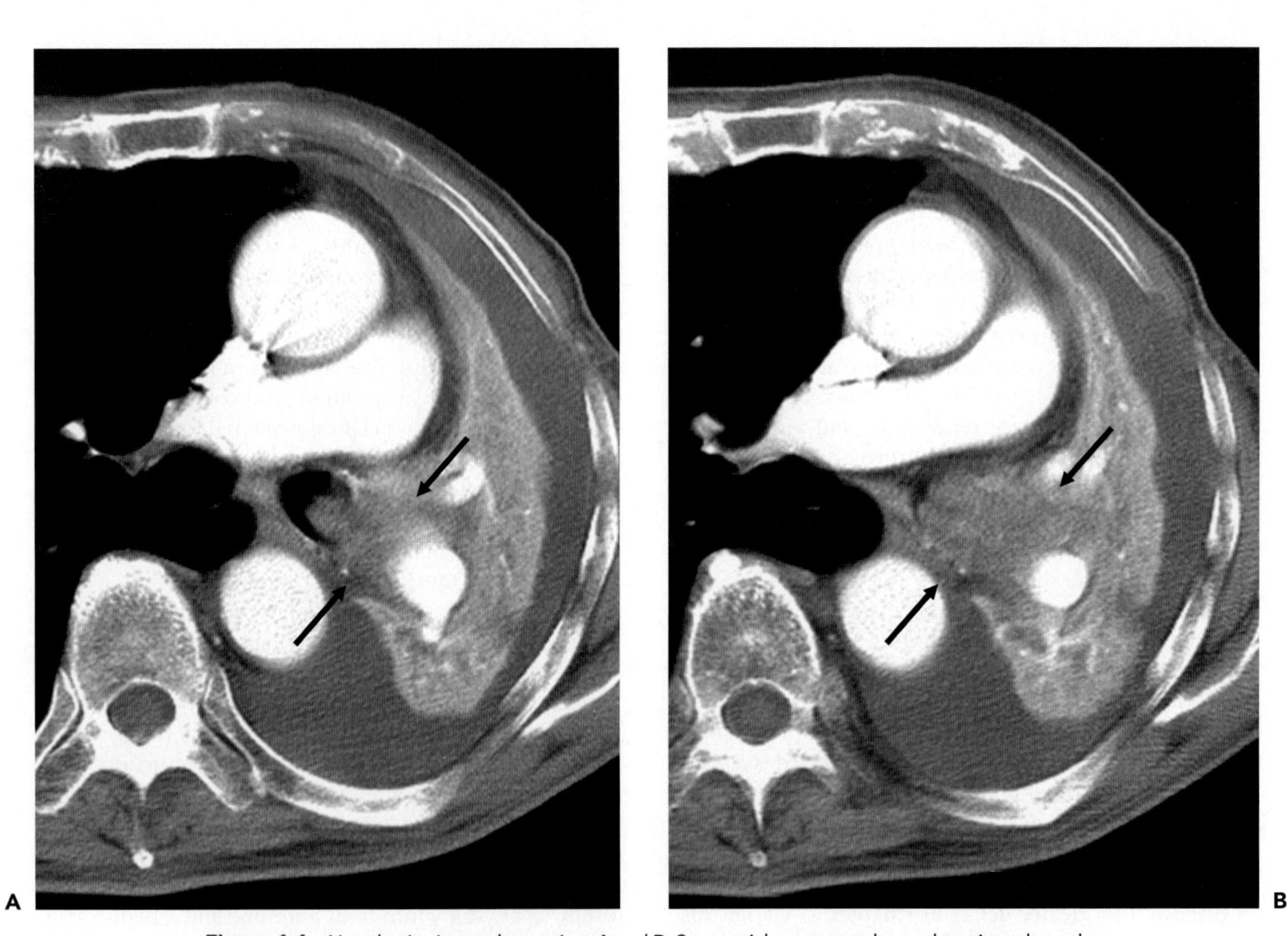

Figure 1-1 Neoplastic airway obstruction. **A** and **B:** Sequential contrast-enhanced sections through the left mainstem and distal left upper and lower lobe bronchi, respectively, show a well-defined intraluminal mass obstructing the distal left mainstem bronchus. Following IV contrast administration, note that the tumor enhances differentially from the peripheral collapsed left upper and lower lobes, allowing precise definition of the true extent of disease (*arrows* in **A** and **B**). A moderate-sized left pleural effusion is also evidence. IV contrast optimally should be used to evaluate all patients presenting with radiographic evidence of collapse.

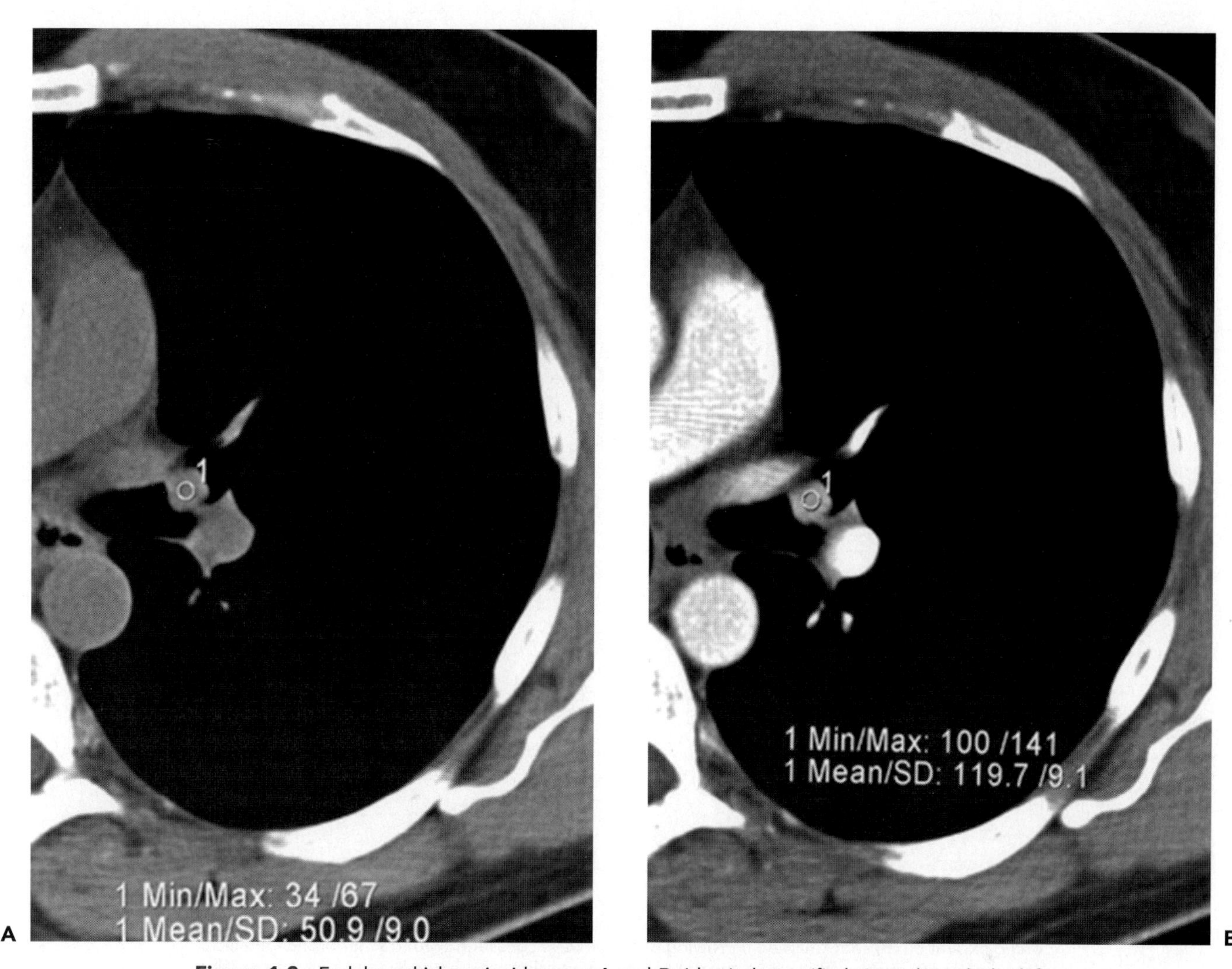

Figure 1-2 Endobronchial carcinoid tumor. **A** and **B:** Identical magnified views through the left upper lobe bronchus first without **(A)** and then following a bolus of IV contrast material **(B).** In this case there is a well-defined soft tissue lesion in the left upper lobe that enhances from 34 to 100 HU. This degree of enhancement is consistent with a highly vascular tumor and is typical of intraluminal carcinoids. (Case courtesy of Dr. Edward Lubat, Hackensack, NJ.)

(Fig. 1-1). Rarely, precontrast- and postcontrast-enhanced images may allow a more precise characterization of abnormalities such as hypervascular tumors (Fig. 1-2) or hypovascular lesions such as bronchogenic or esophageal duplication cysts.

Another technique of considerable value is the addition of select expiratory high-resolution images. As discussed and illustrated throughout this text, high-resolution expiratory images are essential to the diagnosis of a wide range of abnormalities, including, among others, tracheobronchomalacia and obstructive small airway diseases (Fig. 1-3) (25). Although some advocate the routine acquisition of select expiratory images as part of a standard CT examination of the thorax, in our experience this has not proved worthwhile in the vast majority of cases. It should be emphasized that in those cases for which paired inspiratory and forced-expiratory images are required, they should be obtained with a low-dose (40 to 80 mA) technique. As documented by Zhang et al. (22), in a study of tracheal lumen measurements in 10 patients with tracheomalacia, no discernible differences in diagnosis could be identified comparing standard and low-dose techniques.

With the introduction of advanced multidetector CT scanners, interest has also been directed at the potential use of both respiratory and electrocardiogram (ECG) gating to enhance visualization of the tracheobronchial tree. In a recent retrospective study of 25 patients in whom the effect of ECG gating on virtual bronchoscopic images was evaluated, surprisingly image quality proved superior on nongated versus gated images, regardless of the time interval used for reconstructing ECG-gated images (26). Coupled with the substantially higher radiation dose needed to perform ECG gating, this technique should not be used preferentially to study the airways.

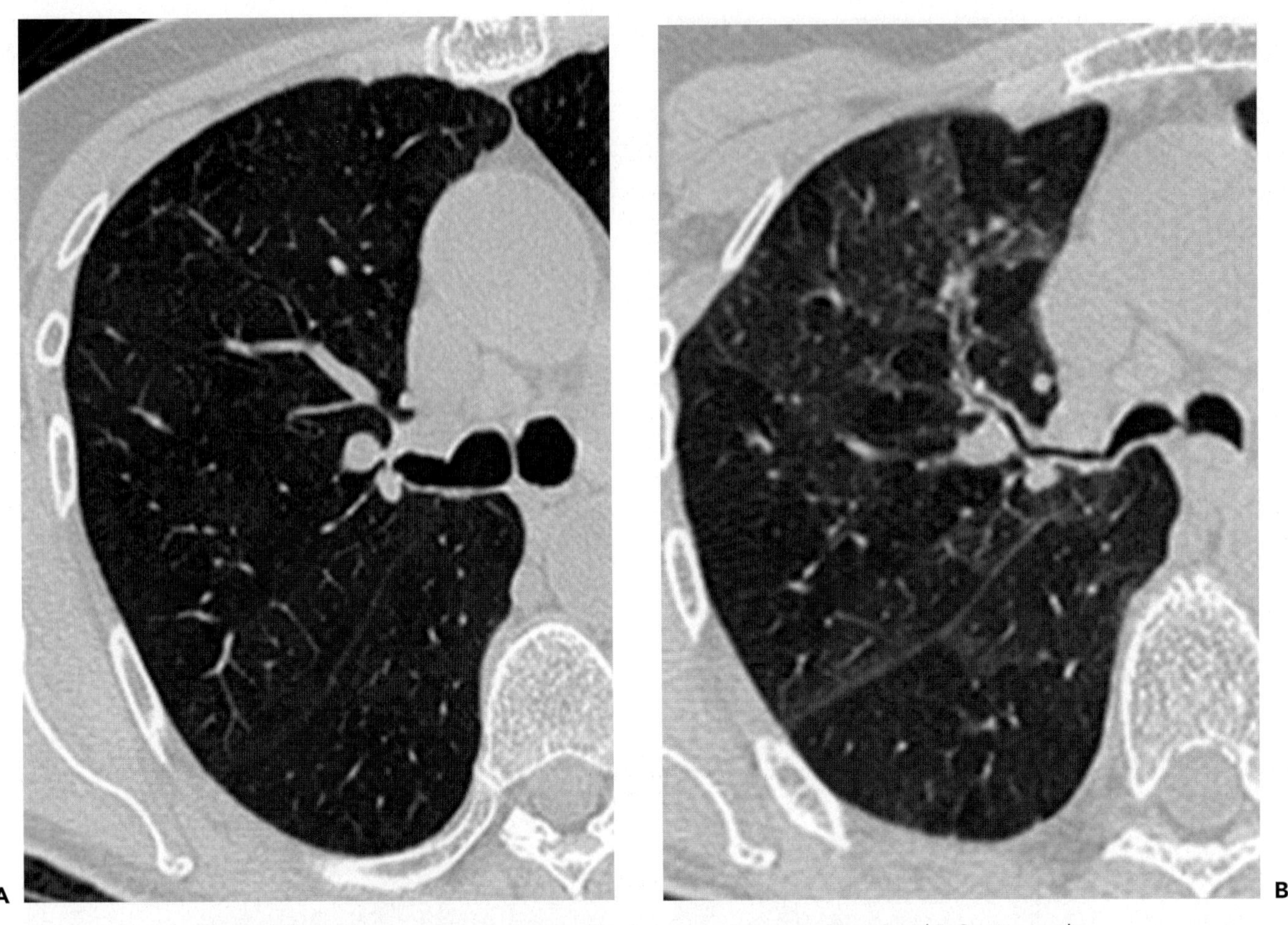

Figure 1-3 Tracheobronchomalacia. Paired inspiratory–expiratory imaging. **A** and **B:** Sections at the level of the carina and proximal right upper lobe bronchus acquired in inspiration **(A)** and following forced expiration **(B)** show marked narrowing of the airways consistent with tracheobronchomalacia. Note mosaic attenuation throughout the right lung in **B,** consistent with peripheral airway obstruction with resultant air trapping. Anterior bowing of the central airways is an important sign that the image was obtained in expiration, and when marked it correlates with bronchoscopic evidence of tracheobronchomalacia.

Advanced Reconstruction Techniques

Although routine axial images remain the standard for identifying airway disease, as discussed in Chapter 2, this method has important limitations, especially in comparison with flexible bronchoscopy. First, CT is limited in its ability to accurately differentiate among mucosal, submucosal, and extrinsic causes of airway narrowing (see Figs. 2-2 and 2-3). Axial CT images also are of notoriously limited value in estimating the length of airway stenoses.

With the recent introduction of multidetector CT scanners capable of generating hundreds of contiguous and/or overlapping high-resolution thin sections throughout the thorax, there has been growing impetus to rely on alternative methods of reconstruction to evaluate the airways and lungs (Fig. 1-4) (27). These include MPRs, maximum intensity projections (MIPs) and minimum intensity projections (MinIPs), external rendering with either 3D shaded-surface displays (SSDs) or volumetric rendering, and internal rendering, or so-called virtual bronchoscopy (VB). Although currently MPRs alone have proved of routine clinical value (23,28), there is still considerable interest in the potential use of the other techniques, especially VB.

Multiplanar Reconstructions

MPRs are typically 1-voxel-thick two-dimensional "tomographic" sections interpolated along an arbitrary plane or, less commonly, a curved surface. Compared with other imaging techniques, MPRs have the advantages of taking little time to reconstruct and requiring no skill. With modern scanners, coronal and sagittal MPRs may be routinely prospectively reconstructed, provided initial volumetric data acquisition is available. The main advantage of MPRs is the ability to allow individual airways to be displayed to best advantage along their nearest long axes. Although variations have been proposed, including double-obliquity MPRs perpendicular to previously reconstructed

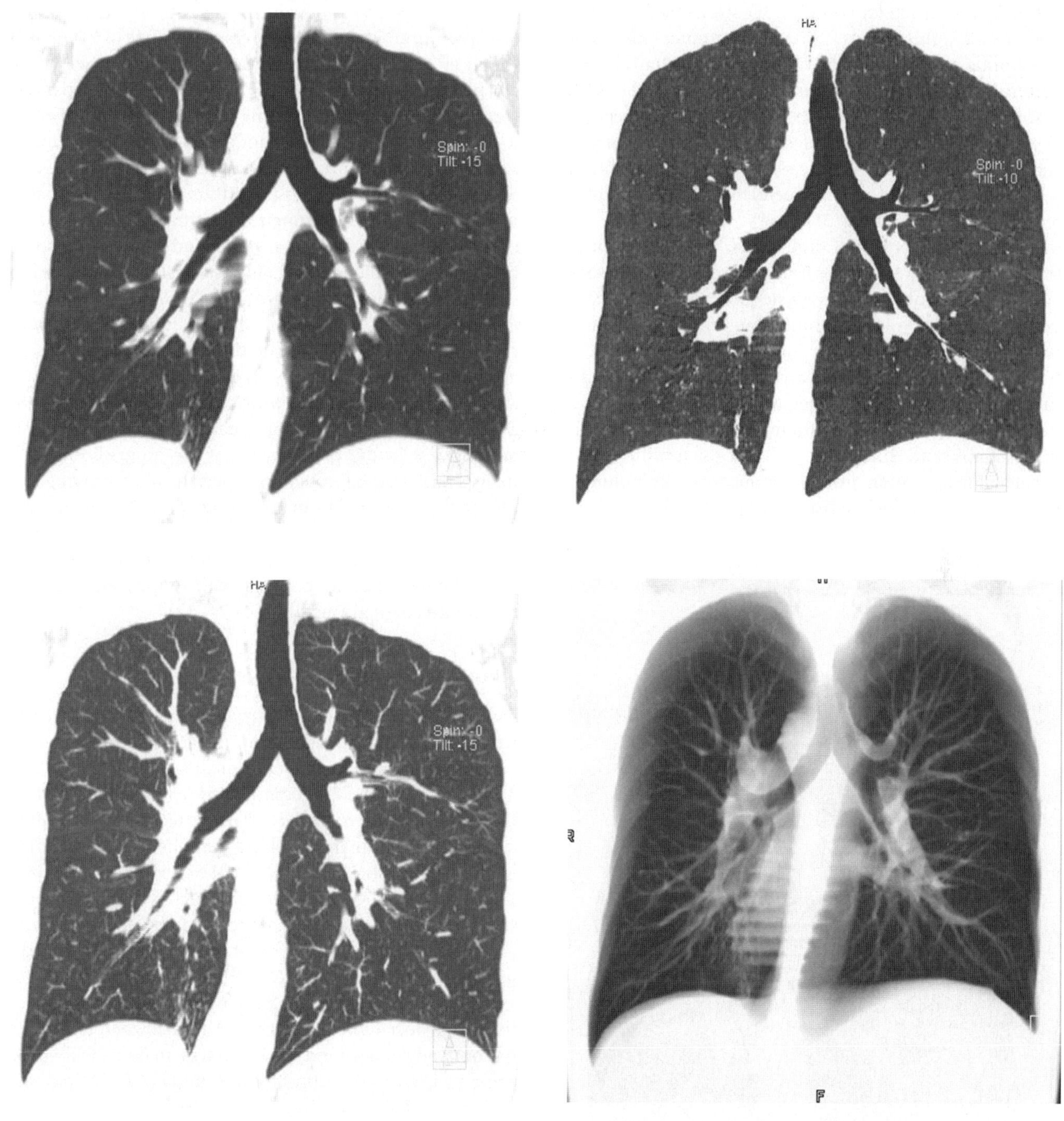

Figure 1-4 Image reconstruction: Kartagener's syndrome. **A** to **D:** Coronal multiplanar reconstruction (MPR) **(A)**, minimum intensity projection image (MinIP) **(B)**, maximum intensity projection image (MIP) **(C)**, and volumetric rendered image **(D)** through the carina in a patient with situs inversus. These images were all reconstructed using five contiguous 1-mm sections obtained from a 16-detector CT scanner using 1-mm collimators. Although MinIPs accentuate the tracheobronchial tree, effectively erasing the pulmonary vasculature and MIPs enhance visualization of the pulmonary vessels at the expense of optimal visualization of the airways, both are 2D representations and therefore lose any perception of depth. In distinction, volumetric rendering preserves depth perception by including all pixels within the volume of interest. MPRs strike an effective balance, equally delineating both vessels and airways, and are most commonly used for obtaining additional views of the airways and lungs.

3D images (29,30) and curved MPRs employing a user-defined trace to render complex 3D structures in a single flat tomographic plane, these techniques are time-consuming and have proved of only limited clinical value. Unfortunately, even with volumetric acquisition, MPRs are susceptible to stair-step artifacts, which limit interpretation. Typically, these artifacts manifest as irregularities along the surfaces of airways that course obliquely. They are directly related to pitch and are independent of collimation or reconstruction algorithm (31).

Despite these potential limitations, MPRs have consistently been shown to be of considerable clinical value, especially for assessing focal airways stenoses such as those that occur following prolonged intubation or lung transplantation (27,32–35). Following lung transplantation, MPRs have been shown to be more accurate than axial images in differentiating normal postoperative changes, such as diverticula resulting from redundant mucosal folds and endoluminal flaps and linear air collections resulting from bronchial invagination, from the more ominous findings of dehiscence and bronchial fistulization (36).

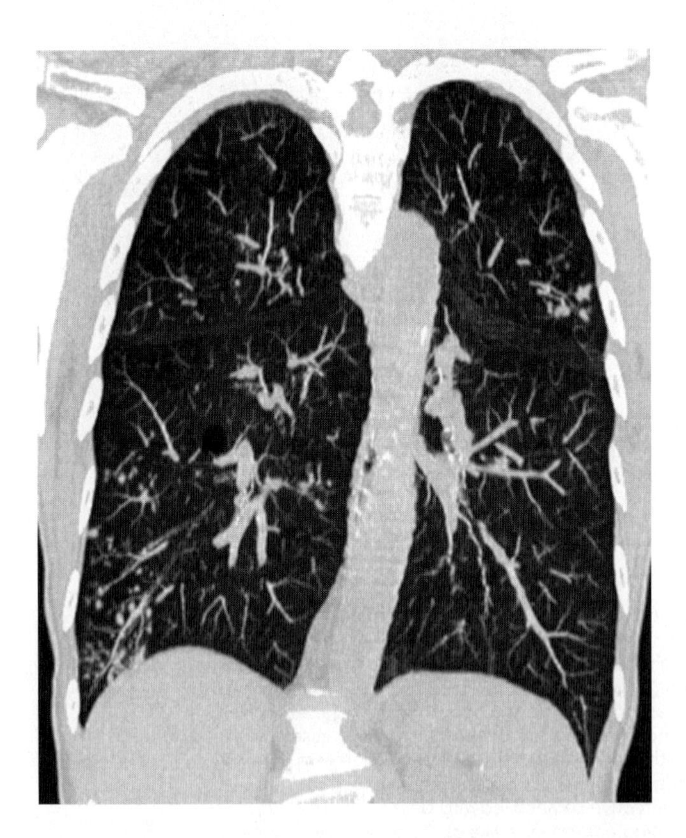

Figure 1-5 Small airway inflammation: MIP coronal section through the posterior portions of the lungs shows multiple clusters of small nodules demonstrating a tree-in-bud configuration. Characteristic of small airway inflammation, in select cases this pattern may be easier to identify with maximum projection images than on routine axial scans.

Maximum and Minimum Projection Images

MIP and MinIP images are 2D representations of 3D data in which either the highest or lowest individual voxel values are projected through a given subvolume along parallel (orthogonal) rays. Although this allows specific density data to be extracted and evaluated independently, this technique sacrifices 3D depth information. Use of the lowest attenuation values within the slab (MinIP imaging) yields images in which the bronchial lumen is accentuated at the expense of the bronchial wall (Figs. 1-4, 3-3, and 3-30A). In distinction, use of the highest available attenuation values within the slab (MIP imaging) accentuates the bronchial wall at the expense of the bronchial lumen (Fig. 1-4). In both cases, the result is to distort the normal cross-sectional appearance of the airways by accentuating only a portion of airway anatomy (37). First introduced by Napel et al. (38) as a technique for improving visualization of blood vessels and airways in the parenchyma of the lung, sliding MIP images have found limited use especially in identifying foci of small airway inflammation (Fig. 1-5). In distinction, although of limited value for evaluating the central airways, MinIP images have proved of use for evaluating the lung parenchyma, both in patients with emphysema and in those with small airway disease (39–42).

External Rendering

External rendering enables visualization of structures from an external vantage point, most often using a simulated light source (see, for example, Figs. 3-5C, 3-10B, and 3-30B). This can be accomplished using either surface thresholding or volume-rendering techniques. In the former, a single binary threshold is applied, rendering only a few voxels visible along the surface of selected structures. These are given the appearance of depth by illuminating the surface with an imaginary source of light. In distinction, volume rendering uses linear or continuous scaling techniques in which every voxel within the original dataset is assigned a proportional value based on the full range of tissue densities represented (43). Although each technique has both advantages and disadvantages, to date, neither has gained widespread routine clinical utility (44). Despite the striking visual appearance of these images, external rendering techniques usually require time-consuming editing to create and rarely allow visualization of airways beyond the mainstem and proximal lobar bronchi. With the shaded-surface technique, in particular, the use of a single threshold also makes these images susceptible to numerous artifacts. When inappropriately selected the result is surface discontinuities or "holes," jagged edges, and "floating pixels." Focal areas of high density including bronchial stents and bronchial cartilage calcifications also may be completely obscured (31).

Analogous to MPRs, 3D surface-rendering techniques have most often been used to identify central bronchial stenoses. Three-dimensional images also have been anecdotally reported of value in a wide range of disparate conditions, including tracheal compression resulting from kyphosis (45), congenital airway abnormalities such as cardiac bronchus (46) or those associated with vascular malformations or rings (24), following stent placement (19), even identification of bronchopleural fistulas (47), among others (1,35,48).

Virtual Bronchoscopy

Internal rendering, or VB, allows visualization of the airways from a point source at a finite distance, simulating human perspective as seen through a bronchoscope. Identical to external imaging of the airways, virtual bronchoscopic images can be obtained using either 3D SSDs or volumetric rendering (30,49–52). Although a detailed description of these techniques is outside the scope of this chapter, a few pertinent aspects of these techniques need to be addressed. With 3D surface rendering, a specific attenuation coefficient is chosen as a threshold to define the air–lumen interface. This renders all voxels as representing either air or soft tissue, without an identifiable transition zone. Unfortunately, this technique has the disadvantage of greater susceptibility to noise and partial volume averaging, resulting in surface discontinuities, jagged edges, and floating pixels. Furthermore, no optimal threshold has been described; instead, thresholds vary, in particular, as a function of the density of the bronchial wall. Using a bronchial phantom, Maniatis et al. (53) have proposed a threshold value of −520 Hounsfield units (HU) as appropriate for visualizing the main central airways, whereas −720 HU has been suggested as requisite for accurate visualization of segmental and subsegmental bronchi.

In distinction, volume rendering makes use of the entire volume of data in which each voxel is classified on the basis of its attenuation value. This allows not only visualization of the endoluminal surface of the airways but real-time visualization of structures through the airway wall, as well. Although this is an advantage over SSTs, it should be noted that this difference has not proved clinically significant. When viewed endoscopically, little distinguishes these techniques (Fig. 1-6). In a recent study comparing the use of ECG gating on evaluation of the bronchial tree, Schertler et al. (26) found no difference in the ability of VB images to visualize all bronchial segments regardless of whether they were reconstructed using an SST or volumetric rendering. It is also noteworthy that nearly all currently available workstations allow simultaneous evaluation of peribronchial tissues through simultaneous annotated displays of corresponding axial, coronal, and sagittal images oriented to conform to any given plane identified from the endoluminal display, further minimizing differences between these techniques. Finally, although it has been suggested that volumetric rendering allows depiction of the bronchial mucosa by including a separate transition zone between air within the lumen and the bronchial wall, it has yet to be shown that this transition zone actually correlates with the appearance of the mucosa at bronchoscopy (54). In this regard, in

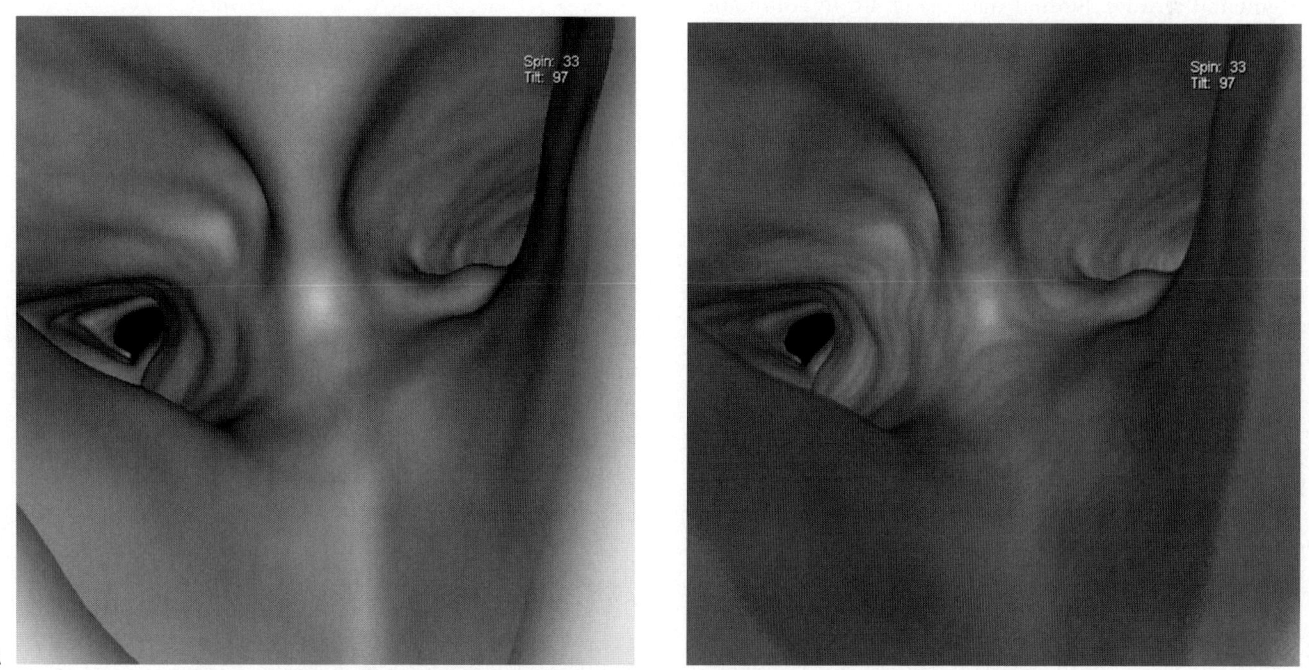

Figure 1-6 Virtual bronchoscopy. **A** and **B:** Virtual bronchoscopic views of the carina in the same patient as Fig. 1-5 reconstructed using shaded-surface **(A)** and volumetric rendering **(B)** techniques. Note that for purposes of routine endoscopic viewing, there is little difference between these techniques.

a study of 44 consecutive patients with thoracic malignancies, although HRCT including VB correctly identified 90% of endoluminal abnormalities (including 100% of obstructive lesions), only 16% of mucosal lesions identified bronchoscopically were correctly identified prospectively (55). It is also worth emphasizing that in this study, although all normal patients were correctly identified by CT, CT demonstrated two false-positive obstructive lesions as well (55).

Other generally available VB tools include orthogonal axes to indicate anterior, posterior, or superior direction and "rearview" imaging, which allows simultaneous depiction of a virtual endoscopic image pointing backward from any given location. This latter technique allows inspection of endobronchial lesions from a vantage point not accessible via routine bronchoscopy (52). It is also possible to measure distances between any fixed points within the airways using "trail markers," which are analogous to the distance markers present on fiberoptic bronchoscopes (52). More recently, attempts have been reported of correlating virtual bronchoscopic images with flexible bronchoscopy in real time, using either sensors attached to the tip of the bronchoscope or external fiduciary markers (56). It has also been shown that augmented endoscopic images combining both real and virtual bronchoscopic information can be created in real time, as the bronchoscopy is being performed, even in the absence of sensors or fiduciary markers (57).

It should be emphasized that the principal parameter in determining the quality of virtual bronchoscopic images is use of thin collimation. In an early study using a single-detector CT scanner with 3-mm sections and a 1-mm reconstruction interval, for example, Summers et al. (30) were only able to identify 82% of lobar and 76% of segmental airways. Similar data using 3-mm collimation have been reported by Lacasse et al. (58), who found that the sensitivity of VB for detecting lobar and segmental bronchial lesions was only 76% and 48%, respectively. Multidetector CT scanners substantially improve the capacity to image the peripheral airways (59). With retrospective target reconstruction using fields-of-view between 16 and 18 cm, spatial resolution now approximates 0.5 mm, allowing routine identification of fifth- to eighth-generation bronchi that were not previously identifiable. The degree to which near-isotropic imaging enhances VB has recently been documented (60). In a comparison of 1.5-mm sections reconstructed q 0.75 mm with 0.75-mm sections reconstructed q 0.4 mm using a 16-row multidetector CT, the use of thinner sections improved visualization of the mean generation of bronchial bifurcations from 4.8 to 6.5 mm ($p < .0003$) (Fig. 2-18); similarly, the diameters of recognizable bronchi improved from a mean of 7.5 to 4.6 mm ($p < .0001$) (60).

To date, indications for VB to evaluate the central airways (extending from the trachea to the proximal lobar bronchi) have been extensively reported. These include assessing tracheal and proximal bronchial stenoses (61–64), including in association with esophageal atresia in neonates and infants (65), as well as in identifying central airway tumors (48,54,58,66–68). VB has been used to evaluate benign bronchial tumors (69), Wegener's granulomatosis (70), suspected foreign body aspiration in children (71), and esophageal carcinoma infiltrating the tracheobronchial tree (72), among others. Unfortunately, none of these indications has received widespread clinical acceptance, largely because nearly identical information regarding the central airways has been available from routine axial and multiplanar reconstructions (54,73,74). Although at least one report has shown VB to be more accurate than MPRs or MIPs for accurately assessing the length of bronchial stenoses, frequent false-positive endobronchial abnormalities have been reported in most series (55).

However, VB does have important potential uses. As discussed in detail in Chapter 2, VB may be of use in determining optimal sites for performing transbronchial needle aspirations and biopsies (see Fig. 2-16) (75). VB has also been successfully used as a means for teaching optimal methods for performing these techniques to inexperienced bronchoscopists (76,77). This potential use of VB is especially promising because, despite excellent results in the reported literature, transbronchial needle biopsy remains generally underutilized (78,79). Another potential area in which VB may come to fill an essential role is in providing a road map for ultrathin bronchoscopic evaluation of peripheral lung lesions (Fig. 1-7). Currently only limited attempts have been made to expand VB to include the peripheral airways (27,80,81).

Advanced Imaging Techniques: Airway Segmentation and CT Bronchography

In addition to the standard advanced image reconstruction methods described previously, it is now possible to automatically segment airways. These images can be used either as virtual bronchographic images (82,83) or as a template for creating virtual bronchoscopic images (Fig. 1-8) (84–86). It is also possible to use automated axis generation to provide a template for the reconstruction of true cross-sectional images through any given airway, regardless of its spatial orientation (Fig. 1-8). This technique has particular potential for the accurate evaluation of bronchial wall dimensions in patients being evaluated for reactive airway disease (87–89). Segmented airways may also be used to obtain visual and quantitative estimates of central airway volume and morphology in both inspiration and expiration (Fig. 1-8).

AIRWAY ANATOMY

Thorough familiarity with the anatomic appearance of the airways, including common variants, is essential for accurate interpretation of thoracic CT images and therefore warrants detailed description.

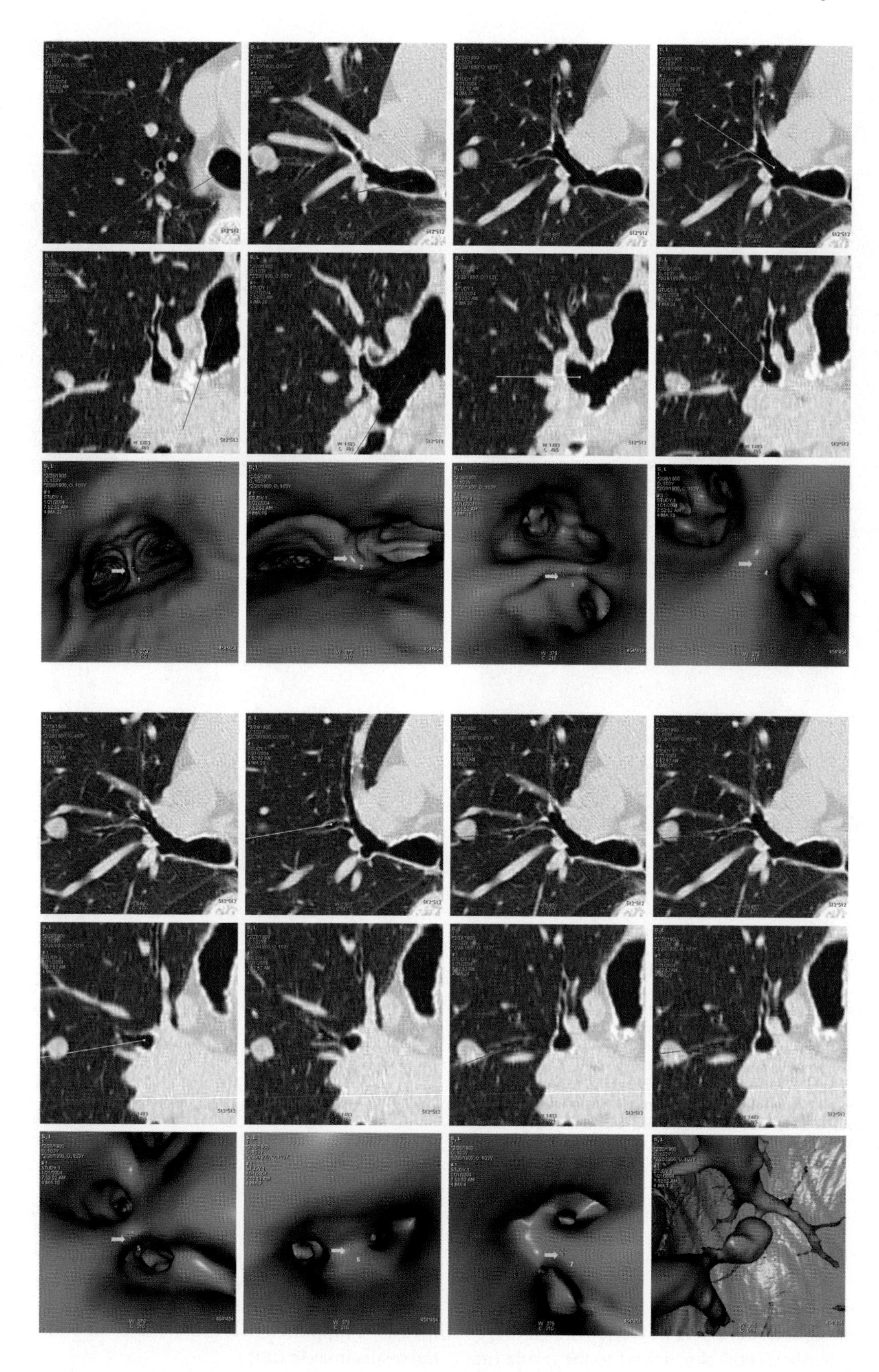

Figure 1-7 Virtual bronchoscopy. **A** and **B:** Sequential high-resolution axial (top row in **A** and **B**) and coronal (middle row in **A** and **B**) sections through the right upper lobe with corresponding virtual bronchoscopic images (bottom row in **A** and **B**) in a patient with a peripheral 2-cm nodule. Multidetector CT scanners capable of obtaining high-resolution images through the entire thorax in a single breath hold have made it possible to image eighth- to ninth-order airways, potentially serving as a road map for both routine and ultrathin bronchoscopy.

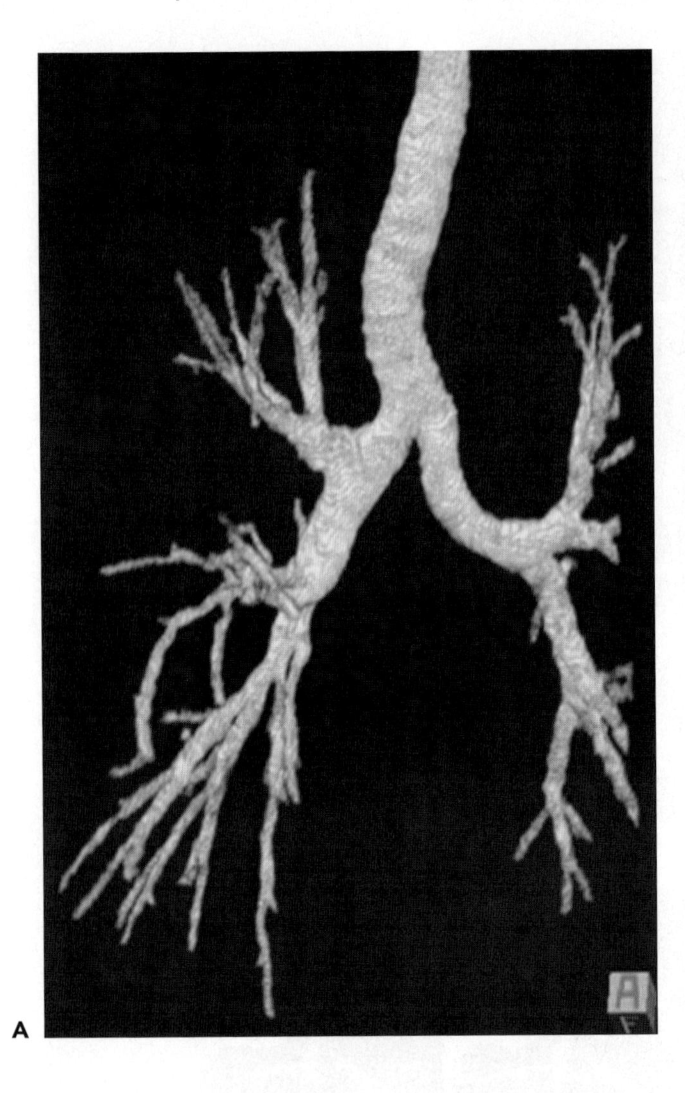

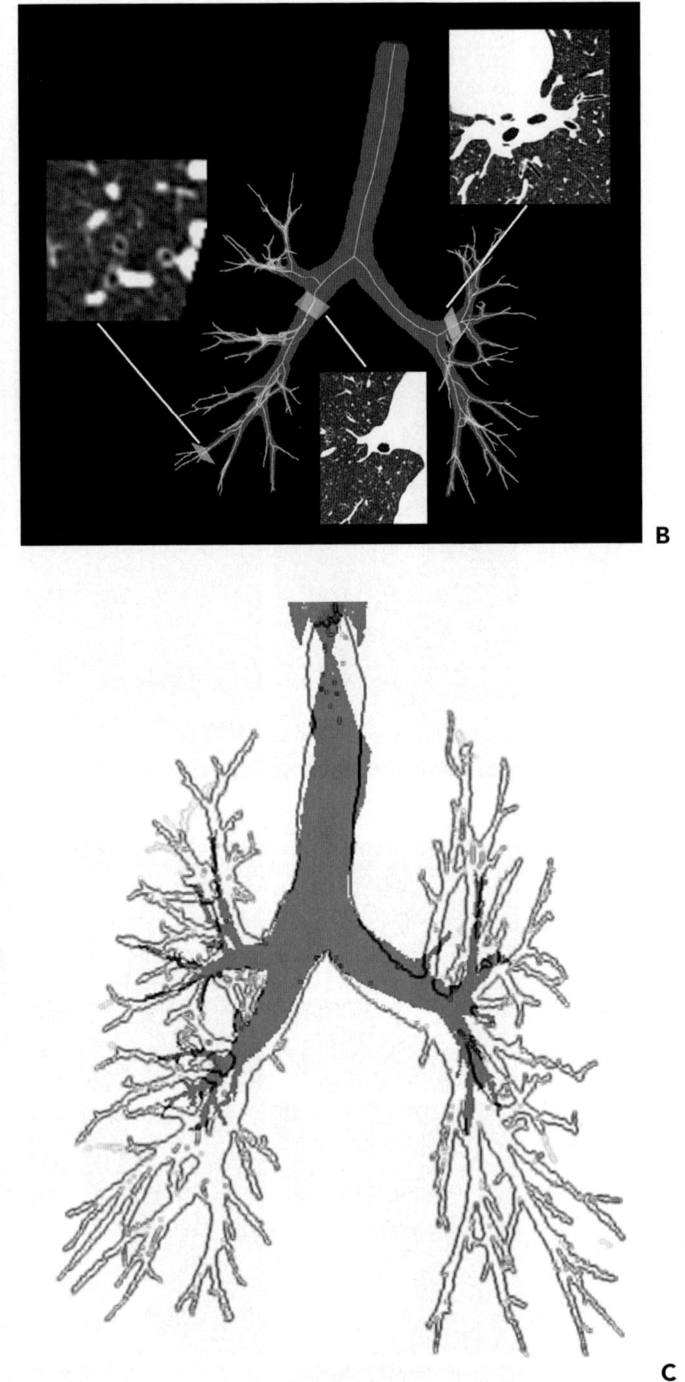

Figure 1-8 Airway segmentation. **A:** 3D Externally rendered view of the segmented tracheobronchial tree rendering a CT bronchographic view of the airways. **B:** Segmented airway tree in a different individual than in **A,** within which the central axes or center lines are delineated. These may serve either as a template for developing automated virtual bronchoscopic images or as a means for obtaining true cross-sectional images through user-selected airways providing precise measurements of luminal area or wall thickness. **C:** Composite view of segmented tracheobronchial tree showing the change in size and morphology between inspiration and forced expiration. (**A** and **C** Courtesy of A.P. Kiraly, Siemens Corporate Research, Princeton, N.J.)

Trachea

The trachea is a cartilaginous and fibromuscular tube extending from the inferior aspect of the cricoid cartilage (at the level of the sixth cervical vertebra) to the carina (at the level of the fifth thoracic vertebra). Typically, the trachea contains 16 to 22 cartilaginous rings that help to support the tracheal wall and maintain an adequate tracheal lumen during forced expiration. From the inside layer out, the tracheal wall includes the mucosa, submucosa, cartilage or muscle, and adventitia (Fig. 1-9). The posterior tracheal wall or membrane lacks cartilage and instead is supported by a thin band of smooth muscle, the trachealis muscle (90).

Overall the trachea measures 10 to 12 cm in length in adults, including both the extrathoracic trachea (measuring 2 to 4 cm in length) and the intrathoracic trachea (beginning at the point where the trachea passes posterior to the manubrium, measuring 6 to 9 cm in length) (91,92). By

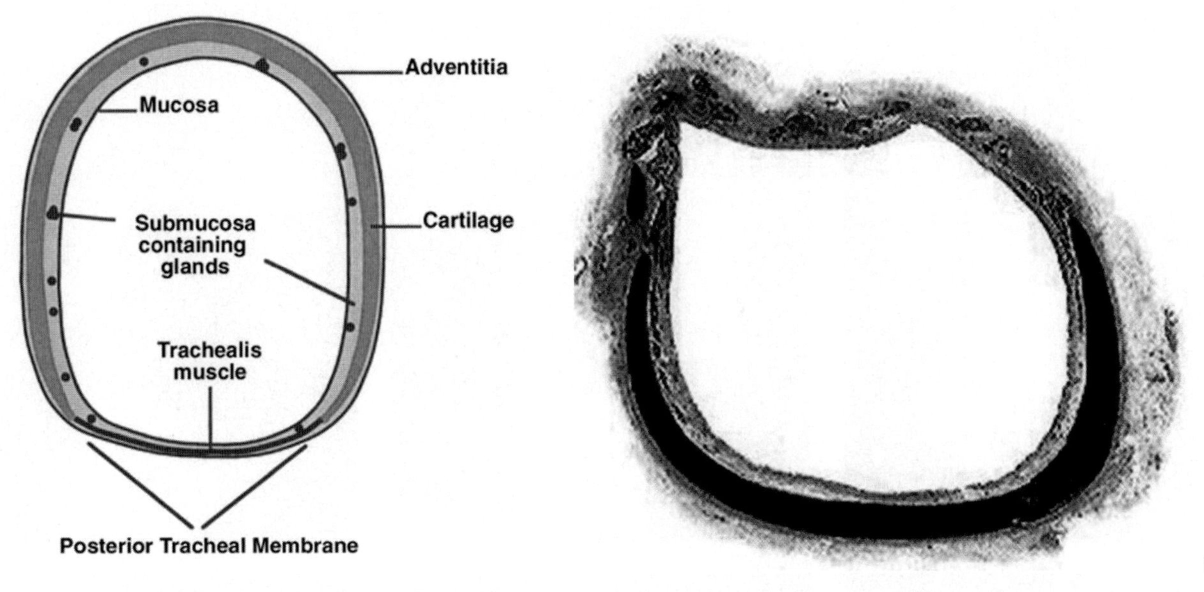

Figure 1-9 Normal tracheal anatomy. **A:** Cross-sectional drawing shows typical appearance of a horseshoe-shaped tracheal cartilage within the anterior and lateral tracheal wall, which is markedly thicker than the posterior tracheal membrane. Although labeled, tracheal mucosa and submucosa are rarely identifiable with CT. **B:** Histopathologic section shows characteristic horseshoe-shaped cartilage *(large arrow)* as dark. The posterior tracheal membrane is bowed anteriorly. (From Webb EM, Elicker BM, Webb WR. Using CT to diagnose nonneoplastic tracheal abnormalities: appearance of the tracheal wall. *AJR Am J Roentgenol* 2000;174:1315–1321, with permission.)

comparison, the trachea measures only approximately 3 cm in length at birth, increasing to 7 to 10 cm in length during childhood. The blood supply to the trachea is supplied superiorly by branches of the inferior thyroid arteries and the extreme right intercostal artery and inferiorly by branches of the bronchial and intercostal arteries (93).

On CT, the tracheal wall appears as a thin 1- to 3-mm stripe (Fig. 1-10). Along its inferior aspect, the right wall of the trachea is in contact with air within the medial aspect of the right upper lobe, resulting in the right paratracheal stripe seen on routine posterior–anterior chest radiographs. Anterolaterally, the trachea lies behind the great vessels and adjacent to the aorta. This position accounts for the frequent finding of focal displacement of the trachea to the left, resulting from marked tortuosity of the brachiocephalic artery, and to the right, resulting from tortuosity of the aortic arch.

On cross section the trachea may appear rounded, oval, or horseshoe shaped. In men tracheal diameters normally vary widely from 13 to 25 mm in the coronal plane (average 19.5 mm) and 13 to 27 mm in the sagittal plane (94). Although the trachea is slightly smaller in women, considerable variability is still noted, with diameters ranging from 10 to 21 mm in the coronal plane (average 17.5 mm) and 10 to 23 mm in the sagittal plane (94). The shape of the intrathoracic trachea can change dramatically with expiration as a result of invagination of the posterior membrane, resulting in a crescent-moon– or horseshoe-shaped lumen (95). As shown on dynamic CT, the mean anteroposterior diameter of the trachea can decrease by as much as 30%. Observation of anterior bowing of the posterior tracheal membrane is of particular value in cases in which there is evidence of mosaic attenuation on high-resolution CT images (Fig. 1-3).

To date, the relationship between tracheal dimensions and respiratory function has yet to be defined. Particular interest has centered on the significance of marked tracheal narrowing in the coronal plane—the so-called saber-sheath trachea (See Fig. 3-20). As originally described, this "anomaly" was seen almost exclusively in emphysematous males (96). In fact, a relationship between tracheal dimensions and the severity of emphysema has been recently established (97). In a study of tracheal morphology in 43 patients before and after lung volume reduction surgery, although the size of the trachea significantly correlated with lung volumes presurgery and postsurgery ($p < .05$), no correlation could be established between tracheal morphology and changes in postsurgical pulmonary function (97). Specifically, following surgery, the intrathoracic trachea decreased in length and increased in axial dimensions, which was likely the result of altered intrathoracic pressure owing to smaller lung volumes. However, as noted, these changes proved to be poor predictors of postoperative lung function, raising doubts concerning a causative relationship between a saber-sheath configuration and emphysema.

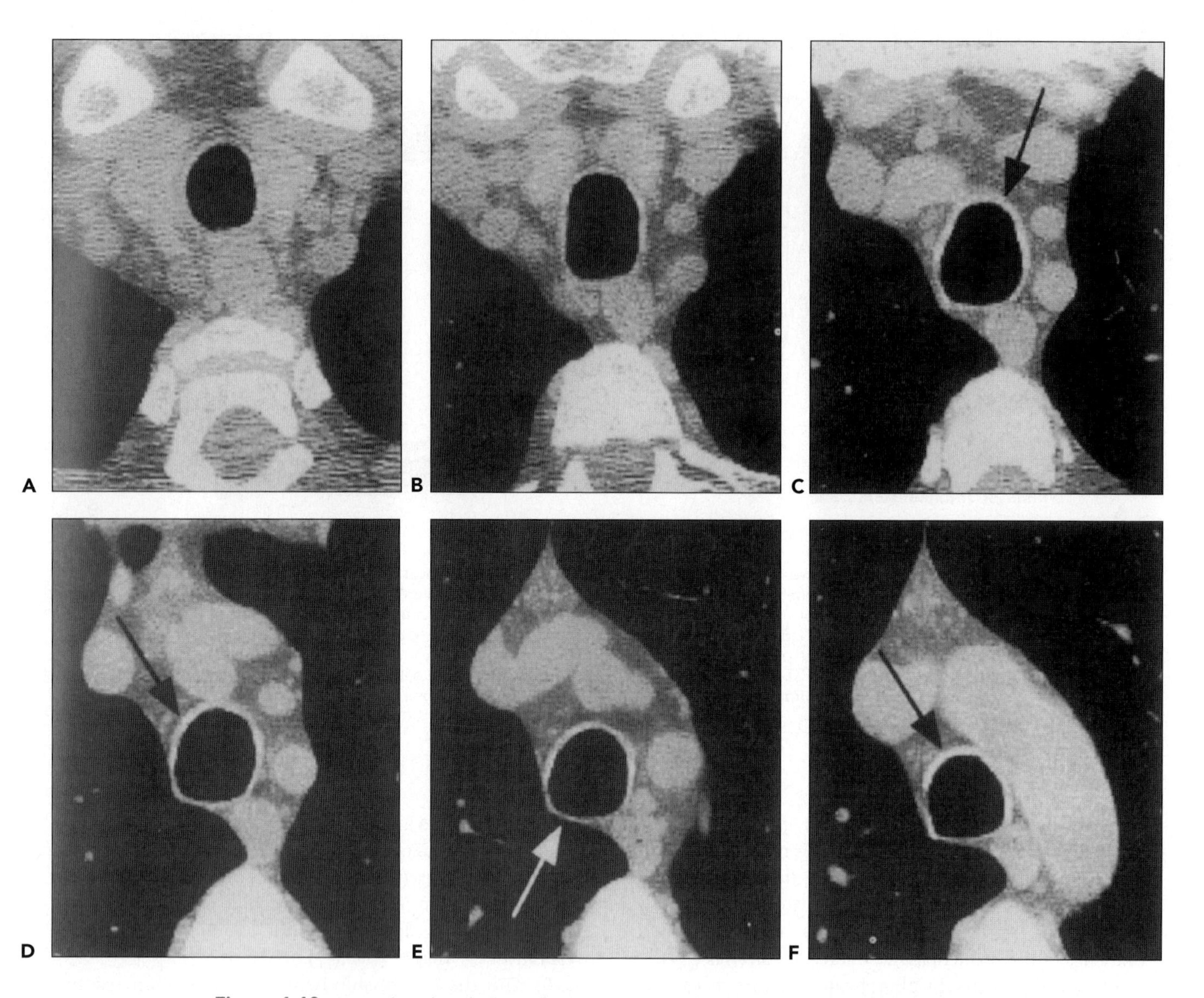

Figure 1-10 Normal trachea: high-resolution CT sections through the trachea, obtained at 1-cm intervals. The tracheal wall is well defined internally by air in the tracheal lumen and is well defined externally by mediastinal fat. Tracheal cartilage within the anterior and lateral tracheal walls appears a few millimeters thick; calcification *(black arrows)* is often present in older patients, more commonly in women. The posterior tracheal wall represents the posterior tracheal membrane *(white arrow)* and is relatively thin. In this patient, it is sharply outlined by lung. The posterior tracheal membrane appears flattened, whereas the cartilage anteriorly gives the trachea a rounded or horseshoe shape.

Mainstem, Lobar, and Segmental Bronchial Anatomy

Principles of Interpretation

Airways divide by dichotomous branching, with approximately 23 generations of branches identifiable from the trachea to the alveoli (Figs. 1-11 and 1-12). Although bronchi are composed of both cartilaginous and fibromuscular elements, distinction between them is less clear-cut than in the trachea, especially the farther the airway lies from the carina. As a rule, for conducting airways distal to the segmental level airway wall thickness is approximately proportional to airway diameter. For airways less than 5 mm in diameter airway walls should measure 1/6 to 1/10 of their diameter (Table 1-1) (98). Consequently, as a general rule, bronchi less than 2 mm in diameter or closer than 2 cm to the pleural surface—the equivalent of seventh- to ninth-generation bronchi—are below the resolution of even HRCT images (99,100).

The ability to visualize airways also reflects the choice of appropriate window settings. As reported by Bankier et al. (101), using three inflation-fixed lungs imaged with high-resolution 1.5-mm images subsequently evaluated with planimetry, optimal evaluation of bronchial walls requires use

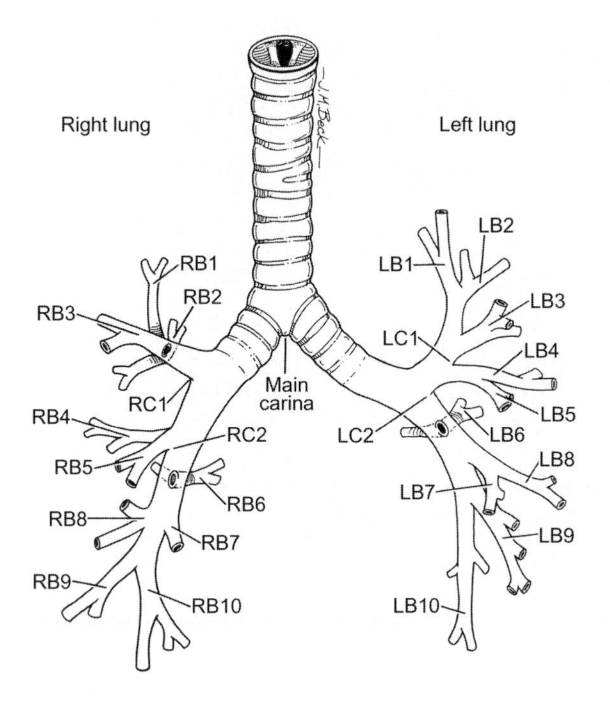

Figure 1-11 Anatomic drawing illustrates terminology of the central airways. (From Prakash UBS. *Bronchoscopy.* New York: Raven Press, 1994, with permission.)

of window centers between −250 and −700 HU, with corresponding window widths between 1,000 and 1,400 HU. Although window widths less than 1,000 HU led to substantial overestimation of bronchial wall thickness, window widths greater than 1,400 HU underestimated wall thickness (Fig. 1-13). In this same study, there was no "interaction" noted between choice of "width" and "center."

Identification of the origin of most bronchi is dependent on recognizing the spurs that separate them. Depending on their angle relative to the CT plane, a spur will appear either as a triangular wedge of soft tissue or, when sectioned along its length, as a linear septum separating adjacent airways. Alternatively, spurs may appear as faint curvilinear densities, especially in airways that course horizontally within the plane of the CT scan. Although the main carina is the most easily identifiable spur, virtually all spurs appear the same. Thickening of these structures, as well as focal peribronchial thickening, may be an early sign of bronchial neoplasia (see Fig. 2-26) (102). Previously, subsegmental bronchi proved especially difficult to identify; basilar airways were identified in only 56% and 35% of patients in the right and left lower lobes, respectively, before volumetric imaging (103). At present, however, nearly all subsegmental bronchi should be routinely identifiable.

CT findings may differ from those seen at bronchoscopy. As a consequence, abnormalities identified by CT should be described using CT-specific terminology. The relationship between CT findings and those identified at bronchoscopy are described in detail in Chapter 2 (see Figs. 2-2 and 2-3).

Bronchial Anatomy: Nomenclature

Although a number of systems for labeling segmental lung anatomy have been proposed, the system described by Jackson and Huber in 1943 (104) has been generally adopted. Bronchi are also designated using a numeric system popularized by Boyden (105). Boyden initially designated upper lobe bronchial segments as B1 (apical segment), B2 (anterior segment), and B3 (posterior segment), with the left apical-posterior segment being B1-3. In 1961 (105), numbers for the anterior and posterior upper lobe segments were switched, and the posterior segment became B2, the anterior segment B3, and the left apical-posterior segment B1-2. Standard nomenclature and 1961 revisions in letter-number codes are used in this book (Table 1–2; Fig. 1-11) (106–108).

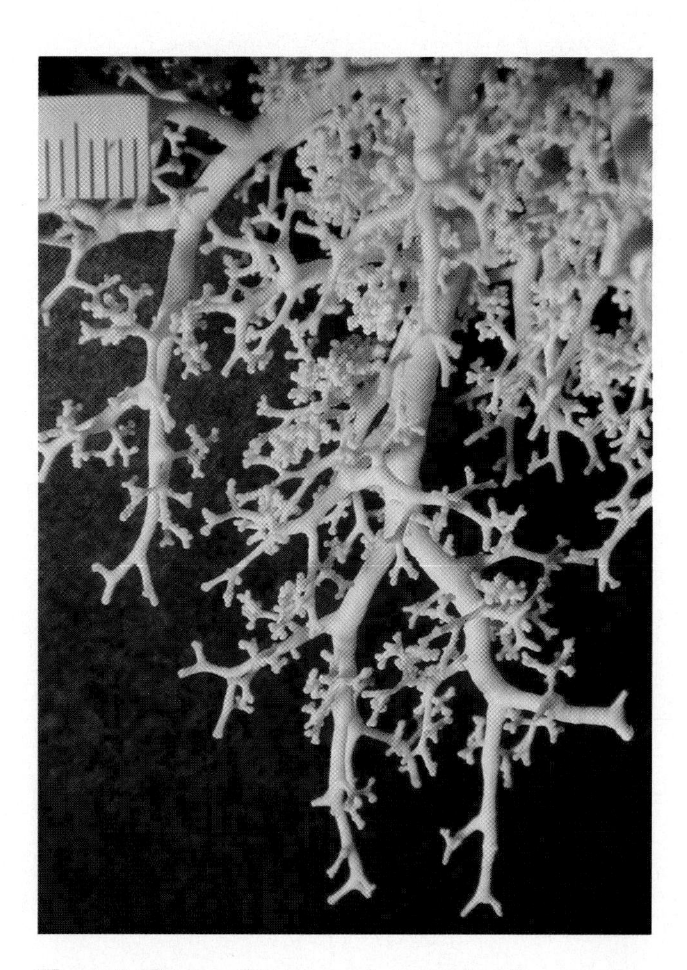

Figure 1-12 Cast of the airways from an inflated autopsy specimen shows to good advantage the true branching nature of the tracheobronchial tree. (Case courtesy of Eugene Weibel, MD, Zurich, Switzerland.)

TABLE 1-1
AIRWAY DIMENSIONS

Airway Division	Generation	Diameter (mm)	Wall Thickness (mm)	Number
Segmental bronchi	2–4	5–8	1.5	30
	6–8	1.5–3	0.3	500
	11	1.0	0.15	2,000
Terminal bronchiole	13	0.7	0.01	8,000
Respiratory bronchiole	15	0.5	0.05	30,000
Intraacinar	16–23	0.3	—	—

Modified from Weibel ER. High resolution computed tomography of the pulmonary parenchyma: anatomical background. Presented at the Fleischner Society Symposium on Chest Disease, Scottsdale, Arizona, 1990, with permission.

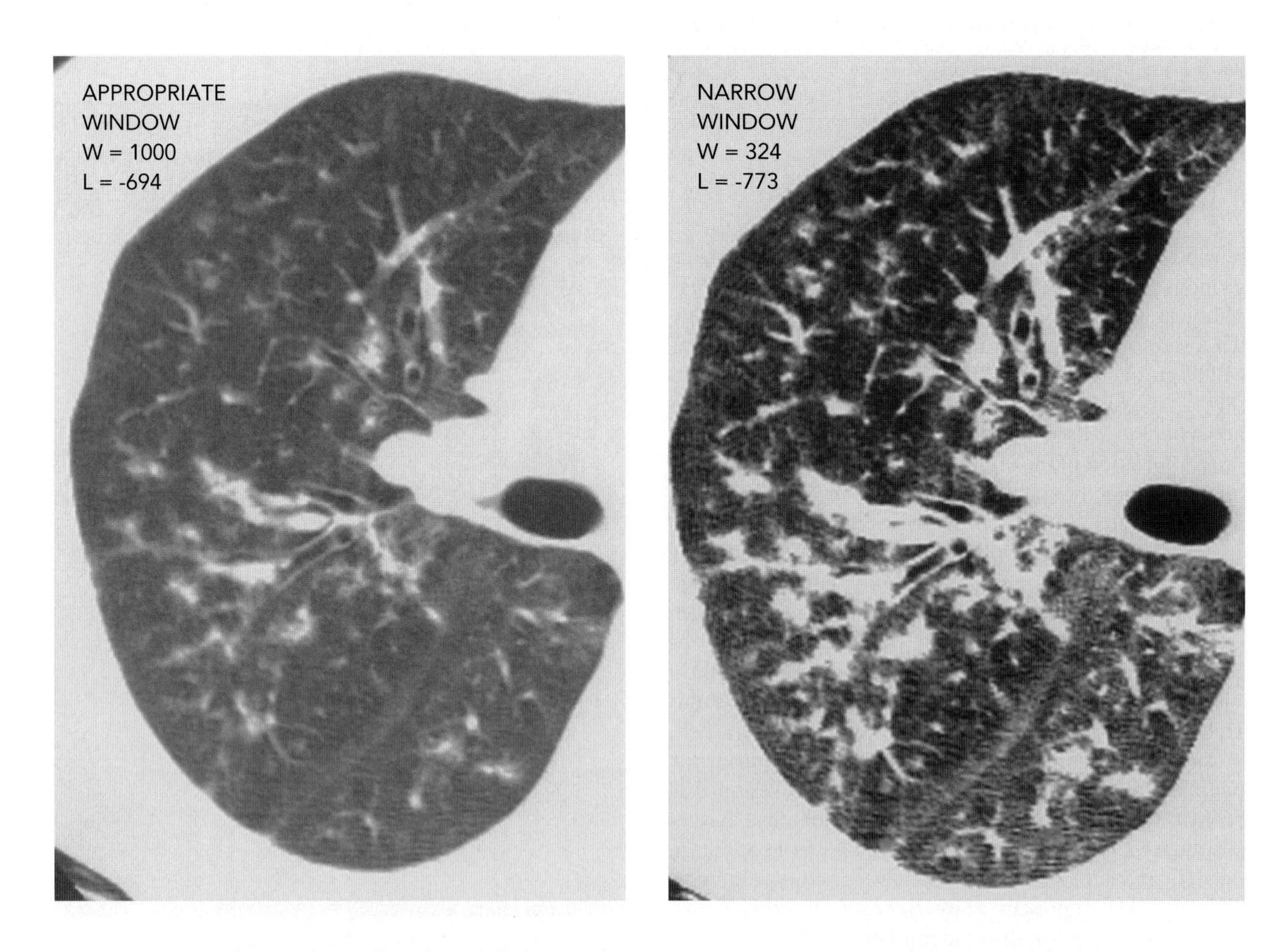

Figure 1-13 Effect of windowing on visualization of anatomic structures. **A**, **B**: Identical magnified sections through the right midlung using window widths and levels as shown. Note that when the window level and width are inappropriately low or narrow (**B**), there is considerable distortion of both normal and abnormal parenchyma. This, in turn, may lead to inappropriate detection or overestimation of the presence or extent of disease. Optimal evaluation of the airways is obtained using window centers between −210 and −700 HU, with corresponding window widths between 1,000 and 1,400.

TABLE 1-2
SEGMENTAL AND SUBSEGMENTAL BRONCHI: NOMENCLATURE AND VARIANTS

Bronchi and Segments	Subsegments	Most Common Variants/Comments[a]
Right lung		
Right upper lobe		
B1, apical	a, apical b, anterior	B1 origin from B3 or less likely B2
B2, posterior	a, apical b, posterior	B2 arising cephalad to B3 (56%), at same level as B2 or B2b (44%)
B3, anterior	a, lateral b, anterior	axillary subsegment formed by B2a and B3b (or both)
Middle lobe		
B4, lateral	a, lateral b, medial	B4 and B5 equivalent in size (44%) trifurcation B4a, B4b, B5 (13%)
B5, medial	a, superior b, inferior	B5 larger than B4 (27%)
Right lower lobe		
B6, superior segmental bronchus	a, medial b, superior c, lateral	B6c, B6a + b bifurcation (60%)
B*, subsuperior bronchus		variable, arises between B6 and B7 (30%)
truncus basalis		bronchial trunk caudal to B6 giving rise to basal segments
B7, medial basilar bronchus	a, anterior b, medial	B7a + b anterior to the right inferior pulmonary vein (60%)
B8, anterior	a, lateral b, basilar	rudimentary B8 (10%)
B9, lateral	a, lateral b, basilar	B8, B9 + 10 bifurcation (60%) B8, B9, B10 trifurcation (15%)
B10, posterior basilar bronchi	a, posterior b, lateral c, basilar	
Left lung		
Left upper lobe		bifurcation into superior (B1 + 2, B3) and inferior trunks (B4, B5) (75%) trifurcation of left upper lobe into B1 + 2, B3, B4 + 5 (16%–25%)
B1 + 2, apicoposterior	a, apical b, posterior c, lateral	 variation in origin of B1 + 2c common
B3, anterior	a, lateral b, medial c, superior	B3 may arise anywhere between B1 + 2 and B4 + 5 B3 poorly defined (25%)
B4, superior lingular bronchus	a, lateral b, anterior	well-developed B4a (40%); size varies depending on distribution of B3
B5, Inferior lingular bronchus	a, superior b, inferior	
Left lower lobe		
B6+, superior bronchus	a, medial b, superior c, lateral	B6a, B6b + c bifurcation (45%)
B*, subsuperior bronchus		variable, arises between B6 and B7, a single stem (30%)
truncus basalis		bronchial trunk giving rise to basal segments, longer than on right
B7 + 8, anteromedial bronchus	B7a, medial B7b, lateral B8a, lateral B8b, basilar	separate origin of B7 (<5%) B7 + 8, B9–10 bifurcation (45%) B7 + 8, 9, 10 trifurcation (15%)
B9, lateral basilar bronchus	a, lateral b, basilar	
B10, posterior basilar bronchus	a, lateral b, basilar	

[a]Percentages shown are approximate.

Right Lung Bronchial Anatomy

Six characteristic axial sections can be routinely identified in most patients, allowing rapid anatomic orientation regardless of individual scan levels (Fig. 1-14). These include (1) the distal trachea/carina and right upper lobe apical segmental bronchus (Fig. 1-14A), (2) the right upper lobe bronchus, including the anterior and posterior segmental bronchi (Fig. 1-14B), (3) the bronchus intermedius (Fig. 1-14C and D), (4) the origin of the middle and lower lobe bronchi, often including the superior segmental bronchus (Fig. 1-14G and H), (5) the trunk of the proximal right lower lobe bronchus—the "truncus basalis" (Fig. 1-14I), and (6) the proximal basilar segmental bronchi (Fig. 1-14J).

Several key points need to be emphasized when evaluating the right-sided airways. The right upper lobe bronchus typically originates at or just below the level of the carina and is termed eparterial because it arises above the right main pulmonary artery. At this point, the posterior wall of the right upper lobe bronchus and, more inferiorly, the bronchus intermedius are in direct contact with air in the right upper lobe; less commonly the apical segment of the right lower lobe is also in direct contact with air, depending on the position of the medial end of the right main fissure.

On occasion, a prominent vein may be identified posterior to these airways draining superiorly into the right superior pulmonary vein. In one study of 280 consecutive patients, a focal round elevation in the posterior wall of the bronchus intermedius was identified in 14 individuals (5%); in 71% this represented a vein originating in the posterior segment of the right upper lobe, whereas in the remaining patients this represented a vein draining the superior segment of the right lower lobe (109). Potential confusion with a true lung nodule can be avoided by noting that this structure is tubular, is identifiable on adjacent sections, and is traceable to the medial aspect of the right superior pulmonary vein.

The origin of the apical segmental bronchus is easily identified by noting the presence of a rounded lucency superimposed on the distal end of the right upper lobe bronchus (Fig. 1-14B). Although posterior displacement (with or without displacement of the right mainstem bronchus or bronchus intermedius) is a sensitive indicator of volume loss within the right upper lobe as a result of scarring, as occurs most often in patients with tuberculosis, anterior displacement is more often seen as a consequence of endobronchial obstruction or following radiation therapy.

Unlike the right upper lobe bronchus, the middle lobe bronchus characteristically has a slightly oblique orientation coursing caudally. As a consequence, it is not uncommon for the distal aspect of the middle lobe bronchus to appear narrowed or triangular in configuration. This simply reflects partial volume averaging and is easily identified as such by evaluating sequential images through the distal middle lobe bronchus and its medial and lateral segments. Although it has been suggested that this airway in particular is best evaluated using an angled gantry, this approach is now seldom used (110), especially when retrospective thin sections can be obtained.

Identification of the basilar segmental airways is facilitated by noting that each subtends a characteristic zone in the lower lobe. Of particular note is the finding that the medial segmental bronchus lies anterior and medial to the inferior pulmonary vein and is the smallest of the basilar airways (Fig. 1-14J). In distinction, the superior segmental and posterobasilar segmental bronchi, respectively, are the largest basilar airways, and they supply the lion's share of the lower lobe.

Left Lung Bronchial Anatomy

Analogous to the right side, six characteristic axial sections can be routinely identified in most patients through the left-sided airways (Fig. 1-14). These include (1) the distal trachea/carina and apical-posterior segmental bronchus of the left upper lobe (Fig. 1-14A to C), (2) the left mainstem bronchus and proximal apical-posterior segmental bronchus (Fig. 1-14D), (3) the distal left mainstem bronchus/proximal left upper lobe bronchus (Fig. 1-14 E), (4) the distal left upper lobe bronchus and proximal lingular bronchus (Fig. 1-14F), (5) the trunk of the proximal left lower lobe bronchus—the "truncus basalis" (Fig. 1-14H), and (6) the proximal basilar segmental bronchi (Fig. 1-14I and J).

Compared with the right-sided airways, a number of salient points must be emphasized. First, the left upper lobe bronchus is a large structure, which allows multiple images to be obtained through both its upper and lower portions. A section through the upper aspect of the left upper lobe bronchus is easily identifiable because the posterior wall of the bronchus at this level is smoothly concave and is further marked by focal increased density compared with the distal left mainstem bronchus owing to a partial volume effect from the left main pulmonary artery as it passes over the left upper lobe bronchus at this point. A rounded lucency is generally identifiable at the distal end of the left upper lobe bronchus at this level, representing the origin of the apical-posterior segmental bronchus (Fig. 1-14E).

In distinction, a section obtained through the lower portion of the left upper lobe bronchus will also include the secondary carina; this is identifiable as a triangular wedge of soft tissue located posterolaterally. The left upper lobe bronchus is marginated laterally at this point by the left interlobar pulmonary artery. A circular lucency at the end of the left upper lobe bronchus at this level indicates the origin of the lingular bronchus (Fig. 1-14F). The superior segmental bronchus is also often seen coursing posteriorly at or near this level (Fig. 1-14F and G). Unlike the superior segmental bronchus, however, the anterior segmental bronchus to the left upper lobe is more unpredictable; most often arising as a trifurcation from the distal end of the left upper lobe bronchus, this same airway may also arise from the apical-posterior segmental bronchus or even the proximal lingular

(*Text continues on page 21.*)

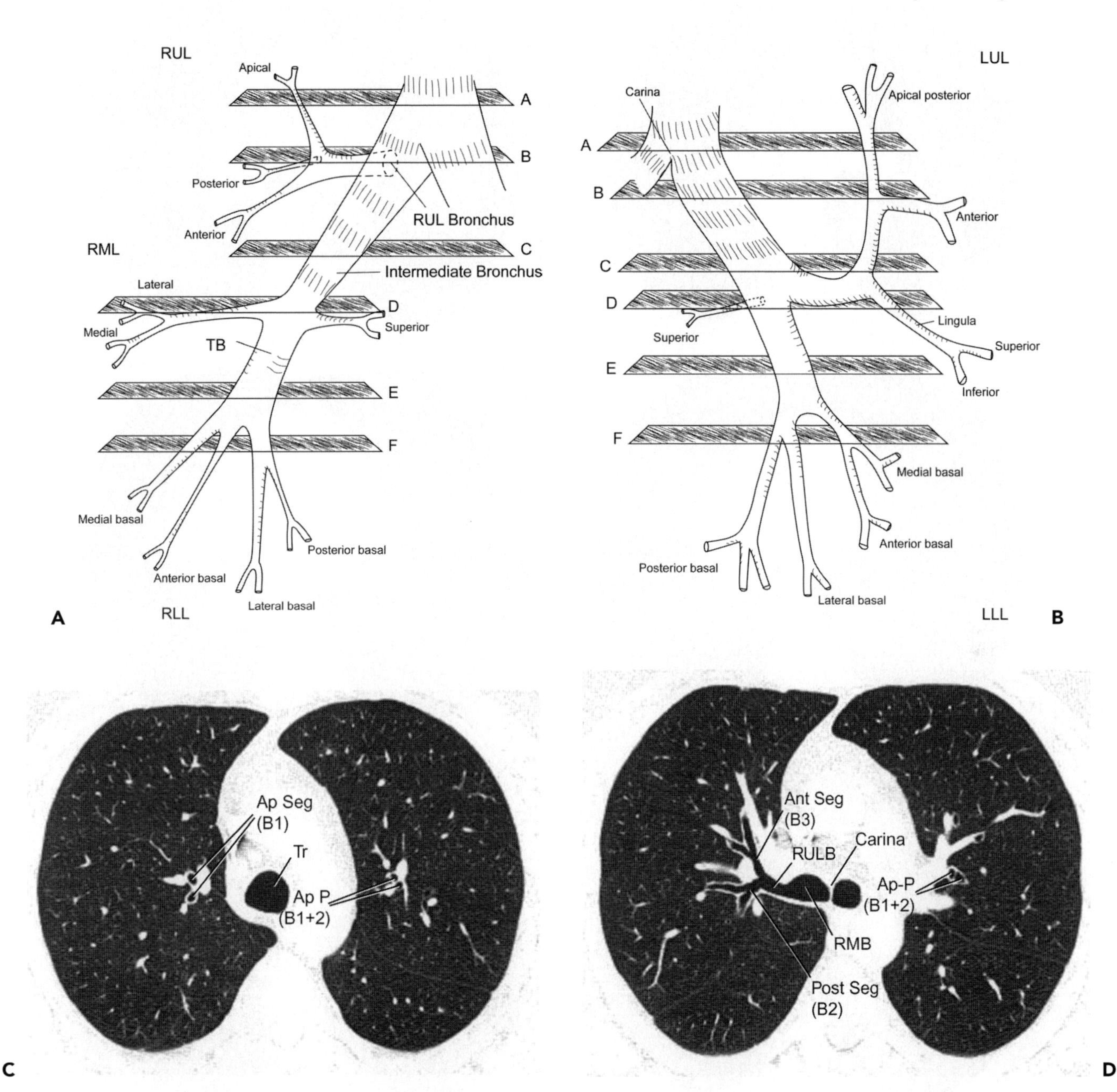

Figure 1-14 Characteristic cross-sectional anatomy of the airways. **A** and **B:** Diagrammatic illustrations of the right and left bronchial trees, respectively, each showing six characteristic axial sections illustrated in **C** to **L. C** to **L:** Axial sections corresponding to the diagrammatic representations in **A** and **B** (see Table 1-2 for correlation). Tr, trachea; Ap Seg (B1), right upper lobe apical segmental bronchus; Ap P (B1 + 2), left upper lobe apical-posterior segmental bronchus; Ant Seg (B2), right upper lobe anterior segmental bronchus; RULB, right upper lobe bronchus; Post Seg (B3), right upper lobe posterior segmental bronchus; BI, bronchus intermedius; LMB, left mainstem bronchus; RMB, right mainstem bronchus; Ant Seg Br (B3), left upper lobe anterior segmental bronchus; Ap-Post (B1 + 2), left upper lobe apical posterior segmental bronchus; LULB, left upper lobe bronchus; LB, lingual bronchus; LLLB, left lower lobe bronchus; MLB, middle lobe bronchus; RLLB, right lower lobe bronchus; Inf LB (B5), inferior lingular bronchus; LLLB, left lower lobe bronchus; Sup LB (B4), superior lingular bronchus; Sup Seg (B6), left lower lobe superior segmental bronchus; Sup Seg Br (B6), right lower lobe superior segmental bronchus; Lat Seg Br (B4), middle lobe lateral segmental bronchus; Med Seg Br (B5), middle lobe medial segmental bronchus; TB-RLL, truncus basalis, right lower lobe; TB-LLL, truncus basialis, left lower lobe; AB-RLL (B8), right lower lobe anterobasilar segmental bronchus; MB-RLL (B7), right lower lobe medial basilar segmental bronchus; LB-RLL (B9), right lower lobe lateral basilar segmental bronchus; PB-RLL (B10), right lower lobe posterobasilar segmental bronchus; AB-LLL (B8), left lower lobe anterobasilar segmental bronchus; MB-LLL (B7), left lower lobe anterobasilar segmental bronchus; LB-LLL (B9), left lower lobe lateral basilar segmental bronchus; PB-LLL (B10), left lower lobe posterobasilar segmental bronchus. *(continued)*

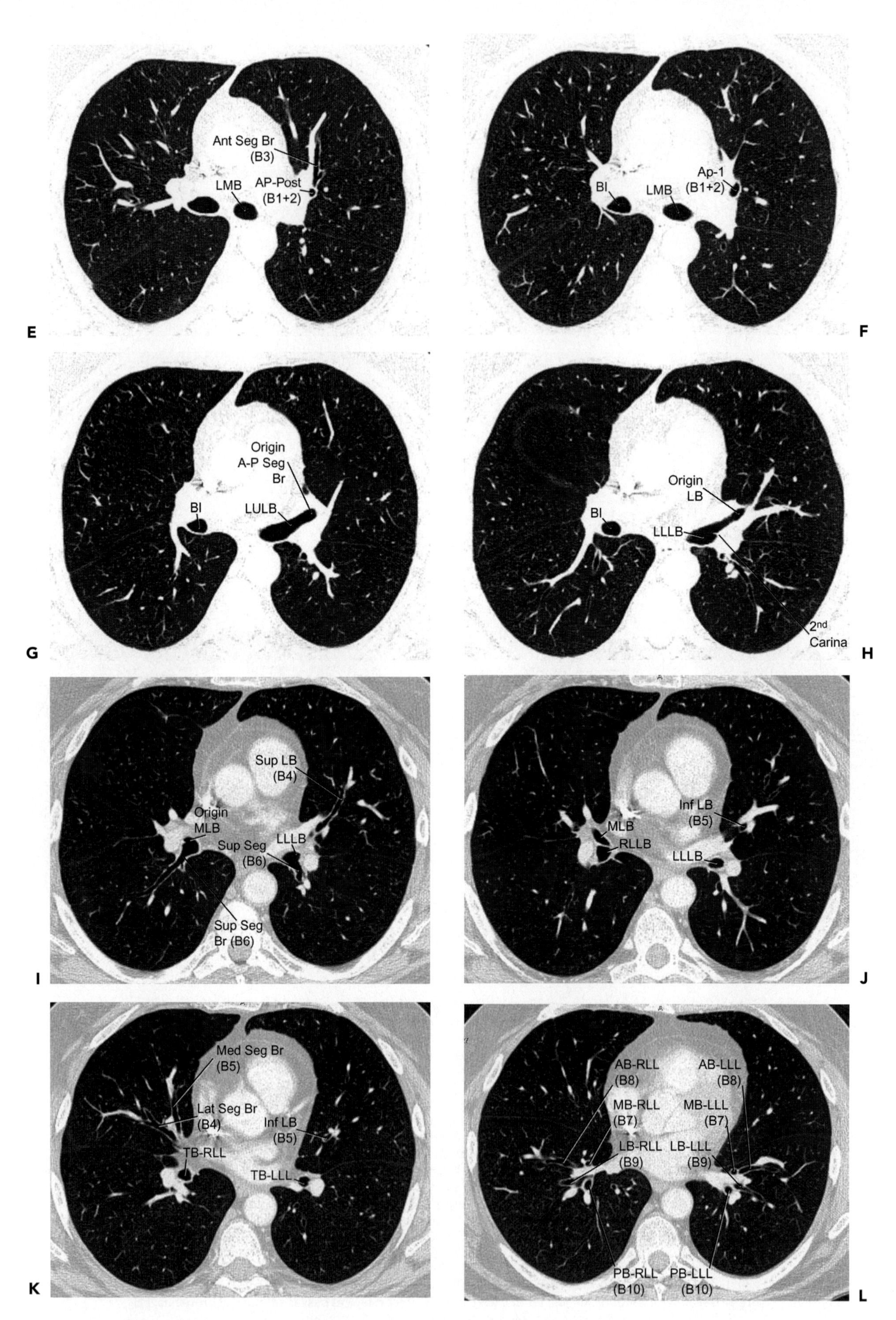

Figure 1-14 *(continued)*

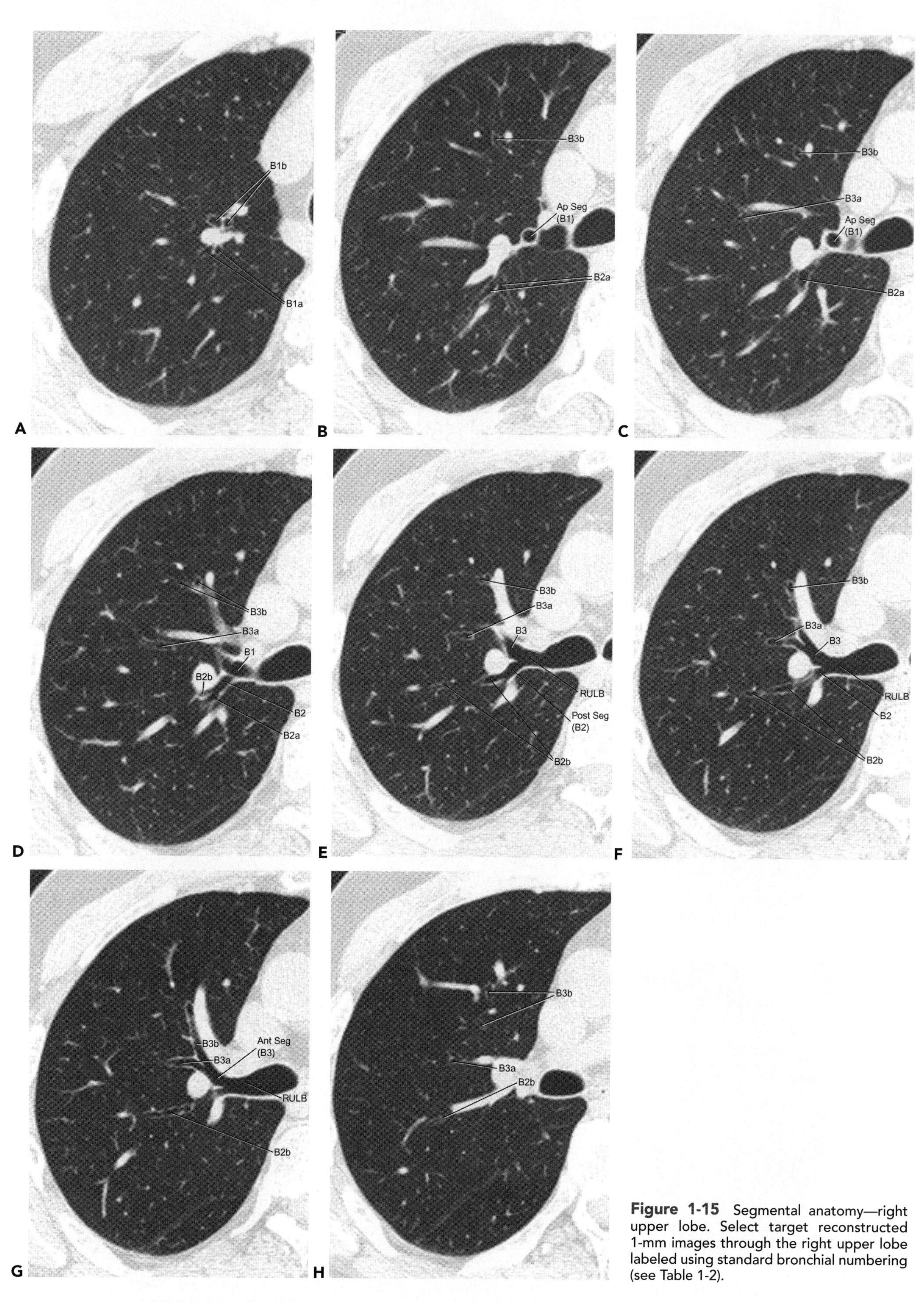

Figure 1-15 Segmental anatomy—right upper lobe. Select target reconstructed 1-mm images through the right upper lobe labeled using standard bronchial numbering (see Table 1-2).

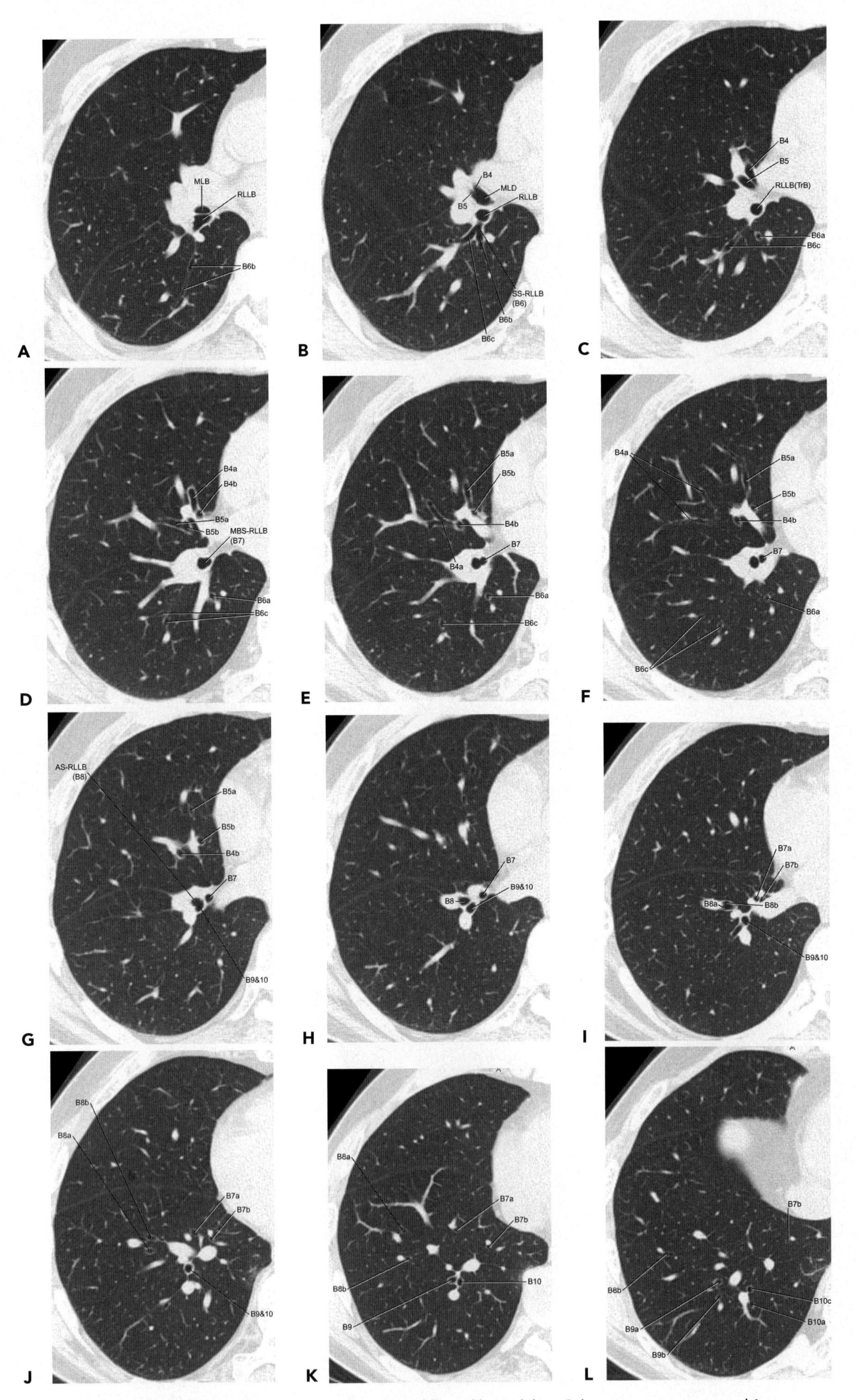

Figure 1-16 Segmental anatomy—right middle and lower lobes. Select target reconstructed 1-mm target images through the middle and right lower lobes labeled using standard bronchial numbering (see Table 1-2).

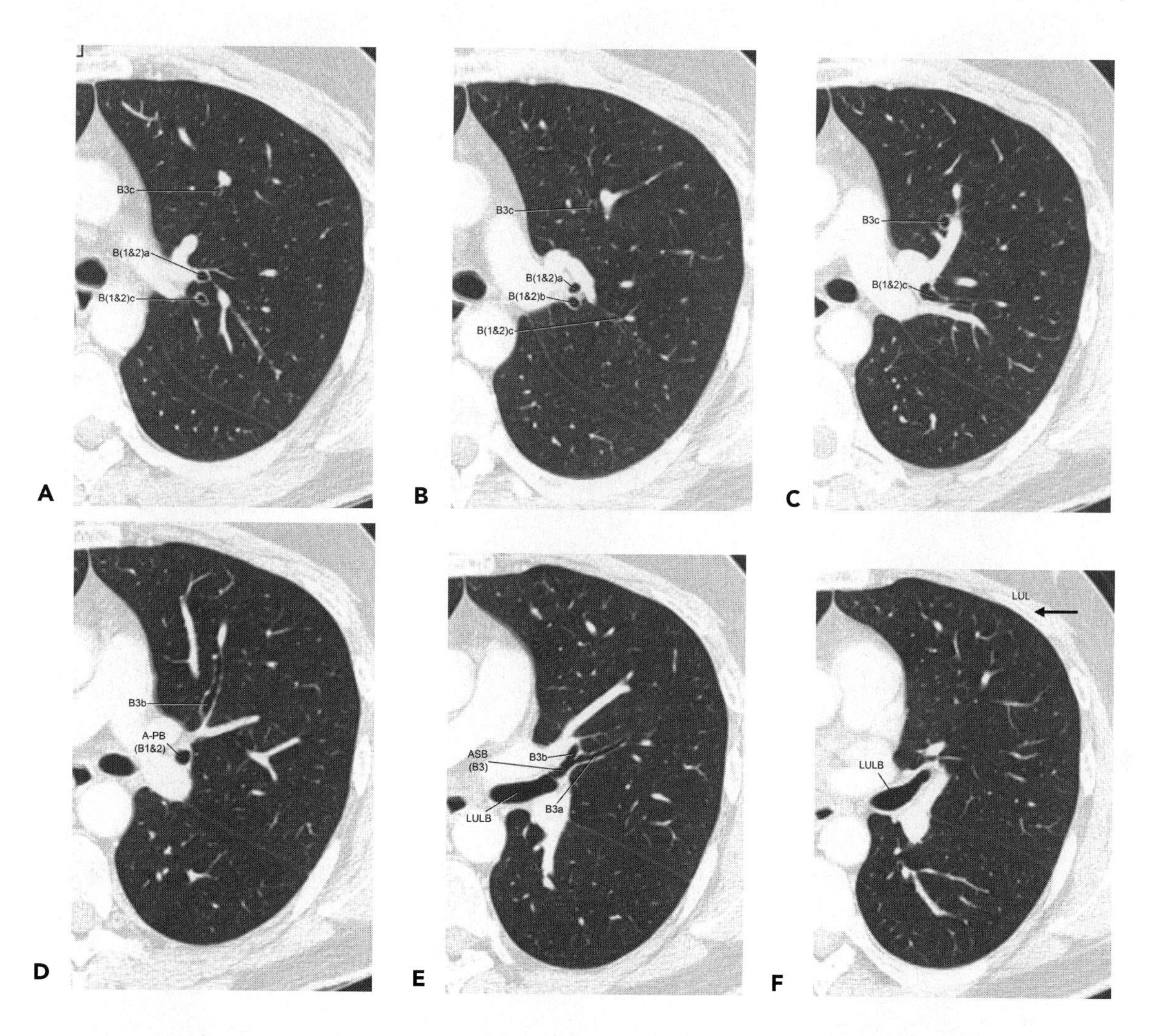

Figure 1-17 Segmental anatomy—left upper lobe. Select target reconstructed 1-mm target reconstructed images through the left upper lobe labeled using standard bronchial numbering (see Table 1-2).

bronchus. Despite this, the anterior segmental bronchus is usually easily identified because it characteristically courses horizontally in the same plane as the CT scan (Fig. 1-14C).

Regarding the basilar airways, the only difference between the right and left sides is that, on the left, the medial and anterobasilar segmental bronchi most often arise from a common trunk (Fig. 1-14I and J). Otherwise, the right and left lower lobe bronchi tend to be mirror images of each other.

Subsegmental Bronchial Anatomy

Unlike lobar and segmental bronchi, in which anatomic variations are generally minor and easily recognized, there is considerable variability in the branching pattern of subsegmental and more peripheral airways. Although they can be identified when sequential or overlapping individual high-resolution images are evaluated, few reliably consistent patterns are identifiable (Figs. 1-15 to 1-18). In fact, no generally accepted terminology exists to describe these airways. Recently, a standard nomenclature was proposed by Suma et al. (111). The impetus was the introduction of ultrathin bronchoscopes (UTBs) with an outer diameter of 2.8 mm. UTBs allow direct visualization of up to tenth-order bronchi and have an inner working channel of 1.2 mm, which allows the use of forceps or brush biopsies. By comparison, routine flexible bronchoscopes typically allow visualization of only fourth- to fifth-order airways.

Although to date only limited use has been made of ultrathin bronchoscopy in the adult population, the potential for coupling virtual bronchoscopic pathway planning with ultrathin bronchoscopy remains of considerable potential (Fig. 1-7). There have been only a few isolated reports to date, mostly in the Japanese literature, of the use of virtual bronchoscopic guidance for directing ultrathin bronchoscopic evaluation specifically of small peripheral lung lesions (81,111–116). In one study using fluoroscopically directed ultrathin bronchoscopy as an adjunct to routine bronchoscopy, a successful diagnosis was established in 11 of 17 patients (64.7%) (116). In the largest

(Text continues on page 24.)

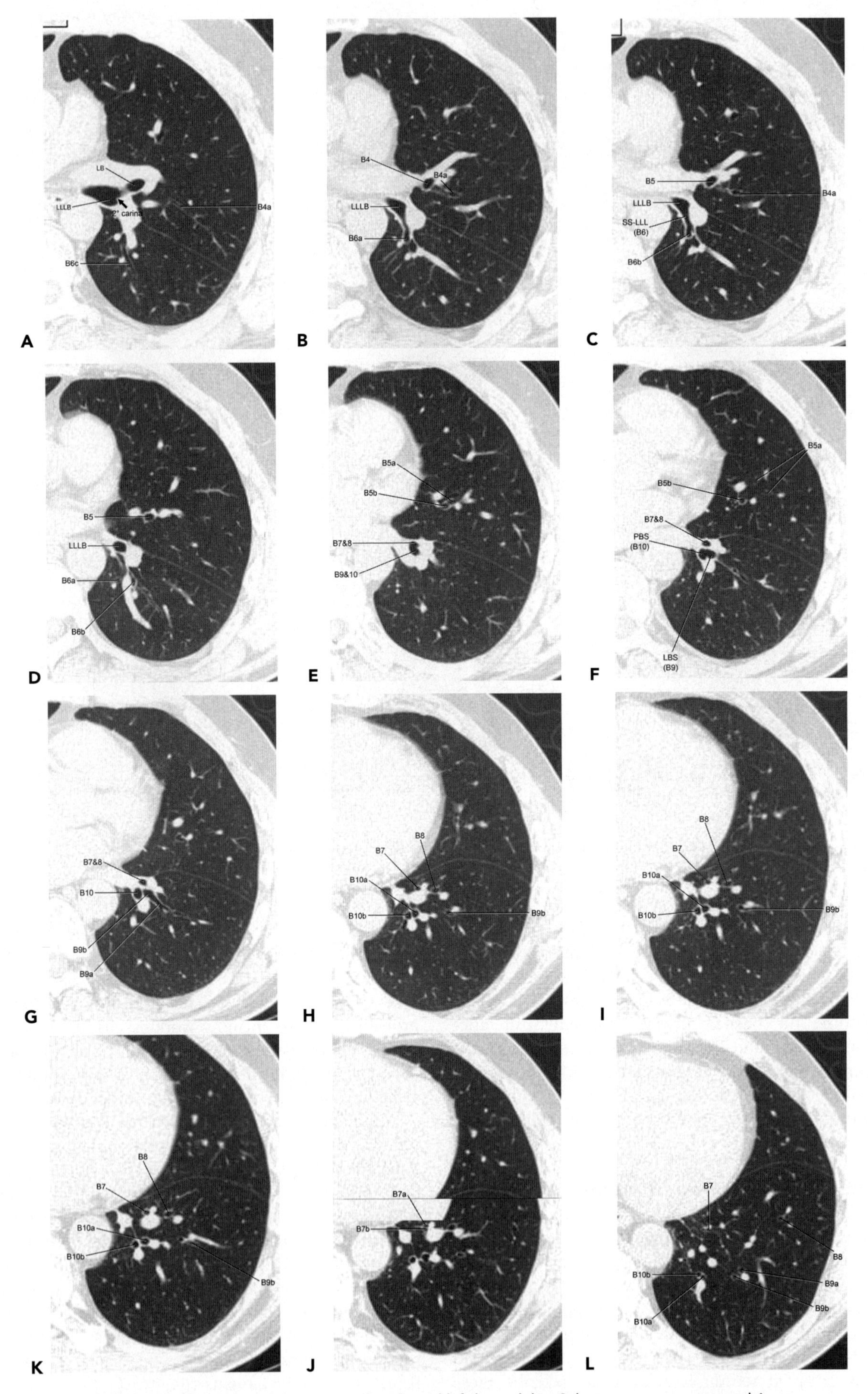

Figure 1-18 Segmental anatomy—lingula and left lower lobe. Select target reconstructed 1-mm target reconstructed images through the left lower lobe labeled using standard bronchial numbering (see Table 1-2).

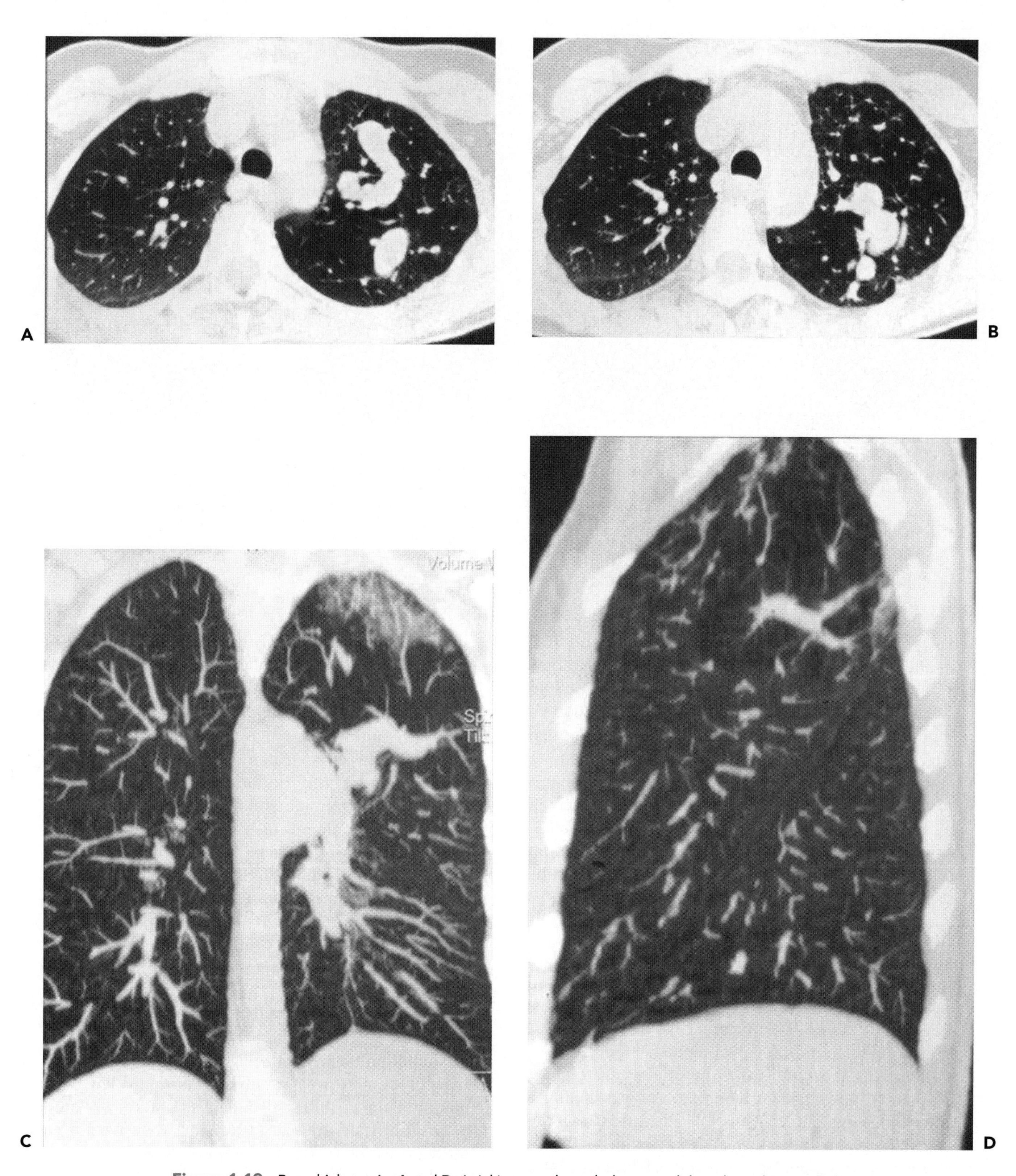

Figure 1-19 Bronchial atresia. **A** and **B:** Axial images through the upper lobes show characteristic branching pattern of mucoid impaction. Note that the peripheral portion of the left upper lobe is emphysematous. **C** and **D:** Volumetrically rendered coronal section and sagittal MIP, respectively, show to better advantage the characteristic branching pattern of a blind-ending, mucoid-impacted left upper lobe bronchus as well as the extent of peripheral emphysema and, in this case, apical consolidation. Involvement of the left upper lobe is characteristic of bronchial atresia.

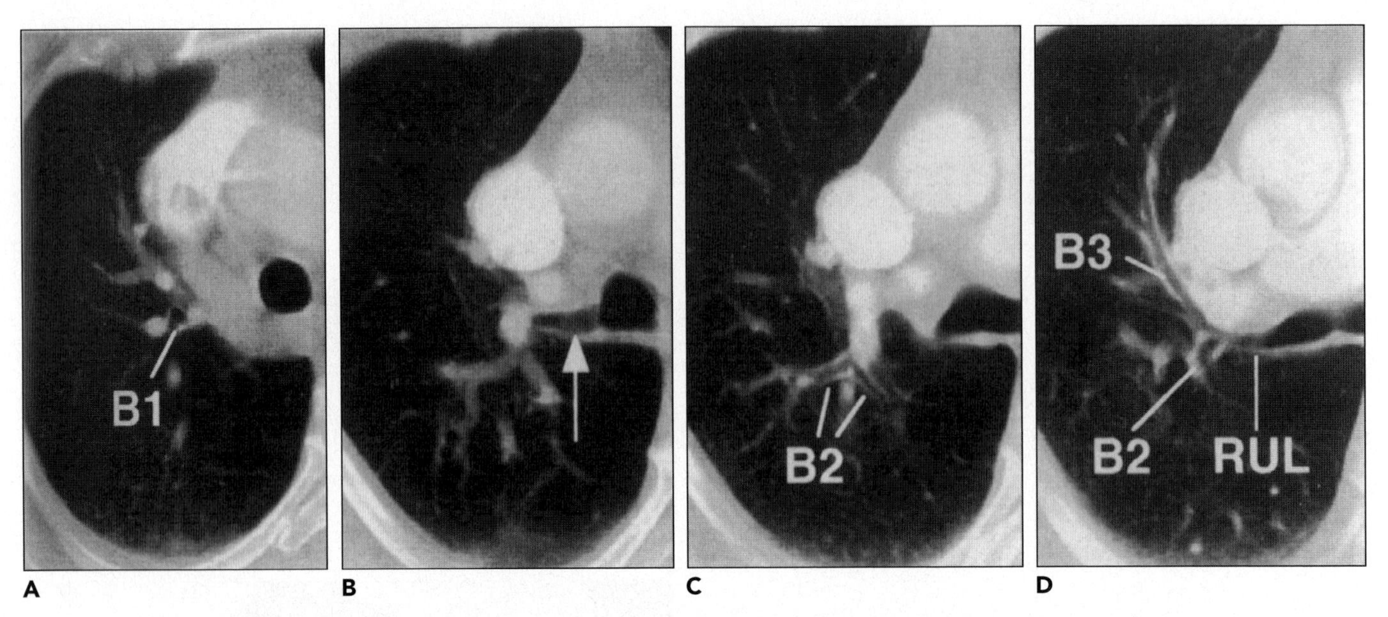

Figure 1-20 Tracheal bronchus. Four images (**A** to **D**) at contiguous levels in a patient with a tracheal bronchus, obtained with spiral technique 7-mm collimation and reconstruction at 7-mm intervals. The tracheal bronchus (*arrow*, **B**) arises from the lateral tracheal wall. It supplies the apical segment of the right upper lobe (B1), seen in cross section in **A**. The right upper lobe bronchus (RUL) gives rise to the anterior (B3) and posterior (B2) segmental bronchi.

series reported to date, Shinagawa et al. (115) performed CT-guided transbronchial biopsy (TBBx) with a UTB. They used virtual bronchoscopic navigation to diagnose peripheral lung lesions smaller than 2 cm in size. Of a total of 26 nodules in 25 patients, these authors successfully biopsied 17 (65%) including 14 neoplasms and 3 benign lesions. For the purposes of this study, virtual bronchoscopic images were obtainable to only fifth-generation airways, likely in part explaining these authors' limited success. Although it is also possible for VB to play a role in directing ultrathin bronchoscopic biopsies in patients with diffuse lung disease by identifying optimal sites for obtaining tissue, this application has yet to be investigated.

Anatomic Variants

Although a wide range of lung bud anomalies have been described, including agenesis, congenital bronchial atresia (Fig. 1-19), congenital lobar emphysema, congenital cystic adenomatoid malformation, and pulmonary bronchogenic cysts, in adults those most often encountered are either anomalous or supernumerary bronchi (117). By definition, a displaced or anomalous bronchus is one that arises at a lower level than normal in the bronchial tree; this same bronchus is considered supernumerary if a normal bronchus also supplies the same lung segment. Although several hypotheses have been proposed to account for these anomalies (118), the following slightly modified classification, as proposed by Wu et al. (119), has proved especially clinically useful:

1. *Anomalies arising from normal higher-order bronchial divisions.* These include, among others, accessory superior segmental bronchi, typically appearing as two closely aligned bronchi both supplying the superior segment of the right lower lobe, and axillary bronchi, identifiable as a supernumerary segmental bronchus supplying the lateral aspect of the right upper lobe.
2. *Anomalies arising from sites typically lacking branches.* Included in this group in particular are tracheal bronchi, accessory cardiac bronchi, and bridging bronchi. The most common example of this anomaly is the tracheal or pig bronchus (Fig. 1-20) (120–123). Identifiable in up to 1% to 2% of normal individuals, tracheal bronchi exclusively arise on the right side and may involve displacement of the entire right upper lobe, the apical segmental bronchus only, or additional supernumerary lobar or separate apical segmental bronchi (124). Although the endoscopic appearance of this anomaly may superficially mimic the rarer entity of tracheal diverticula, CT can readily distinguish these entities (Fig. 1-21) (125). Tracheal bronchi also need to be distinguished from tracheoceles (Fig. 1-22). The latter represent an outpouching or diverticulum involving the posterolateral tracheal wall as a result of focal weakness of the trachealis muscle (126,127). They have been further classified into two groups: those with wide mouths, likely acquired, and those with narrow mouths, likely congenital. These lesions may grow to be quite large and ultimately may serve as reservoirs for debris, leading to recurrent episodes of aspiration pneumonia.

Another commonly encountered bronchial anomaly encountered in up to 0.5% of the population is the so-called accessory cardiac bronchus (Fig. 1-23) (46,128,129). Considered by some to be the only true

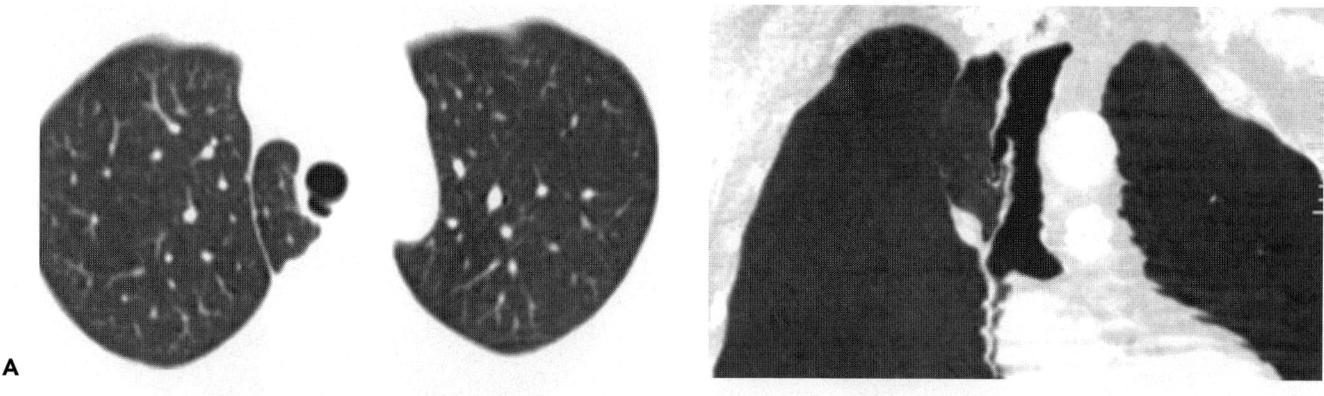

Figure 1-21 Tracheal diverticulum. **A** and **B:** Axial and coronal MPR, respectively, show a well-defined blind-ending tracheal diverticulum originating from the lateral aspect of the midtrachea. This entity should be distinguished from both anomalous bronchi, which typically occur nearer to the carina (see Fig. 1-20), and tracheoceles, which typically originate at a higher level (see Fig. 1-22).

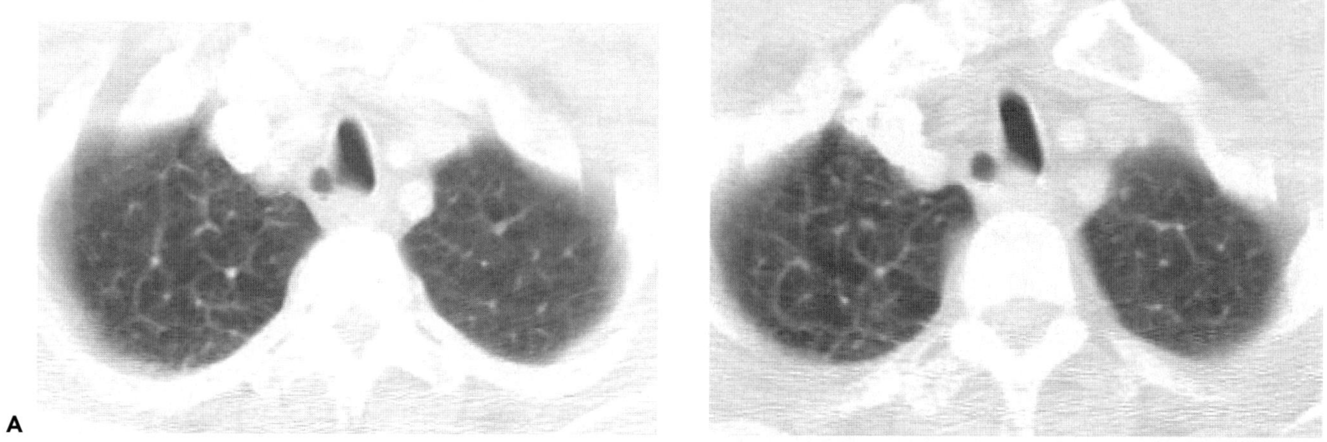

Figure 1-22 Tracheocele. **A** and **B:** Sequential axial images show characteristic outpouching of the posterolateral wall of the intrathoracic trachea at the level of the thoracic inlet.

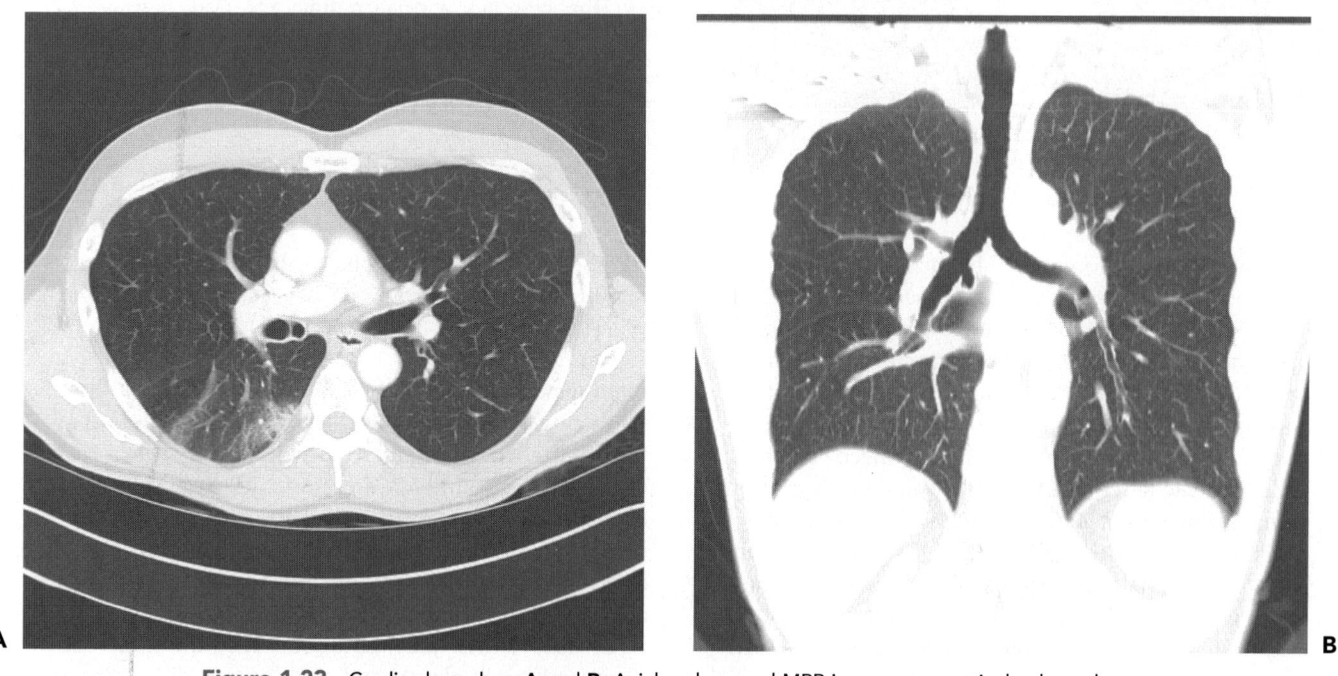

Figure 1-23 Cardiac bronchus. **A** and **B:** Axial and coronal MPR images, respectively, show characteristic appearance of an anomalous bronchus originating from the medial wall of the bronchus intermedius, coursing inferiorly. These may serve as a reservoir for debris, resulting in repeated episodes of aspiration or hemoptysis. In this case note the presence of ill-defined infiltrate in the superior segment of the right lower lobe resulting from aspiration (see also Fig. 2-5).

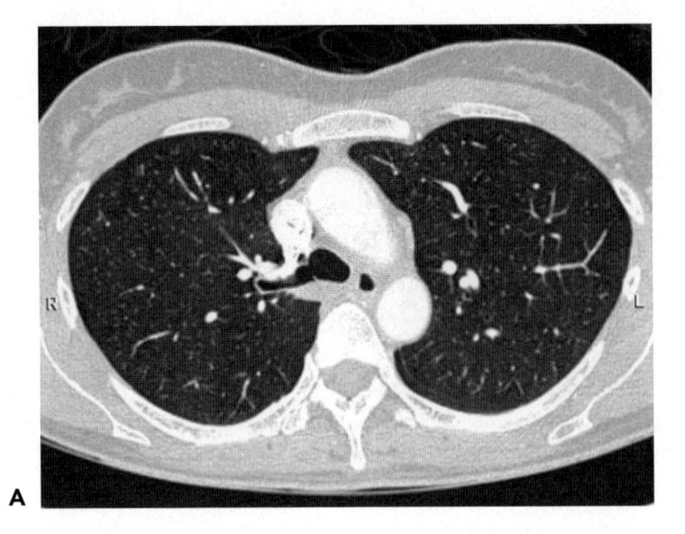

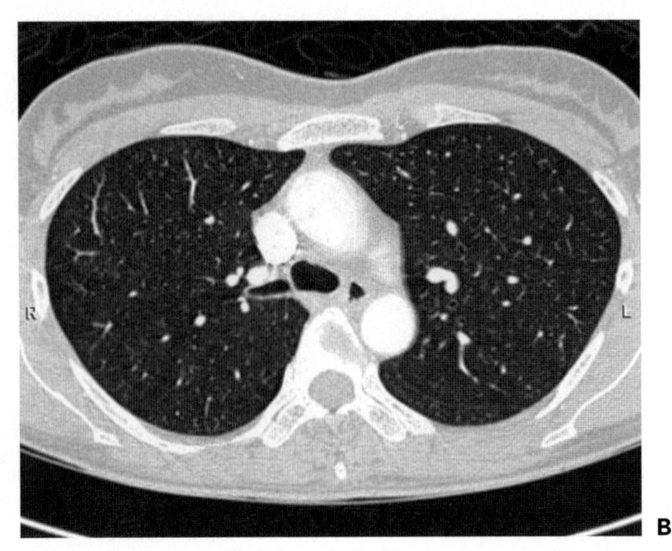

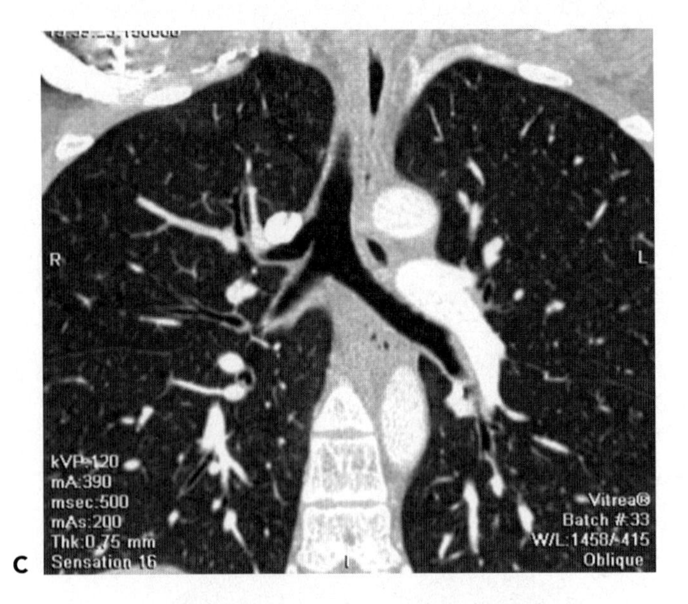

Figure 1-24 Bridging bronchus. **A** and **B:** Sequential axial images at the level of the carina show an unusual configuration of the right upper lobe bronchus originating from the distal trachea. **C:** Coronal reconstruction shows that the right upper lobe bronchus arises separately from the distal trachea, whereas the bronchus intermedius arises from the proximal left mainstem bronchus. This configuration is typical of a so-called bridging bronchus.

supernumerary anomalous bronchus (130), this bronchus always arises from the medial wall of the bronchus intermedius before the origins of the superior segmental and middle lobe bronchi and courses caudally toward the mediastinum, hence the "cardiac" appellation. Of variable length, cardiac bronchi range from short, blind-ending diverticula to longer, branching structures; the latter type are often found in association with rudimentary alveolar tissue, likely representing a rudimentary accessory lobe. Although typically asymptomatic, similar to tracheoceles, cardiac bronchi may serve as a potential reservoir for retained secretions, leading to chronic inflammation and hypervascularity and resulting in recurrent episodes of aspiration pneumonitis or hemoptysis (128,129,131).

Less commonly seen, a bridging bronchus is an anomaly in which the right main bronchus directly supplies the right upper lobe, with the bronchus intermedius originating from the left mainstem bronchus (Fig. 1-24) (132).

3. *Anomalies associated with abnormalities of situs.* Most frequently identified in this category is simple reversal of the right- and left-sided airways (Fig. 1-4). Less commonly encountered are anomalies resulting from bronchial isomerism, in which the pattern of airway branching and pulmonary lobation is identical in the two lungs (119,124). This includes bilateral left-sided airway anatomy (either as an isolated finding or associated with either the venolobar syndrome or, less commonly, polysplenia) and bilateral right-sided airway anatomy. Right-sided airway isomerism is usually associated with asplenia and severe congenital heart disease and is only rarely seen in adults.

REFERENCES

1. Boiselle PM, Ernst A. State-of-the-art imaging of the central airways. *Respiration* 2003;70:383–394.
2. Naidich DP, Funt S, Ettenger NA, Arranda C. Hemoptysis: CT-bronchoscopic correlations in 58 cases. *Radiology* 1990;177:357–362.
3. McGuinness G, Beacher JR, Harkin TJ. Hemoptysis: prospective high-resolution CT/bronchoscopic correlation. *Chest* 1994;105:1155–1162.
4. Corder R. Hemoptysis. *Emerg Med Clin North Am* 2003;21:421–435.
5. McLoud TC. Imaging techniques for diagnosis and staging of lung cancer. *Clin Chest Med* 2002;23:123–136.
6. Kwon KY, Myers JL, Swensen SJ, Colby TV. Middle lobe syndrome: a clinicopathological study of 21 patients. *Hum Pathol* 1995;26:302–307.
7. Molina PL, Hiken JN, and Glazer HS. Imaging evaluation of obstructive atelectasis. *J Thorac Imaging* 1996;11:176–186.
8. Grenier P, Lenoir S, Brauner M. Computed tomographic assessment of bronchiectasis. *Semin Ultrasound CT MR* 1990;11:430–441.
9. Hansell DM. Bronchiectasis. *Radiol Clin North Am* 1998;36:107–128.
10. McGuinness G, Naidich DP. Bronchiectasis: CT/clinical correlations. *Semin Ultrasound CT MRI* 1995;16:395–419.
11. Garg K, et al. Proliferative and constrictive bronchiolitis: classification and radiologic features. *AJR Am J Roentgenol* 1994;162:803–808.
12. Hartman TE, Primack SL, Lee KS, et al. CT of bronchial and bronchiolar diseases. *Radiographics* 1994;14:991–1003.
13. Heyneman LE, Ward S, Lynch DA, et al. Respiratory bronchiolitis, respiratory bronchiolitis-associated interstitial lung disease, and desquamative interstitial pneumonia: different entities or part of the spectrum of the same disease process? *AJR Am J Roentgenol* 1999;173:1617–1622.
14. Ikonen T, Kivisaari L, Harjula AL, et al. Value of high-resolution computed tomography in routine evaluation of lung transplantation recipients during development of bronchiolitis obliterans syndrome. *J Heart Lung Transplant* 1996;15:587–595.
15. Leung AN, Fisher K, Valentine V, et al. Bronchiolitis obliterans after lung transplantation: detection using expiratory HRCT. *Chest* 1998;113:365–370.
16. Ryu JH, Myers J, Swenson SJ. Bronchiolar disorders. *Am J Respir Crit Care Med* 2003;168:1277–1292.
17. Sharma V, Shaaban AM, Berges G, and Gosselin M. The radiological spectrum of small-airway diseases. *Semin Ultrasound CT MRI* 2002;23:339–351.
18. Harkin TJ, Wang K-P. Bronchoscopic needle aspiration of mediastinal and hilar lymph nodes. *J Bronchol* 1997;4:238–249.
19. Ferretti GR, Kocier M, Calaque O, et al. Follow-up after stent insertion in the tracheobronchial tree: role of helical computed tomography in comparison with fiberoptic bronchoscopy. *Eur Radiol* 2003;13:1172–1178.
20. Colice G, Chappel GJ, Frenchman SM, and Solomon DA. Comparison of computed tomography with fiberoptic bronchoscopy in identifying endobronchial abnormalities in patients with suspected lung cancer. *Am Rev Respir Dis* 1985;131:397–400.
21. Haponik F, Britt EJ, Smith PL, and Bleecker ER. Computed chest tomography in the evaluation of hemoptysis. *Chest* 1987;91:80–85.
22. Zhang JB, Hasegawa I, Feller-Kopman D, and Boiselle PM. Dynamic expiratory volumetric CT imaging of the central airways: comparison of standard-dose and low-dose techniques. *Acad Radiol* 2003;10:719–724.
23. Boiselle PM, Dippolito G, Copeland J, et al. Multiplanar and 3D imaging of the central airways: comparison of image quality and radiation dose of single-detector row CT and multi-detector row CT at differing tube currents in dogs. *Radiology* 2003;228:107–111.
24. Siegel MJ. Multiplanar and three-dimensional multi-detector row CT of thoracic vessels and airways in the pediatric population. *Radiology* 2003;229:641–650.
25. Boiselle PM, Feller-Kopman D, Ashiku S, et al. Tracheobronchomalacia: evolving role of dynamic multislice helical CT. *Radiol Clin North Am* 2003;41:627–636.
26. Schertler T, Wildermuth S, Willmann JK, et al. Effects of ECG gating and postprocessing techniques on 3D MDCT of the bronchial tree. *AJR Am J Roentgenol* 2004;183:83–89.
27. Ferretti GR, Bricault I, Coulomb M. Virtual tools for imaging of the thorax. *Eur Respir J* 2001;18:381–392.
28. Grenier PA, Beigelman-Aubry C, Fetita C, and Martin-Bouyer Y. Multidetector-row CT of the airways. *Semin Roentgenol* 2003;38:146–157.
29. Lacrosse M, Trigaux JP, Van Beers BE, and Weynants P. 3D spiral CT of the tracheobronchial tree. *J Comput Assist Tomogr* 1995;19:341–347.
30. Summers RM, Feng DH, Holland SM, et al. Virtual bronchoscopy: segmentation method for real-time display. *Radiology* 1996;200:857–862.
31. Brink JA. Technical aspects of helical (spiral) CT. *Radiol Clin North Am* 1995;33:825–841.
32. Quint LE, Whyte RI, Kazerooni EA, et al. Stenosis of the central airways: evaluation by using helical CT with multiplanar reconstructions. *Radiology* 1995;194:871–877.
33. Schlueter FJ, et al. Bronchial dehiscence after lung transplantation: correlation of CT findings with clinical outcome. *Radiology* 1996;199:849–854.
34. Im JG, et al. Clinical utility of 2D and 3D spiral CT in the evaluation of tracheobronchial disease. *Radiology* 1994;193:261(abst).
35. Salvolini L, Bichi Secchi E, Costarelli L, and DeNicola M. Clinical applications of 2D and 3D CT imaging of the airways—a review. *Eur J Radiol* 2000;34:9–25.
36. McAdams HP, Murray JG, Erasmus JJ, et al. Telescoping bronchial anastomoses for unilateral or bilateral sequential lung transplantation: CT appearance. *Radiology* 1997;203:202–206.
37. Rubin GD, Napel S, Leung AN. Volumetric analysis of volumetric data: achieving a paradigm shift (Editorial). *Radiology* 1996;200:312–317.
38. Napel S, Rubin GD, Jeffrey RB. Technical note. STS-MIP: a new reconstruction technique for CT of the chest. *J Comput Assist Tomogr* 1993;17:832–838.
39. Fotheringham T, Chabat F, Hansell DM, et al. A comparison of methods for enhancing the detection of areas of decreased attenuation on CT caused by airways disease. *J Comput Assist Tomogr* 1999;23:385–389.
40. Yang GZ, Chabat F, Hansell DM. Enhancement of subtle density differences of the lung parenchyma on CT. *Br J Radiol* 1998;71:686–690.
41. Bhalla M, Naidich DP, McGuinness G, et al. Diffuse lung disease: assessment with helical CT—preliminary observations of the role of maximum and minimum projection images. *Radiology* 1996;200:341–347.
42. Rémy-Jardin M, Remy J, Gosselin B, et al. Sliding thin slab, minimum intensity projection technique in the diagnosis of emphysema: histopathologic-CT correlation. *Radiology* 1996;200:665–671.
43. Fishman EK, Magid D, Ney DR, et al. Three-dimensional imaging. *Radiology* 1991;181:321–337.
44. Kauczor HU, Wolcke B, Fischer B. Three-dimensional helical CT of the tracheobronchial tree: evaluation of imaging protocols and assessment of suspected stenoses with bronchoscopic correlation. *AJR Am J Roentgenol* 1996;167:419–424.
45. Moorjani N, Conn G, Rahamim, Ring NJ. Virtual bronchoscopy and 3D spiral CT reconstructions in the management of kyphosis induced tracheal compression. *Thorax* 2004;59:272.
46. Ghaye B, Kos X, Dondelinger RF. Accessory cardiac bronchus: 3D CT demonstration in nine cases. *Eur Radiol* 1999;9:45–48.
47. Vogel N, Wolcke B, Kauczor HU, et al. Detection of bronchopleural fistula with spiral CT and 3D reconstruction. *Aktuelle Radiol* 1995;5:176–178.
48. Schaefer-Prokop C, Prokop M. New imaging techniques in the treatment guidelines for lung cancer. *Eur Respir J* 2002;19:71S–83S.
49. Rubin GD, Beaulieu CF, Argiro V, et al. Perspective volume rendering of CT and MR images: applications for endoscopic imaging. *Radiology* 1996; 199:321–330.
50. Vining DJ, Liu K, Choplin RH, and Haponik EF. Virtual bronchoscopy: relationships of virtual reality endobronchial simulations to actual bronchoscopic findings. *Chest* 1996;109:549–553.
51. Vining DJ, et al. Mediastinal lymph node mapping using spiral CT and three-dimensional reconstructions in patients with lung cancer: preliminary observations. *J Bronchol* 1997;4:18–25.
52. Summers RM. Navigational aids for real-time virtual bronchoscopy. *AJR Am J Roentgenol* 1997;168:1165–1170.
53. Maniatis PN, Triantopoulou CC, Tsalafoutas IA, et al. Threshold selection in virtual bronchoscopy: phantom study and clinical implications. *Acta Radiol* 2004;45:176–183.
54. De Wever W, Vandecaveye, V, Lanciotti S, Verschakelen JA. Multidetector CT-generated virtual bronchoscopy: an illustrated review of the potential clinical indications. *Eur Resp J* 2004;23:776–782.
55. Finkelstein SE, Schrump DS, Nguyen DM, et al. Comparative evaluation of super high-resolution CT scan and virtual bronchoscopy for the detection of tracheobronchial malignancies. *Chest* 2003;124:1834–1840.
56. Higgins WE, et al. Use of integrated virtual-bronchoscopic analysis during live bronchoscopy. *Radiology* 2001;221:P719(abst).
57. Mori K, Deguchi D, Sugiyama J, et al. Tracking of a bronchoscope using epipolar geometry analysis and intensity-based image registration of real and virtual endoscopic images. *Med Image Analysis* 2002;6:321–336.
58. Lacasse Y, Martel S, Hebert A, et al. Accuracy of virtual bronchoscopy to detect endobronchial lesions. *Ann Thorac Surg* 2004;77:1774–1780.
59. Klingenbeck-Regn K, Schaller S, Flohr T. Subsecond multi-slice computed tomography: basics and applications. *Eur J Radiol* 1999;31:110–124.
60. Khan MF, et al. Virtual endoscopy of the tracheo-bronchial system: sub-millimeter collimation with the 16-row multidetector scanner. *Eur Radiol* 2004;14:1400–1405.
61. Hoppe H, Dinkel HP, Walder B, et al. Grading airway stenosis down to the segmental level using virtual bronchoscopy. *Chest* 2004;125:704–711.
62. Hoppe H, Walder B, Sonnenschein M, et al. Multidetector CT virtual bronchoscopy to grade tracheobronchial stenosis. *AJR Am J Roentgenol* 2002; 178:1195–1195.
63. McAdams HP, Palmer SM, Erasmus JJ, et al. Bronchial anastomotic complications in lung transplant recipients: virtual bronchoscopy for noninvasive assessment. *Radiology* 1998;209:689–695.
64. Ferretti GR, Knoplioch J, Bricault I, et al. Central airway stenoses: preliminary results of spiral-CT-generated virtual bronchoscopy simulations in 29 patients. *Eur Radiol* 1997;7:854–859.
65. Lam WW, Tam PK, Chan FL, et al. Esophageal atresia and tracheal stenosis: use of three-dimensional CT and virtual bronchoscopy in neonates, infants, and children. *AJR Am J Roentgenol* 2000;174:1009–1012.
66. Rapp-Bernhardt U, Welte T, Doehring W, et al. Diagnostic potential of virtual bronchoscopy: advantages in comparison with axial CT slices, MPR and mIP? *Eur Radiol* 2000;10:981–988.
67. Summers RM, Selbie WS, Malley JD, et al. Polypoid lesions of airways: early experience with computer-assisted detection by using virtual bronchoscopy and surface curvature. *Radiology* 1998;208:331–337.
68. Summers RM, Shaw DJ, Shelhamer JH. CT virtual bronchoscopy of simulated endobronchial lesions: effect of scanning, reconstruction, and display settings and potential pitfalls. *AJR Am J Roentgenol* 1998;170:947–950.

69. Ferretti GR, Thony F, Bosson JL, et al. Benign abnormalities and carcinoid tumors of the central airways: diagnostic impact of CT bronchography. *AJR Am J Roentgenol* 2000;174:1307–1313.
70. Summers RM, Aggarwal NR, Sneller MC, et al. CT virtual bronchoscopy of the central airways in patients with Wegener's granulomatosis. *Chest* 2002;121:242–250.
71. Haliloglu M, Ciftci AO, Gumus B, et al. CT virtual bronchoscopy in the evaluation of children with suspected foreign body aspiration. *Eur J Radiol* 2003;48:188–192.
72. Rapp-Bernhardt U, Welte T, Budinger M, Bernhardt TM. Comparison of three-dimensional virtual endoscopy with bronchoscopy in patients with oesophageal carcinoma infiltrating the tracheobronchial tree. *Br J Radiol* 1998;71:1271–1278.
73. Naidich DP, Gruden JF, McGuinness G, et al. Volumetric (helical/spiral) CT (VCT) of the airways. *J Thorac Imaging* 1997;12:11–28.
74. Feretti GR, Thony F, Bosson JL, et al. Benign abnormalities and carcinoid tumors of the central airways: diagnostic impact of CT bronchography. *AJR Am J Roentgenol* 2000;174:1307–1313.
75. McAdams HP, Goodman PC, Kussin P. Virtual bronchoscopy for directing transbronchial needle aspiration of hilar and mediastinal lymph nodes: a pilot study. *AJR Am J Roentgenol* 1998;170:1361–1364.
76. Moorthy K, Smith S, Brown T, et al. Evaluation of virtual reality bronchoscopy as a learning and assessment tool. *Respiration* 2003;70:195–199.
77. Crawford SW, Colt HG. Virtual reality and written assessments are of potential value to determine knowledge and skill in flexible bronchoscopy. *Respiration* 2003;71:269–275.
78. Dasgupta A, Mehta AC. Transbronchial needle aspiration—an underused diagnostic technique. *Clin Chest Med* 1999;20:39–51.
79. Haponik EF, Shure D. Underutilization of transbronchial needle aspiration: experiences of current pulmonary fellows. *Chest* 1997;112:251–253.
80. Grenier PA, Beigelman-Aubry C, Fetita C, et al. New frontiers in CT imaging of the airways. *Eur Radiol* 2002;12:1022–1044.
81. Higgins WE, et al. Progress towards virtual-bronchoscopic guidance of peripheral nodule biopsy. *Am J Respir Crit Care Med* 2003 167:A535.
82. Rémy-Jardin M, Rémy J, Artaud D, et al. Volume rendering of the tracheobronchial tree: clinical evaluation of bronchographic images. *Radiology* 1998;208:761–770.
83. Fetita CI, et al. 3D Bronchoview: a new software package for investigating airway disease. *Eur Radiol* 2002;12(Suppl 1):394.
84. Deschamps T, Cohen LD. Fast extraction of minimal paths in 3D images and applications to virtual endoscopy. *Med Image Analysis* 2001;5:281–289.
85. Kiraly AP, Higgins WE, McLennan G, et al. Three-dimensional human airway segmentation methods for clinical virtual bronchoscopy. *Acad Radiol* 2002;9:1153–1168.
86. Swift RD, Kiraly AP, Sherbondy AJ, et al. Automatic axis-generation for virtual bronchoscopic assessment of major airway obstructions. *Comput Med Imaging Graph* 2002;26:103–118.
87. Herold CJ, Brown RH, Mitzner W, et al. Assessment of pulmonary airway reactivity with high-resolution CT. *Radiology* 1991;181:369–374.
88. Wood S, Zerhouni EA, Hoford JD, et al. Measurement of three-dimensional lung tree structures by using computed tomography. *J Appl Physiol* 1995; 79:1687–1697.
89. Brown RH, Zerhouni E. New techniques and developments in physiologic imaging of airways. *Radiol Clin North Am* 1998;36:211–230.
90. Webb EM, Elicker BM, Webb WR. Using CT to diagnose nonneoplastic tracheal abnormalities: appearance of the tracheal wall. *AJR Am J Roentgenol* 2000;174:1315–1321.
91. Gamsu G, Webb WR. Computed tomography of the trachea: normal and abnormal. *AJR Am J Roentgenol* 1982;139:3321–3326.
92. Gamsu G, Webb WR. Computed tomography of the trachea and mainstem bronchi. *Semin Roentgenol* 1983;18:51–60.
93. Zwischenberger JB, Sankar AB. Surgery of the thoracic trachea. *J Thorac Imaging* 1995;10:199–205.
94. Breatnach E, Abbott GC, Fraser RC. Dimensions of the normal human trachea. *AJR Am J Roentgenol* 1984;141:903–906.
95. Stern EJ, Graham CM, Webb WR, and Gamsu G. Normal trachea during forced expiration: dynamic CT measurements. *Radiology* 1993;187:27–31.
96. Greene R. "Saber sheath" trachea: relation to chronic obstructive pulmonary disease. *AJR Am J Roentgenol* 1978;130:441–445.
97. Leader JK, Rogers RM, Fuhrman CR, et al. Size and morphology of the trachea before and after lung volume reduction surgery. *AJR Am J Roentgenol* 2004;183:315–321.
98. Weibel ER, Taylor CR. Design and structure of the human lung. In: Fishman AP, ed. *Pulmonary diseases and disorders*. New York: McGraw-Hill, 1988:11–60.
99. Murata K, Khan A, Rojas KA, and Herman PG. Optimization of computed tomography technique to demonstrate the fine structure of the lung. *Invest Radiol* 1988;23:170–175.
100. Webb WR, Stein MG, Finkbeiner WE, et al. Normal and diseased isolated lungs: high-resolution CT. *Radiology* 1988;166:81–87.
101. Bankier AA, Fleischmann D, Mallek R, et al. Bronchial wall thickness: appropriate window settings for thin-section CT and radiologic-anatomic correlation. *Radiology* 1996;199:831–836.
102. Foster WL, Roberts L Jr, McLendon RE, and Hill RC. Localized peribronchial thickening: a CT sign of occult bronchogenic carcinoma. *AJR Am J Roentgenol* 1985;144:906–908.
103. Naidich SP, Zinn WL, Ettenger NA, et al. Basilar segmental bronchi: thin-section CT evaluation. *Radiology* 1988;169:11–16.
104. Jackson CL, Huber JF. Correlated applied anatomy of the bronchial tree and lungs with a system of nomenclature. *Dis Chest* 1943;9:319–326.
105. Boyden EA. The nomenclature of the bronchopulmonary segments and their blood supply. *Dis Chest* 1961;39:1–6.
106. Ferry RM, Boyden EA. Variations in the bronchovascular patterns of the right lower lobe in fifty lungs. *J Thorac Cardiovasc Surg* 1951;22:188–201.
107. Pitel M, Boyden EA. Variations in the bronchovascular patterns of the left lower lobe in fifty lungs. *J Thorac Cardiovasc Surg* 1953;26:633–653.
108. Yamashita H. *Roentgenologic anatomy of the lung*. Stuttgart: Thieme Medical Publishers, 1978.
109. Kim JS, Choi D, Lee KS. CT of the bronchus intermedius: frequency and cause of a nodule in the posterior wall on normal scans. *AJR Am J Roentgenol* 1995;165:1349–1352.
110. Rémy-Jardin M, Remy J. Comparison of vertical and oblique CT in evaluation of the bronchial tree. *J Comput Assist Tomogr* 1988;12:956–962.
111. Suma Y, et al. Practical methodology for bronchial route analysis using virtual bronchoscopy. *Am J Respir Crit Care Med* 2003;167:A527.
112. Asano F, et al. Case report. Transbronchial diagnosis of a pulmonary peripheral small lesion using and ultrathin bronchoscope with virtual bronchoscopic navigation. *J Bronchosc* 2002;9:108–111.
113. Asano F, et al. Transbronchial diagnosis of a pulmonary peripheral small lesion using an ultrathin bronchoscope with virtual bronchoscopic navigation. *J Bronchol* 2002;9:108–111.
114. Moriya H, Hashimoto N, Honjo H. Visibility of peripheral bronchi in virtual bronchoscopy with 0.5 mm collimation multidetector CT (in Japanese). *Jpn J Clin Radiol* 2001;46:1–7.
115. Shinagawa N, Yamazaki K, Onodera Y, et al. CT-guided transbronchial biopsy using an ultrathin bronchoscope with virtual bronchoscopic guidance. *Chest* 2004;125:1138–1143.
116. Rooney CP, Wolf K, McLennan G. Ultrathin bronchoscopy as an adjunct to standard bronchoscopy in the diagnosis of peripheral lung lesions: a preliminary report. *Respiration* 2002;69:63–68.
117. Zylak CJ, Eyler WR, Spizamy DL, and Stone CH. Developmental lung anomalies in the adult: radiologic-pathologic correlation. *Radiographics* 2002;22:S25–S43.
118. Ghaye B, Szapiro D, Fanchamps JM, and Dondelinger RF. Congenital bronchial anomalies revisited. *Radiographics* 2001;21:105–119.
119. Wu JW, White CS, Meyer CA, et al. Variant bronchial anatomy: CT appearance and classification. *AJR Am J Roentgenol* 1999;172:741–744.
120. Morrison SC. Demonstration of a tracheal bronchus by computed tomography. *Clin Radiol* 1988;39:208–209.
121. Freeman SJ, Harvey JE, Goddard PR. Demonstration of supernumerary tracheal bronchus by computed tomographic scanning and magnetic resonance imaging. *Thorax* 1995;50:426–427.
122. O'Sullivan BP, Frassica JJ, Rayder SM. Tracheal bronchus: a cause of prolonged atelectasis in intubated children. *Chest* 1998;113:537–540.
123. Shipley RT, McLoud TC, Dedrick CG, and Shepard JA. Computed tomography of the tracheal bronchus. *J Comput Assist Tomogr* 1985;9:53–55.
124. Landing BH, Dixon LG. Congenital malformation and genetic disorders of the respiratory tract. *Am Rev Respir Dis* 1979;120:151–185.
125. Karcaaltincaba M, Haliloglu M, Ekinci S. Partial tracheal duplication: MDCT bronchoscopic diagnosis. *AJR Am J Roentgenol* 2003;183:290–292.
126. Moller GM, ten Berge EJFM, Stassen CM. Tracheocele: a rare cause of difficult endotracheal intubation and subsequent pneumomediastinum. *Eur Resp J* 1994;7:1376–1377.
127. Tanaka H, Mori Y, Kurokawa K, and Abe S. Paratracheal air cysts communicating with the trachea: CT findings. *J Thorac Imaging* 1997;12:38–40.
128. McGuinness G, Naidich DP, Garay SM, et al. Accessory cardiac bronchus: computed tomographic features and clinical significance. *Radiology* 1993; 189:563–566.
129. Keane MP, Meaney JF, Kazerooni EA, et al. Accessory cardiac bronchus presenting with haemoptysis. *Thorax* 1997;52:490–491.
130. Mangiula VG, Razvzn VS. The accessory cardiac bronchus; bronchologic aspect and review of the literature. *Chest* 1968;54:35–38.
131. Bentala M, Grijim K, van der Zee JH, and Kloek JJ. Cardiac bronchus: a rare cause of hemoptysis. Case report. *Eur J Cardiothorac Surg* 2002;22:643–645.
132. Gonzalez-Crussi F, et al. "Bridging bronchus," a previously undescribed airway anomaly. *Am J Dis Child* 1976;130:1015–1018.
133. Weibel ER. High resolution computed tomography of the pulmonary parenchyma: anatomical background. Presented at the Fleischner Society Symposium on Chest Disease, Scottsdale, Arizona, 1990.
134. Prakash UBS. *Bronchoscopy*. New York: Raven Press, 1994.

2

Bronchoscopic Evaluation of the Airways with CT Correlations

In parallel with advances in multidetector computed tomography (CT) technology, including the ability to acquire volumetric datasets with near isotropic resolution coupled with advanced reconstruction techniques, similar improvements have occurred in the field of bronchoscopy. These include both improved diagnostic capabilities with sophisticated bronchoscopes coupled with video monitors and striking progress in the ability to perform therapeutic bronchoscopic interventions, (1,1a). It cannot be overemphasized that accurate assessment of the status of these techniques to evaluate the airways requires direct comparison of their capabilities and limitations (2). For this purpose, following a brief review of basic bronchoscopic technology, both rigid and flexible, basic principles of CT interpretation are discussed supplemented by a series of representative cases emphasizing CT–bronchoscopic correlations. The role of CT in guiding interventional bronchoscopic techniques is also reviewed, with particular emphasis placed on transbronchial needle aspiration and biopsy (TBNA) for assessing mediastinal and hilar disease as well as transbronchial biopsy (TBBx) of peripheral lung nodules. Current indications for CT versus bronchoscopy in patients presenting with hemoptysis are discussed. Finally, the application of new technologies to bronchoscopy including autofluorescence and endobronchial ultrasound (EBUS) is addressed.

BRONCHOSCOPY

Since its introduction by Gustave Killian (3) in 1896, the field of bronchoscopy has evolved into an indispensable tool for evaluating, diagnosing, and treating a wide variety of pulmonary and airway disorders.

Rigid Bronchoscopy

The rigid bronchoscope, which underwent many adaptations in the past century, remains remarkably true to Killian's original design. This technique used a hollow metal tube, inserted through the mouth with the patient's neck fully extended, to directly visualize the trachea and mainstem bronchi. Adequate illumination was challenging but sufficiently provided by indirect reflected artificial light; when small electric light bulbs became available, they could be attached at the proximal or distal ends of the bronchoscope for better illumination.

The modern rigid bronchoscope has easily overcome the problem of illumination by means of a light transmitted to the distal tip via fiberoptic bundles. Viewing the airway may be accomplished simply by looking through the tube from the proximal end as Killian did or, more commonly, by means of an optical "telescope" inserted through the bronchoscope to transmit the image to the viewer. Subsequent technologic advances permitted digital images obtained to be transmitted to a digital monitor for exceptionally sharp images of the airways.

In viewing the airways, the rigid bronchoscope still suffers from one of its original drawbacks: its rigidity limits the extent to which it can be advanced into the airways. In practice, no further than the truncus basalis of the right lower lobe and left lower lobe can be reached by a standard rigid bronchoscope. This allows the bronchoscopist to view the proximal lower lobe airways as well as the proximal right middle lobe directly thorough the bronchoscope. Because insertion of the bronchoscope bypasses the upper lobes of each lung, the ability to view these airways through the rigid bronchoscope is limited. This is overcome to some extent by the use of the telescope, even more so if a "side-viewing" telescope is used. The latter provides the view of objects 90 degrees to the long axis of the telescope, in contrast to the "straight ahead" view of the standard telescope. In practice, the rigid telescope can be replaced by the passage of a flexible bronchoscope through the rigid bronchoscope, allowing easy access to airways not in the axis of the rigid bronchoscope.

A major advantage of the rigid bronchoscope over its flexible counterpart is its large inner diameter relative to that of the instrument channel of the flexible bronchoscope. Rigid bronchoscopes range in diameter from 3 to 9 mm, whereas the instrument channel of standard flexible bronchoscopes range in diameter from 1.2 to 3.2 mm. The rigid bronchoscope thus permits the passage of larger instruments such as forceps. In addition, large-bore suction tubes to aspirate secretions and blood can be passed through the rigid bronchoscope, whereas the suction capability of the flexible bronchoscope is governed by the diameter of the instrument channel. Massive hemorrhage, pathologic or iatrogenic, is therefore more easily managed with a rigid bronchoscope. The ability (indeed, the necessity) to ventilate through the rigid bronchoscope affords greater control over the airway to the bronchoscopist than does the flexible bronchoscope, although flexible bronchoscopy (FB) through an endotracheal tube approximates this action. Some bronchoscopists argue that this characteristic may make the rigid bronchoscope more suitable for certain interventional procedures, which is the subject of some debate.

The discomfort of both the necessary degree of neck extension and the passage of the large-caliber rigid bronchoscope through the pharynx, vocal cords, and trachea requires general anesthesia so that the patient can tolerate the bronchoscopy, which adds to the risk of the procedure.

Flexible Bronchoscopy

Shigeto Ikeda introduced FB in 1968. The first flexible bronchoscopes used fiberoptic bundles to transmit light from an external source to the distal tip of the bronchoscope and allowed the resultant view of the illuminated airways at the eyepiece at the proximal end of the bronchoscope. FB permits examination of virtually all bronchi large enough to admit the bronchoscope. Standard flexible bronchoscopes have an outer diameter (OD) range of 4.9 to 6.4 mm, which permit, in adult patients, entry into the fifth- or sixth-generation bronchus. Although only one practitioner at a time can look through the eyepiece, as with the original rigid bronchoscopes, the attachment of a lecture bronchoscope or "teaching head" with its own fiberoptic bundle leading to a second eyepiece permits others to see the bronchoscopic image.

The advent of digital technology provided Ikeda with the means for the next major advance in the capability of FB to provide airway images. He replaced the fiberoptic bundle with a charge-coupled device (CCD) at the distal tip of the flexible bronchoscope, which was wired to a television monitor. This provided several advantages to the bronchoscopist. The monitor obviously allows assistants and others to view the procedure, enhancing performance and its educational value. Recording of images was also simplified, and the recording options increased (see later discussion). Furthermore, the absence of an eyepiece moved the bronchoscopist's face further from the bronchoscope, its instrument channel orifice, and the face of the patient. This decreased the risk of blood, secretions, or aspirated material accidentally splashing the bronchoscopist, significantly reducing the risk of transmission of infections that can penetrate mucous membranes.

Recent advances in digital technology have led to the acquisition of extremely detailed and accurate endobronchial images. Although it is intuitive to believe that such sharply rendered images will enhance the diagnostic and therapeutic abilities of FB, this theory remains to be borne out by formal investigation. In fact, perhaps a greater benefit of current technology lies in its educational value; the ease with which detailed bronchoscopic images can now be reproduced in journals and textbooks, shown in lectures, and transmitted via the Internet around the world could hardly have been imaginable when Ikeda invented FB.

LIMITATIONS OF STANDARD BRONCHOSCOPY

The limitations of airway imaging by the various modalities of bronchoscopy are both shared and unique. Depth of field is a major limiting factor for all bronchoscopic imaging. It is determined by the optical characteristics of the viewing mechanism. Depth of field for standard flexible bronchoscopes and video bronchoscopes is 3 to 100 mm.

Other limitations are related to the diameter of the bronchoscope, which limits the size of the airway that can be entered. Furthermore, airways that are acutely angled may be difficult to enter with the bronchoscope; this is particularly true in more peripheral airways, including the apical segments of both upper lobes. Even the ultrathin bronchoscope (discussed later), which is of a small enough diameter to reach the extreme periphery of the lung, may be difficult to pass into relatively proximal airways if the route requires multiple angulations. Finally, even large, bronchiectatic airways are often not visualized because the bronchoscopic route involves a more proximal airway too small to admit the bronchoscope.

In addition, the small size of the bronchoscope, the distal viewing area, and the instrument channel mean that the bronchoscope's visibility may be relatively easily overcome by mucus, blood, or purulent material that may be difficult to clear from the tip of the bronchoscope.

IMAGE RECORDING AND STORAGE

Older versions of rigid and flexible bronchoscopes could be attached to somewhat cumbersome still and movie cameras, which nonetheless produced excellent pictures of the bronchoscopic views. As noted earlier, the advent of digital technology has vastly simplified the acquisition, management, storage, and sharing of bronchoscopic images. Both analog and digital movies of entire bronchoscopic procedures can be readily obtained. Still images can be taken during the procedure with the touch of a button located near the fingers of the hand controlling the bronchoscope or when reviewing the movies made during the procedure. Computerized databases are now available to provide an electronic record of a procedure, into which digital images can be incorporated to generate printed or stored reports. With appropriate security precautions to protect patient privacy, the electronic records may be integrated into hospitalwide electronic medical records, allowing all privileged users to access the bronchoscopic images on-site or (via the Internet) off-site.

ULTRATHIN BRONCHOSCOPY

Examination of the airways by standard flexible bronchoscopes is generally limited to the fourth- to sixth-generation airways because of the OD of the bronchoscope (4.9 to 6.2 mm). Recently so-called ultrathin bronchoscopes have been developed with ODs ranging from 3.6 to 2.2 mm. The smallest of these bronchoscopes permits visual examination of airways as distal as the tenth generation and beyond.

Ultrathin bronchoscopes with ODs of 3.8 to 2.7 mm and with instrument channels of 1.2 mm are now commercially available. With the exception of one 3.8-mm model that uses a CCD at the tip, all of these bronchoscopes are fiberoptic. This is a reflection of current technology that limits the smallest CCD that can be placed in a functioning bronchoscope. A hybrid model with a 2.8-mm OD uses fiberoptics to obtain the image at the distal tip and transmit the image to a CCD in the body of the bronchoscope, enhancing the image and obviating the attachment of a videocamera to the bronchoscope to transmit images to a video monitor.

Although the size of ultrathin bronchoscopes allows the routine examination of airways in the periphery of the lung, practical limitations accompany the advantages of their small OD. Ultrathin bronchoscopes are less stiff than standard bronchoscopes, so they may be difficult to maneuver if a particularly tortuous route is taken in the peripheral airways. The necessarily small diameter of the instrument channel severely limits the suction capability of ultrathin bronchoscopes, so that even tiny amounts of blood or secretions in the airways can significantly impair visibility. This potential problem is compounded by the nature of peripheral airways to readily collapse when suction is applied within, further impairing visibility. The smallest size ultrathin bronchoscope (2.2 mm) achieves its narrowness by eliminating the instrument channel altogether, thereby providing the bronchoscopist with no means to deal with blood or secretions.

Most early reports of the use of ultrathin bronchoscopes involved their use in the evaluation of large airways in a neonatal and pediatric population, in whom FB had not been feasible. Wood, (4,4a) found that the ultrathin bronchoscope was useful in facilitating endotracheal intubation, and Fan et al. (5) found it useful in evaluating sources of persistent wheezing. Monrigal and Granry (6) used a 2.2-OD bronchoscope to monitor the patency of the trachea and mainstem bronchi during the surgical removal of compressive subcarinal bronchogenic cysts in two very young children. The more recent introduction of an ultrathin bronchoscope with an instrument channel enhanced the diagnostic and therapeutic capabilities of ultrathin bronchoscopy in infants by allowing bronchoalveolar lavage (BAL), suctioning of mucus plugs causing atelectasis, and even selective bronchography (7). Stenotic central airways in adults present challenges to FB similar to those posed by normal airways in infants, so it is not surprising that the role of ultrathin bronchoscopy has been investigated in this setting. Schuurmans et al. (8) used a 2.8-mm ultrathin bronchoscope to examine 24 patients with central airway obstruction due to both benign and malignant causes, with a mean degree of occlusion of 84%. The ultrathin bronchoscope was able to pass through the obstruction in all but three patients, allowing assessment of distal airways and assisting in the planning of appropriate management in 87%.

Kikawada et al. (9) recently described their findings in the peripheral airways of patients with chronic obstructive pulmonary disease. Passage of an ultrathin bronchoscope to the eleventh- or twelfth-generation airway revealed frequent obstruction and granular mucosal changes in patients with chronic bronchitis and "net-like" changes and obstruction in patients with emphysema.

The excitement over the expansion of bronchoscopic capability to a new array of peripheral airways in adults is tempered by practical limitations imposed by the tracheobronchial tree itself. The examination of every branch of the tracheobronchial tree accessible by an ultrathin bronchoscope would surely test the patience of both the bronchoscopist and the patient. In addition, each subsequent branching of the airways makes it easier for the bronchoscopist to become confused as to the particular airway into which the bronchoscope is inserted. For these reasons most studies of the utility of ultrathin bronchoscopes in peripheral airways in adults have focused on the ability of the bronchoscope to access a particular airway, usually one leading to a focal lung lesion, and the optimal means of guiding the bronchoscope to that airway.

One study investigated the use of an ultrathin bronchoscope to identify airways leading to parenchymal lung lesions suspicious for malignancy to aid in immediately subsequent standard bronchoscopy with TBBx (10). The lesions ranged in size from 1.5 to 7.0 mm and were visible on fluoroscopy, which was used to guide the ultrathin bronchoscope to the lesion. Lesions were directly visualized by ultrathin bronchoscope in 4 of 17 patients. After removal of the ultrathin bronchoscope, a standard bronchoscope was inserted to follow the pathway of the ultrathin bronchoscope, and TBBx was performed. TBBx established a diagnosis in 11 of 17 patients (65%) (10). More recent studies investigated the use of ultrathin bronchoscopy in the diagnosis of nodules detected by CT that were too small to be visualized by fluoroscopy. As discussed in greater detail later, this approach is feasible only because of the introduction of virtual bronchoscopic evaluation of peripheral airways.

CT–BRONCHOSCOPIC CORRELATIONS

Diagnostic Correlations: Central Airway Disease

The accuracy of CT to evaluate the central airways was well established even before the introduction of multidetector CT scanners (11–16). Its exceedingly high sensitivity, especially for lesions greater than 5 mm, is easily explicable because air represents a perfect natural contrast agent for CT: Combined with intrinsic high-contrast resolution provided by the interface between luminal air and adjacent mediastinal soft tissues, CT allows the precise location and extent of disease both within and surrounding the central airways.

Nonetheless, despite our current ability to obtain near isotropic images of the airways in a single breathhold period with submillimeter resolution, important limitations remain. CT is of limited value, for example, in the detection of endobronchial lesions smaller than 2 to 3 mm (Fig. 2-1). In a prospective study of 105 lesions in 98 patients with

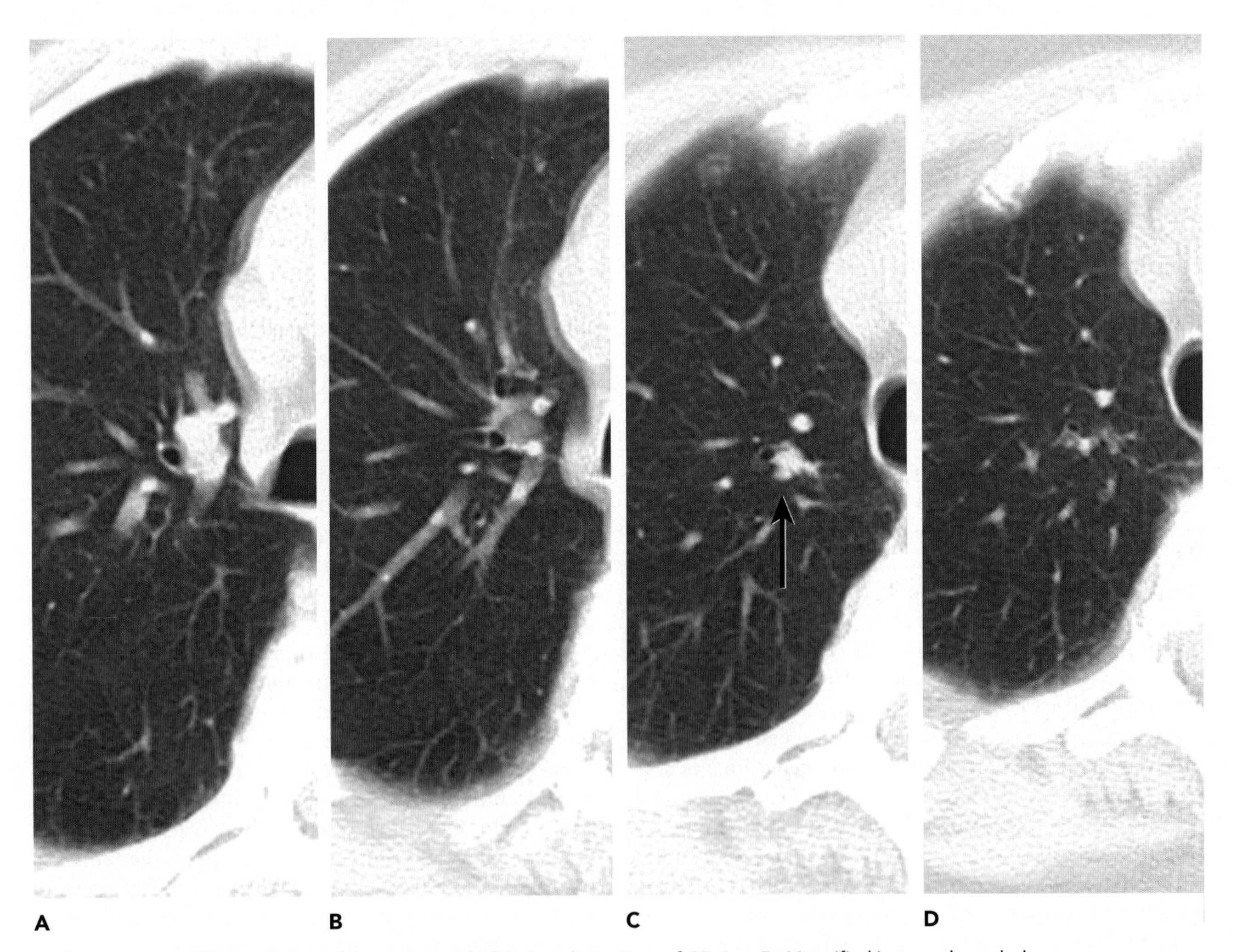

Figure 2-1 Subtle endobronchial lesions: limitations of CT. **A** to **D:** Magnified images through the medial aspect of the right upper lobe. There is subtle deformity of the apical segmental bronchus (*arrow* in **C**). This was initially overlooked. *(continued)*

radiographically occult squamous cell carcinomas identified on the basis of positive sputum cytology, Usuda et al. (17) showed that 27 lesions (26%) proved to be smaller than 2 mm, whereas 23 (22%) were endoscopically invisible, being identified by bronchial brushing alone. It is unlikely that CT would have been of value in detecting these lesions. That CT is limited in the detection of subtle endobronchial lesions is also documented by the results of low-dose CT screening trials. To date, CT has proved ineffective in diagnosing central endobronchial lesions in this population (18–20). Finally, subtle irregularities of the airway walls, often the result of prominent bronchial cartilage, or partial volume averaging in airways coursing obliquely also limit diagnostic accuracy.

In addition, with rare exceptions CT is unable to distinguish between mucosal and submucosal disease (1). CT evidence of smooth airway narrowing, for example, may be associated bronchoscopically with endobronchial, submucosal, or peribronchial disease (Fig. 2-2). Exceptions may be found. Although specific identification of lesions restricted to the airway mucosa remains elusive, lesions that lie internal to tracheal or bronchial cartilages, for example, may be characterized as either mucosal and/or submucosal in location (Fig. 2-3). Other exceptions include the finding of a discrete calcific endobronchial filling defect, as may occur, for example, in patients with an aspirated foreign body (Fig. 2-4) or broncholiths (21). In the latter case, CT may prove more sensitive than bronchoscopy by identifying both intraluminal and peribronchial calcifications distal to inflamed and narrowed airways rendered inaccessible to bronchoscopy. Also included are endobronchial hamartomas within which fat may rarely be identified (22). However, these abnormalities are unusual.

In comparing CT findings with abnormalities identified at bronchoscopy, it is essential to use appropriate descriptive terminology. This requires that a specific CT classification be used to describe abnormalities identified on routine axial images or multiplanar reconstructions (Fig. 2-2) (15). CT–bronchoscopic correlation using virtual bronchoscopy, although promising, remains a specialized technique for

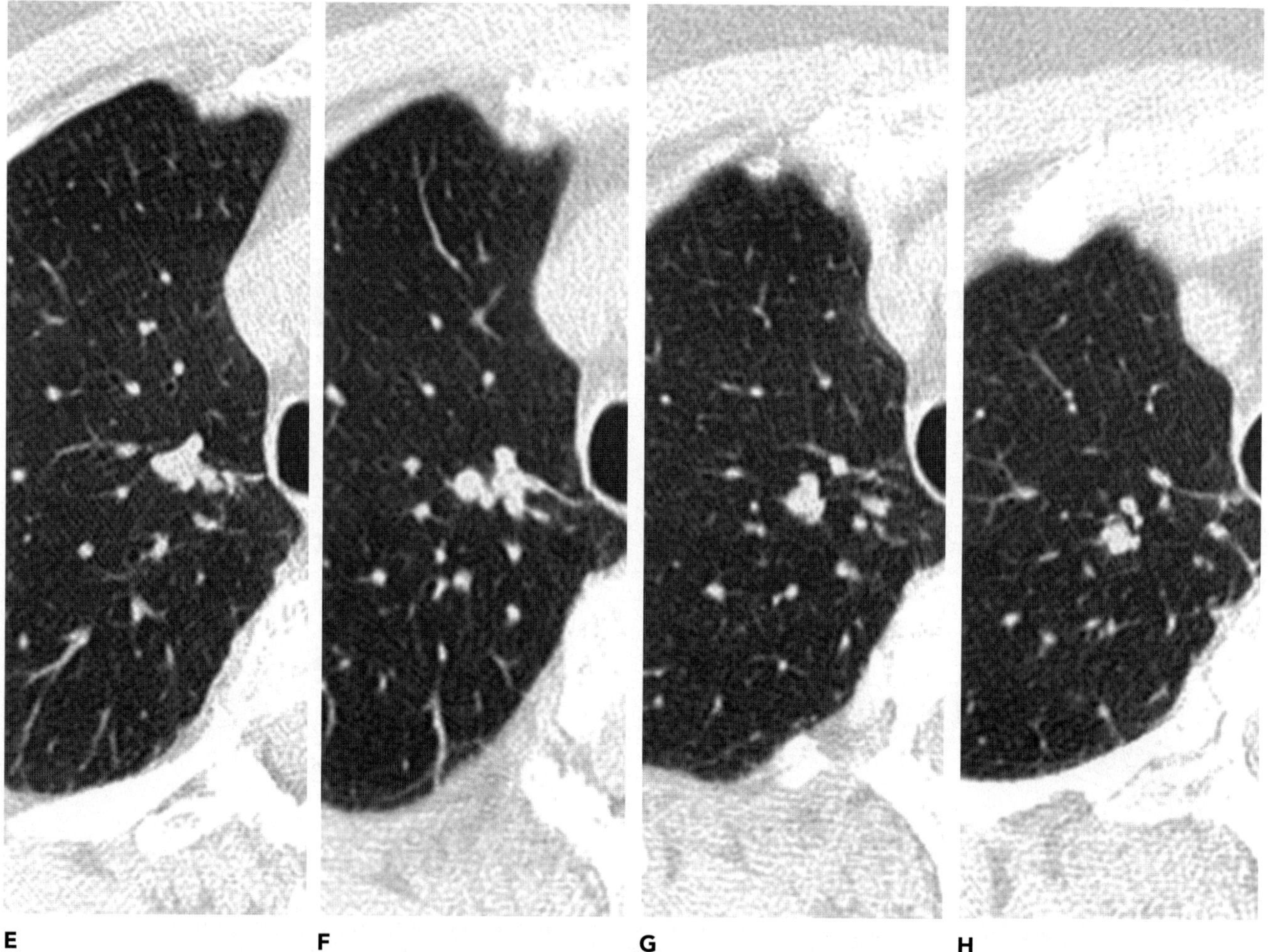

Figure 2-1 *(continued)* **E** to **H:** Magnified images at the same level as shown in **A** to **D**, obtained several months later. This case illustrates the difficulty in identifying small endobronchial lesions in the lobar and segmental airways in particular.

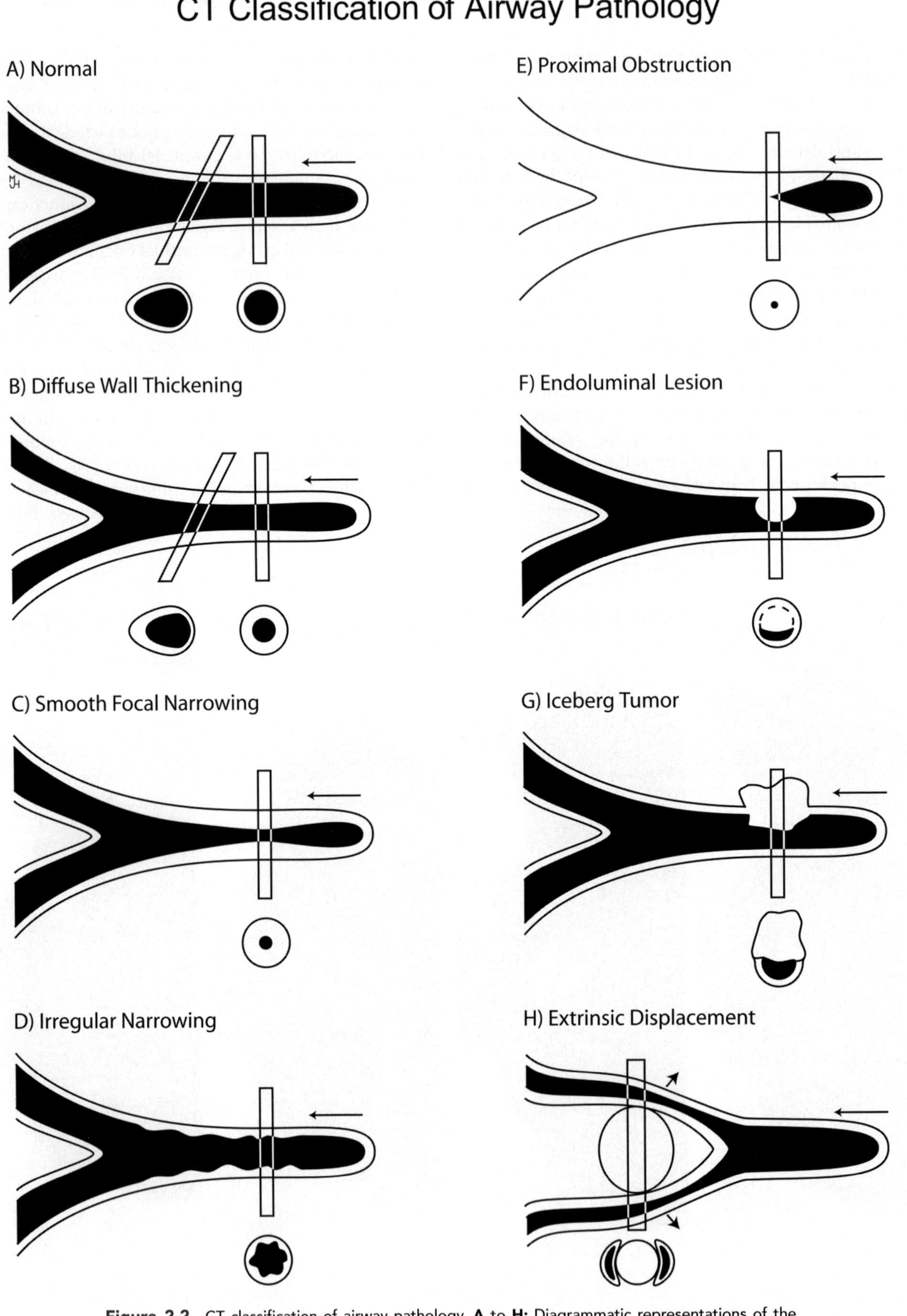

Figure 2-2 CT classification of airway pathology. **A** to **H:** Diagrammatic representations of the appearance of various airway abnormalities as seen on CT sections. In each case, abnormalities are represented as they would appear in axial, oblique (**A, B**), and sagittal planes. Note that this classification makes no attempt to correlate CT findings with a diagnosis of mucosal or submucosal disease. With rare exception, this distinction is typically impossible to establish (See Fig. 2-3).

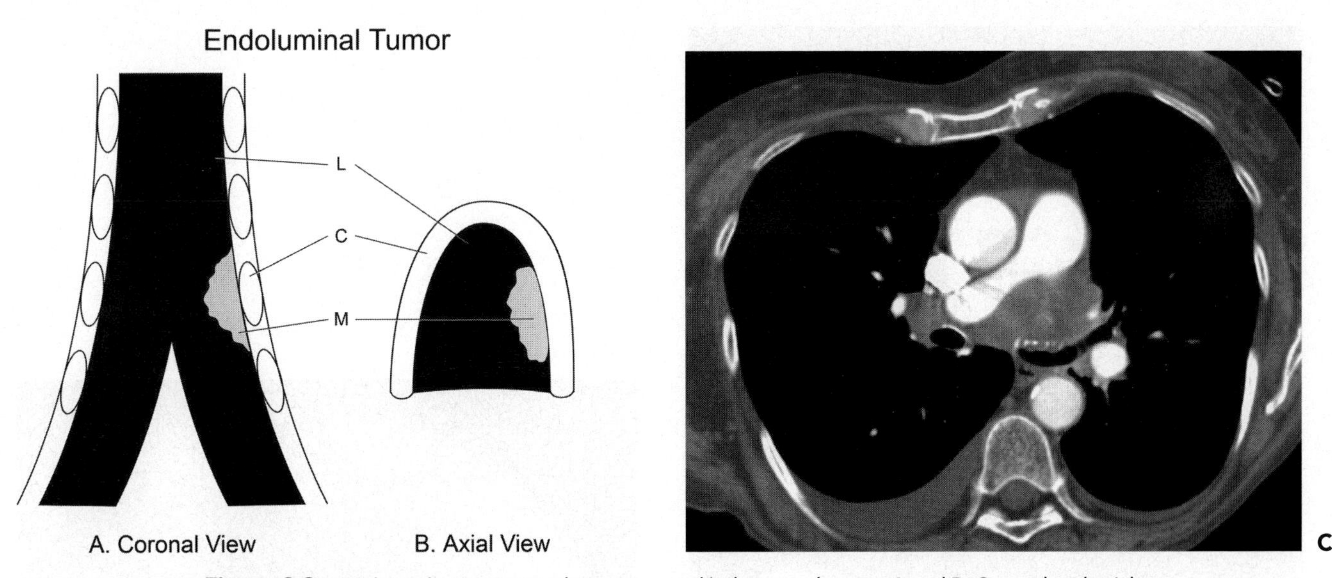

Figure 2-3 CT–bronchoscopic correlation: mucosal/submucosal tumor. **A** and **B:** Coronal and axial drawings, respectively, showing a schematic representation of endoluminal mucosal/submucosal tumor. Although CT does not typically allow a specific diagnosis of mucosal or submucosal disease (Fig. 2-1), one exception is the presence of tumor internal or central to calcified tracheobronchial cartilage. C, cartilage; L, lumen; M, endoluminal mass. **C:** Contrast-enhanced CT section shows extensive mediastinal tumor. In this case, tumor can be identified interior to the left mainstem bronchial cartilage *(arrow)*, allowing accurate mucosa/submucosal localization, subsequently verified endoscopically.

which a specific terminologic classification has yet to be devised (see Chapter 1). With these caveats in mind, the advantages and limitations of CT–bronchoscopic correlations for identifying airway pathology are well illustrated in a series of cases presented in Figs. 2-4 to 2-11.

Diagnostic Correlations: TBNA

The use of CT in lymph node "mapping" to aid in the planning and performance of TBNA may be considered a paradigm for the integration and correlation of CT and bronchoscopic imaging.

The current state of TBNA is largely the result of the pioneering efforts of Ko-Pen Wang (23–25) in the development of both the technique and the instruments. Over the past two decades, numerous reports have documented the value of this procedure (26–34).

TBNA allows cytologic and/or histologic sampling, most often of mediastinal and hilar tissue, in select cases obviating more invasive surgical procedures including mediastinoscopy or thoracotomy. TBNA can access more lymph node stations than any other biopsy technique and has the lowest complication rate as well (35). CT may also be of particular value by identifying cases in which TBNA is not indicated. This includes patients with negative CT scans, for whom the yield has proved sufficiently low to obviate this procedure (28). As important, CT can also help to avoid potentially false-positive biopsies by identifying parenchymal tumors that abut the central airways and making TBNA staging unreliable, as may occur in patients with tumors in the medial portion of the right upper lobe simulating right paratracheal adenopathy (36).

To date, TBNA has most often been used to evaluate patients with suspected intrathoracic neoplasia. In most series, TBNA has resulted in a yield of 60% to 80% sensitivity for diagnosing and staging lung cancer. In one recent multicenter trial TBNA resulted in an overall yield of 48% in 279 patients with non–small cell lung cancer (NSCLC), and 62% in 81 patients with small cell carcinoma among four institutions. As important, TBNA also provided the only bronchoscopic specimen diagnostic for lung cancer in 18% of patients (37). In an assessment of 123 patients with documented malignancy evaluated by TBNA, Sharafkhaneh et al. (31) reported a sensitivity of 69%, with significant correlations noted between a positive TBNA and cell type ($p < .001$) and nodal size ($p < .05$). Consistent with similar previous reports, this study also found that TBNA was most often successful in diagnosing small cell carcinoma compared with NSCLC and least successful for diagnosing lymphoma. Similar results have been reported by Khoo et al. (33) and Cetinkaya et al. (34). In a study of 45 consecutive cases evaluated over a 2-year period by a group of researchers with relatively less experience, TBNA provided an overall diagnosis in 65% of cases (33). Similarly, Hermens et al. (32), in a study of 106 consecutive patients with suspected lung cancer considered eligible for TBNA that were evaluated by six different pulmonologists in a non-university teaching hospital, reported an overall sensitivity of 65%, with malignancy demonstrated in 63 (59%) of 106 cases. Importantly, in this same study, a total of 10 mediastinoscopies were avoided because TBNA demonstrated contralateral N3 disease, leading these investigators to conclude that TBNA is a cost-effective method for staging lung cancer.

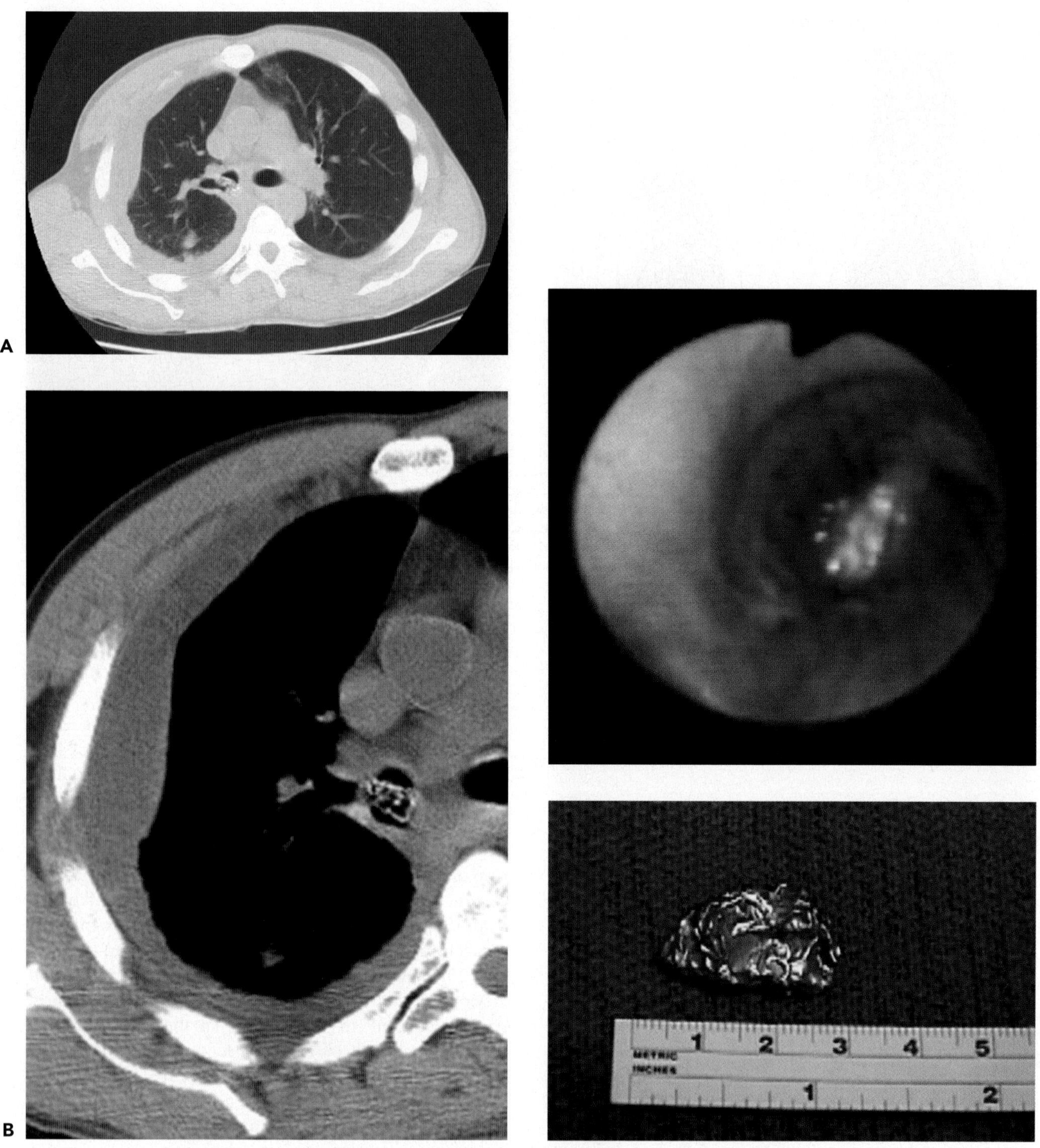

Figure 2-4 CT–bronchoscopic correlation: endobronchial foreign body. **A** and **B:** Magnified CT sections through the right mainstem–right upper lobe bronchus imaged with wide and narrow windows, respectively, show an unusual-appearing intraluminal filling defect in a patient presenting with bacterial pneumonia and empyema. **C:** Endoscopic view revealing a foreign body coated with secretions partially obstructing the right main bronchus. This was successfully removed by forceps. **D:** Image of the same foreign body following removal revealing this to be an aluminum foil packet. The patient subsequently admitted accidentally aspirating the packet containing crack cocaine that he had hidden in his mouth while fleeing the police a month earlier. In this case, the unchanging nature of the endobronchial density on sequential CT scans several days apart prompted the suspicion of a foreign body rather than the initial impression of retained secretions.

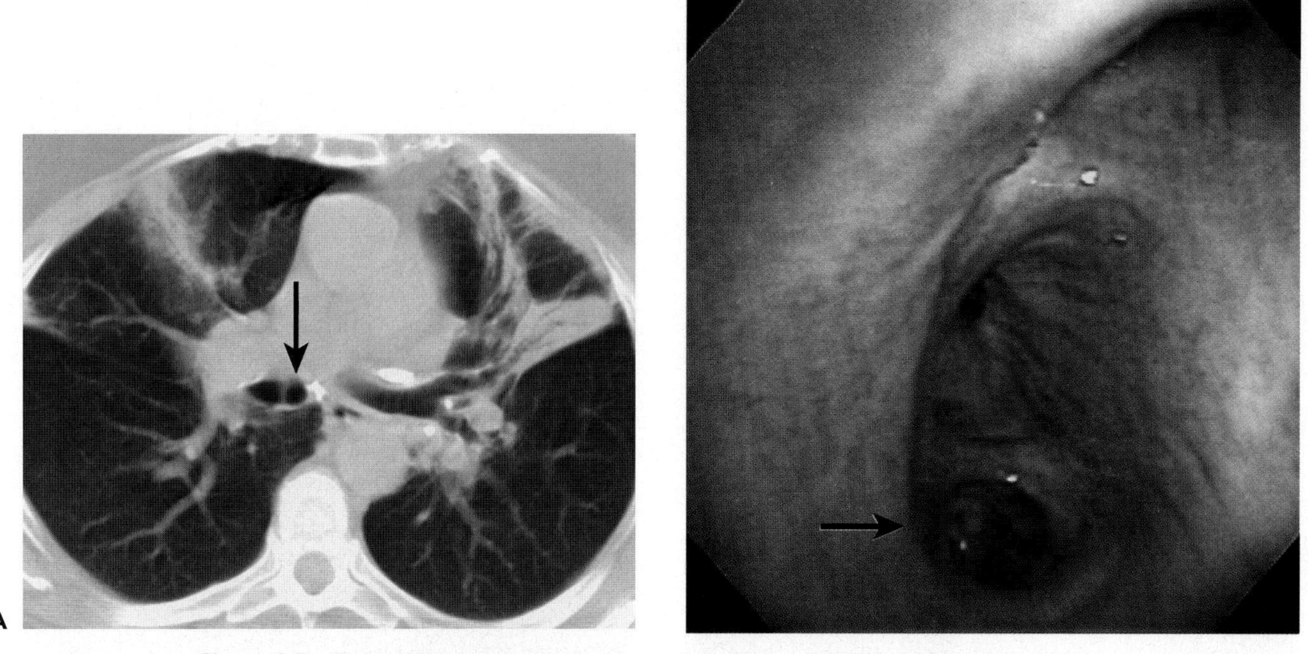

Figure 2-5 CT–bronchoscopic correlations: anomalous airways. **A:** CT of a patient with prior tuberculosis and focal infiltrates demonstrates an anomalous airway *(arrow)* medial to the normal right main bronchus. **B:** Flexible bronchoscopic image confirms the presence of a "cardiac bronchus" (*arrow*), a normal variant. Normal bronchus intermedius and right upper-lobe bronchus are also visible. CT is of particular value in demonstrating anomalous and distorted airways, providing a road map for bronchoscopy in potentially difficult cases.

Although TBNA is most often performed to diagnose and/or stage patients with suspected intrathoracic neoplasia, it cannot be overemphasized that TBNA is also of great utility for diagnosing benign diseases as well, especially tuberculosis (TB) and sarcoidosis (38,39). Cetinkaya et al. (34), for example, used a 22-gauge Wang cytology needle to evaluate 60 consecutive patients with mediastinal or hilar adenopathy. TBNA successfully diagnosed TB in 13 of 20 cases (65%) and provided the sole means of diagnosis in 8 (40%). In this same study, TBNA also provided the only means of diagnosis in 13 (62%) of 21 patients with documented sarcoidosis. Use of TBNA for establishing a diagnosis of TB may be of particular value in patients with AIDS (39). Especially in the setting of immunocompromised patients, active tuberculous nodes have been noted to characteristically appear as low density on CT with an enhancing rim following intravenous administration of contrast media (40). As documented by Harkin et al. (39), TBNA proved diagnostic in 23 (51%) of 45 procedures performed in 41 human immunodeficiency virus (HIV)-positive patients with mediastinal adenopathy, including identification of 21 of 23 documented cases of mycobacterial infection. In this latter group TBNA provided the only diagnostic specimen in 13 (57%). More recently, Bilaceroglu et al. (41) similarly found TBNA to have a sensitivity and specificity for TB of 83% and 100%, respectively, in 76 HIV-negative patients. A rapid diagnosis was obtained in 78%, with TBNA providing the exclusive diagnostic specimen in 68% of cases.

Nearly identical data have also been reported recently by Trisolini et al. (30). In this study of 55 patients with CT evidence of enlarged mediastinal or hilar nodes with clinically suspected sarcoidosis, TBNA showed nonnecrotizing granulomas in 23 (72%) of 32 patients with subsequently documented sarcoidosis. Importantly, of 15 patients undergoing both TBNA and TBBx, TBNA provided the sole means of diagnosis in 7, improving the diagnostic rate by 47%. Similar results have previously been reported by Morales et al. (38) who found that of 51 consecutive patients with suspected sarcoidosis undergoing both TBNA and TBBx, 23% of patients with stage 1 disease and 10% of patients with stage 2 disease had their diagnoses established only by TBNA. Overall, combined TBNA and TBBx yielded a diagnosis in 83% of documented cases.

Although most investigators have argued for routine use of TBNA, regrettably this procedure remains underused by most bronchoscopists. In a survey of 871 North American bronchoscopists, only 12% used TBNA routinely in bronchoscopies for malignancy and only 2% used TBNA in benign disease (42). One of the primary reasons cited for the grudging acceptance of TBNA is the low yield that many practitioners have experienced. This may be the result of two primary factors: unfamiliarity with the technique and the inability to localize unseen lymph nodes relative to bronchoscopically visualized airways. Although the technique generally requires some degree of hands-on training, relating lymph node location to endobronchial anatomy remains an ongoing concern. TBNA was originally designed

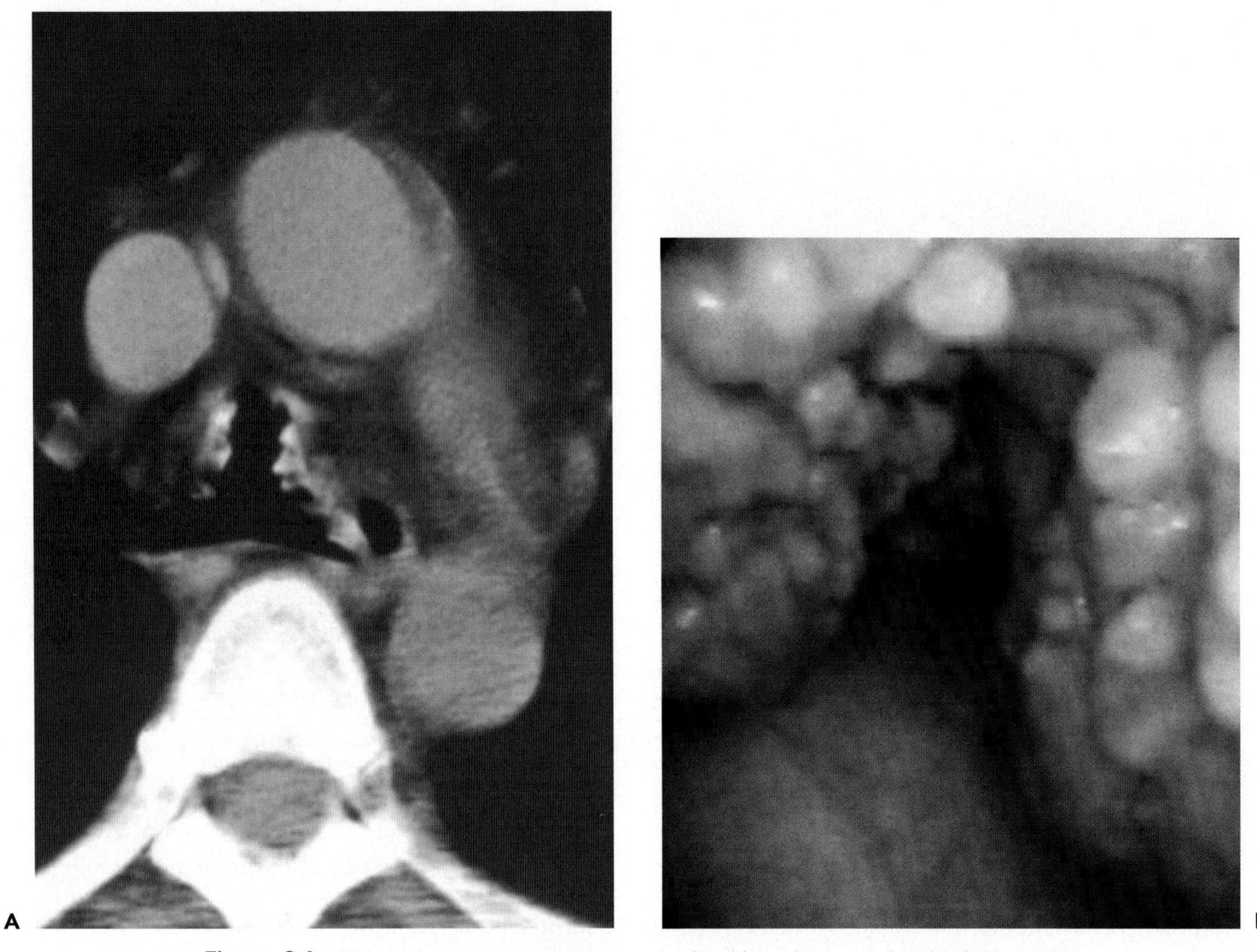

Figure 2-6 CT–bronchoscopic correlations: tracheobronchopathia osteochondroplastica (TO). **A:** Magnified view of the midtrachea imaged with narrow windows shows characteristic appearance of calcified nodules resulting in mild narrowing of the tracheal lumen. Note the absence of involvement of the posterior membranous tracheal wall. This proved to be an incidental finding. **B:** Corresponding flexible bronchoscopic evaluation demonstrates precise CT–endoscopic correlation with characteristic nodular excrescences protruding into airway, pathognomonic of this disease. Spirometry and flow-volume loop revealed minimal obstructive dysfunction (see, in addition, Fig. 3-33).

as a blind technique, that is, using imagination, the bronchoscopist had to visualize the location of enlarged lymph nodes using previously obtained CT images. Wang (43) carefully related lymph nodes in standard locations adjacent to the airways to standard endobronchial landmarks and correlated this to American Thoracic Society (ATS) lymph node staging of NSCLC. In our experience, intimate knowledge of the lymph node map proposed by Wang and its correlation to CT findings is essential for TBNA to be successful when performed as a blind procedure, as is true of the overwhelming majority of cases.

CT–Bronchoscopic Reference Points for TBNA

The nomenclature and endobronchial landmarks for the nodal stations are oriented to the bronchoscopist's perspective. The best use of this system is not to replace the standard ATS staging system (44), which is oriented to surgical and radiologic staging, but to identify those ATS nodal stations that are accessible from within the airways. In our opinion, familiarity with these CT–bronchoscopic correlations is essential for improving the diagnostic yield of TBNA. There are four bronchoscopic sites from which 11 lymph node stations can be sampled: the carina, the right upper lobe bronchus, the bronchus intermedius, and the left-sided secondary carina (Figs. 2-12 to 2-15) (35,43a). The reference point for the first six nodal stations is the carina (Fig. 2-12). Viewing the circumference of the trachea as a clockface, the carina is oriented in a 12 o'clock to 6 o'clock direction. The anterior carina lymph node is sampled by puncturing the carina at the 12 to 1 o'clock position and the posterior carina lymph node at the 5 to 6 o'clock position. The anterior carina nodes are commonly called pretracheal or precarinal by radiologists. The posterior carina position should be punctured only in the setting of adenopathy demonstrated on CT, because a pneumothorax may otherwise result. The right paratracheal lymph node corresponds

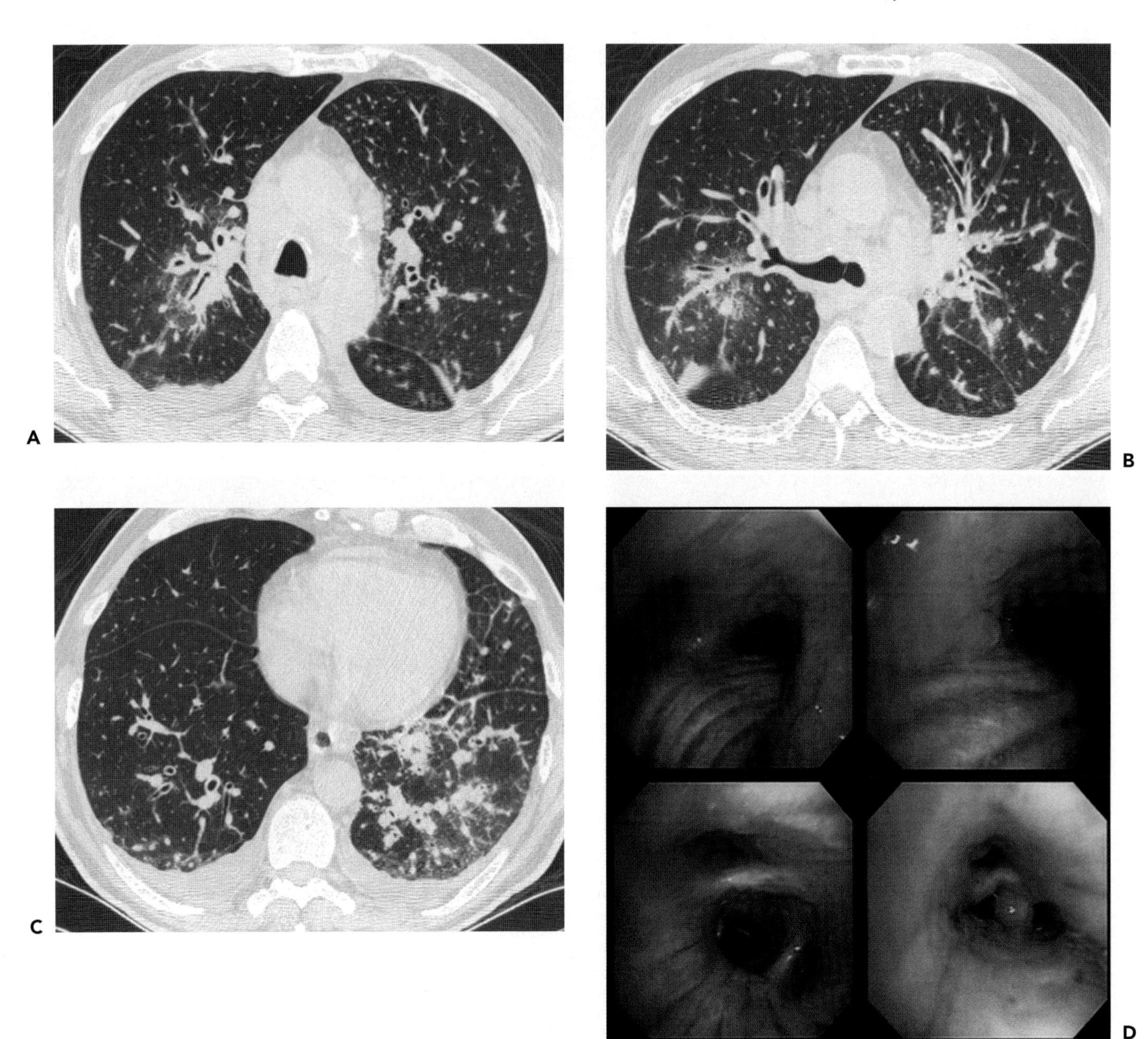

Figure 2-7 CT–bronchoscopic correlation: diffuse squamous cell carcinoma. **A** to **C:** Sequential axial CT images through the carina, right upper lobe bronchus, and lower lobe bronchi, respectively, imaged with lung windows in a patient presenting with a chronic cough show diffuse thickening of the airway walls (*arrows* in **A** to **C**), associated with extensive mediastinal and hilar adenopathy identifiable even with wide windows, and small bilateral effusions. This appearance is nonspecific and compatible with a diffuse infiltrative or inflammatory process involving the entire tracheobronchial tree. **D:** Flexible bronchoscopic images in this same case demonstrate diffuse mucosal thickening and nodular irregularity covering most of the surface of the airways. Forceps biopsy revealed diffusely infiltrative squamous cell carcinoma. In this case, CT and bronchoscopy proved complementary by disclosing different aspects of this patient's clinically unsuspected unresectable tumor.

to ATS station 4R and is sampled through the second, third, or fourth intercartilaginous space of the lower trachea (counting proximally from the carina) at 1 o'clock. The left paratracheal lymph node is designated 4L in the ATS system and is punctured at the 9 o'clock position in the trachea at about the level of the carina or the tracheobronchial angle. The aorta or the pulmonary artery may be inadvertently punctured at this site, if the needle is placed too proximally or distally, respectively. The right and left main bronchus stations correspond to ATS stations 10R and 10L, respectively. These nodes may be sampled by puncturing the bronchus at 12 o'clock in the first intercartilaginous space distal to the carina. All these nodal stations are mediastinal in location, and a positive aspirate indicates at least N2 staging.

The next two stations use the right upper lobe bronchus as a reference. The right upper hilar node, ATS station 11R,

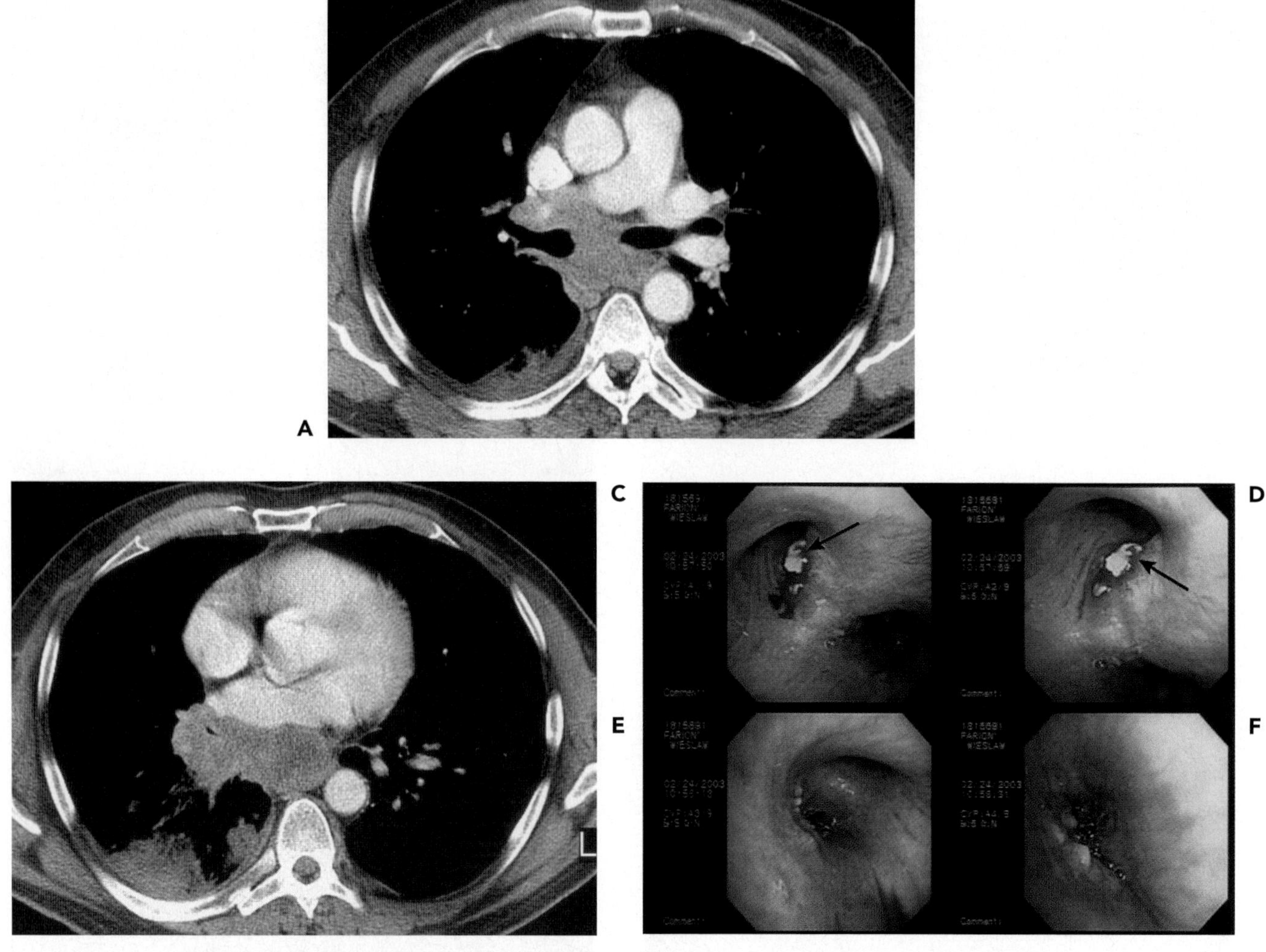

Figure 2-8 CT–bronchoscopic correlation: tumor localization—adenocarcinoma of the lung. **A** and **B:** Sequential contrast-enhanced CT images through the subcarinal space and aortic root, respectively, imaged with narrow windows, in a 48-year-old ex-smoker presenting with two episodes of scant hemoptysis, show extensive tumor throughout the mediastinum. Note that the carina is splayed, and there is slight deformity of the medial and posterior aspect of both the right and left mainstem bronchi (*arrows* in **A**) as well as marked narrowing of the middle lobe bronchus (*arrowhead* in **B**) and apparent obstruction of the proximal right lower lobe bronchus (*arrow* in **B**). This appearance is nonspecific but most often indicative of diffuse extrinsic compression of the airways by extensive malignant adenopathy. Note, as well, marked irregularity of the posterior wall of the left atrium (*curved arrow* in **B**). Although these findings are all suggestive of unresectable tumor, evaluation requires more definitive confirmation. **C** to **F:** Sequential images obtained at the time of bronchoscopy in this same patient reveals extrinsic compression of the bronchus intermedius resulting from enlarged adjacent nodes. In this case there is also evidence of eruption of malignant subcarinal lymph node through the wall of the left main bronchus (*arrows* in **C** and **D**), resulting in endobronchial tumor. Forceps biopsy in the left main bronchus revealed adenocarcinoma. Although the presence of malignant subcarinal lymph nodes staged this patient as at least IIIA (based on an N2 node), confirmation of involvement of the (contralateral) left main bronchus confirmed that there was T4 unresectable tumor. This case points out both the complementary and the competing nature of CT and bronchoscopy for assessing the true extent of tumor.

is punctured through the anterior part of the carina between the right upper lobe and the bronchus intermedius. The superior pulmonary vein may be punctured at this site, and reference to CT ensures that the node is anterior to the airway (Fig. 2-13). The subcarinal station, level 7 in the ATS system, is accessed at 9 o'clock within the right main bronchus proximal to the right upper lobe orifice.

The next reference point is the bronchus intermedius (Fig. 2-14). The right lower hilar node is punctured at the 3 o'clock, and the sub-subcarina is sampled at 9 o'clock. These nodes are often extensions of those sampled higher in the right mainstem, although they can be solely enlarged. The right lower hilar and sub-subcarinal nodes may extend below the level of the right middle lobe orifice. Nonetheless, right lower hilar nodes represent N1 classification, while the sub-subcarinal nodes represent N2 classification.

The last node in the endobronchial map is the left hilar node—ATS station 11L—which is located at the carina

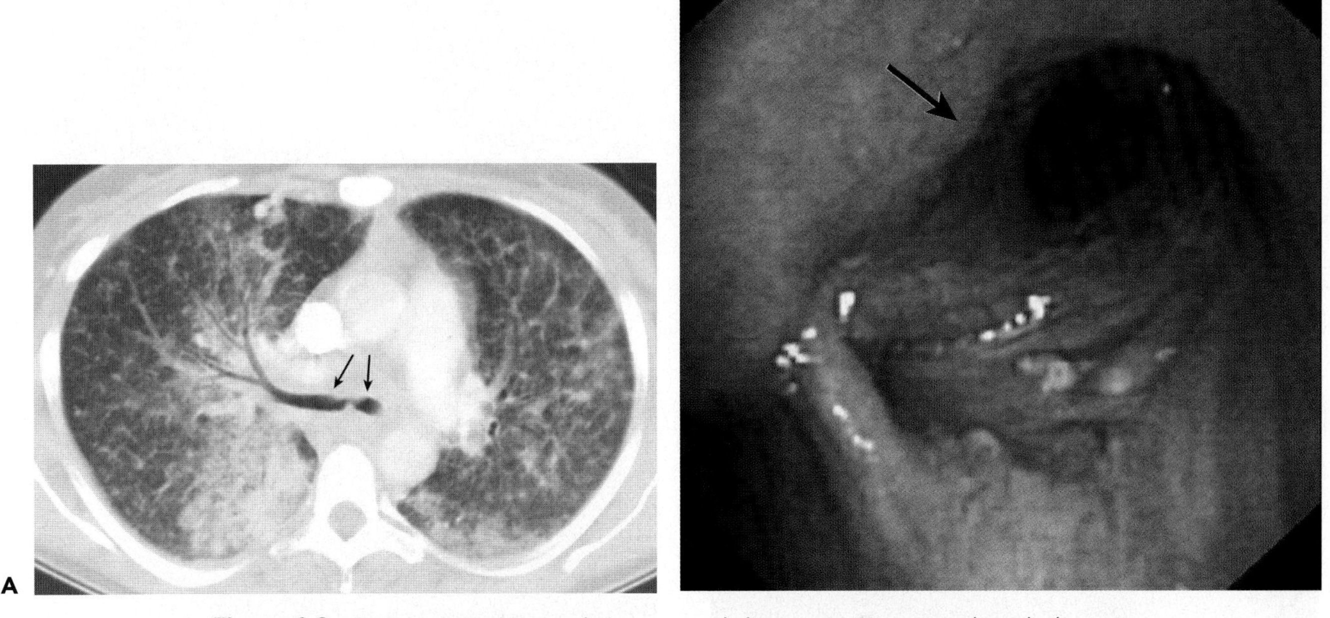

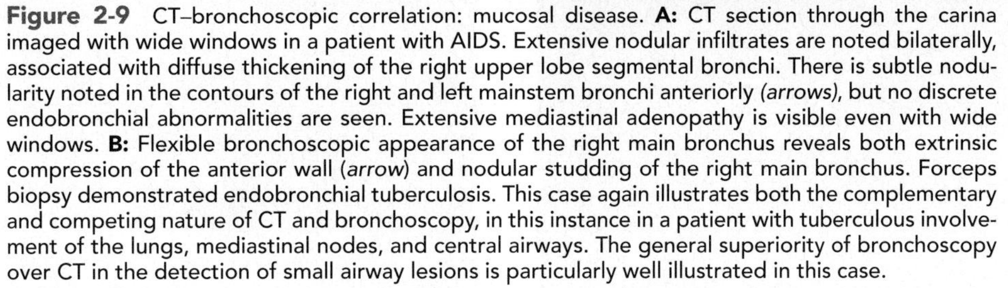

Figure 2-9 CT–bronchoscopic correlation: mucosal disease. **A:** CT section through the carina imaged with wide windows in a patient with AIDS. Extensive nodular infiltrates are noted bilaterally, associated with diffuse thickening of the right upper lobe segmental bronchi. There is subtle nodularity noted in the contours of the right and left mainstem bronchi anteriorly *(arrows)*, but no discrete endobronchial abnormalities are seen. Extensive mediastinal adenopathy is visible even with wide windows. **B:** Flexible bronchoscopic appearance of the right main bronchus reveals both extrinsic compression of the anterior wall (*arrow*) and nodular studding of the right main bronchus. Forceps biopsy demonstrated endobronchial tuberculosis. This case again illustrates both the complementary and competing nature of CT and bronchoscopy, in this instance in a patient with tuberculous involvement of the lungs, mediastinal nodes, and central airways. The general superiority of bronchoscopy over CT in the detection of small airway lesions is particularly well illustrated in this case.

between the left upper and lower nodes (Fig. 2-15). This node is best approached from the origin of the lower lobe bronchus at about the 9 o'clock position.

It is important to emphasize again that selection of the optimal puncture site is based on combining the knowledge of endobronchial landmarks with the location of enlarged lymph nodes on CT. In mentally planning the procedure, it is often helpful to flip the CT scan (which is imaged as if looking up from the patient's feet) right to left, so that the view corresponds to the bronchoscopist's viewpoint looking down from the patient's head.

Alternative Methods for Performing TBNA

In an attempt to overcome dissatisfaction with the frequently blinded nature of standard TBNA, various imaging strategies have been used. These include direct CT guidance—with and without the use of CT fluoroscopy—as well as virtual bronchoscopic and endosonographic guidance (Fig. 2-16). Although the importance of these newer approaches may be limited for experienced bronchoscopists, for whom yields in the range of 85% to 90% have been reported, considerable promise for their use may result for less experienced bronchoscopists.

One method that may aid in increasing the yield of TBNA is CT guidance, that is, performing TBNA with the patient in the CT scanner to confirm puncture of the targeted lymph node. Rong and Cui (45) found this technique improved their yield to 60%, compared with their prior experience of 20% yield using the blind technique. One drawback of the use of direct CT guidance is that it is not performed in real time: Using this technique, additional images must be obtained and reconstructed following placement of the needle, during which time the patient may move. In distinction, CT–fluoroscopy provides real-time cine visualization of the tip of the needle, allowing more confident localization. Cytologic and/or histologic material is then aspirated under direct visualization. It has been demonstrated by CT–fluoroscopy that 41% of 116 needle passes were improperly positioned, whereas subsequent passes established diagnoses in enlarged lymph nodes in all 12 patients studied (46). All patients in this group had previously undergone a nondiagnostic TBNA by the conventional method. Mean fluoroscopic exposure time was 20.5 ± 12.7 seconds. Another group reported a yield for CT–fluoroscopy guided TBNA of 83% in 12 patients, all of whom had also undergone a nondiagnostic TBNA by the conventional method (47). Although these are excellent results for patients with nondiagnostic TBNA by experienced bronchoscopists, CT–fluoroscopy is not readily available and adds considerable expense to the procedure. It has

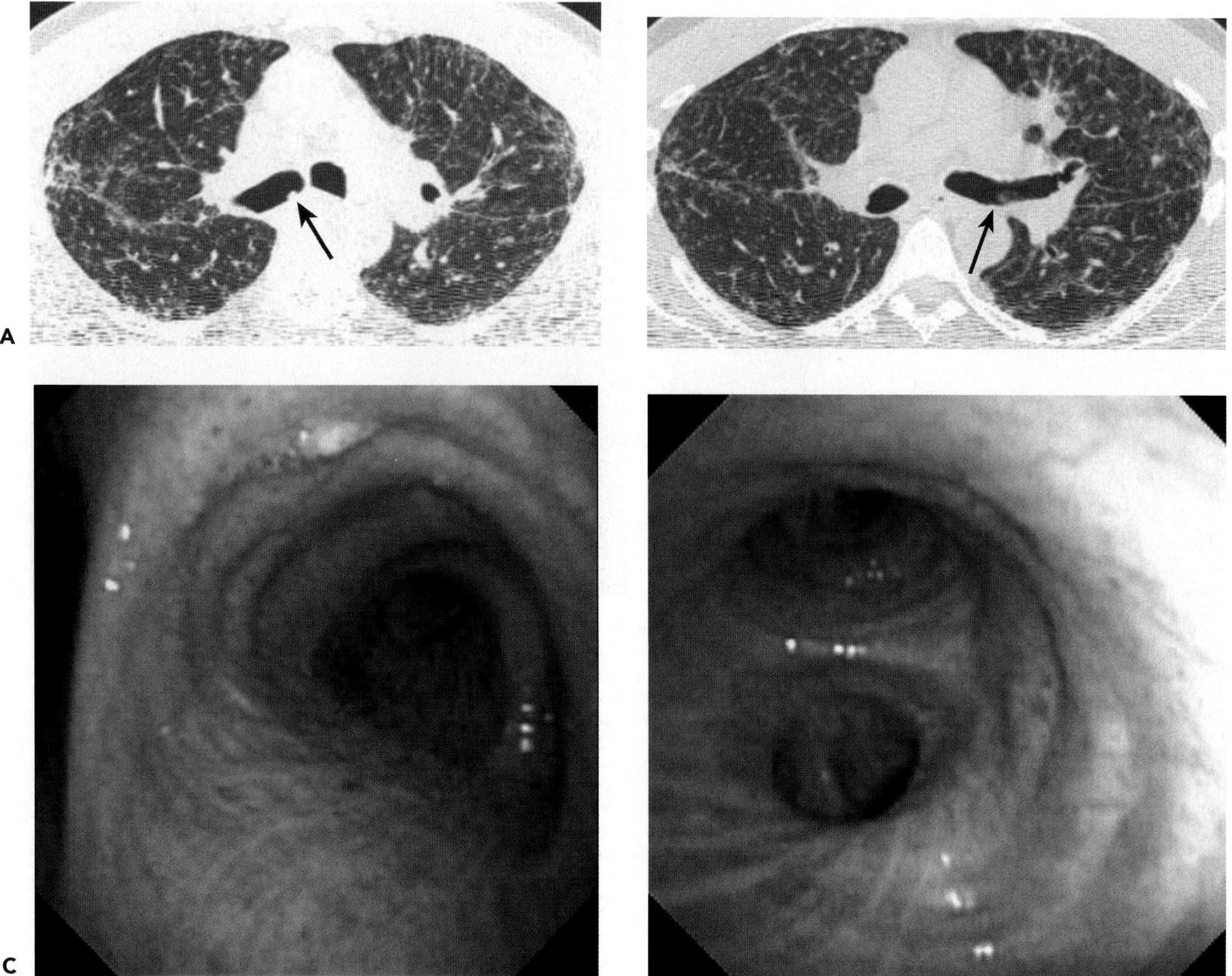

Figure 2-10 CT–bronchoscopic correlation: sarcoidosis. **A** and **B:** CT sections through the right and left mainstem bronchi, respectively, imaged with wide windows show well-defined focal lesions protruding into the proximal right main (**A**) and proximal and distal left main (**B**) bronchi, respectively. Note the presence of diffuse nodular infiltrates in both lungs with a predominantly perilymphatic distribution. **C** and **D:** Bronchoscopic images obtained the next day revealed no evidence of focal endobronchial lesions in the right (**C**) or left (**D**) main bronchi but did show focal areas of fine mucosal nodularity unsuspected from the CT (not shown). Presumably the large "lesions" shown by CT represented secretions that were no longer present by the time of bronchoscopy, although the mucosal nodularity was too subtle to be detected by CT. In this case, although CT disclosed findings characteristic of parenchymal sarcoidosis, apparent endobronchial lesions proved to represent retained secretions. In the setting of focal endobronchial lesions, performing a repeat CT following strenuous coughing may be of value by minimizing the number of false-positive examinations.

not yet been compared head-to-head with conventional TBNA.

More recently, it has been proposed that virtual bronchoscopy may be an aid in planning and performing TBNA (Fig. 2-16) (48,49). As reported by McAdams et al. (50), in a preliminary investigation of virtual bronchoscopic guidance, TBNA was performed in 17 patients, including 16 patients without prior TBNA and one with two previous nondiagnostic TBNAs (50). Using manual tracings of enlarged nodes on every third axial image, endoluminal simulations were created showing the position of nodes relative to virtual bronchoscopic images and displayed in green. These were available for review before TBNA. Altogether, 18 nodes ranging from 1.0 to 5.0 cm were aspirated in 17 patients: Of these, 14 (77%) were positive for malignancy, with diagnoses ranging from metastatic breast cancer to well-differentiated lymphocytic lymphoma (50). Two false-negative aspirates were also noted, including one patient with nodular sclerosing Hodgkin's disease ultimately diagnosed surgically and one patient with metastatic melanoma.

In addition, virtual bronchoscopy has been reported to play a role in the preplanning stage to improve the yield of TBNA (51,52). In one recent study (53), volumetric

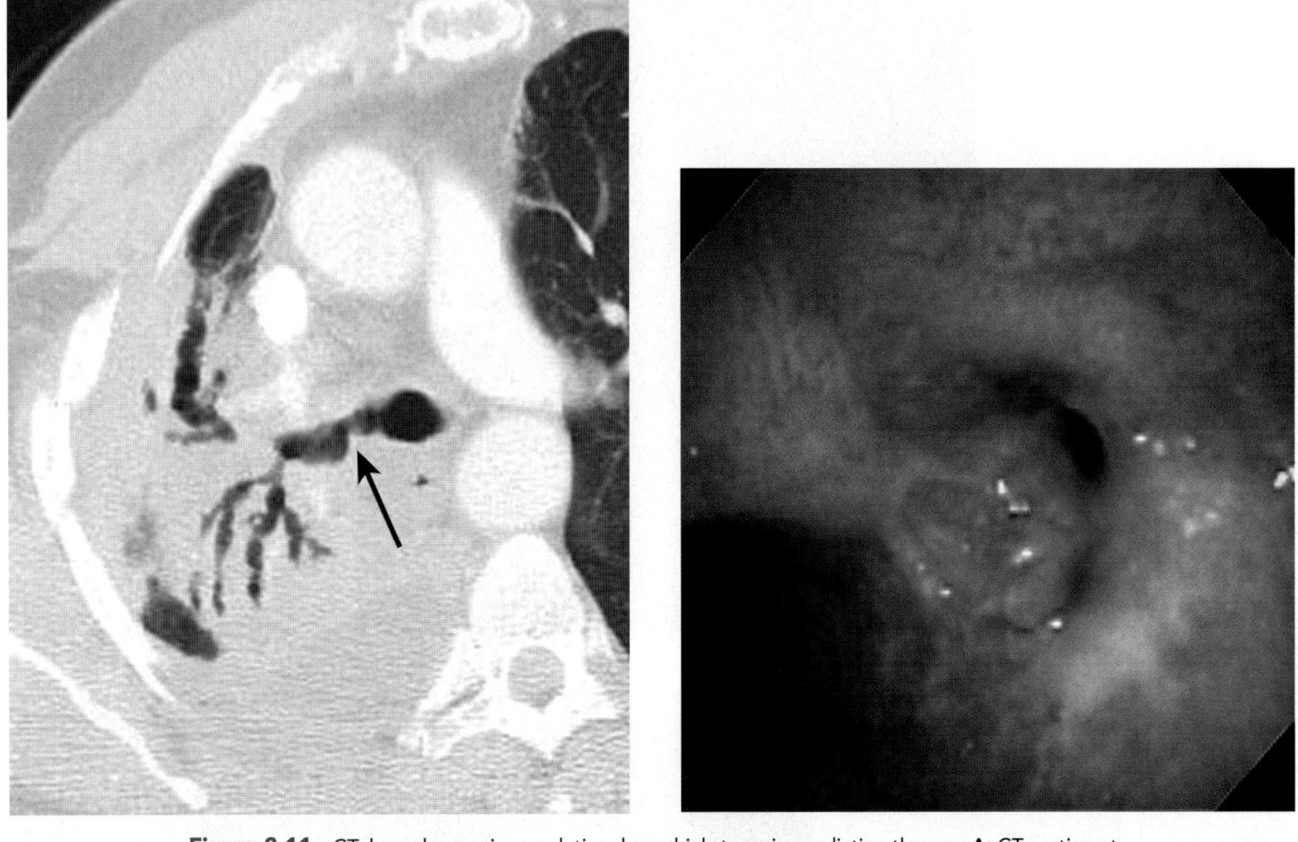

Figure 2-11 CT–bronchoscopic correlation: bronchial stenosis—radiation therapy. **A:** CT section at the level of the main carina imaged with lung windows shows marked nodularity and narrowing of the right mainstem bronchus (*arrow*) in a patient with a previous right upper lobectomy followed by external beam radiation for non–small cell lung cancer. This appearance was considered suspicious for recurrence of malignancy. **B:** Flexible bronchoscopic image confirming nodular right main bronchial stenosis, suspicious for tumor recurrence. Multiple forceps biopsies of this area, however, demonstrated only benign fibrosis. A chest CT obtained 1 year earlier was subsequently recovered and showed no significant interval change. This case demonstrates that close concordance between CT and bronchoscopic appearances may still be nondiagnostic, requiring further histologic evaluation of focal airway pathology.

rendering was used to first highlight a total of 36 sites in 14 patients in whom enlarged nodes could be identified on routine 3-mm axial images: Two separate sets of virtual bronchoscopic images—one without and one with and without nodal highlighting—were subsequently created and viewed by three experienced pulmonologists. Although virtual bronchoscopy added little to the choice of biopsy site for subcarinal nodes and did not significantly alter the selection of optimal sites for sampling aorticopulmonary window nodes, use of virtual bronchoscopic imaging with nodal highlighting increased the successful choice of biopsy sites for hilar nodes (from 37% to 83%; $p = .001$) and for pretracheal nodes (from 59% to 85%; $p = .07$), respectively.

Although a variety of newer techniques are being developed to provide a real-time interface between virtual bronchoscopy and TBNA, including the use of internal and external fiduciary markers and external electromagnetic guidance, among others, these currently remain largely experimental (54–57). The role of endoscopic ultrasonography for performing transbronchial needle aspiration is discussed separately in a later section.

Diagnostic Correlations: Peripheral Disease–Pulmonary Nodules

Clinical assessment of patients with parenchymal nodules presents an important problem in pulmonary diagnosis. It is estimated that nearly 130,000 individuals, or 52 per 100,000 people present yearly with radiographic evidence of focal parenchymal disease, nearly half of which will prove to be malignant (58). Despite the efficacy of flexible FB to identify and diagnose central endobronchial lesions, bronchoscopy is generally not considered as indicated for assessing peripheral nodules. It has been shown that in those cases in which a bronchus can be identified leading to a nodule—a "positive bronchus sign"—the yield of routine FB can be significantly improved (Fig. 2-17) (59–62). Still better results have been reported when detailed bronchographic road maps are first acquired (60,63,64).

Although standard FB is of documented utility in assessing central endobronchial lesions within the visual range of the bronchoscope, it has proved less valuable in

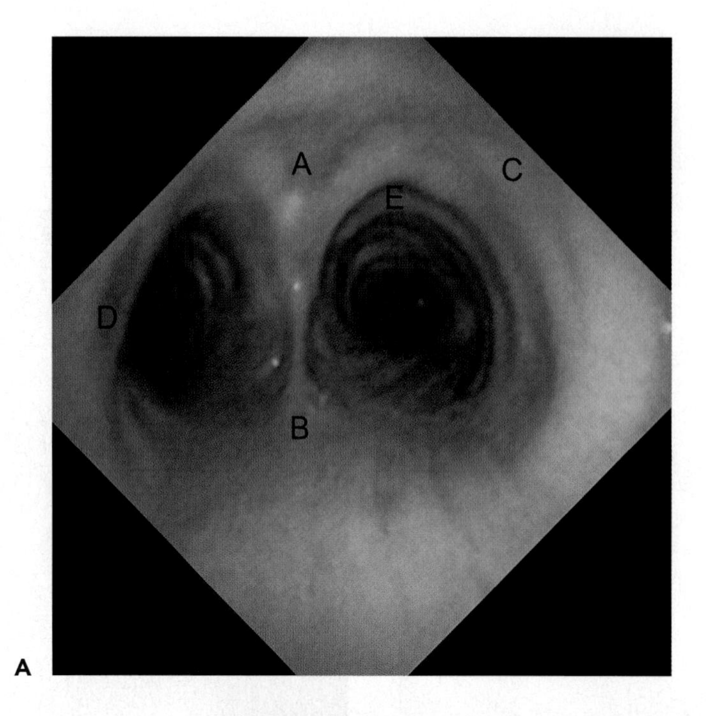

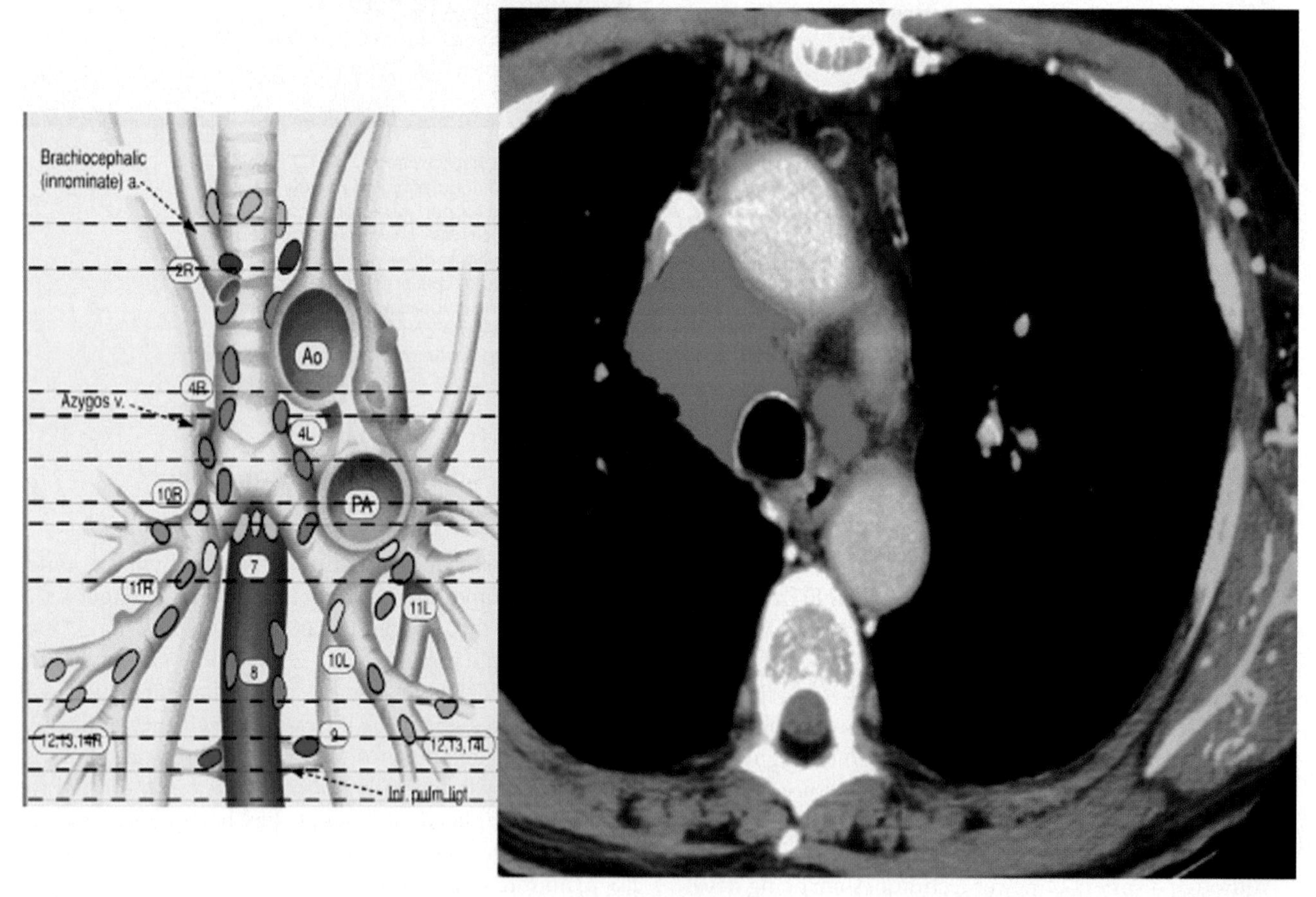

Figure 2-12 Transbronchial needle aspiration (TBNA). Key bronchoscopic landmarks with CT correlation. (1) Main carina **A:** Bronchoscopic image of the main carina. Six landmarks are identifiable in this area, with the main carina considered to be oriented in a 12 o'clock to 6 o'clock direction. These are labeled: (A) anterior carina lymph node, (B) posterior carina lymph node, (C) right paratracheal lymph node, (D) left paratracheal lymph node, (E) right main bronchus lymph node, and (F) left main bronchus lymph node. **B:** CT section through the lower trachea showing right and left paratracheal nodes corresponding to Fig. 2-12A landmarks C and D, outlined in orange. (From Ko JP, et al. CT depiction of regional nodal stations for lung cancer staging. *AJR Am J Roentgenol* 2000;174:775–782, with permission.) *(continued)*

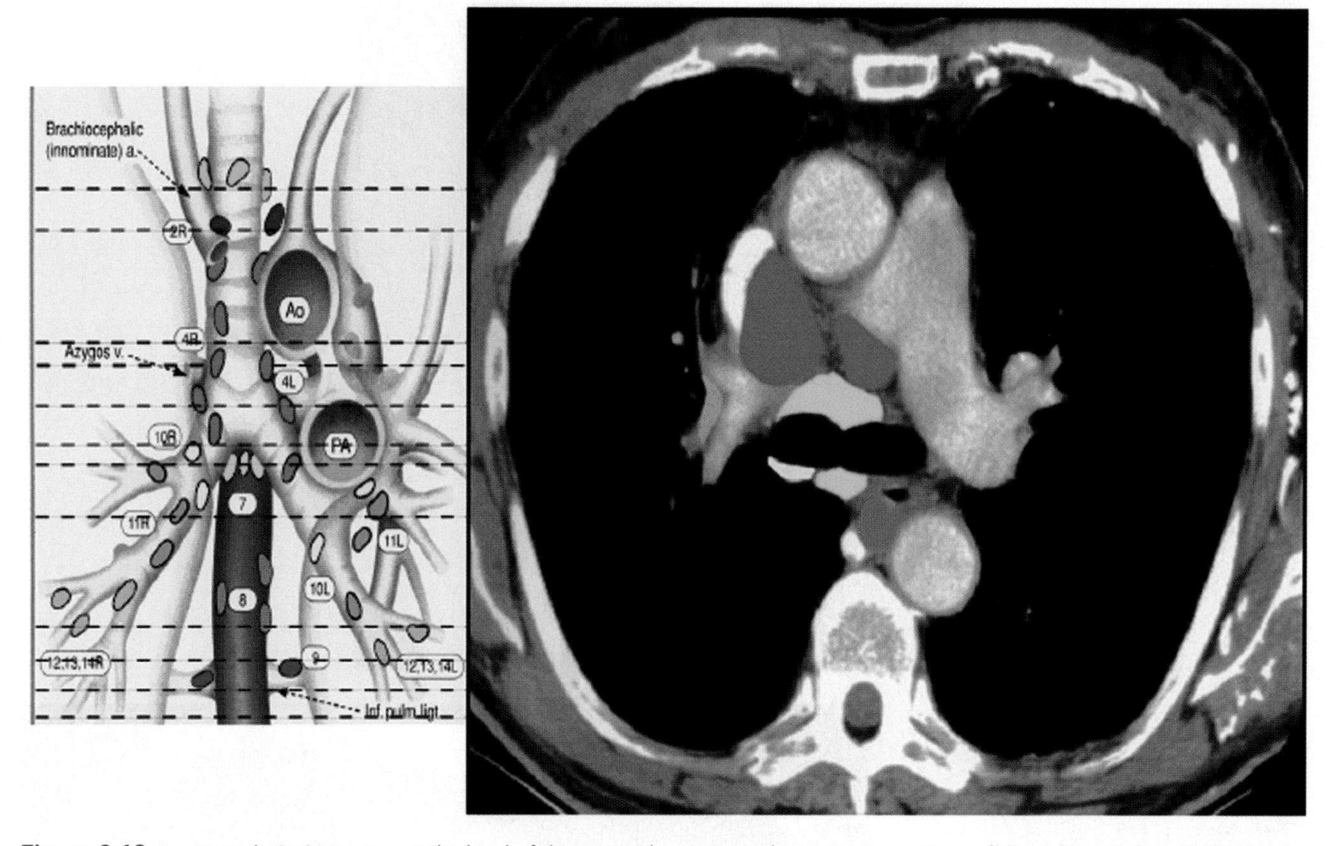

Figure 2-12 *(continued)* **C:** CT section at the level of the carina showing conglomerate appearance of the right main bronchial, anterior carinal, and left main bronchial nodes, respectively, anterior to the carina, and posterior carinal lymph node behind the carina, both outlined in turquoise. Note that all other colored nodes should be considered inaccessible with TBNA performed at the level of the carina.

assessing peripheral lung nodules. Overall the yield of bronchoscopic biopsy of peripheral nodules has generally been reported to range between 40% and 80% (58). A number of factors account for this discrepancy, including small size, location (central vs. peripheral), benign versus malignant disease, the type of procedure performed (BAL, bronchial brushing, or bronchial needle vs. forceps biopsy), whether FB is performed under fluoroscopic guidance, and interbronchoscopist variability (65). Numerous studies have shown that size is the most important determinant of success of TBBx. The poorest results are consistently obtained in patients with peripheral lesions smaller than 2 cm (66–68). In a recent survey of 30 studies evaluating the performance characteristics of bronchoscopy for diagnosing peripheral lung nodules, Schreiber et al. (69) noted that FB proved 62% sensitive for lesions larger than 2 cm but only 33% sensitive for lesions smaller than 2 cm. Although the results of TBBx for lung nodules may be improved when performed under ultrasonographic guidance, this technique is not generally available, is expensive, and still requires clinical validation (70,71). Although the yield of FB is greater for malignant nodules, this likely reflects the fact that benign lesions tend to be smaller (67). It should be noted that there is wide variation in the manner in which "peripheral" is defined (66,72–76). Using CT criteria, Baaklini et al. (67) reported significant differences in FB yield when lesions of less than 2 cm were further divided into those in the peripheral one third of the lung compared with those in the middle third.

Despite these limitations, it has been shown that the yield of FB can be improved by obtaining biopsies when a bronchus can be identified in relation to a nodule (a positive CT bronchus sign) (59–62). Gaeta et al. (60), in a study of 33 consecutive cases of documented peripheral lung cancers, found that FB provided a definitive diagnosis in 13 (59%) of 22 lesions with a positive bronchus sign versus 2 (18%) of 11 without ($p = .29$). Although the prevalence of a positive bronchus sign has varied considerably in the few reported series published to date, this likely is a reflection of CT technique. Using high-resolution 1.5-mm sections, a positive bronchus sign is seen in approximately 60% of cases (59,60). More recently, in a prospective study of 100 consecutive patients in whom a positive bronchus sign could be established, a diagnostic accuracy of 91% by curette biopsy was reported, including 18 of 22 lesions smaller than 2 cm. Importantly, in this study, multiplanar reconstructions enabled identification of leading bronchi in 38 cases in which routine axial images showed no such relationship (62). These findings suggest that enhanced CT visualization techniques will have a positive impact on the yield of TBBx. That precise delineation of the relationship between peripheral lung nodules and bronchi may improve

(Text continues on page 48.)

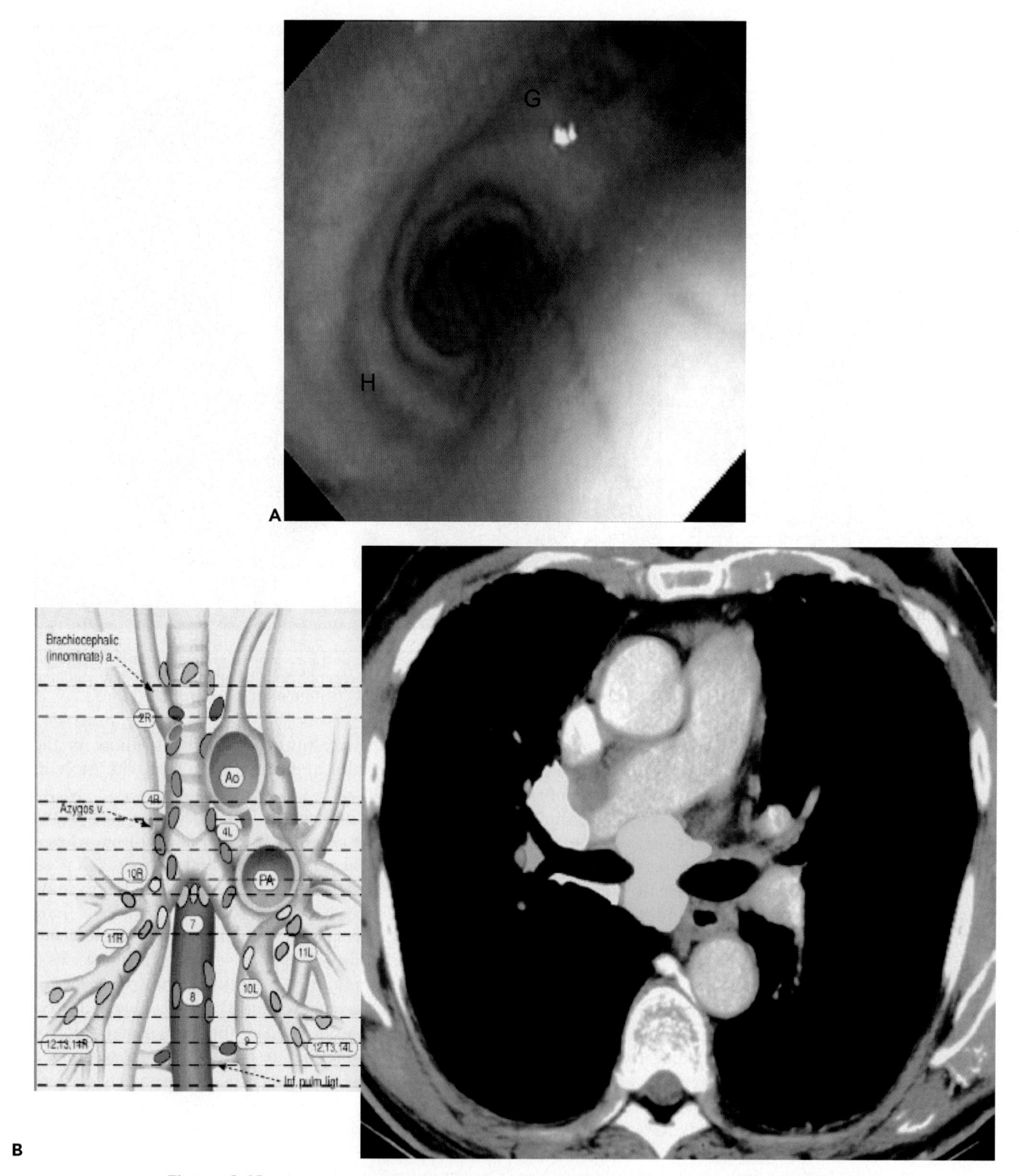

Figure 2-13 TBNA. Key bronchoscopic landmarks with CT correlation. (2) Right upper lobe bronchus **A:** Bronchoscopic image of the right upper lobe bronchus: two landmarks reference the carina between the bronchus intermedius *(left)* and the right upper lobe bronchus (*right*). (G) Right hilar lymph node, (H) subcarinal lymph node. **B:** CT section below the carina at the level of the right upper lobe bronchus shows characteristic cross-sectional appearance of the right hilar and subcarinal nodes, respectively, outlined in yellow and turquoise, respectively, corresponding to Fig. 2-13A, landmarks G and H. (From Ko JP, et al. CT depiction of regional nodal stations for lung cancer staging. *AJR Am J Roentgenol* 2000;174:775–782, with permission.)

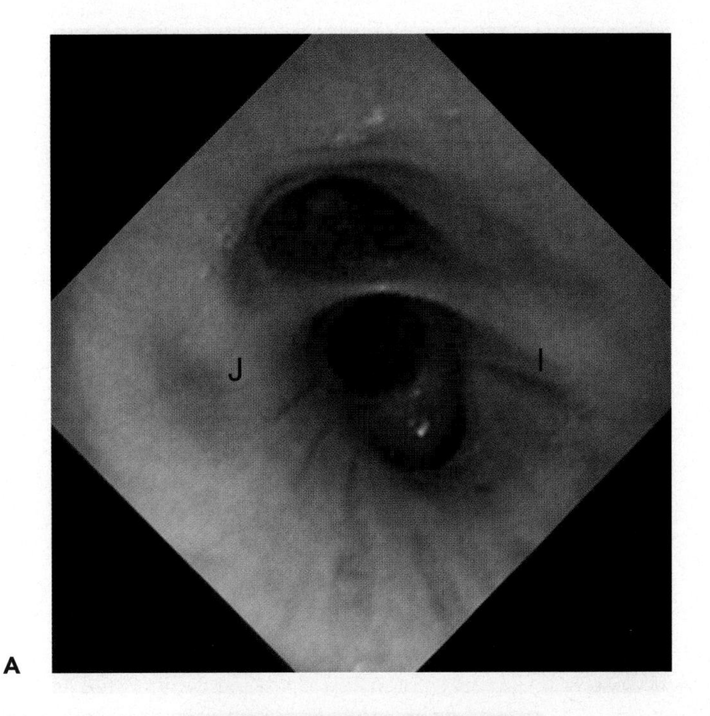

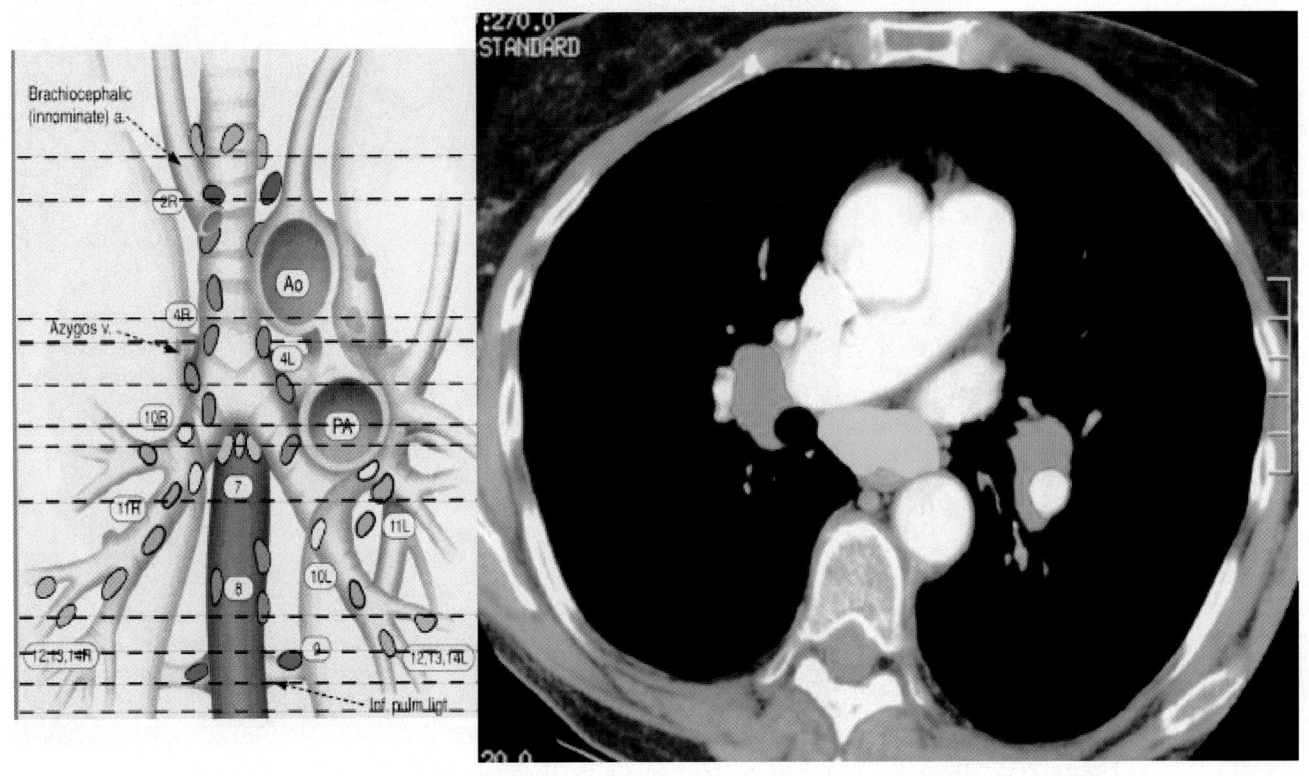

Figure 2-14 TBNA. Key bronchoscopic landmarks with CT correlation: (3) Bronchus intermedius **A:** Bronchoscopic image of the distal bronchus intermedius (BI): two landmarks are in the area of the bifurcation between the right middle lobe *(top)* and the right lower lobe (*bottom*). (I) Right lower hilar lymph node, (J) sub-subcarinal lymph node. **B:** CT section through the bronchus intermedius showing the appearance of right hilar and sub-subcarinal nodes, outlined in green and turquoise, respectively, corresponding to Figs. 2-14A and B, and 2-15A. (From Ko JP, et al. CT depiction of regional nodal stations for lung cancer staging. *AJR Am J Roentgenol* 2000;174:775–782, with permission.)

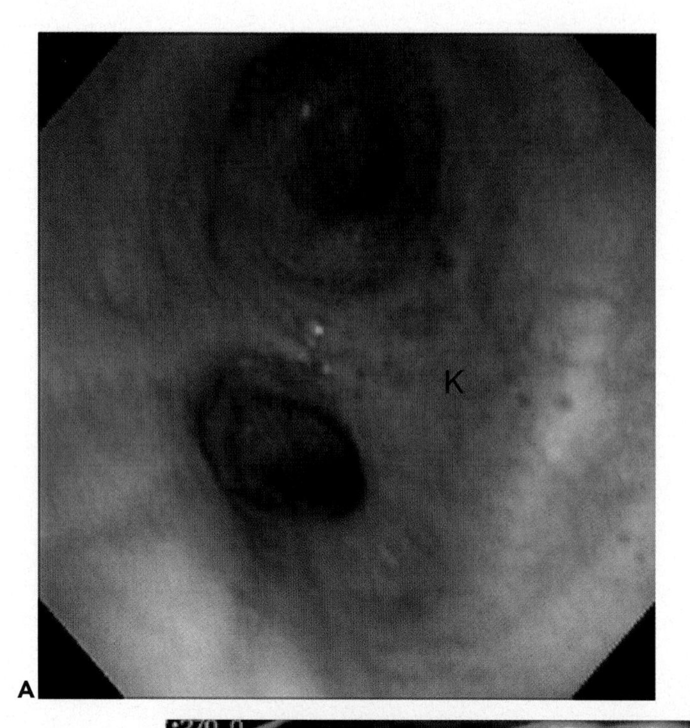

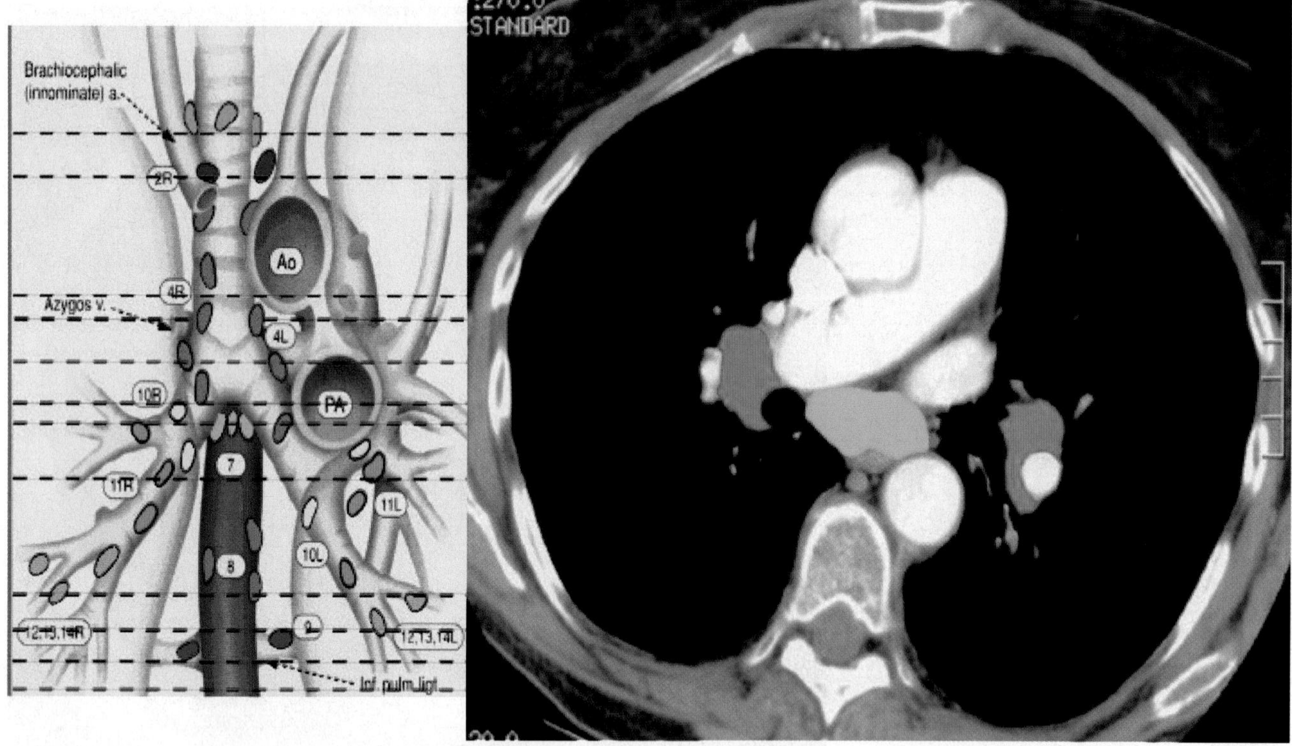

Figure 2-15 TBNA. Key bronchoscopic landmarks with CT correlation: (4) Secondary left-sided carina. **A:** Bronchoscopic image of the bifurcation between the left upper lobe (*top*) and left lower lobe (*bottom*), the secondary carina. This corresponds to CT section shown in Fig. 2-14B. (K) Left hilar lymph node.

the efficacy of TBBx has also been shown in studies in which positive contrast bronchography has been used to provide a preliminary road map (60,63,64). Using transbronchial curettage, Mori et al. (63) reported the yield of TBBx to be as high as 88.5% for tumors of 1.5 to 2 cm when biopsies were preceded by selective bronchography.

In a further attempt to assess the significance of a positive bronchus sign for diagnosing solitary lung nodules, Bilaceroglu et al. (77) prospectively evaluated the use of multiple diagnostic procedures, including bronchial washings, brushings, and TBNA, in 92 patients with solitary nodules or masses between 2 and 5 cm that were within reach of routine fiberoptic bronchoscopy. Using 2-mm sections to define the relationship between nodules and airways, these authors noted that a significant difference

(*Text continues on page 50.*)

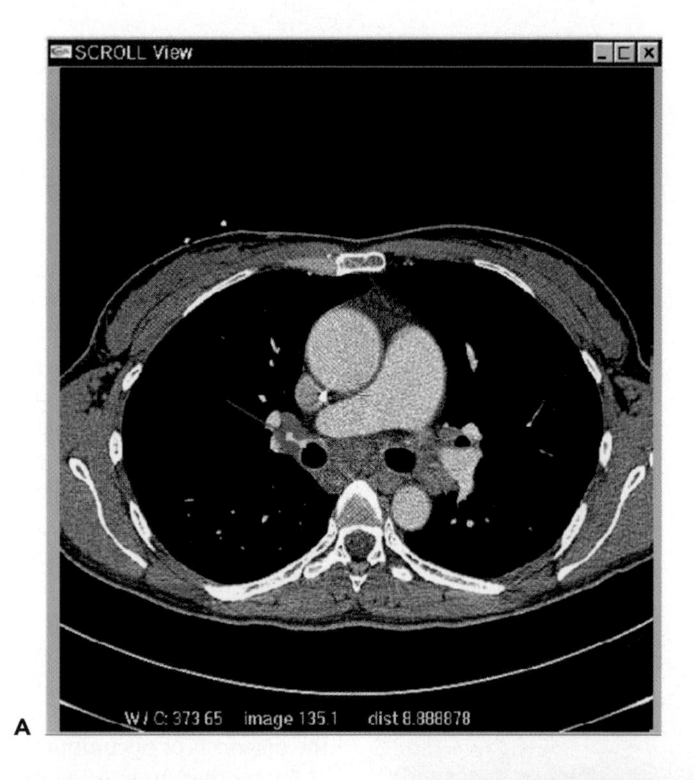

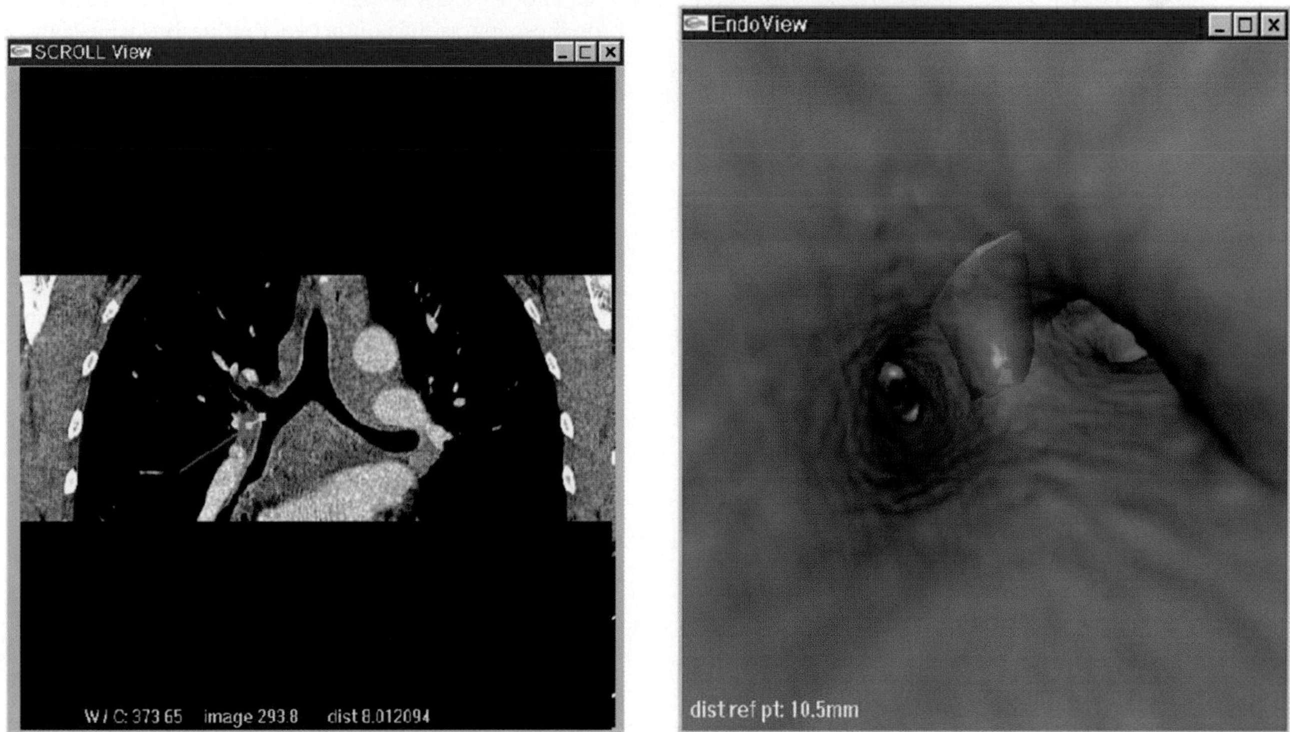

Figure 2-16 TBNA: virtual bronchoscopic guidance. **A** and **B:** Axial and coronal CT sections, respectively, imaged with narrow windows at the level of the bronchus intermedius show enlarged right hilar and subcarinal nodes. In this case, right hilar nodes have been semiautomatically outlined and appear in color. Note that the most optimal angle for accessing these nodes is also presented (yellow lines in A and B). **C:** Virtual bronchoscopic image looking inferiorly from the distal bronchus intermedius showing the bifurcation of the right upper lobe bronchus and bronchus intermedius. The exact location of the right hilar nodes outlined in **A** and **B** are now superimposed on the virtual bronchoscopic image. In this case, virtual bronchoscopy serves as a road map assisting TBNA in accessing nodes in locations less frequently biopsied.

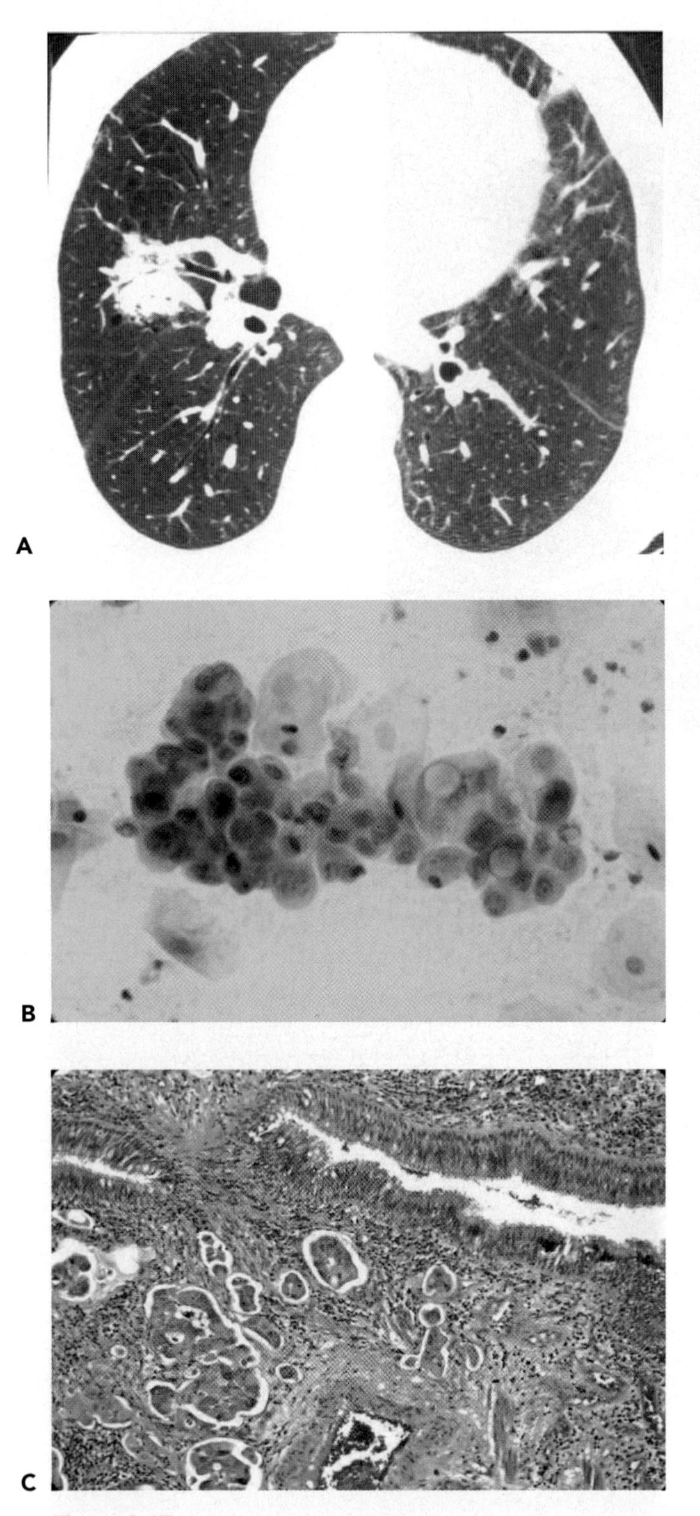

Figure 2-17 CT–bronchoscopic correlation. The positive bronchus sign. **A:** Magnified view through the middle lobe showing an irregular nodule. A branch of the middle lobe bronchus can clearly be traced to this lesion, which is causing irregular narrowing of the airway. **B** and **C:** Cytologic and histologic correlation. Cytologic specimens (**B**) revealed malignant cells, a finding that was further confirmed by transbronchial biopsy showing extensive submucosal tumor (**C**). In cases in which a close relationship between nodules and airways can be established, cytologic and histologic specimens obtained bronchoscopically are likely to be positive. (From Naidich DP, et al. *CT and MRI of the thorax*, vol 3. Philadelphia: Lippincott, 1999, with permission.)

with bronchoscopy providing the diagnosis in 40 (82%) of 49 cases with a positive bronchus sign versus only 19 (44%) of 43 without ($p < .01$). These data further confirm the added value of CT in first delineating the relationship between nodules and airways before bronchoscopy.

With the recent introduction of high-quality virtual bronchoscopy, the possibility that CT may provide detailed road maps leading to peripheral nodules is just beginning to be explored (10,78–83). This includes the potential use of peripheral branches of the pulmonary arteries as substitute markers for peripheral airways less than 2 mm in size (83a). As discussed previously, the impetus for this method is the relatively recent development of ultrathin bronchoscopes, which allow direct visualization of sixth- to eleventh- or twelfth-order bronchi. This was first described in one patient by Asano et al. (79). This group used virtual bronchoscopy images to guide an ultrathin bronchoscope to a peripheral lesion that was 18 by 14 mm. CT was then used during the bronchoscopy to confirm the approach of the ultrathin bronchoscope to the lesion and the placement of a bioptome into the lesion. Examination of the biopsy specimen established the diagnosis of pneumonia.

In another study using *fluoroscopically* directed ultrathin bronchoscopy as an adjunct to routine bronchoscopy, a successful diagnosis was established in 11 (64.7%) of 17 patients (10). In the largest series reported to date, Shinagawa et al. (83) performed CT-guided TBBx with an ultrathin bronchoscope using virtual bronchoscopic navigation to diagnose peripheral lung nodules smaller than 2 cm. Of a total of 26 nodules in 25 patients, these authors successfully biopsied 17 (65%), including 14 neoplasms and 3 benign lesions. However, it should be noted that, in this study, virtual bronchoscopic images were obtainable to only fifth-generation airways, which probably in part explains these authors' limited success (83). Figure 2-18 illustrates that virtual bronchoscopy, using high-resolution images obtained from multidetector CT scanners, may provide detailed road maps and allow successful biopsy of peripheral lung nodules under CT guidance with the use of ultrathin bronchoscopes.

Figure 2-18 Virtual bronchoscopic CT-guided ultrathin bronchoscopy. **A** to **H:** Select magnified axial (A to D) and corresponding sagittal (E to H) images beginning at the secondary carina and proceeding caudally in a patient with a left lower lobe nodule. **I** to **L:** Virtual bronchoscopic views corresponding to the axial and sagittal views shown in **A** to **H. M** to **P:** Bronchoscopic views obtained using ultrathin bronchoscopy. These correspond precisely with the virtual bronchoscopic views at the same levels shown in **I** to **L. Q:** CT scanogram obtained at the time of bronchoscopy showing the extremely peripheral position of the ultrathin bronchoscope. **R:** Magnified view of the left lower lobe showing the tip of the ultrathin bronchoscope within the left lower lobe nodule. These images confirm that virtual bronchoscopy may be indispensable by providing a road map to guide ultrathin bronchoscopes into regions of the lung previously difficult to access by bronchoscopists. (See Fig. 1-7 as well.)

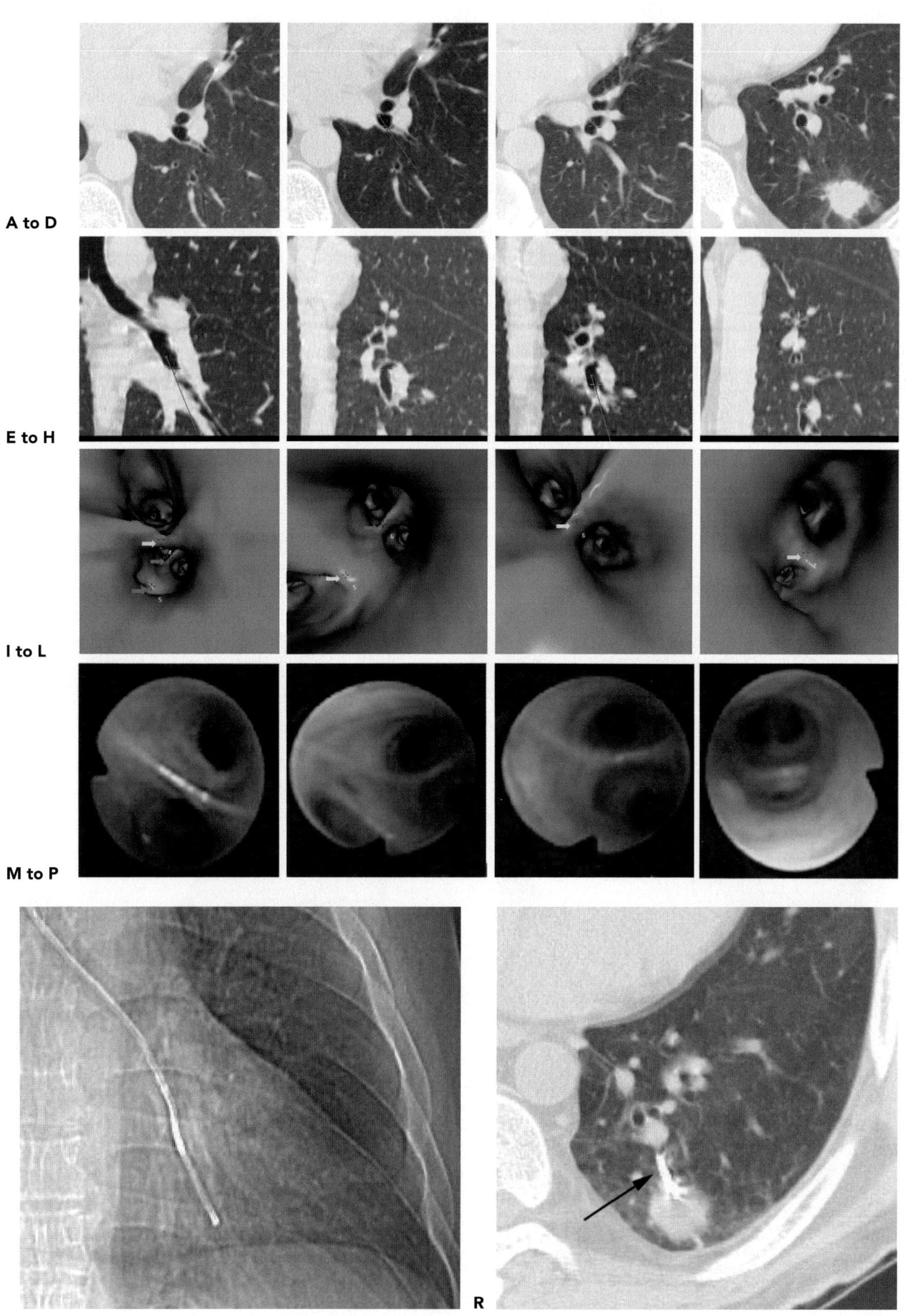
A to D
E to H
I to L
M to P
Q
R

Despite these early promising results and the impressive correlation between airway anatomy mapped by virtual bronchoscopic means and that observed by ultrathin bronchoscopy as distal as tenth-generation airways, the technique is far from ideal. In addition to the earlier descriptions of limitations of the ultrathin bronchoscopes, the size of the instrument channel limits the size of the instruments that can be passed into a peripheral lesion. The small forceps currently available frequently provide specimens inadequate for pathologic diagnosis. The current technique also requires real-time CT confirmation of ultrathin bronchoscope and biopsy position, entailing additional radiation exposure to the staff and patient and occupation of the CT scanner for significant periods. Shinagawa et al. (83) found the average total time of the examination to be just under 30 minutes, although the CT room was occupied for about an hour per procedure. Despite these limitations, the potential for virtual bronchoscopic guidance of ultrathin bronchoscopy to expand the range of current clinical indications for biopsy of peripheral nodules remains undefined. In our judgment, the ultimate clinical value of ultrathin bronchoscopy for evaluating peripheral nodules will depend on several factors, among them the development of automated methods of generating virtual bronchoscopic pathways, thus eliminating the need for time-consuming image processing.

Therapeutic Correlations

In addition to its ability to identify bronchial lesions, both centrally and peripherally, CT may play an essential role in treatment planning (Figs. 2-19 to 2-23). In addition to allowing direct visualization of the central airways enabling identification of subtle mucosal, submucosal, and endobronchial abnormalities and providing bacteriologic, cytologic, and histologic material from endobronchial, peribronchial, and parenchymal sites (84), an increasing number of therapeutic interventions may now be performed bronchoscopically (1). In patients with central airway obstruction, CT allows distinction between central tumor and peripheral atelectasis (85,86). In most cases for which therapeutic interventions are planned, CT plays an essential role by accurately assessing the true extent of extra-

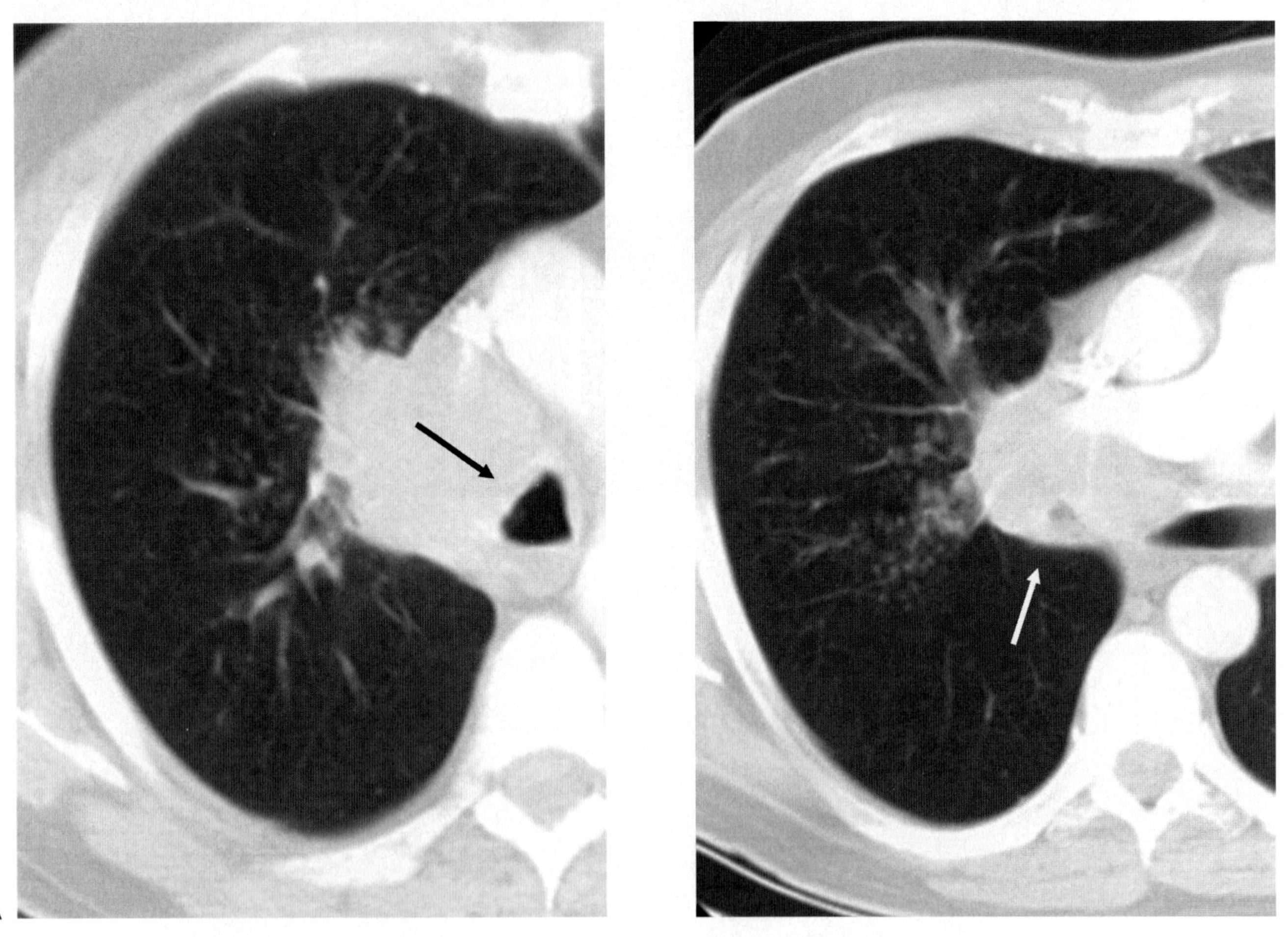

Figure 2-19 CT–bronchoscopic correlation: use in therapeutic planning—bronchogenic carcinoma. **A** and **B:** CT sections through the distal trachea and right mainstem bronchus, respectively, imaged with wide windows demonstrate extensive mediastinal adenopathy causing eccentric nodular compression of the anterolateral wall of the distal trachea and marked nodularity and near complete occlusion of the right main bronchus in a patient with known non–small cell lung cancer. Note patency of airways beyond the occluded right mainstem bronchus (*arrow* in **A**). *(continued)*

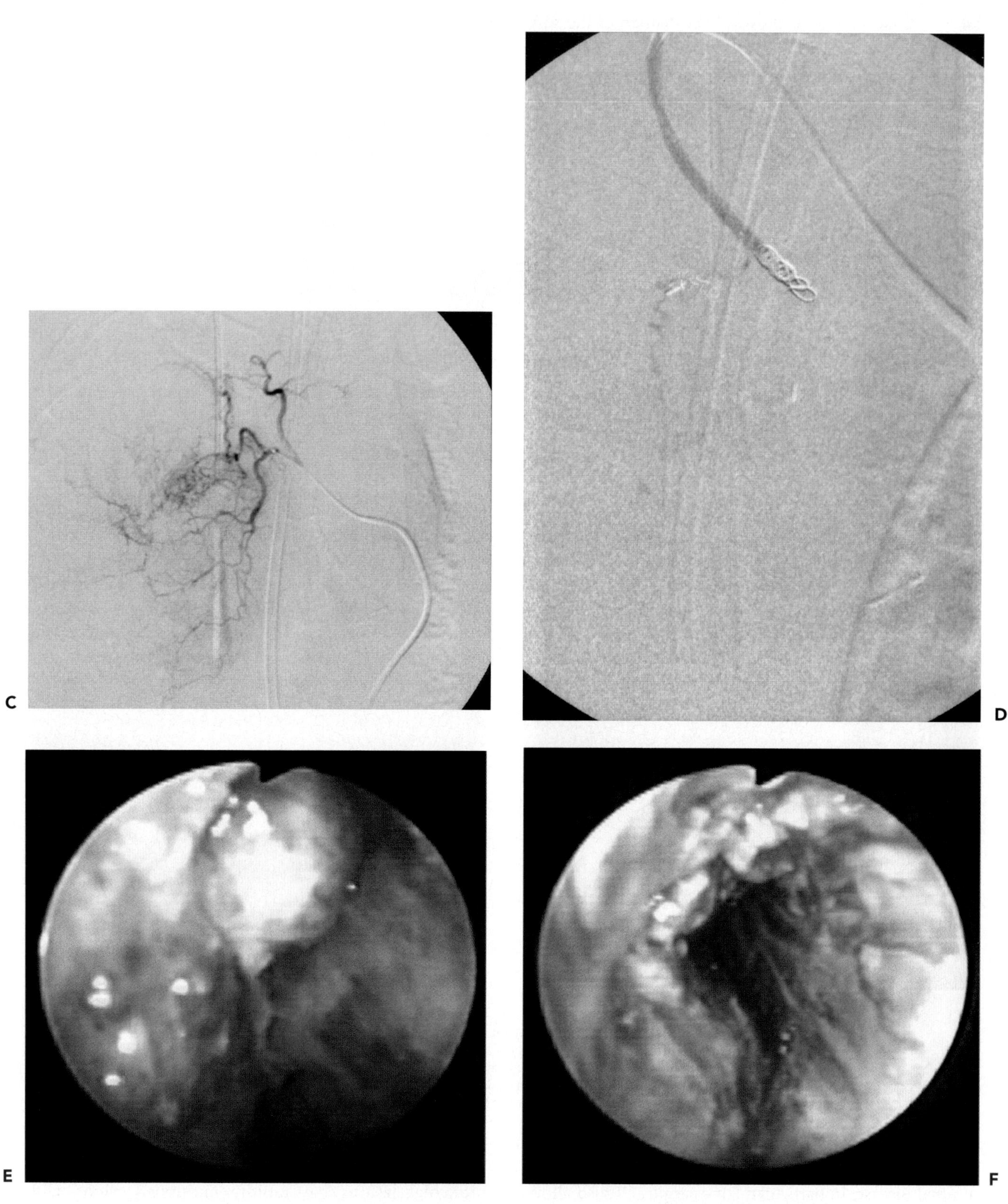

Figure 2-19 *(continued)* **C** and **D:** Magnified subtraction views prebronchial and postbronchial artery embolization. Note that in **C** there is massive extravasation of contrast media from hypertrophied bronchial arteries that is successfully extinguished following bronchial arterial embolization (**D**). **E:** Flexible bronchoscopy shows presence of tumor within the distal trachea with extensive submucosal invasion and obstruction of right main bronchus. **F:** Appearance of right main bronchus after removal of obstructing tumor by electrocautery through the flexible bronchoscope. Although the right upper lobe remained obstructed, the airways distal to the right upper lobe were patent as indicated by CT. This case again illustrates the complementary nature of CT and bronchoscopy. In this case, the combination of the findings of unresectable lung cancer (T4N2M0), mainstem bronchus occlusion, and patent airways distal to the occlusion identifiable by CT were indications for an interventional bronchoscopic procedure such as electrocautery to maintain airway patency.

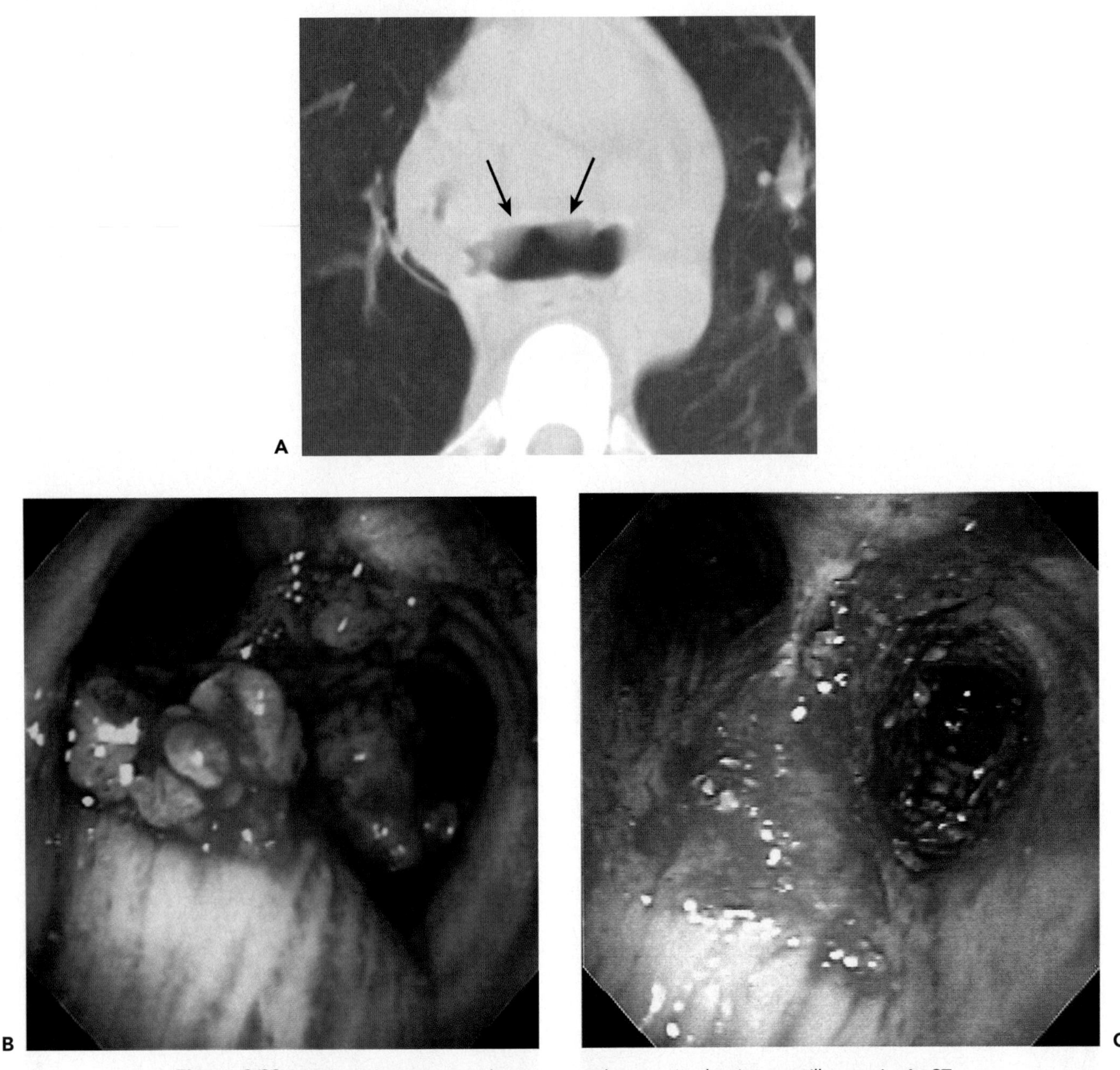

Figure 2-20 CT–bronchoscopic correlation: use in therapeutic planning—papillomatosis. **A:** CT section through the carina in a patient with recurrent respiratory papillomatosis presenting with worsening dyspnea demonstrates irregular nodularity of the carina and proximal right and left mainstem bronchi *(arrows)*. **B:** Flexible bronchoscopy confirms the presence of large papillomatous lesions, photographed at full inspiration. On forced exhalation and coughing, the orifice to each main bronchus was almost totally obstructed. **C:** Flexible bronchoscopic appearance of the same airways after removal of papillomas by electrocautery.

luminal disease, in particular. For example, CT also allows visualization of distal airways that otherwise cannot be evaluated bronchoscopically because of proximal airway obstruction (Fig. 2-19). Similarly, CT can identify patients' otherwise unresectable tumors resulting from direct mediastinal invasion or unsuspected parenchymal, osseous, or adrenal metastases.

Since the mid-1990s, the number of novel interventional techniques that can be applied to the treatment of endobronchial lesions has rapidly multiplied: along with surgery, radiation, and chemotherapy, interventional bronchoscopy now legitimately forms one of the mainstays for treating endobronchial malignancy. Although a detailed assessment of the various techniques now available is outside the intended scope of this chapter, a short summary of these procedures is worthwhile. As extensively reviewed by Chan et al. (1,1a), recent advances in interventional bronchoscopy include the following procedures.

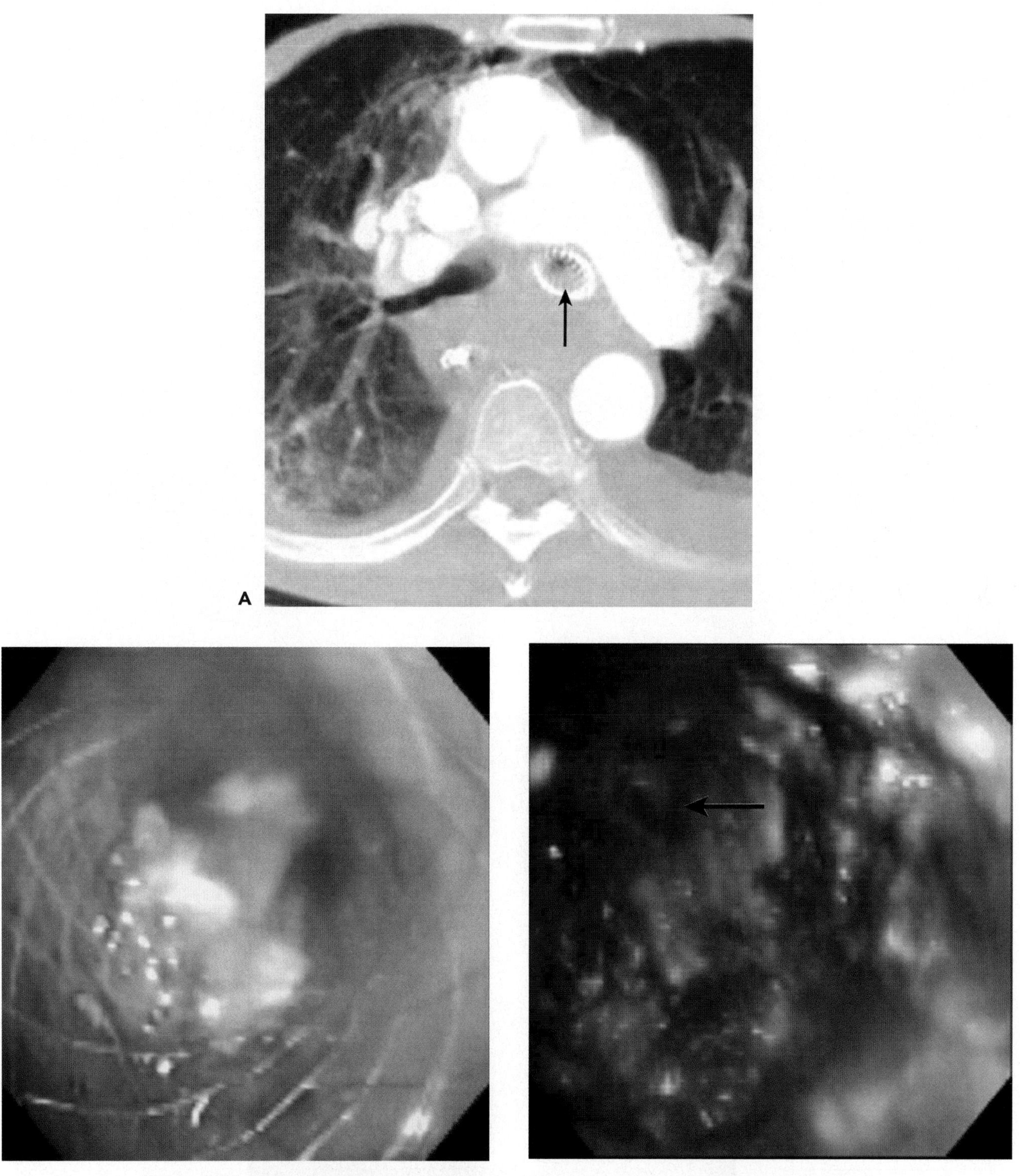

Figure 2-21 CT–bronchoscopic correlation: use in therapeutic planning—stent evaluation. **A:** CT of a patient with esophageal carcinoma who had previously required endobronchial stent placement in the left main bronchus resulting from extrinsic compressive obstruction of the bronchus by the primary tumor. CT was obtained to evaluate dyspnea 4 weeks after an uncovered self-expanding metal stent had been placed within the left mainstem bronchus. Note that in addition to extensive posterior mediastinal tumor, there is soft tissue density filling the lumen of the stent *(arrow)*. **B:** Flexible bronchoscopy confirmed the presence of tissue obstructing the stent. Forceps biopsy revealed invasive esophageal carcinoma. **C:** Flexible bronchoscopic appearance of the left main bronchus after removal of the obstructing tumor by argon plasma coagulation via the flexible bronchoscope. Patent distal airways are seen *(arrow)*. Because of the electroconductive nature of metal stents, this technique is safer than electrocautery within the lumen of a stent and is much less likely to damage the stent than is the Nd:YAG laser.

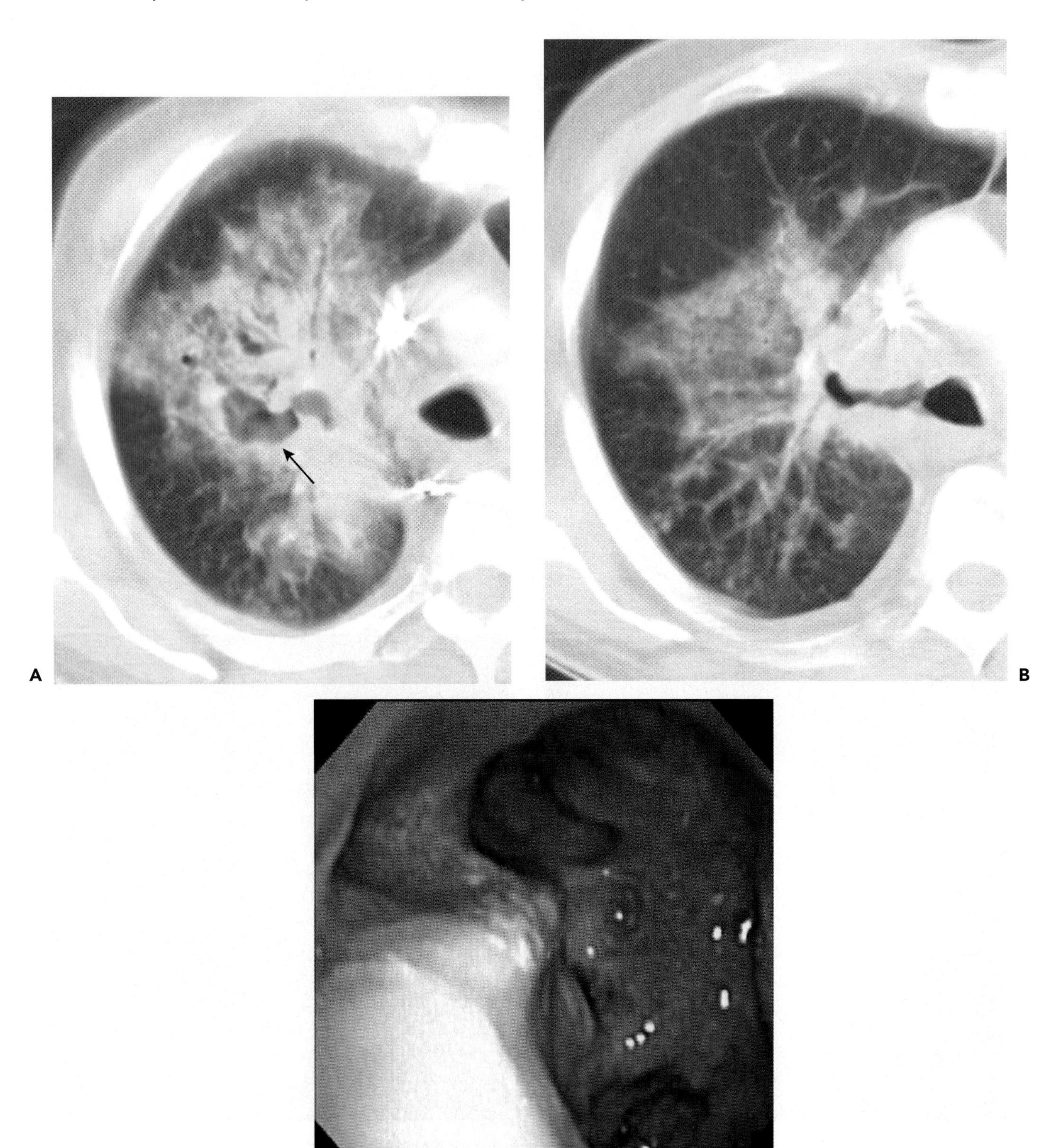

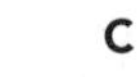

Figure 2-22 CT–bronchoscopic correlation: use in therapeutic planning—cavitary lung disease. **A** and **B:** Magnified views through the right upper lobe at the level of the distal carina and right upper lobe bronchus, respectively, in the same patient shown in Fig. 2-11. Despite embolization and combined radiation and chemotherapy, however, this patient subsequently developed fever, productive cough, and a right upper lobe cavity (*arrow* in **A**). Clinically suspected diagnoses included cavitary bacterial pneumonia, tuberculosis, invasive aspergillosis, and recurrent tumor. **C:** Image obtained at the time of flexible bronchoscopy shows the tip of the bronchoscope extending directly into the cavity. Biopsy showed only necrosis and bacteria, without evidence of tumor. Subsequent clinical improvement followed antimicrobial therapy alone. In this case, the CT finding of an accessible airway leading directly into a focal lesion predicted a high likelihood for a successful diagnostic bronchoscopy.

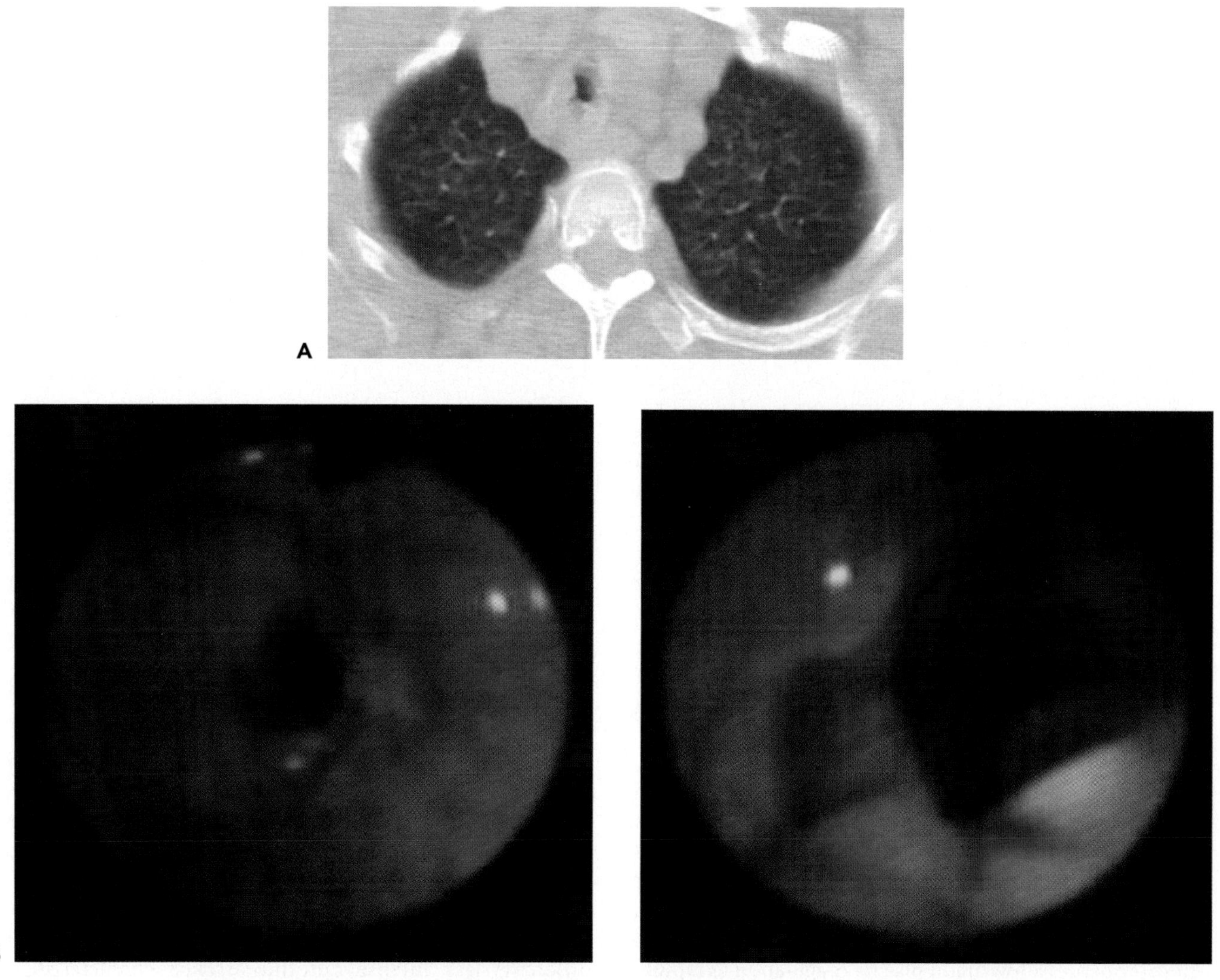

Figure 2-23 Ultrathin bronchoscopy: tracheal stenosis **A:** CT section through the midtrachea showing a severe stenosis secondary to previous longstanding intubation. **B** and **C:** Images obtained with ultrathin bronchoscopy in the same patient in **A**. Ultrathin bronchoscopy is especially helpful in determining the extent of obstruction from the most proximal (**B**) to most distal and narrowest level of tracheal stenosis (**C**). In this case, the ultrathin bronchoscope was capable of passing through the most stenotic point to confirm the patency of the distal trachea (not shown).

Neodymium:Yttrium-Aluminum-Garnet Laser Phototherapy

Neodymium:yttrium-aluminum-garnet (Nd:YAG) laser phototherapy uses light energy to vaporize and coagulate endobronchial lesions and can be used with either flexible or rigid bronchoscopes (87,88). It is often the procedure of choice for providing rapid, symptomatic palliation of airway obstruction, with success depending on both the location and especially the length of airway involvement. Complications include airway perforation and rarely fire (89).

Photodynamic Therapy

Photodynamic therapy (PDT) involves the use of photosensitizing drugs administered intravenously that preferentially localize to tumors allowing their subsequent activation by monochromatic light of an appropriate wavelength (87,90,91). PDT is less commonly used than Nd:YAG laser phototherapy, in part because of a lack of immediate effect and in part because of the development of intense photosensitivity necessitating avoidance of sunlight.

Cryotherapy

Using a variety of agents, including nitrous oxide or carbon monoxide, endobronchial lesions are alternately exposed first to freezing and then to thawing, resulting in intracellular and extracellular crystallization and tissue necrosis. Lesions are treated by direct contact of the tip of the cryoprobe with the tumor. Although cryotherapy is associated with fewer complications, especially airway perforation, than is laser phototherapy, the maximal effects of cryotherapy occur 7 to 10 days after its application. Cryotherapy requires follow-up bronchoscopy to clear debris and assess results and often requires one or two repeat attempts to obtain maximum effectiveness in relieving bronchial obstruction. These qualities make cryotherapy inadequate for rapid relief of tracheobronchial obstruction. Still, cryotherapy remains a safe and inexpensive alternative to laser phototherapy (92).

Electrocautery

In distinction to photodynamic laser therapy, electrocautery techniques, as the name implies, use high-frequency alternating current to generate thermal energy as a method for coagulating or vaporizing endobronchial lesions (Fig. 2-20) (93). Complications include potential airway perforation, hemorrhage, and occasional fire. Electrocautery is safe and effective and can be used with either a flexible or a rigid bronchoscope.

Brachytherapy

With brachytherapy, tumors are treated by local endobronchial radiation with ^{192}iridium, enabling the delivery of approximately 3,000 rads directly to lesions (92,93). Typically used in combination with external radiation or laser phototherapy, brachytherapy has approximately the same success rate as other interventional procedures for providing palliation. Similar to other interventional techniques, complications include hemorrhage and perforation. Additional side effects include radiation-induced bronchitis and stenosis.

Argon Plasma Coagulation

Argon plasma coagulation involves the passage of argon gas through a probe with an electrode at its tip, which ionizes the gas into plasma. The ionized plasma seeks out conducting tissue and desiccates, coagulates, and devitalizes it. Penetration is to the depth of approximately 3 to 4 mm. These properties allow argon plasma coagulation to rapidly remove tumor analogous to laser phototherapy, with a lower incidence of complications such as airway perforation and fire (94), which permits safe use inside a metallic stent (Fig. 2-21).

Airway Stents

The use of stents, including those made of metal and silicone, has gained widespread acceptance for relieving both benign and malignant central airway obstructions (95–98). Although silicone stents generally require the use of rigid bronchoscopy, self-expanding metallic stents are readily placed by FB. Proper placement of either type necessitates careful planning. As with other methods of interventional bronchoscopy for which CT facilitates delineation of the extent of airway obstruction, CT plays an especially important role before stenting by predetermining the optimal diameter and length of the stent (see Fig. 3-11, Chapter 3). Reconstruction of helical CT images into three-dimensional or virtual bronchoscopic images can be used for this purpose (99). Miyazawa et al. (100) used a combination of spirometry, ultrathin bronchoscopy, 3D reconstruction of CT images, and EBUS to evaluate the choke point of flow limitation in malignant tracheobronchial stenosis before and after stent placement to evaluate the functional need for further stenting. CT has also proved beneficial in the follow-up of stent placement (101). Complications include stent migration, obstruction resulting from the development of excessive granulation tissue, and tumor recurrence (Fig. 2-21). Another complication is the added potential of fire in patients with silicone stents undergoing laser phototherapy. In addition to the use of stents, focal airway stenoses may be treated with balloon dilatation or bronchoplasty. Similar to angioplasty, this technique, which requires that balloons be introduced by either flexible or rigid bronchoscopes, is most often successful in dilating short-segment stenoses (102).

AUTOFLUORESCENCE BRONCHOSCOPY

Lung cancer remains the leading cause of death resulting from cancer, in large part because of the advanced nature of the disease at presentation in the overwhelming majority of patients. The fact that lung cancer is curable in its early stages has driven intensive efforts to reliably detect early lung cancer. However intuitively attractive this logic may be, large trials of screening for lung cancer have not demonstrated a mortality benefit in at-risk patients. These trials used some combination of serial sputum cytology and chest radiograph, and the methodology and interpretation of these studies have been the subject of some debate. The magnitude of the problem has led investigators to explore the capability of new technologies to detect early lung cancer.

The nature of normal tissue to autofluoresce when illuminated by light of particular wavelengths and the slightly different, less intense autofluorescence characteristics emitted by dysplastic or malignant tissue was discovered in the early part of the last century. The phenomenon of autofluorescence is due to the presence in tissue of fluorophores including NAD/NADH, flavines, and tryptophane. These substances may be present in lower concentrations in abnormal tissue, which, in combination with increases in epithelial thickness and blood flow, alter autofluorescence (103). The distinction between autofluorescence emissions by normal endobronchial mucosa and that of dysplastic and carcinomatous lesion in the visualizable airways is the basis of the development of autofluorescence bronchoscopic techniques.

Early efforts in this area focused on the use of hematoporphyrin derivatives to enhance the weak natural autofluorescence of abnormal tissue in the airways, which could then be observed by FB (90). These efforts were based on the observation that certain fluorescent compounds were concentrated by malignant tissue. However, because the hematoporphyrin derivatives were administered systemically, their use was complicated by severe photosensitivity in the recipients (104).

Recent technologic advances have led to techniques by which the weak natural autofluorescence is enhanced by digital means, allowing the bronchoscopist to view the

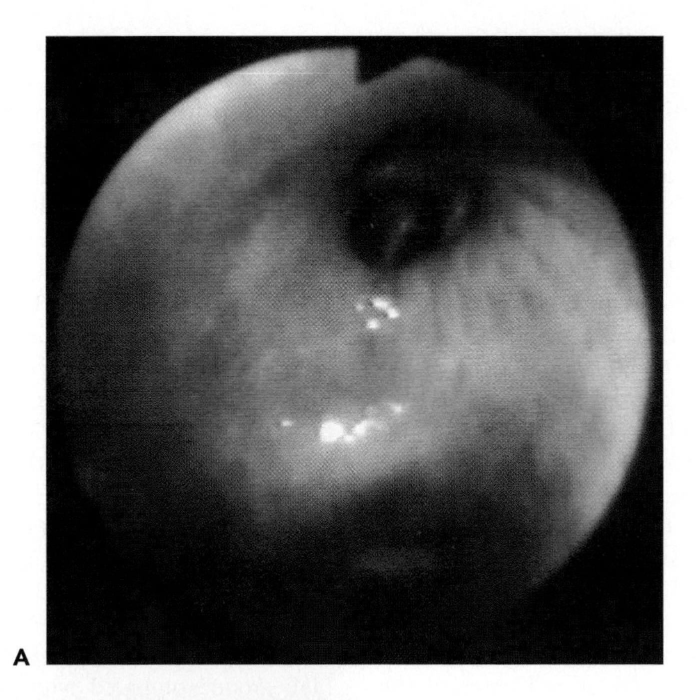
A

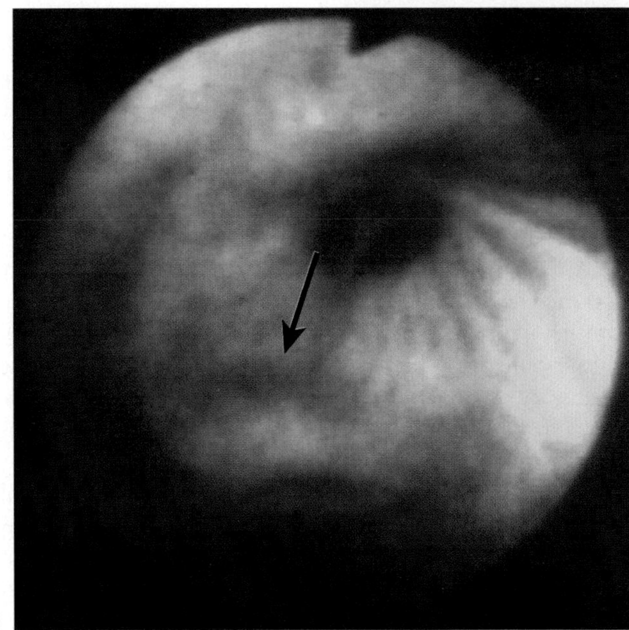
B

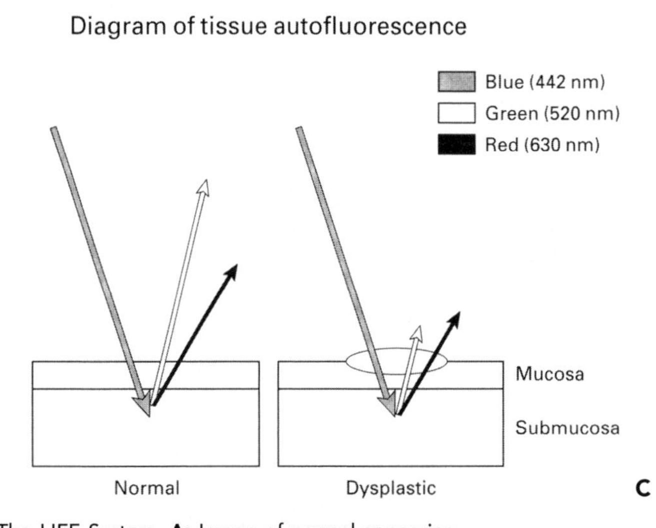

C

Figure 2-24 Autofluorescence bronchoscopy: The LIFE System. **A:** Image of normal-appearing carina obtained by standard white-light bronchoscopy through a fiberoptic bronchoscope. **B:** The same carina observed using the Xillix LIFE System. Normal tissue appears green, and dysplastic or carcinomatous tissue has a reddish-brown color *(arrow)*. Forceps biopsy revealed severe dysplasia. **C:** Schematic representation of tissue autofluorescence. With blue light of 442 nm normal tissue appears to autofluoresce more intensely in the green spectrum compared with red. In distinction, the intensity of autofluorescence of dysplastic tissue is greatly diminished, although less so in the red spectrum than the green. The result is that dysplastic tissue is recognizable by a reddish-brown hue, whereas normal tissue appears green (see **A** and **B**).

changes with the naked eye. When illuminated by blue light of 442-nm wavelength, the normal endobronchial tissue autofluoresces in both the green and red spectrums, with the emitted red light of lesser intensity. Dysplastic and carcinomatous endobronchial lesions will autofluoresce with less intensity but with the red light of greater intensity than the green.

The Xillix Technologies Corporation developed the light-induced fluorescence endoscopy (LIFE) system to take advantage of the autofluorescence phenomenon. A helium-cadmium laser light source emitting blue light of 442 nm illuminates the airways through a fiberoptic bronchoscope. A camera attached to the bronchoscope contains two CCDs, which detect the red and green emissions, respectively, from the mucosa. This information is transmitted to a motherboard that enhances the difference between the spectra emitted by normal and abnormal tissue and integrates the data into a single, real-time image. Normal tissue appears green, and dysplastic and carcinomatous tissue appears reddish-brown (Fig. 2-24).

The development of the LIFE system came about largely through the efforts of Dr. Stephen Lam. An early report of the use of LIFE in subjects who were smokers or patients with suspected or prior resected lung cancer found approximately a doubling in the detection of endobronchial carcinoma in situ (CIS) and dysplasia compared with white-light bronchoscopy (WLB) (105). A large North American multicenter trial of the LIFE system in 173 patients with known or suspected lung cancer found a 6.3-fold increase in the detection of dysplasia and CIS compared with WLB. However, there was a high false-positive rate for LIFE-directed biopsies (0.34), and the positive predictive value was only 0.39 for LIFE and WLB combined (106).

Success in the detection of early lung cancer and premalignant lesions with LIFE has varied from study to study. The lowest success rate was reported by Kurie et al. (107) in 1998, in a study performed in 92 subjects with a smoking history of at least 20 pack-years as a component of a chemoprevention trial. These investigators found no increase in abnormal pathology in biopsies taken from sites that exhibited normal autofluorescence compared with those that appeared abnormal or when LIFE was compared with WLB. The degree of lung cancer risk in this study group has been questioned given the overall low number of abnormalities found on biopsy (108) although one third of the subjects had had prior NSCLC or a head and neck cancer (107).

To avoid the possible bias of performing WLB before LIFE, as was done in the North American multicenter trial, Venmans et al. (109) randomized the order in which the two techniques were performed in 33 high-risk patients. They found that sensitivity and specificity for the detection of dysplasia and CIS were comparably high for the two techniques. Hirsch et al. (110) randomized 55 subjects to the order of LIFE and WLB and to individual bronchoscopists. All were at high risk for lung cancer based on a smoking history of at least 30 pack-years, evidence of airflow obstruction, and either abnormal sputum cytology or previous or suspected lung cancer. Fifty-eight percent of the patients were found to have at least one biopsy with moderate or severe dysplasia. The relative sensitivity of LIFE to WLB was 3.1, and LIFE was not significantly less specific than WLB (70% vs. 78%, respectively) (110).

Another system for the detection of early lung cancer based on tissue autofluorescence, the D-Light system, was developed by the Karl Storz Company. This system can be used in conjunction with an inhaled photosensitizer 5-aminolevulinic acid (ALA), which minimizes systemic side effects. Herth et al. (111) recently reported a comparison of LIFE with D-Light in 332 patients in a crossover-design study. These investigators found both systems to be comparable in the detection of 62 areas of metaplasia or dysplasia, 11 CIS, and 127 invasive carcinomas. Based on a three-point classification of normal, abnormal, or suspicious appearance, there was a disparity in classification between the two systems in only 5 of 1,117 areas biopsied (2 normal, 2 dysplasias, 1 invasive carcinoma). The authors did find that the mean examination time was significantly different, 11.7 minutes for LIFE compared with 7.4 minutes for D-Light (111).

The optimal use of autofluorescence bronchoscopy remains to be determined. It is impractical to use either of the current systems in all individuals at risk for lung cancer, but certain subgroups may benefit if they are at particularly high risk. Perhaps the most well-defined risk group comprises those patients in lung cancer screening trials who are found to have abnormal sputum cytology from a radiographically occult source. Shibuya et al. (112) compared LIFE in a group of 64 patients with sputum cytology suspicious or positive for malignancy to WLB in 48 historical controls with similar findings who had bronchoscopy before the availability of LIFE. They found that the diagnosis of preinvasive lesions was greatly improved in the LIFE group compared with the WLB controls (70% vs. 15%). Others have found autofluorescence bronchoscopy to be useful in patients with known NSCLC, both preoperatively to detect unsuspected synchronous lung cancer (3 of 48 patients reported by van Rens [113]) and postoperatively to detect unsuspected recurrence (3 of 51 patients reported by Weigel [114]). Autofluorescence has also been used in the evaluation of response of dysplastic lesions to chemopreventive agents such as retinol (114a).

Although the high false-positive rates commonly reported have been a concern in the use of autofluorescence bronchoscopy, recent studies suggest that abnormal autofluorescence may predict malignant potential even in the setting of normal histology. Using comparative genomic hybridization, one study found chromosome aberrations (most commonly in chromosome 3) in 81% of specimens demonstrating abnormal autofluorescence and normal histology (115). Another group reported alteration in *p53* gene expression in 28% of samples with abnormal autofluorescence and normal histology, compared with 42% in invasive carcinoma (116).

Subsequent modifications to the LIFE design are currently undergoing clinical investigation, including replacement of the laser light source with a blue filter and automatic measurement of the red-green autofluorescence ratio to complement the subjective judgment of color by the bronchoscopist. These changes are intended to make the equipment less expensive and less bulky and improve the speed and ease of the procedure. Whether the yield is improved will need to be investigated.

ENDOBRONCHIAL ULTRASOUND

Until recently, bronchoscopic examination of the airways was limited to the endobronchial appearance of the accessible areas of the tracheobronchial tree. Interest in allowing the bronchoscopist to "see" the layers of the walls of airways and beyond, to extraluminal structures, has promoted the adaptation of ultrasound technology to bronchoscopy (117).

As with all forms of ultrasonography, intimate contact is needed between the probe and adjacent structures to successfully propagate sound waves. EBUS suffers potential limitations because of the presence of intervening air between the probe and the bronchial wall, which results in considerable image degradation. The tracheobronchial tree is air-filled, which has necessitated innovative probe design to permit the realization of EBUS. Investigators began to pass ultrasound probes designed for intravascular or endoscopic use through bronchoscopes (118,119). The field of view was limited to extraluminal structures adjacent to the point of contact of the probe with the airway wall, with airway secretions acting as coupling agents. Promising though limited experience with these catheters led to the development of ultrasound probes specifically designed to be used endobronchially. To provide the necessary sound-conducting interface with the curved airway wall, the probes were fitted with balloons that were inflated with water. The enhancement of sound conduction by the water-filled balloon on 20-MHz probes yields high definition of structures as deep as 4 cm. If the balloon obstructs the airway, 360-degree images of the wall and surrounding structures can be obtained.

Early investigators of EBUS quickly learned to identify the components of the walls of normal airways and the appearance of surrounding structures such as blood vessels and lymph nodes. Up to seven layers within the wall of large airways have been reported to be identifiable: two of the inner mucosa, three of cartilage, and two of the outer adventitia (Fig. 2-25). Vessels can be easily identified by their pulsation and low internal echo density. In distinction, lymph nodes as small as 2 mm can be identified by their high echo density.

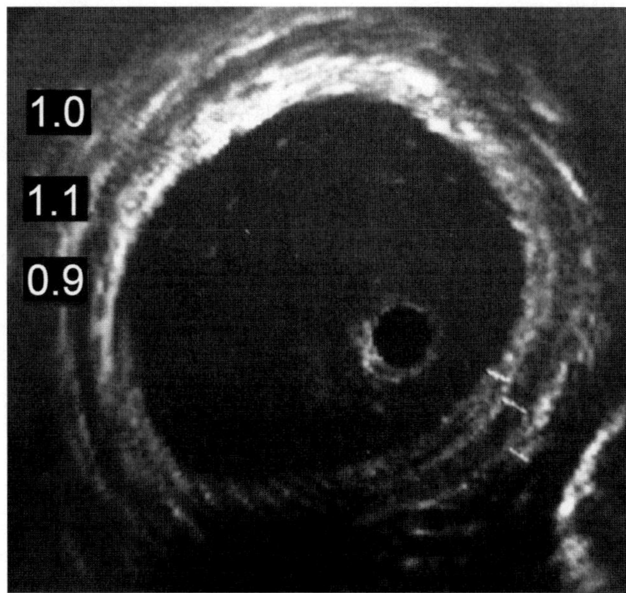

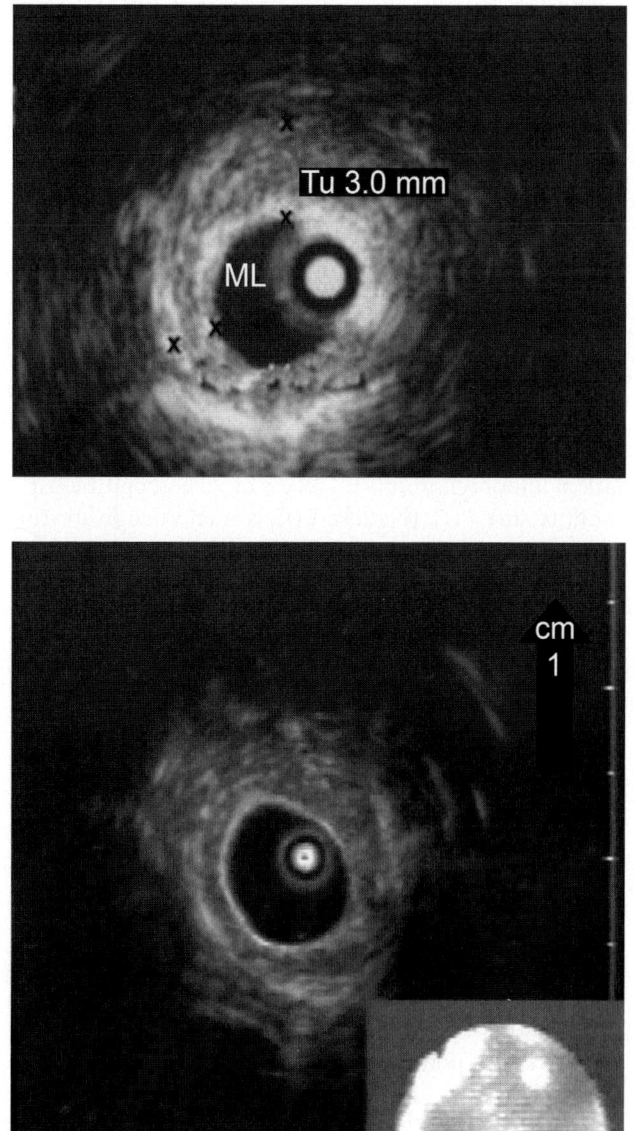

Figure 2-25 Endobronchial ultrasound **A:** *In vitro* endobronchial ultrasound appearance of the normal trachea showing five identifiable portions of the airway wall. From inside out these include one hyperechoic layer representing mucosa and submucosa, a second anechoic layer representing cartilage, and a third echogenic layer representing the adventitia. As illustrated in this figure, these layers measure 1, 1.1, and 0.9 mm, respectively. Note that the endobronchial probe lies eccentrically within the tracheal lumen and that the definition of the tracheal wall is nonuniform, resulting from lack of uniform contact between the probe and the mucosa. **B:** Endobronchial ultrasound in a different patient than shown in **A**, showing early tumor infiltration of the bronchial wall, causing loss of the normal airway levels shown in **A**. (Tu 3.0 mm = tumor defined by x's in the upper portion of the image; ML, lumen; x's in the lower left portion of the image, normal-uninvolved portion of the bronchial wall. **C:** Endobronchial ultrasound in a third patient, showing focal destruction of the bronchial wall resulting in loss of definition of the normal airway layers *(arrows)*. (Parts **A** and **B** from Herth F, et al. Endobronchial ultrasound improves classification of suspicious lesions detected by autofluorescence bronchoscopy. *J Bronchol* 2003;10:249–252, with permission; Part **C** courtesy of Dr. Armin Ernst, Boston, Massachusetts.)

EBUS Evaluation of Airway Wall Involvement by Malignancy

Baba et al. (120) attempted to correlate EBUS images with airway histopathology in 61 patients with intrathoracic malignancies who underwent pneumonectomy, lobectomy, or bronchoscopic forceps biopsy. EBUS was performed in 21 patients with endobronchially visible tumors with subsequent ultrasonographic evaluation performed *ex vivo* in resected specimens for the remaining 40 patients. These investigators found correlation between the thickness of cartilage as determined by EBUS and the actual histologic thickness measured with calipers. Malignant tissue was characterized by hypoechoic areas, and invasion of the cartilage layer was readily identified as well (120). EBUS has also been shown to be of use in evaluating tracheobronchial invasion by esophageal carcinoma, a diagnosis typically difficult to establish definitively by other imaging methods. Nishimura et al. (121) performed EBUS in 59 patients with newly diagnosed esophageal carcinoma and compared the findings with those of endoscopic ultrasound, bronchoscopy, and CT. All patients tolerated completion of EBUS, but a complete endoscopic examination was obtained in only 44%. The accuracy of the diagnosis of tracheobronchial invasion by esophageal carcinoma by EBUS was 91%, superior to bronchoscopy, endoscopic ultrasound, and CT with accuracies of 78%, 85%, and 58%, respectively (121).

Takahashi et al. (122) used EBUS to evaluate the depth of tumor invasion of airway walls in 22 radiographically occult lesions detected by sputum cytology. Lesions were characterized as either not reaching the cartilaginous layer (group A) or invading the cartilaginous layer (group B). The patients were then treated by irradiation, PDT, or surgical resection. Accuracy of the EBUS category was determined either by histologic examination of surgical specimens or by lack of tumor cells found on repeat bronchoscopic biopsy 2 months after PDT (because PDT is ineffective in treating malignancy invading to the depth of cartilage). This group reported that EBUS had a sensitivity of 86%, specificity of 67%, and accuracy of 80% for the diagnosis of malignant invasion not reaching the cartilaginous layer (122). Similarly, Herth et al. (123) evaluated the capability of EBUS to distinguish airway compression by tumor from invasion in 105 patients who underwent chest CT followed by bronchoscopy with EBUS and subsequent surgery. Compared with CT, EBUS had a surgically confirmed superior sensitivity (89% vs. 75%), specificity (100% vs. 28%), and accuracy (94% vs. 51%). This compared favorably with a previous report of 93% accuracy for endobronchial ultrasonographic evaluation of tracheobronchial invasion by tumor in 15 surgically resected patients (124). In addition to assessing malignant disease, the usefulness of EBUS in the diagnosis of benign tracheobronchial damage resulting from relapsing polychondritis in two patients has also been reported (125).

Herth et al. (126) investigated the benefit of adding EBUS examination to the findings of LIFE in the tracheobronchial tree in 74 patients in whom histologic correlation also was obtained. Although malignancy was correctly diagnosed by LIFE in 69%, this increased to 97% with the addition of EBUS. As striking, whereas LIFE proved correct in diagnosing 55% of benign lesions, this number increased to 97% with the addition of endoscopic ultrasonography. Not surprisingly, these authors concluded that EBUS should be added to LIFE because it increased the probability of detecting early neoplasms (126).

EBUS in Guiding TBNA

As discussed, numerous attempts have been made to overcome the blind nature of TBNA using a variety of complementary imaging techniques. Unfortunately, with one exception (127), many reports have documented that the echogenic properties of mediastinal and hilar lymph nodes are not sufficiently distinctive to allow reliable differentiation between benign and malignant adenopathy (128). As a consequence, interest has largely focused on the use of EBUS to direct TBNA. The first comparison of TBNA guided by the standard endobronchial landmarks established by Wang to EBUS-guided TBNA was reported by Shannon et al. (129). In this study, 80 patients with known or suspected lung cancer and suspicious lymph nodes identified by CT were randomized to TBNA either with or without ultrasound guidance. No statistically significant difference was noted: standard TBNA proved positive in 22 of 24 patients (91%) with cancer and EBUS-guided TBNA proved positive in 25 of 30 cases (83%). Ultrasound guidance, however, did decrease the number of aspirates required to diagnose malignancy in paratracheal lymph nodes with the presence of an on-site cytologist (129). It should be noted that this group used an intravascular ultrasound probe.

A more recent study using a dedicated EBUS probe reported successful sampling by EBUS-guided TBNA of lymph nodes ranging from 8 to 43 mm in 207 of 242 patients (86%) with malignancy confirmed in 72% (130). This same group subsequently performed a randomized trial of conventional TBNA versus EBUS-guided TBNA. Although they found no significant difference in yield in the subcarinal lymph node station, EBUS-guided TBNA proved significantly better than conventional TBNA in all other lymph node stations combined (84% vs. 58%) (131). Despite these findings, EBUS-guided TBNA suffers the important limitation that it is necessary to remove the ultrasound probe from a standard bronchoscope to pass the TBNA catheter. Consequently, anatomic landmarks first identified sonographically must then be visually remembered by the bronchoscopist during the performance of biopsies. Furthermore, the rotational nature of the current probes provides no consistent orienting landmarks for the observer, and the planes of view change repeatedly as the tracheobronchial tree is traversed, causing further potential disorientation. To overcome these issues, a prototype bronchoscope with an ultrasound probe built in at the tip has been investigated (132). Other models are now undergoing clinical trials. In the meantime, as recently reported, use of an existing dual-channel bronchoscope and a TBNA catheter to observe the needle entering lymph nodes suggests a means of dealing with these limitations using currently available instruments (133). The first use of a new dedicated convex probe ultrasound bronchoscope developed by the Olympus Corporation to guide real-time TBNA has recently been reported. This bronchoscope has at its tip a curved linear array transducer that scans parallel to the axis of the bronchoscope. The resulting direction of view is 30 degrees forward oblique. The 2.0-mm instrument channel admits a 22-gauge aspirating needle, which can be observed puncturing the airway wall into adjacent lymph nodes by ultrasound in real-time. The authors used this bronchoscope to guide TBNA of mediastinal and hilar lymph nodes in 70 patients, of whom 45 had malignant disease (133a). Using this bronchoscope, they found that TBNA demonstrated a sensitivity, specificity, and accuracy for distinguishing benign from malignant disease of 96%, 100%, and 97%, respectively. However, 8 of 45 patients with malignancy (18%) and 21 of 25 patients (84%) with benign etiologies required surgical confirmation of TBNA findings.

EBUS in Assessing Peripheral Lesions

Goldberg et al. (119) were the first to report on the use of EBUS to identify airways leading to small peripheral lesions. Subsequently, Kurimoto et al. (134) reported characterization of six classes of peripheral nodules by preoperative EBUS according to their echogenic patterns; they compared these with surgical pathology specimens and found strong correlation between select sonographic patterns and both benign and malignant nodules. These studies raise the possibility of using EBUS to identify airways not ordinarily visualized by routine bronchoscopy and thereby to allow biopsy of peripheral lesions typically considered endoscopically inaccessible. To date, at least one preliminary report has documented that EBUS-guided TBBx of lesions smaller than 2 cm provided a histologic diagnosis in 54% of patients, in whom all initial routine transbronchial biopsies had proved nondiagnostic (134a).

EBUS in Guiding Therapeutic Procedures

Reports of EBUS assisting in the planning and performance of interventional bronchoscopic techniques including mechanical tumor removal and stent placement are appearing with increasing frequency (135,136). In one study, EBUS guided or changed therapy in 43% of 1,174 instances of therapeutic bronchoscopy, the majority for malignant airway compromise. Changes included adjustment of stent dimensions, termination of tumor debridement as vessels were approached, and deferment of bronchoscopic procedures in favor of surgical management (135). Studies in rabbits (137) and pediatric patients (138) have suggested a role for EBUS in the accurate measurement of subglottic diameters in pediatric disorders, which may also lead to a role in therapy.

HEMOPTYSIS

Hemoptysis is a common manifestation of numerous diseases, both pulmonary and extrapulmonary in origin (Table 2-1). Given the need for careful analysis of the airways in this setting, not surprisingly hemoptysis represents the ideal subject for evaluating the individual and combined roles of bronchoscopy and CT. Traditionally, management has been guided by the quantity of bleeding; massive hemoptysis usually is defined as 600 mL per 24 hours, reflecting the observation that oxygen transfer is impaired when approximately 400 mL of blood fills the alveolar space (139). Bleeding may originate from several sources within the lungs, including the bronchial and pulmonary arteries as well as the pulmonary capillary bed. In 90% of cases, massive hemoptysis originates from high-pressure bronchial arteries; however, as noted by Coreder, this accounts for only 1.5% of all patients presenting with hemoptysis (139a,139b).

Management of patients with massive hemoptysis remains controversial, especially regarding the indications and timing of surgery. Dividing patients into three categories, based on whether or not immediate surgery, delayed surgery, or no surgery was performed in a retrospective study of 43 patients presenting with massive hemoptysis, Jougon et al. (140) reported that mortality was highest in the immediate surgical group (19%) and those treated by only nonsurgical means (26%). In distinction, no deaths were reported in the group in which surgery was delayed following nonsurgical interventions, including four of five patients treated by percutaneous bronchial arterial embolization.

The role of CT in assessing patients with hemoptysis is controversial (141) despite the fact that from the outset nearly all studies evaluating the role of HRCT in patients with hemoptysis have reported excellent results (Fig. 2-26) (14,16,142–145). In particular, CT has proved of value in establishing the etiology in patients in whom no prior diagnosis could be established by fiberoptic bronchoscopy, and in particular in patients with radiographically occult peripheral cancers and bronchiectasis. Millar et al. (142), for example, found that CT provided a diagnosis in 20 of 50 patients (40%) with otherwise unexplained hemoptysis. Set et al. (16) in a comparison of the utility of FB and HRCT in 91 patients found that CT detected all 27 tumors seen bronchoscopically as well as an additional 7, 5 of which were beyond bronchoscopic range. Similarly, McGuinness et al. (14), in a prospective study of 57 consecutive patients presenting with hemoptysis who were evaluated with both CT and FB, found that CT identified all cancers. Furthermore, the overall diagnostic yield of bronchoscopy was documented to be less than that of CT (47% versus 61%, respectively).

Although most patients, especially those with recurrent hemoptysis, are currently evaluated with some combination of CT and bronchoscopy, the sequence in which these studies are performed remains especially controversial

(146–148). Tak et al. (148), for example, in a recent study of 50 patients presenting with hemoptysis and a normal or nonlocalizing radiograph, were able to establish a definitive diagnosis in 17 (34%) patients: Of these, the etiology was established by HRCT in 30% of cases, whereas bronchoscopy proved diagnostic in only 10%. Importantly, CT identified all patients with focal airway pathology established by FB. These findings led these investigators to conclude that CT should be performed as the initial test in patients presenting with hemoptysis. Others disagree (149). Lenner et al. (146), for example, in a recent review of the diagnosis and management of patients presenting with hemoptysis concluded that following an initial chest radiograph, bronchoscopy should remain the next step in the diagnostic algorithm. However, the investigators acknowledged that the overall diagnostic accuracy of CT exceeds that of bronchoscopy and that a preliminary CT might be of value by directing the bronchoscopist to areas of abnormality for the purposes of both diagnosis and staging. Recently, a role for CT before bronchoscopy has even been suggested for patients presenting with massive hemoptysis (141). In their study of 80 patients with massive hemoptysis who were admitted to an intensive care unit, Revel et al. (141) showed that CT proved more efficient than bronchoscopy by identifying the source of bleeding in 77% versus 8% of cases but comparable in identifying site of bleeding (70% versus 73%).

It should be noted that the role of bronchoscopy in the evaluation of patients with hemoptysis is in itself controversial. This is especially true for establishing a diagnosis of lung cancer. Although bronchoscopy is of proved efficacy in evaluating patients with central endobronchial disease, its overall diagnostic accuracy in patients presenting with hemoptysis in most reported series is surprisingly low; this is especially true in patients presenting with normal or nonlocalizing radiographs (150–153). Poe et al. (154), in a classic study of 196 patients with normal or nonlocalizing chest radiographs, found that in only 33 cases (17%) were specific causes established bronchoscopically. Similarly, Sharma et al. (153) reported normal FB examinations in 81% of 53 patients with hemoptysis. Although the site of bleeding was localized in five patients, no specific diagnoses were made, and carcinoma was not detected in any patient during the procedure or at follow-up.

The value of bronchoscopy for establishing a diagnosis of lung cancer in patients presenting with hemoptysis and normal or nonlocalizing chest radiographs, in particular, is disputed. To date, most studies have concluded that there is a low incidence of bronchogenic carcinoma in patients presenting with normal or nonlocalizing chest radiographs with or without normal sputum results (150,152,153, 155,156). Adelman et al. (157), in an attempt to determine the clinical significance of a negative bronchoscopic exam-

TABLE 2-1
CONDITIONS ASSOCIATED WITH HEMOPTYSIS

COMMON	UNCOMMON	RARE
Neoplasia Bronchogenic carcinoma, carcinoid tumors	Alveolar hemorrhage syndromes Goodpasture syndrome	Cardiac disease (mitral stenosis/heart failure)
Acute infection Active tuberculosis Bacterial and fungal pneumonia Lung abscess	Vasculitis (Wegener's granulomatosis)	Arteriovenous malformations
	Broncholithiasis	Hematologic disorders
	Foreign body aspiration	
Chronic airway infection and inflammation Bronchitis		
Bronchiectasis Cystic fibrosis Mycetomas in preexisting cavities		
Trauma		
Pulmonary infarction		
Iatrogenic		
Lung biopsy (transbronchial/percutaneous)		
Anticoagulation		
Pulmonary artery catheterization		
Sarcoidosis		
Cryptogenic		

ination in patients at risk for lung cancer, reviewed the clinical outcome over a 3-year period of 67 patients with cryptogenic hemoptysis after nondiagnostic bronchoscopy. Although 85% of these patients remained well, nine died of nonpulmonary conditions; only one patient was subsequently diagnosed with lung cancer 20 months after bronchoscopy, without recurrence of hemoptysis. These results suggest a tenuous relationship between hemoptysis and early carcinoma. More recently, in an assessment of the cost-effectiveness of thoracic CT and bronchoscopy in patients referred for evaluation of hemoptysis, Law et al. (147) evaluated 56 patients of whom 39 had CT examinations and 42 were evaluated by FOB (with the others excluded for a variety of reasons, including obvious diagnoses by history and physical findings, poor patient condition, and lack of patient compliance) and found that in none of these patients did either procedure result in a diagnosis of lung cancer (147). Furthermore, in comparing the incidence of carcinoma before and after 1992, a time when combined bronchoscopy and CT were widely used, the incidence of lung cancer was noted to decrease, leading these investigators to conclude that both bronchoscopy and CT are overused.

These findings are contradicted by another recent retrospective study of the long-term outcome of patients with hemoptysis of unknown etiology (158). Of a retrospective evaluation of 135 patients with hemoptysis of unknown origin who were initially evaluated with both chest radiography and bronchoscopy, follow-up data were available for 115; of these, lung cancer developed in 7 (6%), all of whom were smokers over the age of 40, and proved unresectable at the time of presentation. Although these findings suggest a

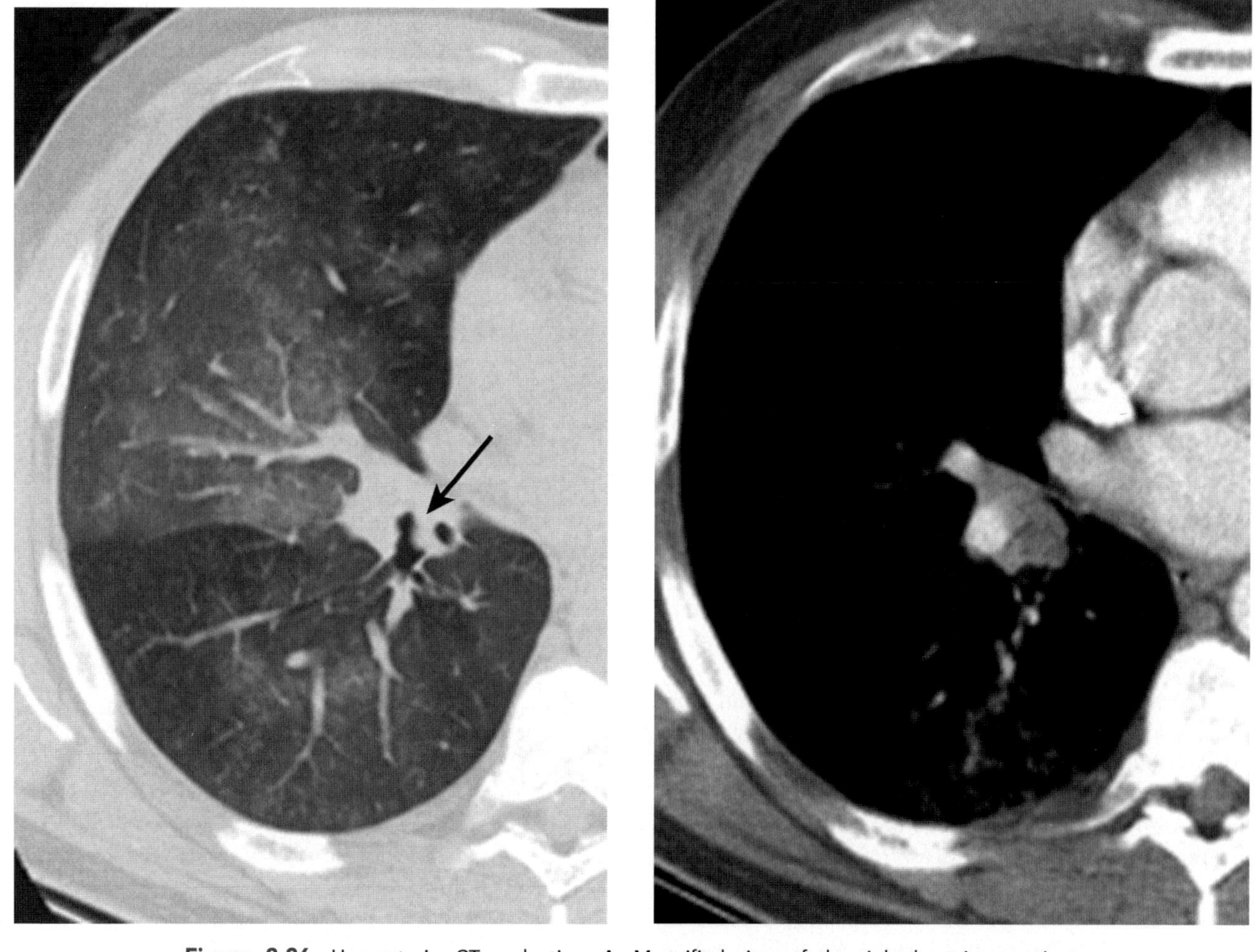

Figure 2-26 Hemoptysis. CT evaluation. **A:** Magnified view of the right lung in a patient presenting with hemoptysis shows patchy ground-glass infiltrates in both the middle and right lower lobes. Note that there is a well-defined filling defect in the right lower lobe bronchus just at the origin of the superior segmental bronchus *(arrow)*. **B:** Magnified view at a slightly different level than shown in **A**, imaged with narrow windows, confirms the presence of airway obstruction as well as focal hilar adenopathy. As shown by this case, CT reliably identifies endobronchial tumors large enough to cause hemoptysis of this degree, while additionally providing the bronchoscopist with an accurate road map complementary evaluation of the extraluminal extent of tumor. In this case, the lesion was restricted to the airways and right hilum, thereby allowing resection. Biopsy proved non–small cell lung cancer.

possible role for CT surveillance in assessing smokers with otherwise unexplained hemoptysis, this remains to be established.

Any assessment of hemoptysis requires consideration of changing patterns in disease prevalence over the past several decades (14,16,145,150,159–161) as well as consideration of marked differences depending on geographic location and demographics (148,162,163). Worldwide, TB remains the commonest cause of hemoptysis. Perhaps the most important determinant of etiologic variability is the addition of newer diagnostic techniques, including FB and high-resolution CT (14,16,142). Before 1970, for example, in addition to TB, the commonest established causes of hemoptysis included bronchiectasis (usually granulomatous in origin) and lung cancer. Following the introduction of flexible fiberoptic bronchoscopy, chronic bronchitis became the commonest cause along with bronchogenic carcinoma, with TB and bronchiectasis considered unlikely causes, clearly reflecting the widespread reports of the use of FOB predominantly in advanced industrialized countries (150,153,159). With the introduction of CT, and in particular the use of high-resolution CT techniques in the 1990s, it quickly became apparent that bronchiectasis, far from being a vanishing disease, was often the commonest cause of hemoptysis in most series (14,164). That bronchiectasis remains a common cause of hemoptysis has been confirmed by numerous recent reports as well (146). Fidan et al. (162), for example, in a recent retrospective study of 108 patients referred for evaluation, reported that although lung cancer was the commonest cause of hemoptysis, occurring in 34% of cases, bronchiectasis was the second most common cause, identified in 25%. In a similar recent report, Abal et al. (163) prospectively evaluated 52 patients with hemoptysis and found that bronchiectasis was the commonest cause, occurring in 21% of cases, followed by bronchiectasis associated with prior granulomatous disease in another 17%. These data support the need for close evaluation of the peripheral airways in all patients with otherwise unexplained hemoptysis.

In summary, in the setting of hemoptysis, CT and bronchoscopy should be considered complementary procedures. HRCT cannot replace bronchoscopy, especially in its ability to provide biopsy specimens for histologic or cytologic examination or emergent control of bleeding. FB may be more specific in bilateral disease, for example, in patients with tuberculosis, bronchiectasis, or aspergillomas. In turn, bronchoscopy is limited in detecting peribronchial abnormalities, as well as in diagnosing parenchymal disease, especially bronchiectasis. Given these considerations, in our experience CT is generally obtained before bronchoscopy for the following reasons: (a) In patients with normal or nonlocalizing chest radiographs, CT is valuable in detecting otherwise occult tumors, including both subtle endobronchial lesions and occult peripheral lung tumors. CT is especially valuable in patients with peripheral tumors by providing a road map to lesions beyond the limit of bronchoscopic visualization. (b) In cases in which TBNA may be of value, CT may play an indispensable role by assisting in the selection of optimal biopsy sites. (c) Similarly, in patients in whom therapeutic intervention may be indicated, CT can assist in the selection of appropriate candidates and in the optimization of technique. (d) Finally, CT is also indispensable for diagnosing bronchiectasis as well as other causes of diffuse lung disease associated with hemoptysis, including sarcoidosis, for example. In the appropriate clinical setting, this may obviate bronchoscopy altogether.

BRONCHOSCOPY: FUTURE DIRECTIONS

The feasibility of the adaption of new technologies such as optical coherence tomography (OCT) and confocal microendoscopy to bronchoscopy is currently under investigation, particularly in the area of early detection of lung cancer (165). OCT uses infrared light to detect tissue microstructure (166). It can penetrate as deep as 2 mm into *in vitro* pig airways, with a spatial resolution of 10 μm (167). Yang et al. (167) found that OCT could distinguish structures such as epithelium, mucosa, cartilage, and glands in *in vitro* human airways. Good correlation with OCT images and histopathology was also demonstrated. However, although technically feasible, such techniques remain to be tested for clinical applicability and utility in humans.

REFERENCES

1. Chan AL, et al. Advances in the management of endobronchial lung malignancies. *Curr Opin Pulm Med* 2003;9:301–308.

1a. Ernst A, Feller-Kopman D, Becker HD, et al. Central airway obstruction. *Am J Respir Crit Care Med* 2004;169:1278–1297.

2. Naidich DP, Harkin TJ. Airways and lung: correlation of CT with fiberoptic bronchoscopy. *Radiology* 1995;197:1–12.

3. Killian G. Uber direkte Bronchoskopie. *Munch Med Wochenschr* 1898;27: 844–847.

4. Wood RE. Clinical applications of ultrathin flexible bronchoscopes. *Pediatr Pulmonol* 1985;1:244–248.

4a. Kosucu P, Ahmetoglu A, Koramaz I, et al. Low-dose MDCT and virtual bronchoscopy in pediatric patients with foreign body aspiration. *AJR* 2004;183;1771–1777.

5. Fan LL, Sparks LM, Dulinski JP. Applications of an ultrathin flexible bronchoscope for neonatal and pediatric airway problems. *Chest* 1986;89: 673–676.

6. Monrigal JP, Granry JC. Excision of bronchogenic cysts in children using an ultrathin fibreoptic bronchoscope. *Can J Anaesth* 1996;43:694–696.

7. Hasegawa S, et al. Development of an ultrathin fiberscope with a built-in channel for bronchoscopy in infants. *Chest* 1996;110:1543–1546.

8. Schuurmans MM, et al. Use of an ultrathin bronchoscope in the assessment of central airway obstruction. *Chest* 2003;124:735–739.

9. Kikawada M, et al. Peripheral airway findings in chronic obstructive pulmonary disease using an ultrathin bronchoscope. *Eur Respir J* 2000;15:105–108.

10. Rooney CP, Wolf K, McLennan G. Ultrathin bronchoscopy as an adjunct to standard bronchoscopy in the diagnosis of peripheral lung lesions: a preliminary report. *Respiration* 2002;69:63–68.

11. Mayr B, et al. Comparison of CT with MR imaging of endobronchial tumors. *J Comput Assist Tomogr* 1987;11:43–48.

12. Davis AL, Salzman SH, eds. Bronchiectasis. In: Cherniack NS, ed. *Chronic obstructive pulmonary disease.* Philadelphia: WB Saunders, 1991:316–338.

13. Henschke CI, Davis SD, Auh PR. Detection of bronchial abnormalities: comparison of CT and bronchoscopy. *J Comput Assist Tomogr* 1987;11: 432–435.

14. McGuinness G, Beacher JR, Harkin TJ. Hemoptysis: prospective high-resolution CT/bronchoscopic correlation. *Chest* 1994;105:1155–1162.

15. Naidich SP, et al. Comparison of CT and fiberoptic bronchoscopy in the evaluation of bronchial disease. *AJR Am J Roentgenol* 1987;148:1–7.

16. Set PAK, et al. Hemoptysis: comparative study of the role of CT and fiberoptic bronchoscopy. *Radiology* 1993;189:677–680.
17. Usuda K, et al. Relation between bronchoscopic findings and tumor size of roentgenographically occult bronchogenic squamous cell carcinoma. *J Thorac Cardiovasc Surg* 1993;106:1098–1103.
18. Henschke CI, Naidich DP, Yankelevitz DF. Early lung cancer action project: initial findings on repeat screenings. *Cancer* 2001;1:1533–159.
19. Henschke CI, Yankelevitz DF, McCauley DI. Early lung cancer action project: overall design and findings from baseline screenings. *Lancet* 1999;354:99–105.
20. Swensen SJ, et al. Lung cancer screening with CT: Mayo Clinic experience. *Radiology* 2003;226:756–761.
21. Conces DJ, Tarver RD, Vix VA. Broncholithiasis: CT features in 15 patients. *AJR Am J Roentgenol* 1991;157:249–253.
22. Cosio BG, et al. Endobronchial hamartoma. *Chest* 2002;122:202–205.
23. Wang KP, et al. Flexible transbronchial needle aspiration for staging of bronchogenic carcinoma. *Chest* 1983;84:571–576.
24. Wang KP, Terry PB. Transbronchial needle aspiration in the diagnosis and staging of bronchogenic carcinoma. *Rev Respir Dis* 1983;127:344–347.
25. Wang K-P. Staging of bronchogenic carcinoma by bronchoscopy. *Chest* 1994;106:588–593.
26. Harrow EM, Oldenburg FA. Transbronchial needle aspiration in clinical practice: a five-year experience. *Chest* 1985;96:1268–1272.
27. Mehta AC, et al. Transbronchial needle aspiration for histology specimens. *Chest* 1989;96:1228–1232.
28. Schenk DA, Bower JH, Bryan CL. Transbronchial needle aspiration staging of bronchogenic carcinoma. *Am Rev Respir Dis* 1986;134:146–148.
29. Schenk DA, Strollo PJ, Pickard JS. Utility of the Wang 18-gauge transbronchial histology needle in the staging of bronchogenic carcinoma. *Chest* 1989;96:272–274.
30. Trisolini R, et al. The value of flexible transbronchial needle aspiration in the diagnosis of stage I sarcoidosis. *Chest* 2003;124:2126–2130.
31. Sharafkhaneh A, et al. Yield of transbronchial needle aspiration in diagnosis of mediastinal lesions. *Chest* 2003;124:2131–2135.
32. Hermens FHW, et al. Diagnostic yield of transbronchial histology needle aspiration in patients with mediastinal lymph node enlargement. *Respiration* 2003;70:631–635.
33. Khoo KL, et al. Transbronchial needle aspiration: initial experience in routine diagnostic bronchoscopy. *Respir Med* 2003;97:1200–1204.
34. Cetinkaya E, et al. Diagnostic value of transbronchial needle aspiration by Wang 22-gauge cytology needle in intrathoracic lymphadenopathy. *Chest* 2004;125:527–531.
35. Harkin TJ, Wang K-P. Bronchoscopic needle aspiration of mediastinal and hilar lymph nodes. *J Bronchol* 1997;4:238–249.
36. Cropp AJ, DiMarco AF, Lankerani M. False-positive transbronchial needle aspiration in bronchogenic carcinoma. *Chest* 1984;85:696–697.
37. Harrow EM, et al. The utility of transbronchial needle aspiration in the staging of bronchogenic carcinoma. *Am J Respir Crit Care Med* 2000;161: 601–607.
38. Morales CF, et al. Flexible transbronchial needle aspiration in the diagnosis of sarcoidosis. *Chest* 1994;106:709–711.
39. Harkin TJ, Ciotoli C, Addrizzo-Harris DJ, et al. Transbronchial needle aspiration (TBNA) in patients infected with HIV. *Am J Respir Crit Care Med* 1998;157:1913–1918.
40. Pastore SM, et al. Intrathoracic adenopathy associated with pulmonary tuberculosis in patients with human immunodeficiency virus infection. *Chest* 1993;103:1433–1437.
41. Bilaceroglu S, et al. Transbronchial needle aspiration in diagnosing intrathoracic tuberculous lymphadenitis. *Chest* 2004;26:259–67.
42. Prakash UBS, Offord KP, Stubbs SE. Bronchoscopy in North America: the ACCP survey. *Chest* 1991;100:1668–1675.
43. Wang KP. Staging of bronchogenic carcinoma by bronchoscopy. *Chest* 1994;106:588–593.
44. Ko JP, et al. CT depiction of regional nodal stations for lung cancer staging. *AJR Am J Roentgenol* 2000;174:775–782.
45. Rong F, Cui B. CT scan directed transbronchial needle aspiration biopsy for mediastinal nodes. *Chest* 1998;114:36–39.
46. Goldberg SN, et al. Mediastinal lymph node biopsy: diagnostic yield of transbronchial mediastinal lymph node biopsy with CT fluoroscopic guidance—initial experience. *Radiology* 2000;216:764–767.
47. White CS, et al. Transbronchial needle aspiration—Guidance with CT fluoroscopy. *Chest* 2000;118:1630–1638.
48. Fleiter T, et al. Comparison of real-time virtual and fiberoptic bronchoscopy in patients with bronchial carcinoma: opportunities and limitations. *Am J Roentgenol* 1997;169:1591–1595.
49. Haponik EF, Aquino SL, Vining DJ. Virtual bronchoscopy. *Clin Chest Med* 1999;20:201–217.
50. McAdams HP, Goodman PC, Kussin P. Virtual bronchoscopy for directing transbronchial needle aspiration of hilar and mediastinal lymph nodes: a pilot study. *AJR Am J Roentgenol* 1998;170:1361–1364.
51. Crawford SW, Colt HG. Virtual reality and written assessments are of potential value to determine knowledge and skill in flexible bronchoscopy. *Respiration* 2003;71:269–275.
52. Moorthy K, et al. Evaluation of virtual reality bronchoscopy as a learning and assessment tool. *Respiration* 2003;70:195–199.
53. Hopper KD, et al. Transbronchial biopsy with virtual CT bronchoscopy and nodal highlighting. *Radiology* 2001;221:531–536.
54. Bricault I, Ferretti G, Cinquin P. Registration of real and CT-derived virtual bronchoscopic images to assist transbronchial biopsy. *IEEE Trans Med Imaging* 1998;17:703–714.
55. Sherbondy AJ, et al. Virtual bronchoscopic approach for combining 3-D CT and endoscopic video. In: Medical imaging 2000: physiology and function from multidimensional images. *Proc SPIE* 2000;3978:104–116.
56. Schwarz Y, et al. Electromagnetic navigation during flexible bronchoscopy. *Respiration* 2003;70:516–522.
57. Mori K, et al. Tracking of a bronchoscope using epipolar geometry analysis and intensity-based image registration of real and virtual endoscopic images. *Med Image Analysis* 2002;6:321–336.
58. Tan BB, et al. The solitary pulmonary nodule. *Chest* 2003;123:89S–96S.
59. Naidich DP, et al. Solitary pulmonary nodules: CT–bronchoscopic correlation. *Chest* 1988;93:595–598.
60. Gaeta M, et al. Bronchus sign on CT in peripheral carcinoma of the lung: value in predicting results of transbronchial biopsy. *AJR Am J Roentgenol* 1991;157:1181–1185.
61. Gaeta M, et al. Carcinomatous solitary pulmonary nodules: evaluation of the tumor-bronchi relationship with thin-section CT. *Radiology* 1993;187: 535–539.
62. Bandoh S, et al. Diagnostic accuracy and safety of flexible bronchoscopy with multiplanar reconstruction images and ultrafast Papanicolaou stain—evaluating solitary pulmonary nodules. *Chest* 2003;124: 1985–1992.
63. Mori K, et al. Diagnosis of peripheral lung cancer in cases of tumors 2 cm or less in size. *Chest* 1989;95:304–308.
64. Ono R, Loke J, Ikeda S. Bronchofiberscopy with curette biopsy and bronchography in the evaluation of peripheral lung lesions. *Chest* 1981;79:162–166.
65. Minami H, et al. Interbronchoscopist variability in the diagnosis of lung cancer by flexible bronchoscopy. *Chest* 1994;105:1658–1662.
66. Fletcher EC, Levin DC. Flexible fiberoptic bronchoscopy and fluoroscopically guided transbronchial biopsy in the management of solitary pulmonary nodules. *West J Med* 1982;136:477–483.
67. Baaklini WA, et al. Diagnostic yield of fiberoptic bronchoscopy in evaluating solitary pulmonary nodules. *Chest* 2000;117:1049–1054.
68. Westcott JL. Diagnostic approach to solitary pulmonary nodule. *J Bronchol* 1996;3:316–323.
69. Schreiber G, McCrory DC. Performance characteristics of different modalities for diagnosis of suspected lung cancer—summary of published evidence. *Chest* 2003;123:115S–128S.
70. Herth FJF, Ernst A, Becker HD. Endobronchial ultrasound-guided transbronchial lung biopsy in solitary pulmonary nodules and peripheral lesions. *Eur Respir J* 2002;20:972–974.
71. Turner JF. Endobronchial ultrasound and peripheral pulmonary lesions—localization and histopathologic correlates using a miniature probe and the flexible bronchoscope. *Chest* 2002;122:1874–1875.
72. Stringfield JT, et al. The effect of tumor size and location on diagnosis by fiberoptic bronchoscopy. *Chest* 1977;72:474–476.
73. Cortese DA, McDougall JC. Biopsy and brushing of peripheral lung cancer with fluoroscopic guidance. *Chest* 1979;75:141–145.
74. Radke JR, et al. Diagnostic accuracy in peripheral lung lesions. Factors predicting success with flexible fiberoptic bronchoscopy. *Chest* 1979;76: 176–179.
75. Lai RS, et al. Diagnostic value of transbronchial lung biopsy under fluoroscopic guidance in solitary pulmonary nodule in an endemic area of tuberculosis. *Respir Med* 1996;90:139–143.
76. Chechani V. Bronchoscopic diagnosis of solitary pulmonary nodules and lung masses in the absence of endobronchial abnormality. *Chest* 1996;109: 620–625.
77. Bilaceroglu S, et al. CT bronchus sign-guided bronchoscopic multiple diagnostic: procedures in carcinomatous solitary pulmonary nodules and masses. *Respiration* 1998;65:49–55.
78. Asano F, et al. CT-guided transbronchial diagnosis using ultrathin bronchoscope for small peripheral pulmonary lesions (English abstract). *Nihon Kokyuki Gakkai Zasshi* 2002;40:11–16.
79. Asano F, et al. Case report. Transbronchial diagnosis of a pulmonary peripheral small lesion using and ultrathin bronchoscope with virtual bronchoscopic navigation. *J Bronchosc* 2002;9:108–111.
80. Moriya H, Hashimoto N, Honjo H. Visibility of peripheral bronchi in virtual bronchscopy with 0.5 mm collimation multidetector CT [in Japanese]. *Jpn J Clin Radiol* 2001;46:1–7.
81. Higgins WE, et al. Progress towards virtual-bronchoscopic guidance of peripheral nodule biopsy. *Am J Respir Crit Care Med* 2003;167:A535.
82. Suda Y, et al. Practical methodology for bronchial route analysis using virtual bronchoscopy. *Am J Respir Crit Care Med* 2003;167:A527.
83. Shinagawa N, et al. CT-guided transbronchial biopsy using an ultrathin bronchoscope with virtual bronchoscopic guidance. *Chest* 2004;125: 1138–1143.
83a. Onodera Y, Omatsu T, Takeuchi S, et al. Enhanced virtual bronchoscopy using the pulmonary artery: improvement in route mapping for ultraselective transbronchial lung biopsy. *AJR Am J Roentgenol* 2004;183:1103–1110.

84. Shure D. Transbronchial biopsy and needle aspiration. *Chest* 1989;95: 1130–1138.
85. Glazer HS, Anderson DJ, Sagel SS. Bronchial impaction in lobar collapse: CT demonstration and pathologic correlation. *AJR Am J Roentgenol* 1989;153:485–488.
86. Woodring JH, Reed JC. Radiographic manifestations of lobar atelectasis. *J Thorac Imaging* 1996;11:109–144.
87. Cortese DA, Edell ES, Kinsey JH. Photodynamic therapy for early stage squamous cell carcinoma of the lung. *Mayo Clin Proc* 1997;72:595–602.
88. Litle VR, et al. Photodynamic therapy for endobronchial metastases from nonbronchogenic primaries. *Ann Thorac Surg* 2003;76:370–375.
89. Moghissi K, Dixon K. Is bronchoscopic photodynamic therapy a therapeutic option in lung cancer? *Eur Respir J* 2003;22:535–541.
90. Cortese DA, Kinsey JH. Endoscopic management of lung cancer with hematoporphyrin. *Mayo Clin Proc* 1982;57:543–547.
91. Dougherty TJ, Gomer CJ, Henderson BW. Photodynamic therapy. *J Natl Cancer Inst* 1998;90:889–905.
92. Sheski FD, Mathur PN. Cryotherapy, electrocautery, and brachytherapy. *Clin Chest Med* 1999;20:123–138.
93. Lee P, Kupeli E, Mehta AC. Therapeutic bronchoscopy in lung cancer—laser therapy, electrocautery, brachytherapy stents, and photodynamic therapy. *Clin Chest Med* 2002;23:241–256.
94. Morice RC, et al. Endobronchial argon plasma coagulation for treatment of hemoptysis and neoplastic airway obstruction. *Chest* 2001;119:781–787.
95. Bolliger CT. Airway stents. *Semin Respir Crit Care Med* 1997;18:563–570.
96. Mehta AC, Dasgupta A. Airway stents. *Clin Chest Med* 1999;20:139.
97. Wood DE, et al. Airway stenting for malignant and benign tracheobronchial stenosis. *Ann Thorac Surg* 2003;76:167–172.
98. Higgins R, et al. Airway stenoses after lung transplantation—management with expanding metal stents. *J Heart Lung Transplant* 1994;13: 774–778.
99. Ernst A, et al. Central airway obstruction. State-of-the-art. *Am J Respir Crit Care Med* 2004;169:1278–1297.
100. Miyazawa T, et al. Stenting at the flow-limiting segment in tracheobronchial stenosis due to lung cancer. *Am J Respir Crit Care Med* 2004; 169:1096–1102.
101. Ferretti GR, et al. Follow-up after stent insertion in the tracheobronchial tree: role of helical computed tomography in comparison with fiberoptic bronchoscopy. *Eur Radiol* 2003;13:1172–1178.
102. Ferretti G, et al. Benign noninflammatory bronchial stenosis: treatment with balloon dilatation. *Radiology* 1995;196:831–834.
103. Qu J, MacAulay C, Lam S. Laser induced fluorescence spectroscopy at endoscopy: tissue optics, Monte Carlo modeling and in vivo measurements. *Opt Eng* 1995;34:3334–3343.
104. Kato H, Cortese DA. Early detection of lung cancer by means of hematoporphyrin derivative fluorescence and laser photoradiation. *Clin Chest Med* 1985;6:237–253.
105. Lam S, Macaulay C, Leriche JC. Early localization of bronchogenic carcinoma. *Diag Ther Endosc* 1994;1:75–78.
106. Lam S, et al. Localization of bronchial intraepithelial neoplastic lesions by fluorescence bronchoscopy. *Chest* 1998;113:696–702.
107. Kurie JM, et al. Autofluorescence bronchoscopy in the detection of squamous metaplasia and dysplasia in current and former smokers. *J Natl Cancer Inst* 1998;90:991–995.
108. Kennedy TC, Lam S, Hirsch FR. Review of recent advances in fluorescence bronchoscopy in early localization of central airway lung cancer. *Oncologist* 2001;6:257–262.
109. Venmans BJ, van der Linden JC, van Boxem J. Early detection of preinvasive lesions in high risk patients. A comparison of conventional fiberoptic and fluorescence bronchoscopy. *J Bronchol* 1998;5:280–283.
110. Hirsch FR, et al. Fluorescence versus white-light bronchoscopy for detection of preneoplastic lesions: a randomized study. *J Natl Cancer Inst* 2001; 93:1385–1391.
111. Herth FJF, Ernst A, Becker HD. Autofluorescence bronchoscopy—a comparison of two systems (LIFE and D-light). *Respiration* 2003;70: 395–398.
112. Shibuya K, et al. Fluorescence bronchoscopy in the detection of preinvasive bronchial lesions in patients with sputum cytology suspicious or positive for malignancy. *Lung Cancer* 2001;32:19–25.
113. van Rens MT, et al. The clinical value of lung imaging fluorescence endoscopy for detecting synchronous lung cancer. *Lung Cancer* 2001;32:13–18.
114. Weigel TL, et al. Fluorescence bronchoscopic surveillance after curative surgical resection for non-small-cell lung cancer. *Ann Surg Oncol* 2000; 7:176–180.
114a. Lam S, MacAuley C, LeRiche JC, et al. Key issues in lung cancer chemoprevention trials of new agents. *Recent Results Cancer Res* 2003;163:182–195.
115. Helfritzsch H, et al. Differentiation of positive autofluorescence bronchoscopy findings by comparative genomic hybridization. *Oncol Rep* 2002;9:697–701.
116. Martin B, et al. Expression of p53 in preneoplastic and early neoplastic bronchial lesions. *Oncol Rep* 2002;9:223–229.
117. Becker H, Herth F. Endobronchial ultrasound of the airways and the mediastinum. In: Bolliger CT, Mathur P, eds. *Interventional bronchoscopy. Progress in respiratory research*, vol 30. Basel: Karger, 2000:80–93.
118. Hurther TH, Hanrath P. Endobronchial sonography: feasibility and preliminary results. *Thorax* 1992;47:565–567.
119. Goldberg BB, Steiner RM, Liu JB. US-assisted bronchoscopy with use of miniature transducer-containing catheters. *Radiology* 1994;190:233–237.
120. Baba M, et al. Correlation between endobronchial ultrasonography (EBUS) images and histologic findings in normal and tumor-invaded bronchial wall. *Lung Cancer* 2002;35:65–71.
121. Nishimura Y, et al. Bronchoscopic ultrasonography in the diagnosis of tracheobronchial invasion of esophageal cancer. *J Ultrasound Med* 2002; 21:49–58.
122. Takahashi H, et al. A prospective evaluation of transbronchial ultrasonography for assessment of depth of invasion in early bronchogenic squamous cell carcinoma. *Lung Cancer* 2003;42:43–49.
123. Herth F, et al. Endobronchial ultrasound reliably differentiates between airway infiltration and compression by tumor. *Chest* 2003;123: 458–462.
124. Tanaka F, et al. Evaluation of tracheo-bronchial wall invasion using transbronchial ultrasonography (EBUS). *Eur J Cardio Thorac Surg* 2000;17: 570–574.
125. Miyazu Y, et al. Endobronchial ultrasonography in the diagnosis and treatment of relapsing polychondritis with tracheobronchial malacia. *Chest* 2003;124:2393–2395.
126. Herth F, et al. Endobronchial ultrasound improves classification of suspicious lesions detected by autofluorescence bronchoscopy. *J Bronchol* 2003;10:249–252.
127. Okamoto H, et al. Endobronchial ultrasonography for mediastinal and hilar lymph node metastases of lung cancer. *Chest* 2002;121:1498–1506.
128. Becker H, Herth F. Is endobronchial ultrasound indispensable in clinical practice? Pro: endobronchial ultrasound. *J Bronchol* 2002;9:145–151.
129. Shannon JJ, et al. Endobronchial ultrasound-guided needled aspiration of mediastinal adenopathy. *Am J Respir Crit Care Med* 1996;153: 1424–1430.
130. Herth FJ, Becker HD, Ernst A. Ultrasound-guided transbronchial needle aspiration—an experience in 242 patients. *Chest* 2003;123:604–607.
131. Herth F, Beck R, Ernst A. Conventional vs. endobronchial ultrasound-guided transbronchial needle aspiration: a randomized trial. *Chest* 2004;125:322–325.
132. Ono R, Suemasu K, Matsunaka T. Bronchoscopic ultrasonography for diagnosis of lung cancer. *Jpn J Clin Oncol* 1993;23:34–40.
133. Kanoh K, et al. A case of real-time endobronchial ultrasonography-guided bronchial needle aspiration using a double-channel flexible bronchoscope. *J Bronchol* 2002;9:112–114.
133a. Yasufuku K, Chiyo M, Sekine Y, et al. Real-time endobronchial ultrasound-guided transbronchial needle aspiration of mediastinal and hilar lymph nodes. *Chest* 2004;126:122–128.
134. Kurimoto N, et al. Assessment of usefulness of endobronchial ultrasonography in determination of depth of tracheobronchial tumor invasion. *Chest* 1999;115:1500–1506.
134a. Yang MC, Liu WT, Wang CH, et al. Diagnostic value of endobronchial ultrasound-guided transbronchial lung biopsy in peripheral lung cancers. *J Formos Med Assoc* 2004;103:124–129.
135. Herth F, et al. Endobronchial ultrasound in therapeutic bronchoscopy. *Eur Respir J* 2002;20:118–121.
136. Shirakawa T, et al. A case of successful airway stent placement guided by endobronchial ultrasonography. *J Bronchol* 2004;11:45–48.
137. Giguere C, et al. Ultrasound and a new videobronchoscopic technique to measure the subglottic diameter. *J Otolaryngol* 2000;29:290–298.
138. Husein M, et al. Ultrasonography and videobronchoscopy to assess the subglottic diameter in the paediatric population: a first look. *J Otolaryngol* 2002;31:220–226.
139. Corder R. Hemoptysis. *Emerg Med Clin North Am* 2003;21:421–435.
139a. Yoon YC, Lee KS, Jeong YJ, et al. Hemoptysis: bronchial and nonbronchial systemic arteries at 16-detector row CT. *Radiology* 2005;234:292-298.
139b. Yoon W, Kim JK, Kim YH, et al. Bronchial and nonbronchial systemic artery embolization for life-threatening hemoptysis: a comprehensive review. *Radiographics* 2002;22:1395–1409.
140. Jougon J, et al. Massive hemoptysis: what place for medical and surgical treatment. *Eur J Cardio Thorac Surg* 2002;22:345–351.
141. Revel MP, et al. Can CT replace bronchoscopy in the detection of the site and cause of bleeding in patients with large or massive hemoptysis? *Am J Roentgenol* 2002;179:1217–1224.
142. Millar A, et al. The role of computed tomography (CT) in the investigation of unexplained hemoptysis. *Respir Med* 1992;86:39–44.
143. Naidich DP, et al. Hemoptysis: CT–bronchoscopic correlations in 58 cases. *Radiology* 1990;177:357–362.
144. Haponik EF, Chin R. Hemoptysis: clinicians' perspectives. *Chest* 1990;97: 469–475.
145. Hirshberg B, et al. Hemoptysis: etiology, evaluation, and outcome in a tertiary referral hospital. *Chest* 1997;112:440–444.
146. Lenner R, Schilero GJ, Lesser M. Hemoptysis: diagnosis and management. *Comp Ther* 2002;28:7–14.
147. Law GTS, et al. Cost-effectiveness of CT thorax and bronchoscopy in haemoptysis with normal CXR for exclusion of lung cancer. *Australasian Radiol* 2002;46:381–383.

148. Tak S, et al. Haemoptysis in patients with a normal chest radiograph: bronchoscopy—CT correlation. *Australasian Radiol* 1999;43:451–455.
149. Haponik F, et al. Computed chest tomography in the evaluation of hemoptysis. *Chest* 1987;91:80–85.
150. Santiago S, Tobias J, Williams AJ. A reappraisal of the causes of hemoptysis. *Arch Intern Med* 1991;151:2449–2451.
151. Peters J, McClung HC, Teague RB. Evaluation of hemoptysis in patients with a normal chest roentgenogram. *West J Med* 1984;141:624–626.
152. Jackson CV, Savage PJ, Quinn DL. Role of fiberoptic bronchoscopy in patients with hemoptysis and normal chest radiographs. *Chest* 1985;87: 142–144.
153. Sharma SK, et al. Fiberoptic bronchoscopy in patients with haemoptysis and normal chest roentgenograms. *Indian J Chest Dis Allied Sci* 1991; 33:15–18.
154. Poe RH, et al. Utility of fiberoptic bronchoscopy in patients with hemoptysis and a nonlocalizing chest roentgenogram. *Chest* 1988;92:70–75.
155. Poe RH, et al. Use of fiberoptic bronchoscopy in the diagnosis of bronchogenic carcinoma. A study in patients with idiopathic pleural effusions. *Chest* 1994;105:1663–1667.
156. Lederle FA, Nichol KL, Parenti CM. Bronchoscopy to evaluate hemoptysis in older men with nonsuspicious chest roentgenograms. *Chest* 1989;95: 1043–1047.
157. Adelman M, et al. Cryptogenic hemoptysis: clinical features, bronchoscopic findings, and natural history in 67 patients. *Ann Intern Med* 1985;102: 829–834.
158. Herth F, Ernst A, Becker HD. Long-term outcome and lung cancer incidence in patients with hemoptysis of unknown origin. *Chest* 2001;120: 1592–1594.
159. Johnson H, Reisz G. Changing spectrum of hemoptysis: underlying causes in 148 patients undergoing diagnostic flexible bronchoscopy. *Arch Intern Med* 1989;149:1666–1668.
160. DiLeo MD, Amedee RG, Butcher RB. Hemoptysis and pseudohemoptysis: the patient expectorating blood. *Ear Nose Throat* 1995;74:826–828.
161. Reisz G, et al. The causes of hemoptysis revisited: a review of the etiologies of hemoptysis between 1986 and 1995. *Mo Med* 1997;94:633–635.
162. Fidan A, et al. Hemoptysis: a retrospective analysis of 108 cases. *Respir Med* 2002;96:677–680.
163. Abal AT, Nair PC, Cherian J. Haemoptysis: aetiology, evaluation, and outcome—a prospective study in a third-world country. *Respir Med* 2001; 95:548–552.
164. Grenier P, Lenoir S, Brauner M. Computed tomographic assessment of bronchiectasis. *Semin Ultrasound CT MR* 1990;11:430–441.
165. Sutedja TG. New techniques for early detection of lung cancer. *Eur J Cardio Thorac Surg* 2003;39:57s–66s.
166. Pitrus C, et al. High resolution imaging of the upper respiratory tract with optical coherence tomography: a feasibility study. *Am J Respir Crit Care Med* 1998;157:1640–1644.
167. Yang Y, et al. Use of optical coherence tomography in delineating airway microstructure: comparison of OCT images to histopathological sections. *Phys Med Biol* 2004;49:1247–1255.
168. Naidich DP, et al. *CT and MRI of the thorax*, vol 3. Philadelphia: Lippincott, 1999.
169. Colice G, et al. Comparison of computed tomography with fiberoptic bronchoscopy in identifying endobronchial abnormalities in patients with suspected lung cancer. *Am Rev Respir Dis* 1985;131:397–400.

Trachea and Central Bronchi

3

Tracheal disease has traditionally been difficult to identify. It has been described as the radiologic blind spot in the chest (1). Recognition of tracheal disease is notoriously difficult, especially early in its course; it has been estimated that the tracheal lumen must be occluded by more than 75% before symptoms of obstruction develop, and even then patients are frequently mistaken as being asthmatic. In a minority of cases hemoptysis may lead to early diagnosis. Although a relatively rare cause of primary disease, earlier diagnosis is now often possible with the advent of routine computed tomography (CT) imaging.

For descriptive purposes this chapter first addresses focal and then diffuse tracheal abnormalities, with the recognition that this distinction may be arbitrary. A description of tracheal anatomy and normal tracheal variants is presented in Chapter 1.

FOCAL TRACHEAL DISEASE

Tracheal Trauma

Patients suffering tracheal trauma frequently fail to live long enough to be evaluated (2). In patients who do receive medical attention, blunt trauma may also result in pulmonary contusion and/or laceration, thoracic spine injuries, esophageal disruption, or multiple fractures. Extrathoracic organ injury is also frequently encountered (3). Not surprisingly, most reported series are small. Trauma may be either penetrating or, more often, blunt (Figs. 3-1 to 3-4). Although penetrating tracheal injuries typically involve the neck, blunt traumatic injuries usually involve the intrathoracic portions of the trachea and often extend to the mainstem bronchi (4). Most often the result of deceleration or so-called steering wheel injuries, proposed mechanisms of injury include compression of the airways between the sternum and thoracic spine with lateral expansion of the thorax; shearing at fixation points, especially at the carina; and elevated intratracheal pressure, especially against a closed glottis (5). These injuries result in transverse lacerations; disruption of the posterior, membranous portion of the trachea; or, less commonly, shearing of the mainstem bronchi from the carina (Figs. 3-2 and 3-3). Although the entire length of the trachea is vulnerable to injury following blunt trauma more than 80% of cases occur within 2.5 cm of the carina (2). It has been suggested that the left mainstem bronchus is less frequently disrupted, probably because of its longer course through the mediastinum, which offers some extra measure of protection. Additional causes of tracheal rupture include overdistension of endotracheal tubes (Fig. 3-4) and traumatic intubation (6).

Radiographic findings most often include pneumomediastinum and deep cervical emphysema (7). Unfortunately, neither of these signs is specific for tracheal disruption. Pneumomediastinum, for example, most commonly occurs secondary to air leaks originating in the pulmonary interstitium, the so-called Macklin effect (8). Pneumothoraces are also common, presumably the result of disruption of the mediastinal pleura. In those patients in whom the airway is partly occluded by blood clots or compression by an adjacent mediastinal hematoma, the first sign of tracheal rupture may be a persistent air leak following chest tube insertion. In more severe cases, bronchial avulsion may lead to a falling away of the involved lung from the hilum resulting from disruption of central attachments, the so-called fallen lung sign (7).

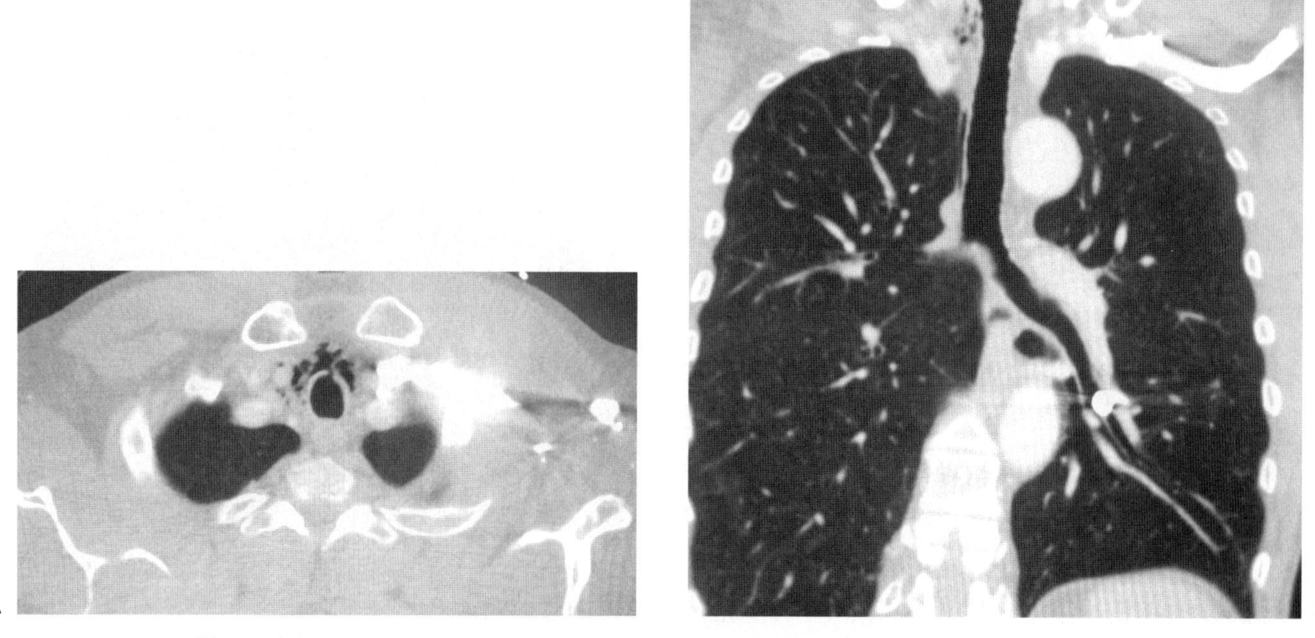

Figure 3-1 Penetrating tracheal trauma. **A:** Axial section through the trachea at the level of the clavicles shows mediastinal air associated with subtle disruption of the anterior tracheal wall following a gunshot wound to the neck. **B:** Coronal MPR shows that the bullet subsequently lodged in the distal left lower lobe bronchus. (Case courtesy of Stuart E. Mirvis, Baltimore, Maryland).

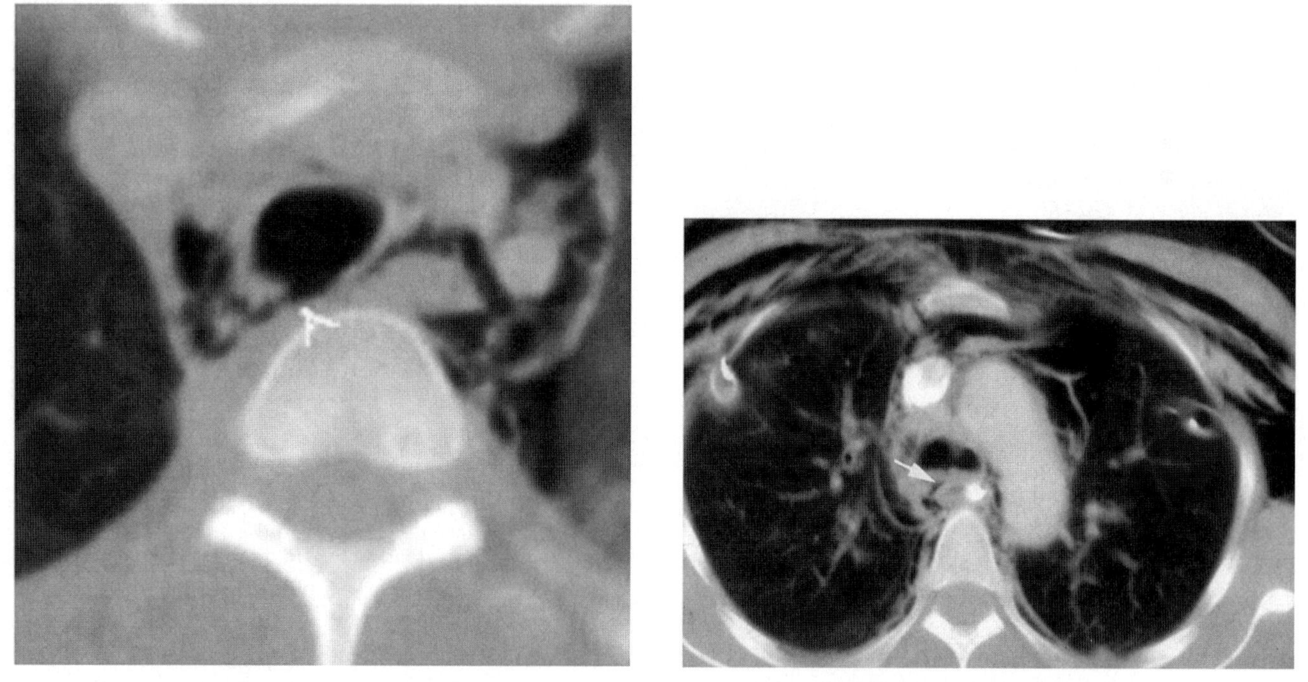

Figure 3-2 Blunt tracheal trauma. **A:** CT scan at the level of the great vessels shows a defect *(arrowhead)* in the posterior membranous trachea. Note extensive mediastinal emphysema and left upper lobe contusion. **B:** CT scan at the level of the aortic arch imaged with mediastinal windows in a different patient than shown in **A.** A defect is clearly identifiable in the membranous trachea with air tracking into the mediastinum *(arrowheads).* Note extensive mediastinal as well as subcutaneous air. A pleural tube is present on the right side. (From Chen J-D, et al. Using CT to diagnose tracheal rupture. *AJR Am J Roentgenol* 2001;176:1273–1280, with permission.)

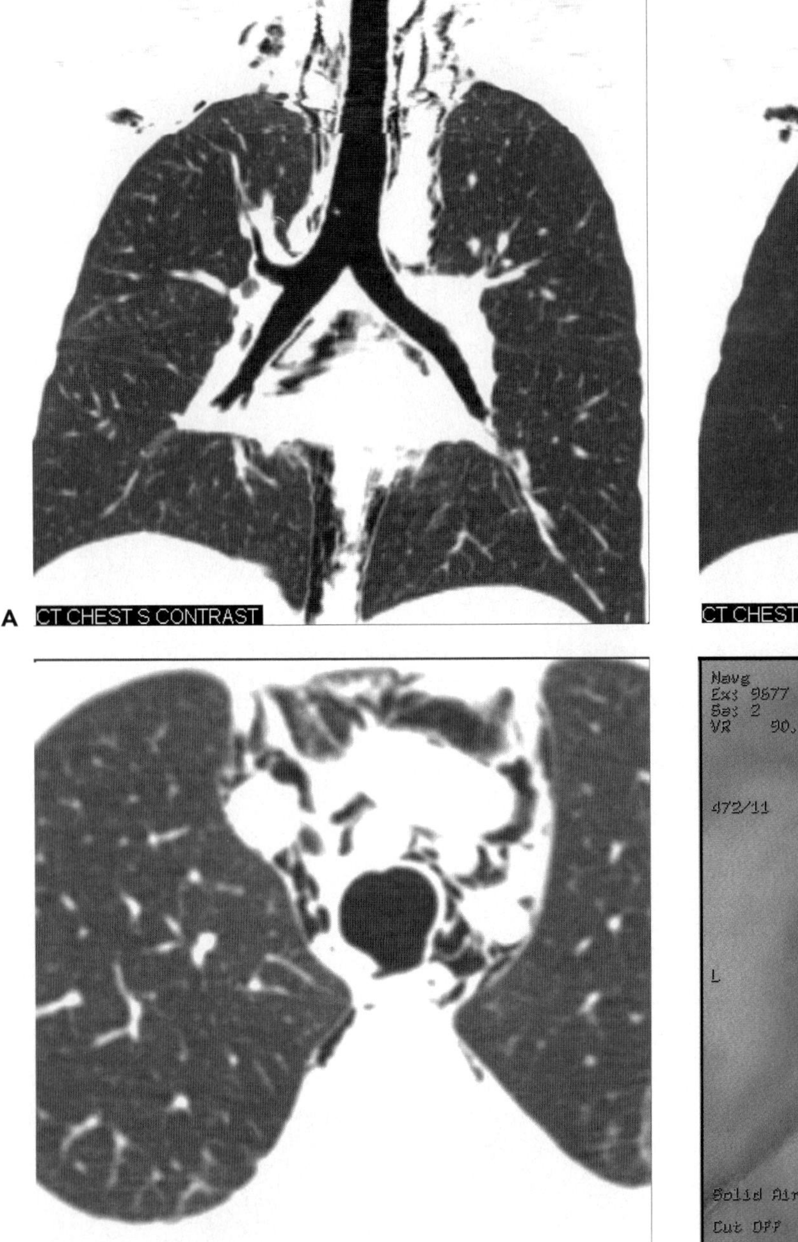

Figure 3-3 Blunt trachea trauma. Imaging techniques. **A** and **B:** Multiplanar (MPR) and minimum projection (MinIP) coronal reconstructions, respectively, through the trachea show extensive mediastinal and deep cervical emphysema. Note the absence of a pneumothorax. **C:** Axial image through the midtrachea shows a focal defect in the posterior membranous trachea with resultant extensive pneumomediastinum. **D:** Virtual bronchoscopic image pointing from within the midtrachea toward the carina shows a deep groove in the posterior membranous trachea *(arrow)* extending toward the origin of the right mainstem bronchus. Subsequent bronchoscopic evaluation confirmed the presence of a membranous tear corresponding anatomically with the virtual bronchoscopic image. (Case courtesy of James Gruden, M.D., Atlanta, Georgia.)

CT findings in patients with blunt trauma have been reported (8–12). In a recent retrospective study of 14 patients with tracheal rupture either resulting from trauma or following intubation, CT proved diagnostic in 85%, providing direct visualization of tracheal tears in 10 patients (71%). Direct signs of tracheal rupture included focal wall defects in more than 50% of patients (Figs. 3-2 and 3-3); less commonly, rupture resulted in a deformed tracheal lumen. In this same series, overdistension of the tube balloon was noted to be particularly common, occurring in five of seven intubated patients. Of particular value was the finding of herniation of the endotracheal tube balloon

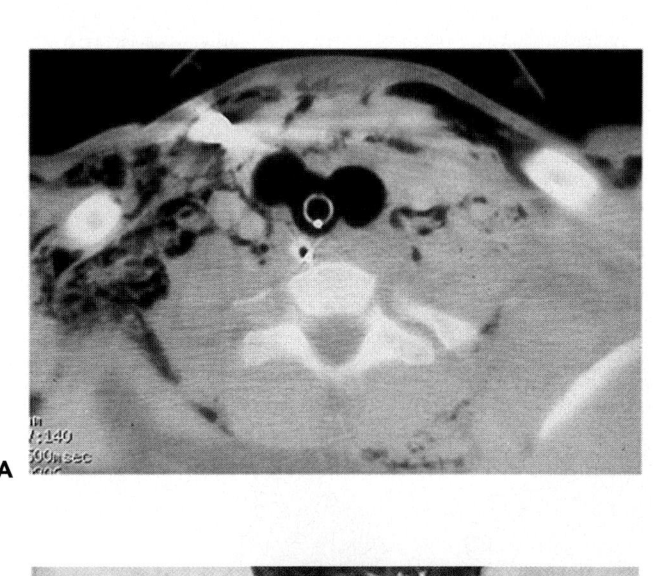

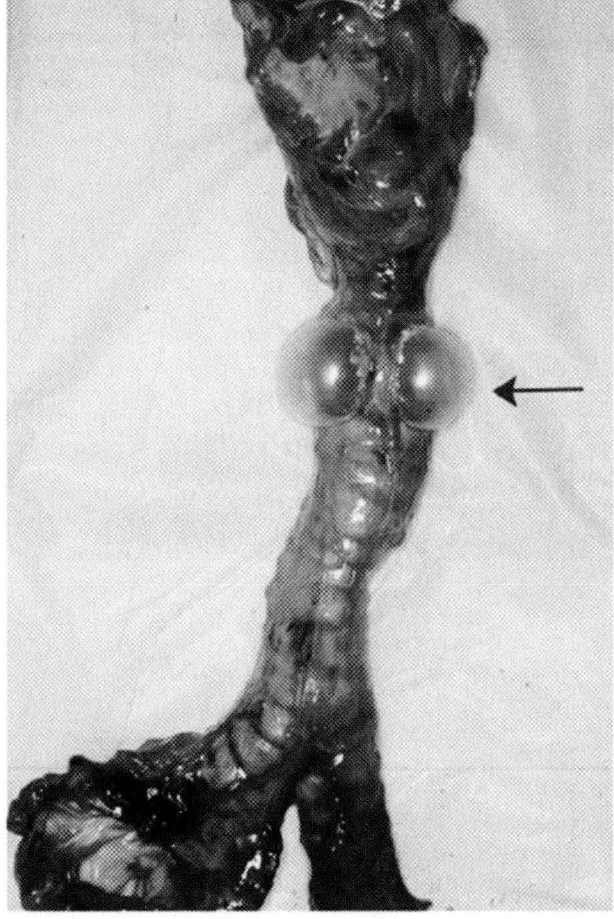

Figure 3-4 Tracheal rupture secondary to overdistention of an endotracheal tube balloon. **A:** Axial image through the lower neck shows extensive deep emphysema. Overdistension of the endotracheal tube balloon resulted in herniation of the balloon through bilateral tears in the anterolateral walls of the trachea producing a "Mickey Mouse" appearance of the balloon *(arrows)*. Note the presence of a feeding tube within the esophagus posteriorly. **B:** Photograph of an experimentally injured trachea showing herniation of the balloon through anterolateral trachea tears mimicking the appearance of the trachea shown in **A.** (From Chen J-D, et al. Using CT to diagnose tracheal rupture. *AJR Am J Roentgenol* 2001;176:1273–1280, with permission.)

outside the confines of the tracheal wall (Fig. 3-4). It should be emphasized that optimal evaluation of tracheal injuries should include use of advanced image processing, especially multiplanar reconstructions. In select cases, visualization of tracheal tears may be most easily identified with virtual bronchoscopy (Fig. 3-3).

Although imaging findings are often suggestive, definitive diagnosis and therapy require bronchoscopy in nearly all patients. Rare exceptions include patients in whom the diagnosis can be made presumptively because of direct observation or evidence of a massive air leak following chest tube placement (13). Although treatment typically involves surgical repair, conservative therapy has been advocated for individuals with postintubation membranous tracheal ruptures if these are less than 2 cm long (6,14). Late manifestations of tracheal rupture include strictures, and patients presenting with wheezing that can be potentially misdiagnosed as asthma.

Tracheal Stenosis

Benign airway strictures may be congenital or acquired. The most common cause of acquired strictures is iatrogenic injury resulting from intubation. Although previous reports have documented complications occurring in up to 10% to 15% of patients following intubation, their incidence has decreased dramatically since the introduction of high-volume/low-pressure balloons (15). In distinction, complications following tracheostomy tube insertion remain common, occurring in approximately 40% of patients. The two principal sites of stenosis following intubation or tracheostomy are at the stoma and at the level of the endotracheal or tracheostomy tube balloon (16). In both cases, strictures result from pressure necrosis, causing ischemia and subsequent scarring. Stenosis also may be the result of inflammation, with subsequent thinning and weakening of the tracheal wall (tracheomalacia) in the segment between the stoma and cuff; narrowing may also be caused by granulation tissue resulting from direct tracheal injury by the endotracheal or tracheostomy tube tip (16). Another complication is tracheal rupture. Rarely, tracheobrachiocephalic artery or tracheoesophageal fistulas may occur, the latter usually developing secondary to combined tracheal and esophageal intubation. Additional causes of tracheal stenosis include strictures resulting from infection, most often tuberculous, and following lung transplantation. After lung transplantation, complications typically occur at the level of the bronchial anastomosis and include dehiscence, necrosis, and stenosis from malacia, fibrous stricture, prominent granulation tissue formation, or a combination of these conditions (17–21).

Regardless of etiology, both CT and magnetic resonance (MR) have proved reliable methods for assessing tracheobronchial strictures (Figs. 3-5 and 3-6). In all cases, accurate evaluation requires that the precise length and degree of stenosis be assessed along with associated peritracheal or bronchial abnormalities. CT with multiplanar

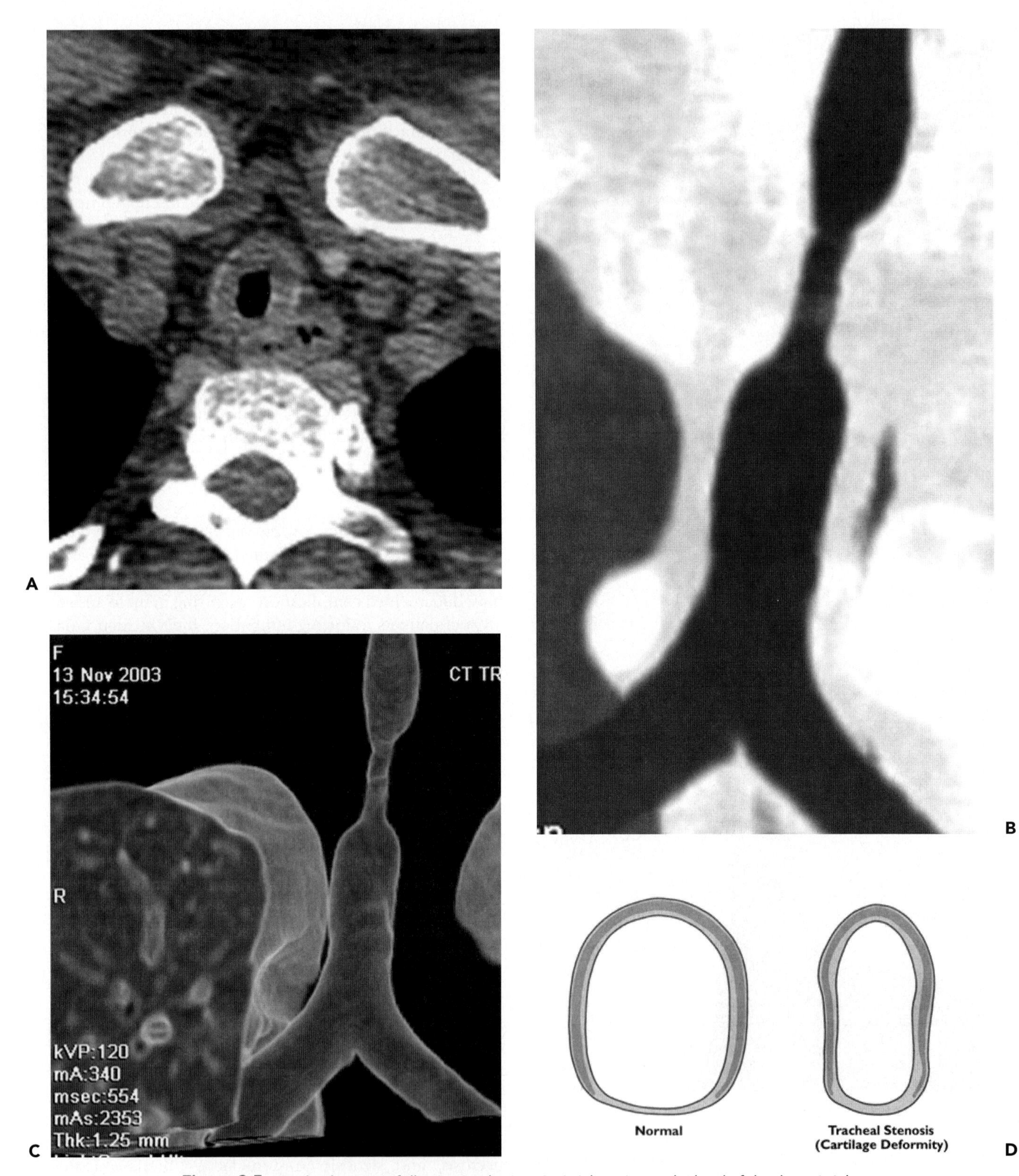

Figure 3-5 Tracheal stenosis following intubation. **A:** Axial section at the level of the thoracic inlet shows markedly increased soft tissue density internal to the tracheal cartilage causing irregular narrowing of the tracheal lumen. **B** and **C:** Multiplanar (MPR) and 3D surface rendered coronal reconstructions, respectively, through the trachea show to good advantage the true extent of the stricture, information essential for optimal surgical planning. **D:** Comparison of the appearance of tracheal stenosis caused by granulation tissue and a normal trachea. Soft tissue internal to the tracheal cartilage is irregularly thickened. (**A** to **C:** courtesy of Phillip Boiselle, M.D., Boston, Massachusetts; **D:** from Webb EM, Elicker BM, Webb WR. Using CT to diagnose nonneoplastic tracheal abnormalities: appearance of the tracheal wall. *AJR Am J Roentgenol* 2000;174:1315–1321, with permission.)

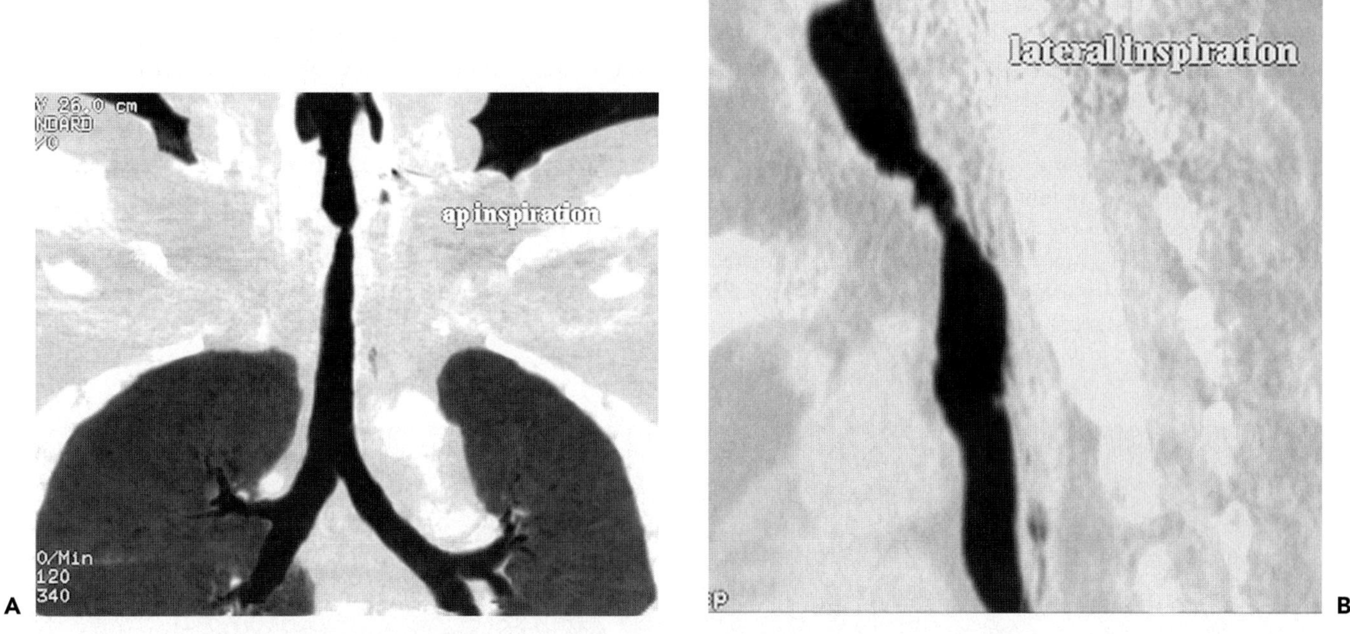

Figure 3-6 Subglottic stenosis. **A** and **B:** Coronal and sagittal multiplanar reconstructions (MPRs) through the neck and upper chest, respectively, show a focal subglottic stenosis. (Case courtesy of Phillip Boiselle, M.D., Boston, Massachusetts.)

reconstructions, in particular, has proved of value with sensitivities of greater than 90% reported (22). It should be noted that in select cases additional certainty in assessing the degree of stenoses may also be attained by use of virtual bronchoscopy (23,24).

Although endoscopic management of tracheal stenoses has been proposed, especially with the use of lasers or stents, these typically provide only temporary benefits. Primary tracheal and laryngotracheal resection and reconstruction remain the optimal methods for treating nonneoplastic stenoses; resection up to 4 cm is feasible, which is the equivalent of eight cartilaginous rings (25). In one series of 58 patients with postintubation or idiopathic stenoses, major complications occurred in 12%, including anastomotic dehiscence and vocal cord paralysis (25).

Primary Tracheal Neoplasia

Primary tumors of the trachea are rare, representing less than 1% of bronchial neoplasms (26–29) To date, a bewildering array of different tracheal tumors, both benign and malignant, have been reported, including both primary epithelial and mesenchymal neoplasms as well as secondary neoplasia resulting from either metastases or, more commonly, direct tracheal invasion by adjacent mediastinal neoplasms (30). In fact, only a few lesions occur with any frequency, and squamous cell carcinoma (SCC) and adenoid cystic carcinoma (ACC) together account for up to 86% of cases (26–29). Other relatively less common malignant lesions encountered include carcinoid and mucoepidermoid tumors, while endobronchial hamartomas and bronchial papillomas are the most common benign lesions. Although these tumors are discussed separately, it should be emphasized that as a group, regardless of their cell type, most patients with endotracheal and proximal bronchial neoplasms present with a limited number of symptoms and signs: cough, wheezing, stridor, hemoptysis, and evidence of either parenchymal consolidation or atelectasis, depending on the site and degree of bronchial obstruction.

Squamous Cell Carcinoma

Squamous cell carcinoma (SCC) almost always occurs in middle-aged male smokers, paralleling the development of

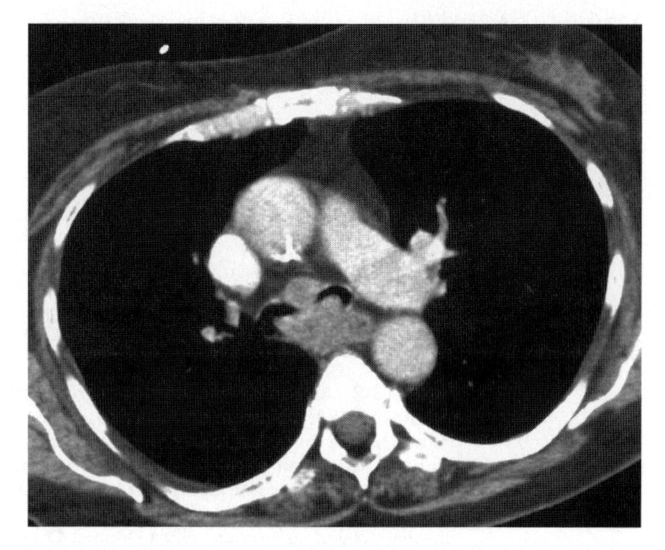

Figure 3-7 Squamous cell carcinoma. Axial section shows soft tissue mass involving the carina resulting in marked narrowing of both the right and especially the left mainstem bronchi. Biopsy proved squamous cell carcinoma. (Case courtesy of Dr. Moulay Meziane, Cleveland, Ohio.)

these tumors in the lung. SCC has been found in association with either a previous history or concurrent or subsequent occurrence of SCC somewhere else in the respiratory tract in up to 40% of patients (27). Spread to adjacent mediastinal lymph nodes is common and carries a worse prognosis. Less often there is extension of tumor into the mainstem bronchi or adjacent esophagus, resulting in malignant esophageal-bronchial fistulas (30). On CT these lesions preferentially involve the trachea and mainstem bronchi (Fig. 3-7). Characteristically they appear as polypoid intraluminal masses; less commonly these tumors appear with eccentric, markedly irregular wall thickening and resultant luminal narrowing. Regardless of their intraluminal appearance, extension into the adjacent mediastinum or subcarinal space is common and easily identified by CT (31). In some patients SCCs may result in tracheoesophageal or bronchoesophageal fistulization. In these patients, determining the site of origin of the tumor may be problematic (Fig. 3-8). Rarely, SCCs may cause diffuse bilateral infiltration of the tracheobronchial tree. In

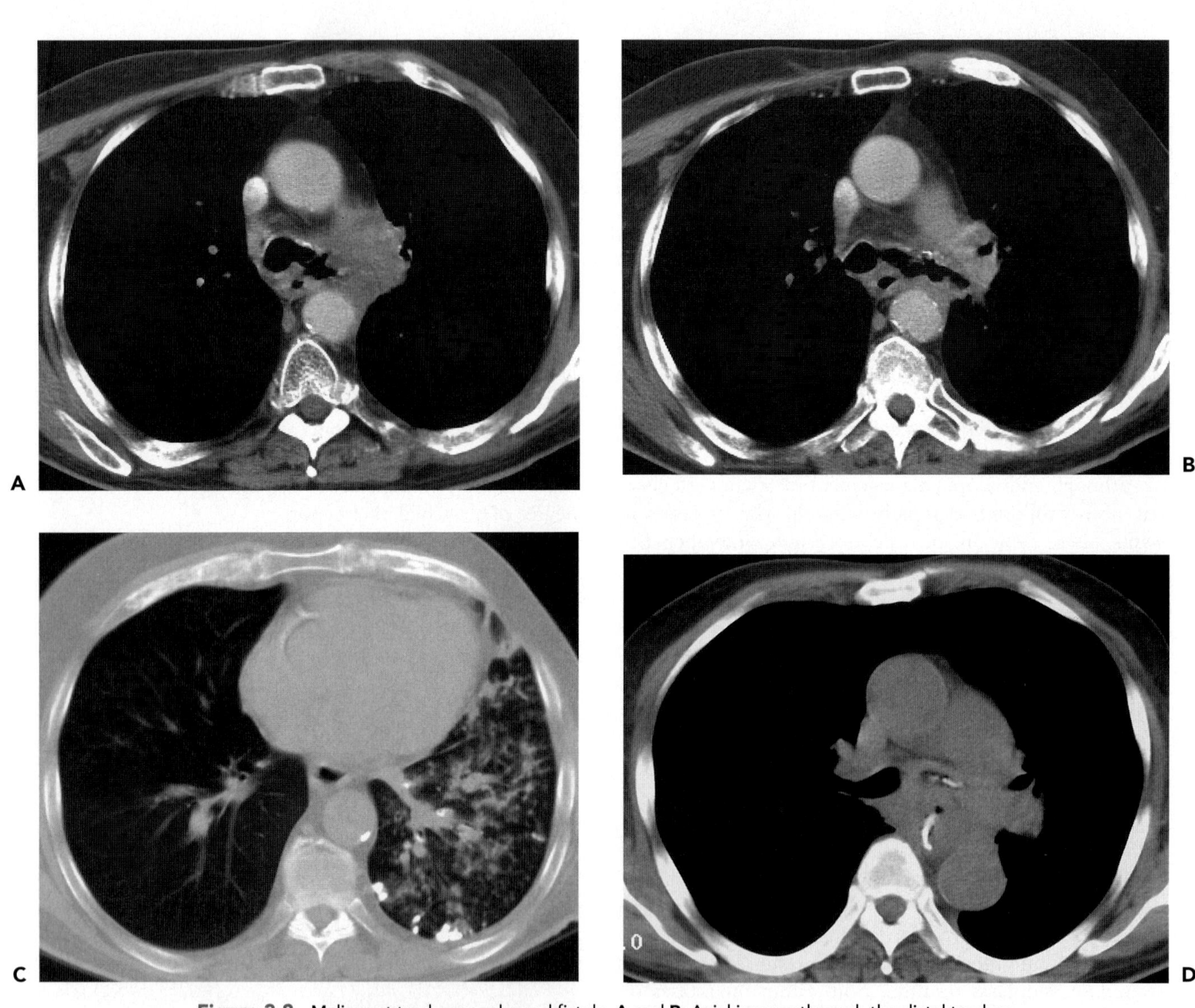

Figure 3-8 Malignant tracheoesophageal fistula. **A** and **B**: Axial images through the distal trachea and proximal left mainstem bronchus, respectively, show an irregular extraluminal air collection posterior and lateral to the left main bronchus, distinct from air within the esophageal lumen (arrows). Note the presence of left paratracheal/aorticopulmonary window soft tissue mass/adenopathy. **C**: Axial image through the lower lobe following a barium swallow showing evidence of aspiration. Fistulization between the bronchial tree and esophagus was subsequently confirmed at bronchoscopy. Histologically proved squamous cell carcinoma. **D**: Axial section through the carina in a different patient than shown in **A** to **C** shows evidence of oral contrast media in both the esophagus and left mainstem bronchus, confirming the presence of a fistula between the airways and esophagus. In this case, this patient had previously documented esophageal carcinoma. In a given case, establishing the origin of a malignant tracheobronchoesophageal fistula may be difficult to determine. (Cases courtesy of Dr. Moulay Meziane, Cleveland, Ohio.)

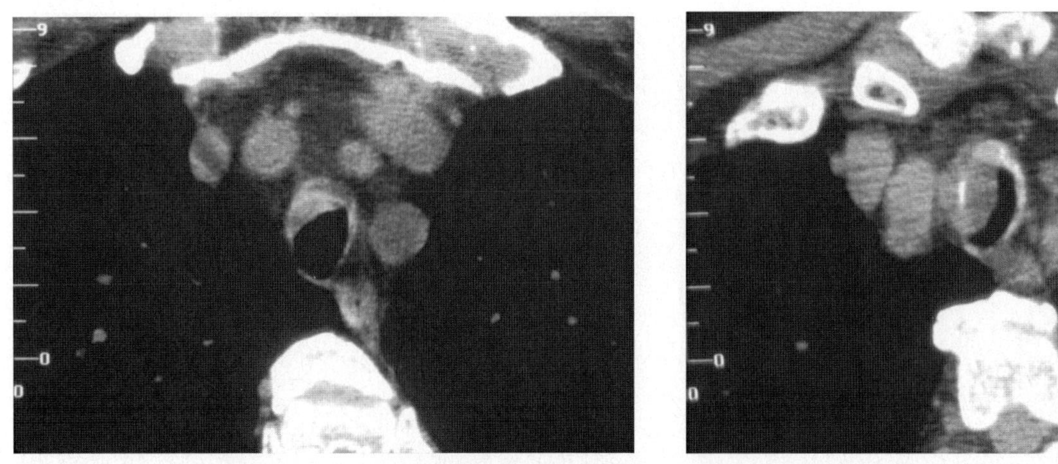

Figure 3-9 Adenoid cystic carcinoma. **A** and **B:** Axial CT sections through the midtrachea in two different patients, both with focal adenoid cystic carcinomas. Note that in each case there is an eccentric soft tissue mass involving only a portion of the tracheal wall with variable degrees of tracheal narrowing and extension into the adjacent soft tissues of the mediastinum. In both cases, CT clearly shows limited extraluminal invasion, confirming that these lesions are resectable.

these patients, prebronchoscopic CT diagnosis requires a high level of clinical suspicion (Fig. 2-7).

Sialadenoid Tumors

Pulmonary analogs of the salivary glands, tumors arising from tracheobronchial mucous glands primarily include cystic ACCs; less often encountered are mucoepidermoid carcinomas, which make up approximately 5% of these tumors. Other rare salivary gland tumors include mucous gland adenomas, pleomorphic adenomas, and acinic cell carcinomas (32); still more rarely reported are pulmonary oncocytomas and myoepitheliomas (33). ACCs represent low-grade malignancies that show a marked propensity for local invasion, especially invasion of submucosal and perineural lymphatics (34). Compared with SCCs, ACCs occur in slightly younger individuals with a mean age of between 40 and 50 years and show no apparent sex predilection. Furthermore, their occurrence is unrelated to cigarette smoking (27). Although lymph node metastases are relatively uncommon, especially in comparison with SCCs, metachronous hematogenous metastases are common, occurring in 44% of patients in one series (34). Most of these tumors arise from the distal trachea or proximal mainstem bronchi and appear as intraluminal polypoid masses causing luminal narrowing with invasion of adjacent mediastinal structures commonly seen (Figs. 3-9 and 3-10) (33). Rarely, they may prove multifocal in distribution (Fig. 3-11).

Unlike ACCs mucoepidermoid tumors most often are identified in segmental bronchi; in one series, they occurred in segmental bronchi in 8 of 12 patients (35). They also tend to occur in younger patients, with half less than 30 years of age (33). On CT although these lesions tend to be smaller and more circumscribed, often identifiable as solitary pulmonary or endoluminal nodules, they are otherwise indistinguishable from ACCs. As with other lesions causing airway obstruction, mucoepidermoid tumors often result in parenchymal consolidation or atelectasis. They may also extend distally to present as foci of mucoid impaction.

Carcinoid Tumors

Carcinoid tumors are neuroendocrine neoplasms that arise within bronchial or bronchiolar epithelium. They are presumed to arise from existing Kulchitsky cells, neuroepithelial bodies, or pluripotential bronchial epithelial stem cells (36). They present a spectrum of histologic subtypes ranging from low- to high-grade neoplasms and are classified as typical carcinoids, atypical carcinoids, and large cell neuroendocrine carcinomas; the highest grades merge with small cell carcinoma (37). In addition to findings related to bronchial obstruction, carcinoid tumors cause hemoptysis in up to 50% of patients, reflecting their hypervascular stroma. In addition, carcinoid tumors are also known to produce a variety of hormones and neuroamines including adrenocorticotropic hormone (ACTH), serotonin, and somatostatin, among others. Cushing syndrome has been reported, although rarely. Carcinoid syndrome may also occur, although only in patients with known liver metastases (37).

Most endobronchial carcinoid tumors are centrally located. Easily identified bronchoscopically, they typically appear as smooth, cherry-red lesions with a propensity to bleed on biopsy. Although massive hemoptysis has been reported, in fact these lesions are usually safely biopsied. They tend to exhibit variable growth patterns, but most often they extend extraluminally, resulting in so-called iceberg lesions. With more peripheral lesions, airway obstruction may result in focal mucoid impaction.

(*Text continues on page 80.*)

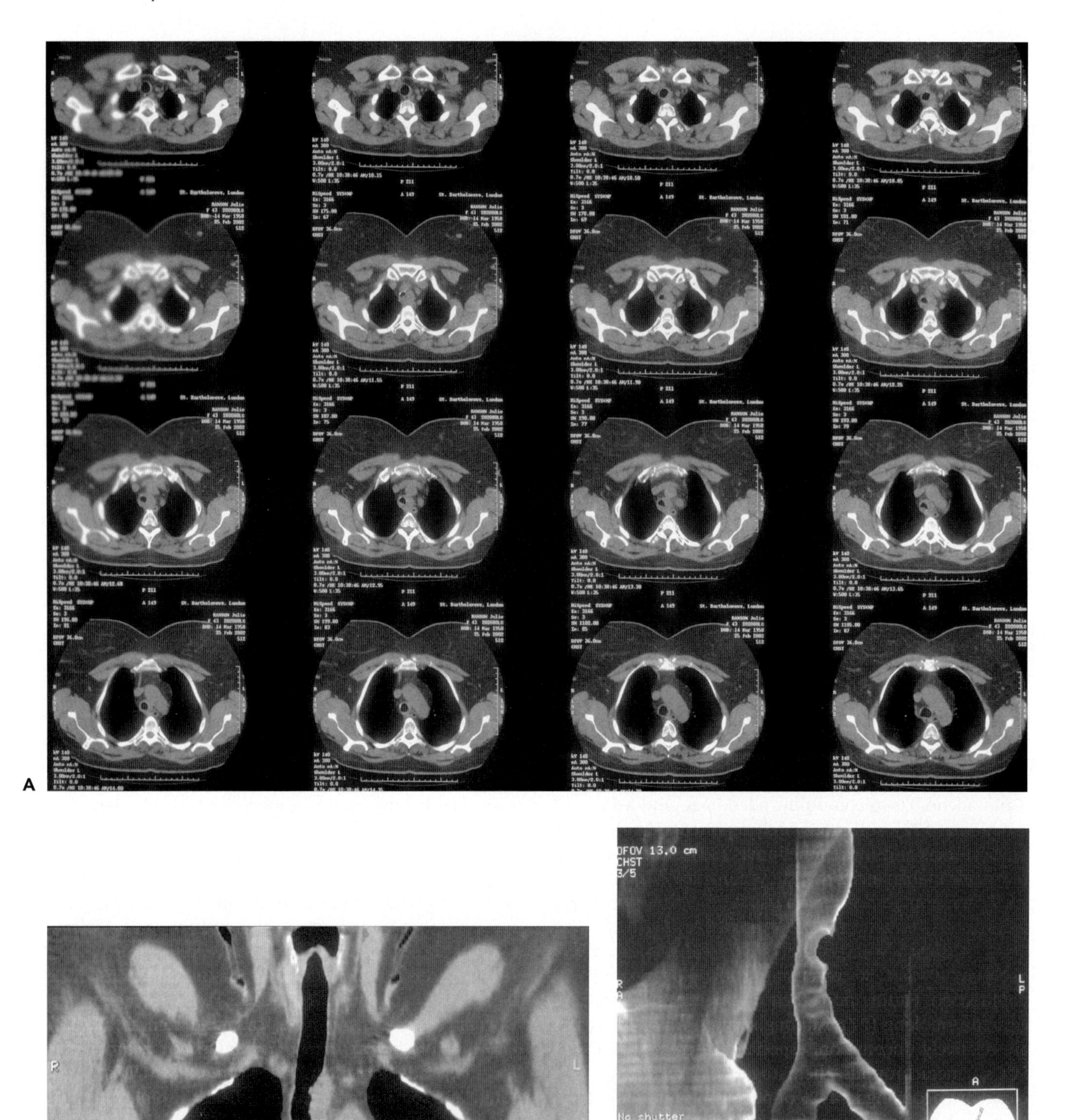

Figure 3-10 Adenoid cystic carcinoma. **A:** CT section through the midtrachea shows irregular soft tissue mass causing marked narrowing and slight lateral displacement of the trachea. In this case there is extensive soft tissue invasion of the adjacent mediastinal fat (compare with Fig. 3-10). Despite this finding, absence of definite encasement of adjacent mediastinal organs indicates that this tumor should still be considered resectable. **B** and **C:** Multiplanar and 3D surface rendering of this lesion, respectively, show to good advantage the true length of tracheal involvement. Note that the MPR is superior for delineating the extraluminal component of the tumor.

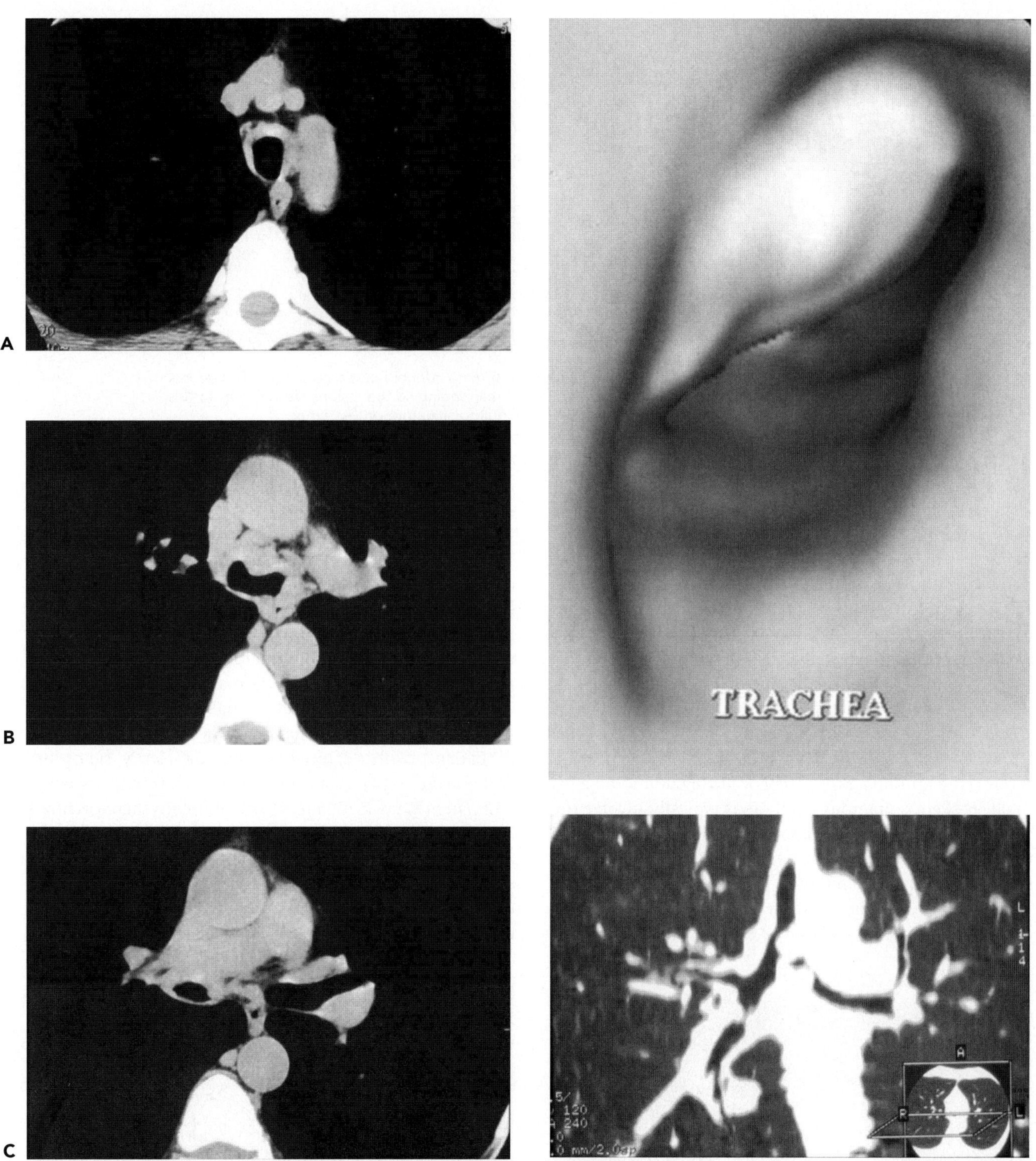

Figure 3-11 Multifocal adenoid cystic carcinoma. **A** to **C:** Axial images through the distal trachea, carina, and subcarinal space, respectively, show multiple foci of both nodular and circumferential bronchial wall thickening, associated with marked focal narrowing of the adjacent airway lumens. Note that in **B** there is also evidence of adjacent mediastinal adenopathy. **D:** Virtual bronchoscopic view of the distal trachea shows a nearly obstructing polypoid lesion arising from the left lateral wall of the trachea. Not surprisingly, endoscopic visualization of the distal airways was limited in this patient. **E:** Coronal MPR shows to good advantage the multiple sites of tumor, including the distal trachea, the proximal left mainstem bronchus, and the bronchus intermedius. *(continued)*

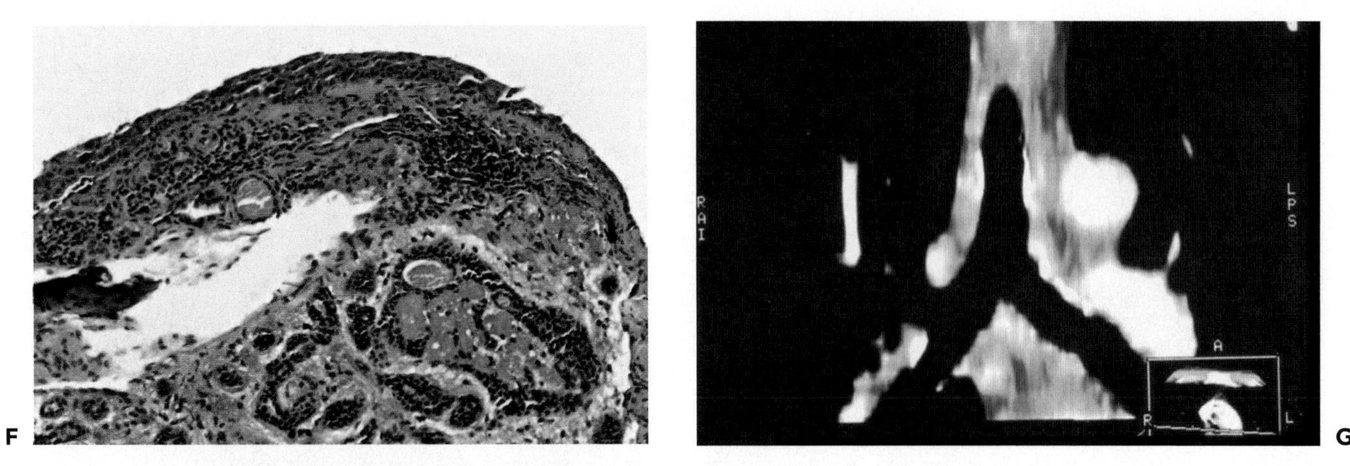

Figure 3-11 *(continued)* **F:** Histologic evaluation confirming adenoid cystic carcinoma. **G:** Coronal MPR showing placement of three separate stents corresponding to the lesions shown in **E.** In this case, surgical resection was not an option, given the multifocal nature of the tumor.

On CT, endobronchial carcinoid tumors most often present either as hilar masses or discrete intraluminal lesions (Figs. 3-12 and 3-13). A characteristic triad of features has been described, including the finding of a well-defined round or slightly lobulated tumor causing narrowing of the adjacent airway, associated with eccentric calcifications (38). These calcifications are identifiable in up to a third of patients (36,39). Carcinoid tumors are also well known to markedly enhance following administration of intravenous contrast media (Fig. 1-2; see also Fig. 3-13).

Benign Tracheal Tumors

The most common benign tracheal neoplasm is a squamous cell papilloma. Most often occurring in middle-aged male smokers, squamous papillomas typically involve the larynx or bronchi. Isolated tracheal involvement is rare and is usually limited to the tracheal wall (30). In addition to solitary neoplasms, papillomas are also classified as either inflammatory or as laryngotracheobronchial papillomatosis (40). Inflammatory polyps can be either solitary or multiple and arise in response to chronic irritation, as occurs with endobronchial foreign bodies or exposure to hot or corrosive gases. Inflammatory polyps have also been associated with broncholithiasis.

Laryngotracheal papillomatosis refers to a condition associated with multiple papillomas. Typically arising in the larynx, these lesions are histologically similar to solitary papillomas, although they most often occur in children under 5 years of age. Papillomatosis is etiologically linked to infection with human papillomavirus, either contracted at birth or acquired through sexual transmission. In this regard, papillomatosis recently has been reported to occur in patients with acquired immunodeficiency syndrome (AIDS) (Fig. 3-14). In a comprehensive literature review of 532 patients, tracheal and bronchial involvement occurred in approximately 5% of patients, whereas pulmonary parenchymal disease occurred in less than 1% (41). Unfortunately, spontaneous remission is unusual, with malignant transformation to SCC reported in adults. The origin of parenchymal disease is controversial. Because tracheobronchial

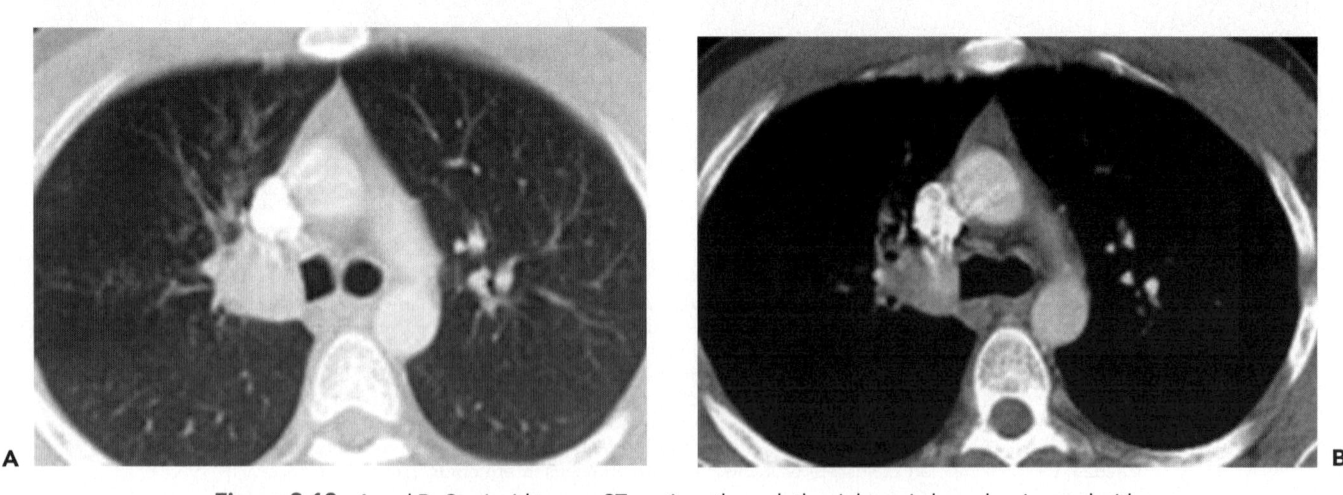

Figure 3-12 **A** and **B:** Carcinoid tumor. CT sections through the right main bronchus imaged with wide and narrow windows, respectively, show a focal soft tissue mass protruding into the bronchial lumen. Note that there is evidence of peribronchial thickening involving the anterior segmental airways in the right upper lobe, a finding consistent with probable chronic airway obstruction resulting in recurrent episodes of infection.

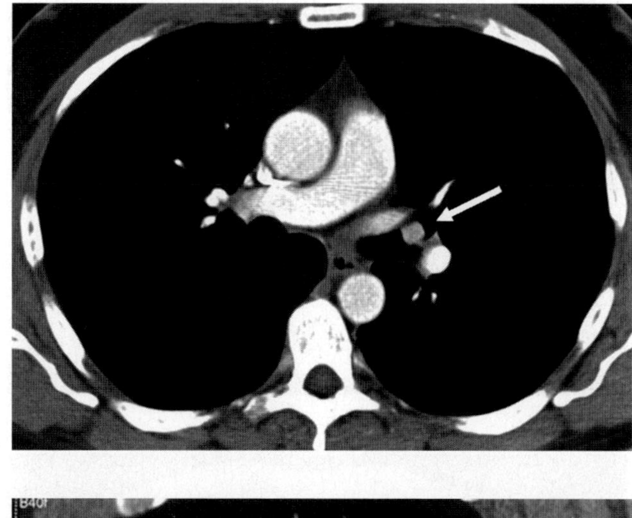

A

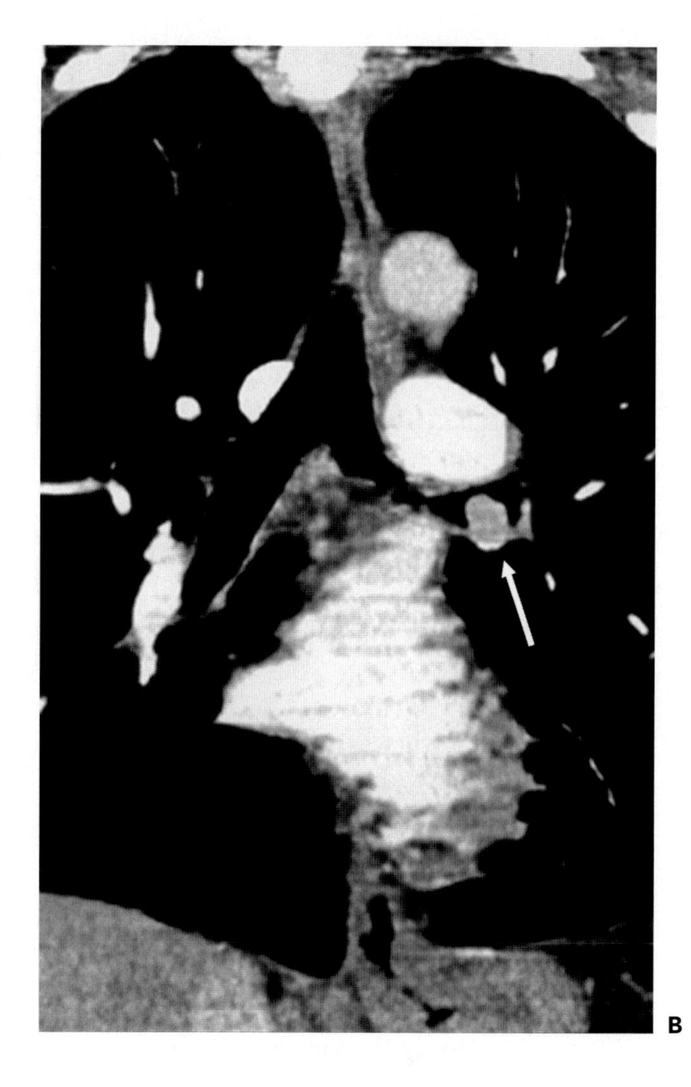

B

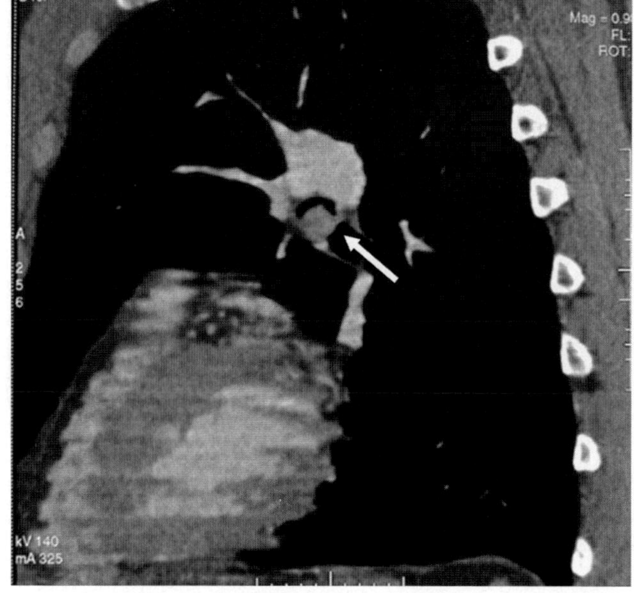

C

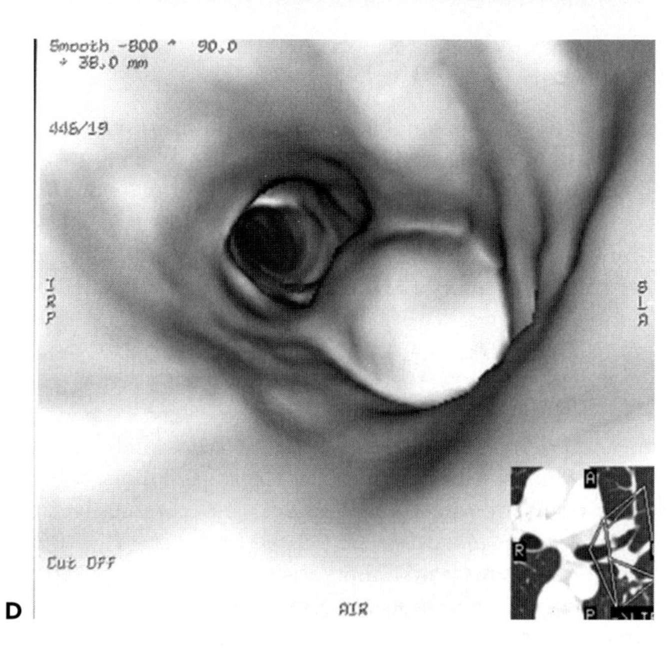

D

Figure 3-13 **A:** Axial image through the distal left upper lobe bronchus shows a well-defined, discrete intrabronchial lesion. **B** and **C:** Coronal and sagittal MPRs, respectively, and **D:** virtual bronchoscopic image show this same lesion to good advantage, again confirming its endobronchial location. This is the same lesion illustrated in Fig. 1-2, showing marked hypervascularity following intravenous contrast administration.

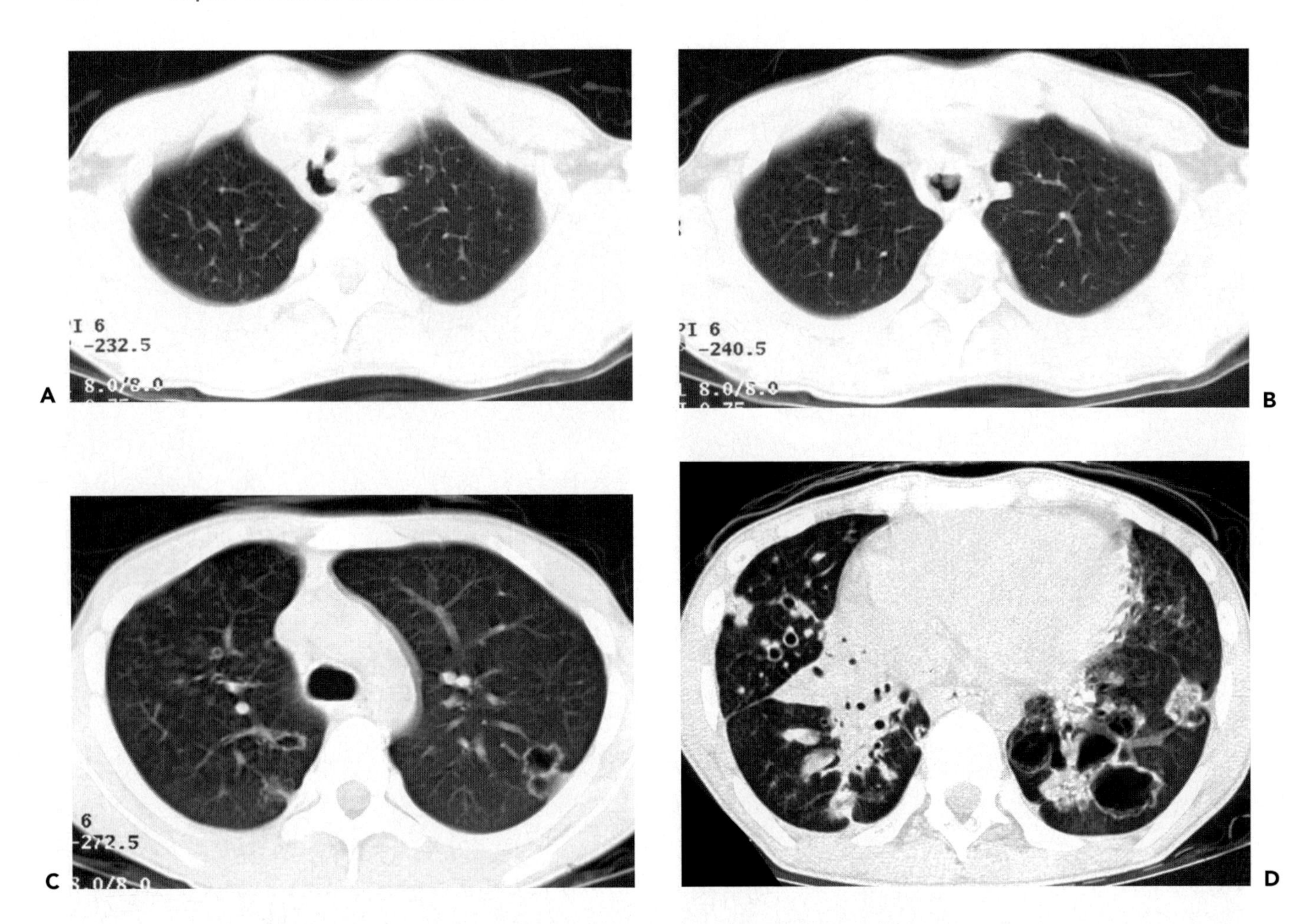

Figure 3-14 Laryngotracheal papillomatosis in a patient with AIDS. **A** and **B:** Axial CT images through the upper and midtrachea, respectively, show marked nodular irregularity of the tracheal lumen resulting from multiple polypoid lesions. **C** and **D:** Axial CT section shows typical appearance of diffuse laryngotracheal papillomatosis resulting in scattered nodules, some of which are cavitary (See also Fig. 2-20).

and parenchymal disease is rarely encountered without coexistent laryngeal disease, it has been assumed that spread occurs by endobronchial dissemination. An association between distal spread and prior tracheostomy further supports this conclusion. Lesions typically appear first as well-defined centrilobular nodules that subsequently undergo central necrosis, resulting in multiple thin-walled cavities (Fig. 3-14). Bronchiectasis, with or without parenchymal consolidation and atelectasis, is often identified in association with nodular densities, presumably the result of bronchial occlusion and subsequent inflammation or infection.

Endobronchial hamartoma is another benign lesion that is occasionally encountered. Although they are the commonest benign cause of a solitary pulmonary nodule, endobronchial hamartomas are rare, estimated to represent between 10% and 20% of intrathoracic hamartomas (42). Hamartomas are mesenchymal lesions composed of a mixture of cartilage, fat, and fibrous tissue (43). They most often occur in segmental bronchi; tracheal involvement is distinctly unusual. In a report of 43 patients with documented endobronchial hamartomas, the most common presenting symptoms were recurrent respiratory tract infections and hemoptysis occurring in 44% and 33% of patients, respectively (42). On CT, although infrequently reported, the presence of fat is considered diagnostic of this entity (Fig. 3-15) (44,45).

Secondary Malignant Neoplasms

In addition to primary tumors, the trachea and central bronchi may also be secondarily involved by tumors, either as a result of direct invasion, or less commonly by hematogenous metastases (Fig. 3-16) (31). Local invasion most often results from tumors arising from the esophagus, larynx, thyroid, and lung. Metastatic disease, although less common, most often results from renal and colonic primary lesions (46). It should be emphasized that assess-

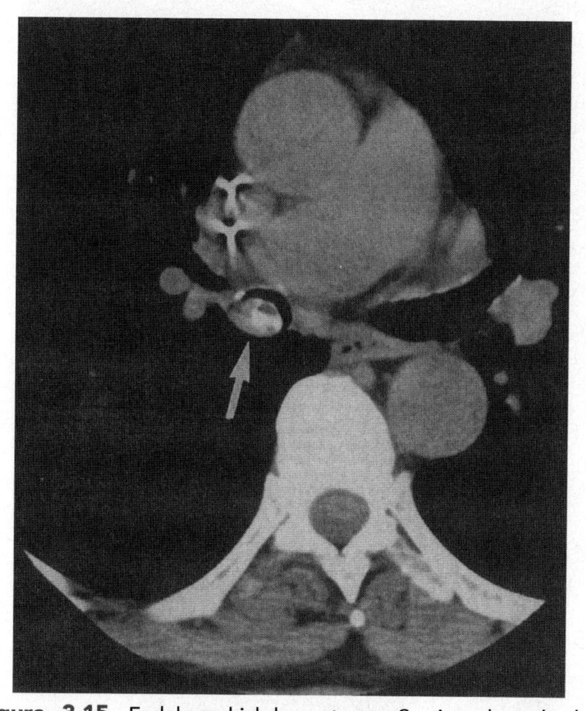

Figure 3-15 Endobronchial hamartoma. Section through the bronchus intermedius shows a well-defined endobronchial mass within which foci of both calcification and fat *(arrow)* can be identified. Histologically proved endobronchial hamartoma.

ment of tracheal invasion may be exceedingly difficult with CT. The finding of a peritracheal soft-tissue mass causing focal displacement of the adjacent tracheal lumen should be interpreted as nonspecific. It cannot be overemphasized that in the absence of a discrete endobronchial mass, evidence of fistulization to adjacent mediastinal structures, or destruction of tracheal cartilage, the diagnosis of tracheal or mainstem bronchial invasion is limited (Figs. 3-17 and 3-18). Definitive evaluation usually necessitates either bronchoscopic or histologic confirmation. Although it has been reported that MR may be preferable to CT in assessing invasion of the tracheal wall (47), to date routine use of MR for this purpose has not gained widespread acceptance

Endobronchial Neoplasms: Management and Prognosis

Given the overlap in both clinical manifestations and CT appearance of most endobronchial lesions, not surprisingly definitive diagnosis requires histologic evaluation in nearly all cases. In addition to the primary tracheal lesions mentioned previously, it should be noted that a bewildering variety of additional rare endobronchial lesions have been reported (27,48,49). Regardless of origin, primary endotracheal lesions are best treated surgically, especially with primary resection and reanastomosis, usually followed by radiation. To date, most large series have primarily focused on patients with SCCs and ACCs. In a series of 20 patients with primary tracheal neoplasms treated surgically, Hazama et al. (29) reported a 5-year survival rate of 72.3% for patients undergoing surgical treatment including segmental tracheal, laryngotracheal, or carinal resections. Nearly identical results have been reported by others (27,50). Overall, approximately three quarters of patients with primary tracheal or carinal lesions will be resectable.

In an evaluation of 198 patients with primary tracheal tumors reported by Grillo et al. (27), 147 (74%) were treated surgically, including 44 with SCCs, 60 with ACCs, and 43 with assorted benign and malignant tumors. Surgical mortality for primary resections was 5%. Patients with ACCs survived longer than those with SCCs, especially when the latter were associated with mediastinal adenopathy. Curiously, in patients with ACCs, survival was similar whether or not there was evidence of mediastinal nodes or residual tumor along the margins at resection. Nearly identical results have been reported by Hazama et al. (29), who also noted that survival in patients with ACCs was independent of the presence of positive margins at surgery. In this setting, it turns out that the benefits of performing primary resection outweigh the potential liability of leaving behind residual microscopic tumor.

Although surgical resection is to be preferred when feasible, an increasing number of nonsurgical options are now available for the treatment, and especially the palliation, of endobronchial tumors. As discussed in depth in Chapter 2, these include neodymium:yttrium-aluminum-garnet (Nd:YAG) laser phototherapy, photodynamic therapy following the intravenous administration of photosensitizing drugs, cryotherapy, electrocoagulation, brachytherapy, and endobronchial stents with or without prior bronchoplasty (Figs. 3-12 and 3-19) (51).

DIFFUSE TRACHEAL DISEASE

A wide variety of inflammatory abnormalities, both infectious and noninfectious, diffusely affect the trachea and mainstem bronchi (31,52). These include both primary and secondary tracheal abnormalities and typically result either in diffuse luminal narrowing or, less commonly, in dilatation. As will be discussed, CT plays an integral role in the evaluation of these conditions by accurately depicting the tracheal wall and surrounding structures as well as by providing physiologic assessment of tracheal mechanics.

Tracheobronchomegaly

Tracheobronchomegaly refers to a heterogeneous group of patients who have marked dilatation of the trachea and mainstem bronchi (53–55). Also referred to as Mournier-Kuhn syndrome, tracheobronchomegaly is a rare disorder marked by diffuse dilatation of the trachea and mainstem bronchi. It is frequently associated with tracheal

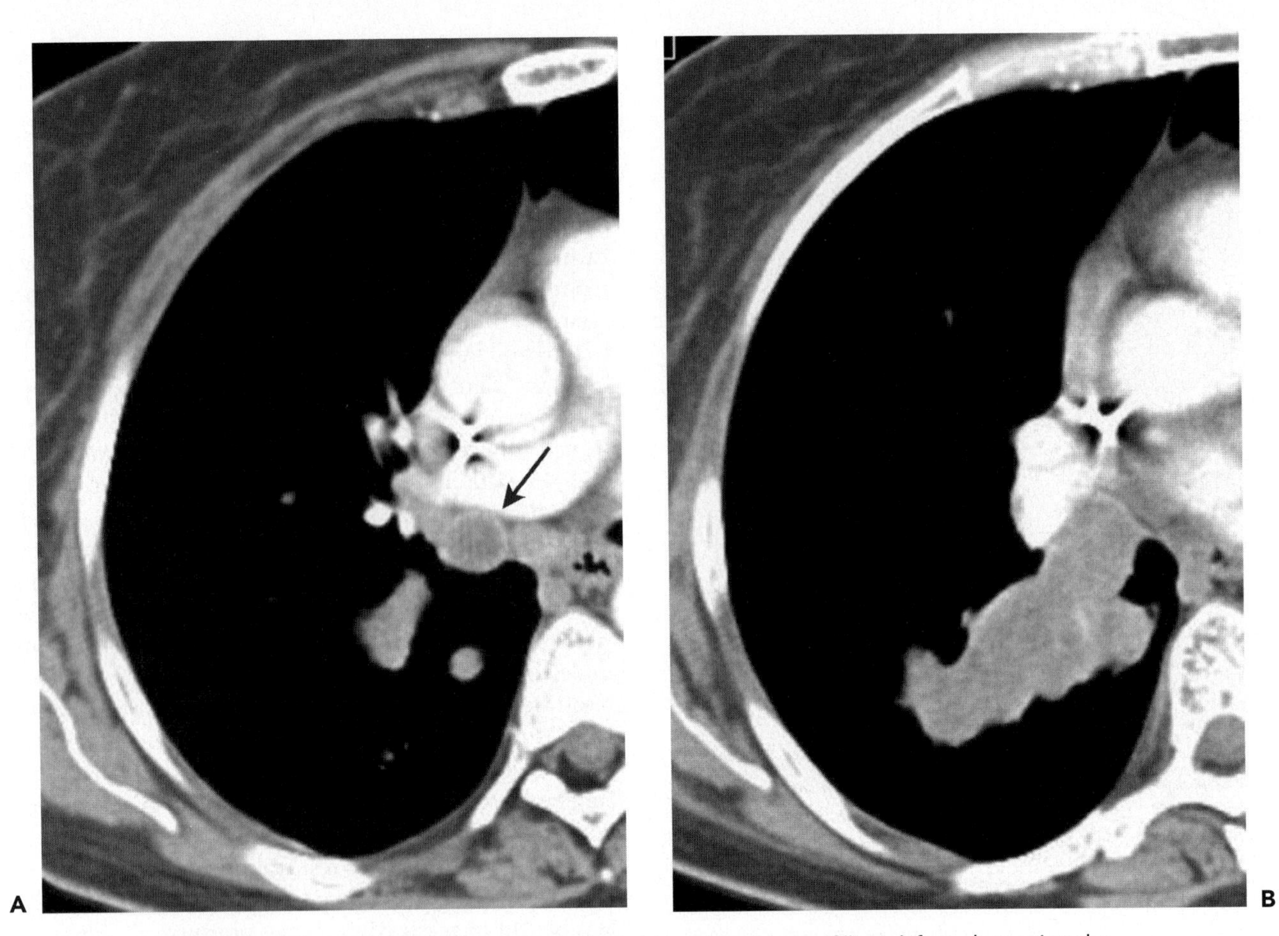

Figure 3-16 Endobronchial metastasis. **A:** Axial section shows a filling defect obstructing the bronchus intermedius *(arrow)*. **B:** Axial image obtained below **A** shows extensive mucoid impaction of the bronchi within the superior segment secondary to proximal endobronchial obstruction. Biopsy proved metastatic colon cancer.

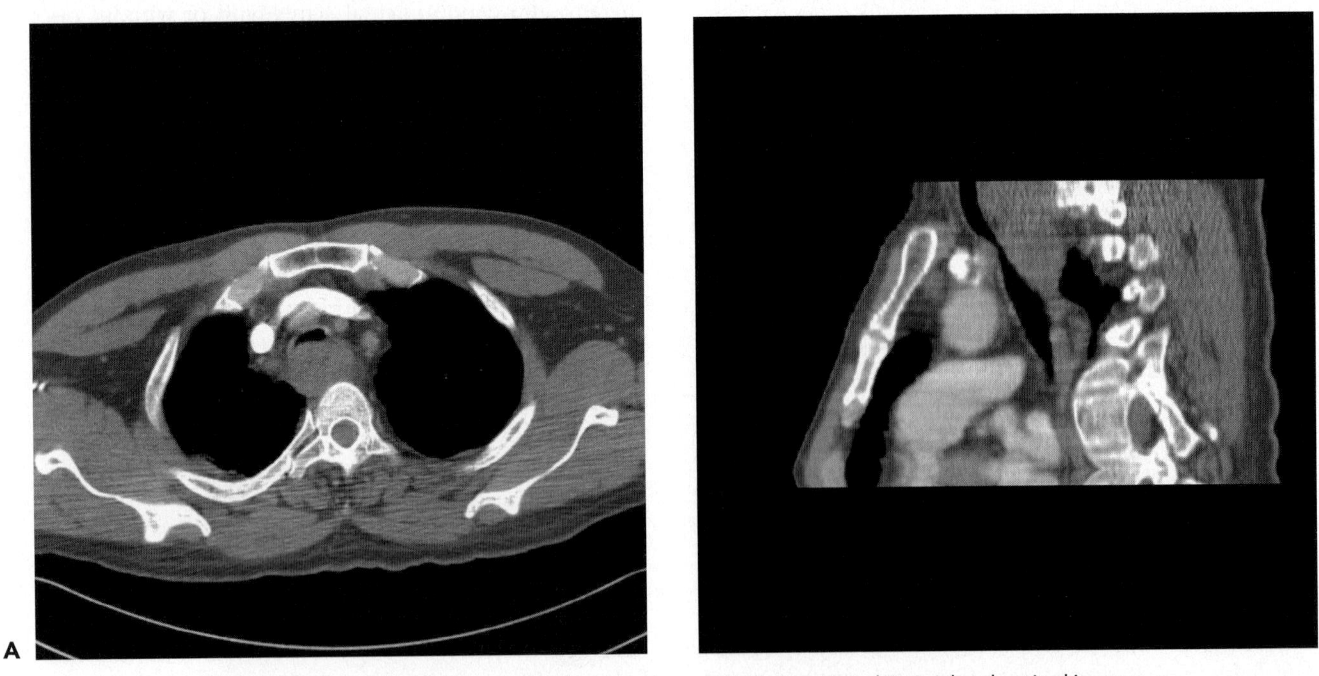

Figure 3-17 Extrinsic compression from esophageal carcinoma. **A** and **B:** Axial and sagittal images through the trachea in a patient with esophageal carcinoma show smooth displacement of the trachea anteriorly causing narrowing of the lumen. Despite the long segment of trachea affected, at bronchoscopy there was no evidence of tracheal invasion.

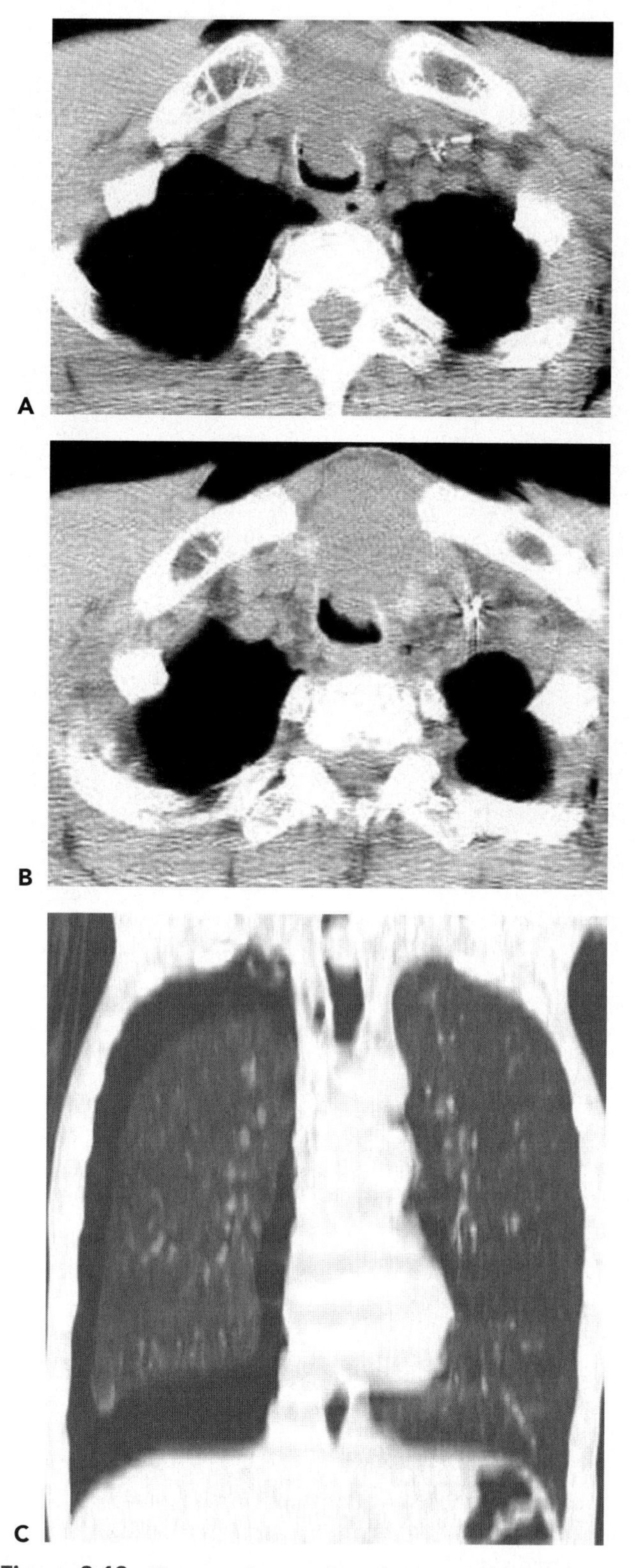

Figure 3-18 Recurrent laryngeal carcinoma; tracheal invasion. **A** and **B:** Contiguous axial sections at the level of the thoracic inlet/upper trachea show evidence of a large soft tissue mass in the anterior mediastinum extending posteriorly and causing direct invasion of the anterior tracheal wall, with disruption of the anterior cartilages resulting in a large, partially obstructing intraluminal polypoid soft tissue mass. Given these findings, CT diagnosis of tracheal invasion is unequivocal (compare with Fig. 3-17). **C:** Coronal reconstruction showing the intraluminal tracheal mass at the level of the thoracic inlet. In this case, partial obstruction of the trachea resulted in bilateral pneumothoraces.

diverticulosis, recurrent lower respiratory tract infections, and bronchiectasis.

The etiology of tracheobronchomegaly remains controversial. Factors favoring a congenital etiology include evidence of deficiency of tracheobronchial muscle fibers and absence of the myenteric plexus. It is frequently found in association with other congential or connective tissue disorders, including ankylosing spondylitis, Marfan's syndrome, cystic fibrosis, Ehlers-Danlos syndrome, and cutis laxa in children (56,57). Factors favoring an acquired etiology include the finding that the disorder most frequently occurs in cigarette-smoking men in their third and fourth decades without an antecedent history of respiratory tract infection (56,57). An association between tracheomegaly and diffuse pulmonary fibrosis also has been reported, presumably the result of increased traction on the tracheal wall resulting from increased elastic recoil pressure in both lungs exerting opposing force (56,57).

CT findings in patients with tracheobronchomegaly include a tracheal diameter of greater than 3 cm, as measured 2 cm above the aortic arch and diameters of 2.4 and 2.3 cm for the right and left main bronchi, respectively (31,58). Additional findings include tracheal scalloping or diverticula, the latter being especially common along the posterior membranous tracheal wall. Of particular interest is the potential relationship between tracheomegaly and bronchiectasis (Fig. 4-38). As noted by Roditi and Weir (56), in a study of 75 consecutive patients referred to rule out bronchiectasis, 12% proved to have tracheomegaly, including 7 (17%) with bronchiectasis. These data suggest that tracheomegaly may play a causative role in the development of bronchiectasis as a result of abnormal mucus clearance because of an inefficient cough resulting in stagnant mucus.

Another key finding is marked expiratory collapse indicative of tracheomalacia (59), also the result of weakened tracheal cartilage. Tracheomalacia may be seen in association with a number of disorders in addition to tracheobronchomegaly, including most causes of diffuse tracheal inflammation, such as relapsing polychondritis, as well as following trauma or especially in patients with chronic bronchitis, among others. Symptoms are typically nonspecific and include chronic cough, dyspnea, and occasionally hemoptysis (60). Tracheomalacia has also been associated with spontaneous tracheal rupture (14). In patients in whom this diagnosis is suspected, additional expiratory scans may be essential. Aquino et al. (60) showed that the probability of tracheomalacia varied between 89% and 100% when the change in the sagittal diameter of the trachea exceeded 289%.

Initially proposed using noncontiguous expiratory high-resolution CT images (59,61), whenever possible the use of high-resolution volumetric acquisition has clear advantages (62). In addition to contiguously imaging the entire length of the trachea, high-resolution volumetric data acquisition also provides invaluable information regarding peripheral

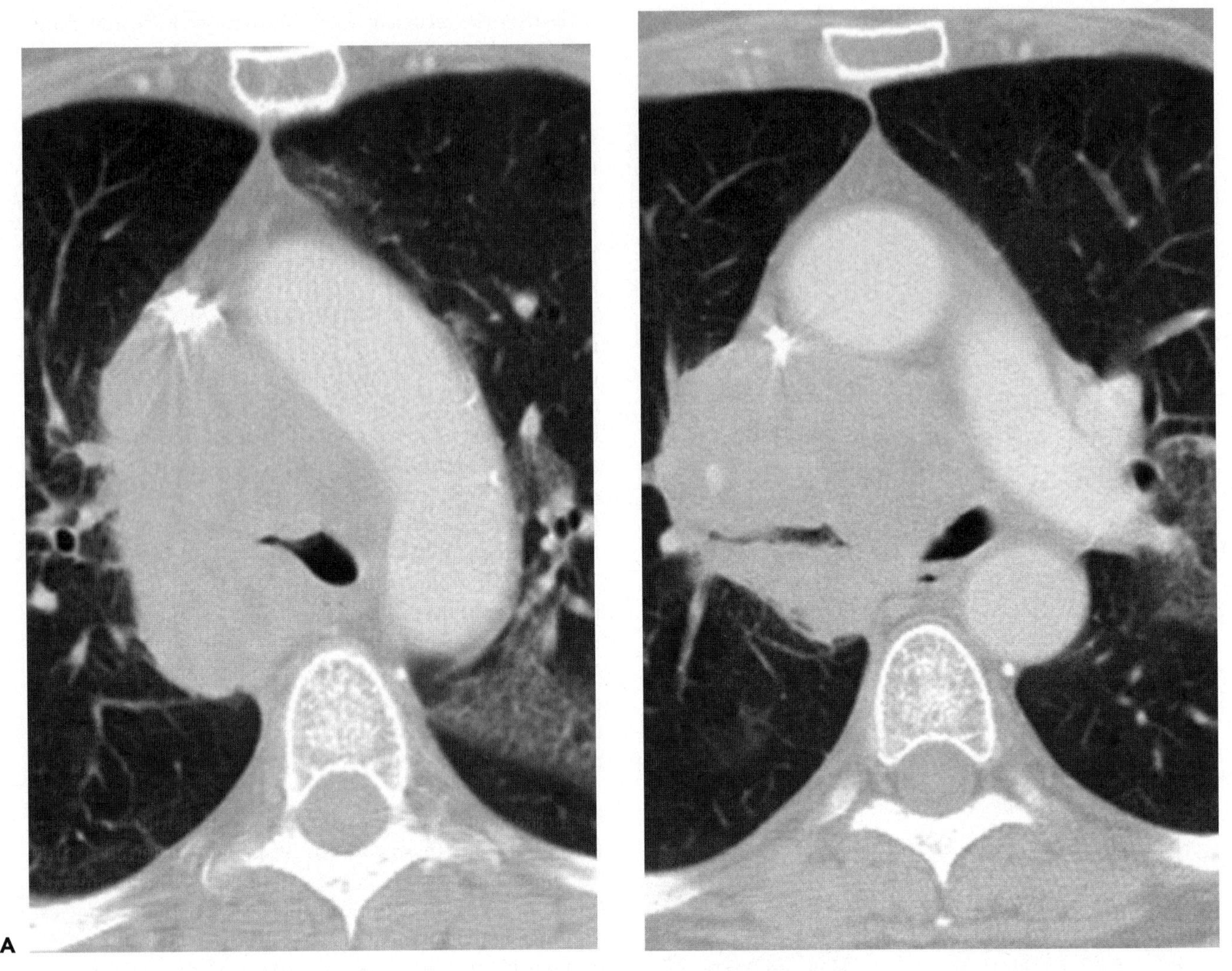

Figure 3-19 Squamous cell carcinoma of the lung: endobronchial stenting. **A** and **B:** Axial CT sections through the distal carina and proximal mainstem bronchi, respectively, show extensive mediastinal tumor causing eccentric narrowing of the distal trachea, near complete obstruction of the right mainstem bronchus, and apparent extrinsic compression of the medial aspect of the left mainstem bronchus. Note that there is also slight nodular irregularity of the anterior wall of the left mainstem bronchus, suggesting possible tumor infiltration. *(continued)*

air trapping, a frequent ancillary finding. Although precise quantitative estimation of the severity of tracheomalacia has also been reported using electron beam CT (EBCT), this technique remains generally less available (63).

Diffuse Tracheal Narrowing

Included in the group of patients with diffuse tracheal narrowing are those with infectious disorders, including bacterial, viral, and fungal infections as well as those with a variety of generally rare, noninfectious disorders including tracheopathia osteochondrolytica, relapsing polychondritis, Wegener's granulomatosis, amyloidosis, sarcoidosis, and ulcerative colitis (31,52). Although differential diagnosis may be limited owing to the similarity of the appearance of these conditions, as will be discussed and illustrated, some have sufficiently distinctive appearances to suggest the correct diagnosis.

Saber-Sheath Trachea

Saber-sheath trachea is a not uncommon cause of diffuse narrowing involving the intrathoracic trachea only. On CT this condition is easily recognized by noting that the internal side-to-side diameter of the trachea is decreased to half or less the corresponding sagittal diameter (Fig. 3-20) (31,52,64). It is almost always associated with chronic obstructive pulmonary disease (COPD) (65). Although this condition is classically described as a static deformity, further narrowing of the tracheal lumen can be documented when patients are examined using CT obtained during forced expiration or a Valsalva maneuver (31,66–68).

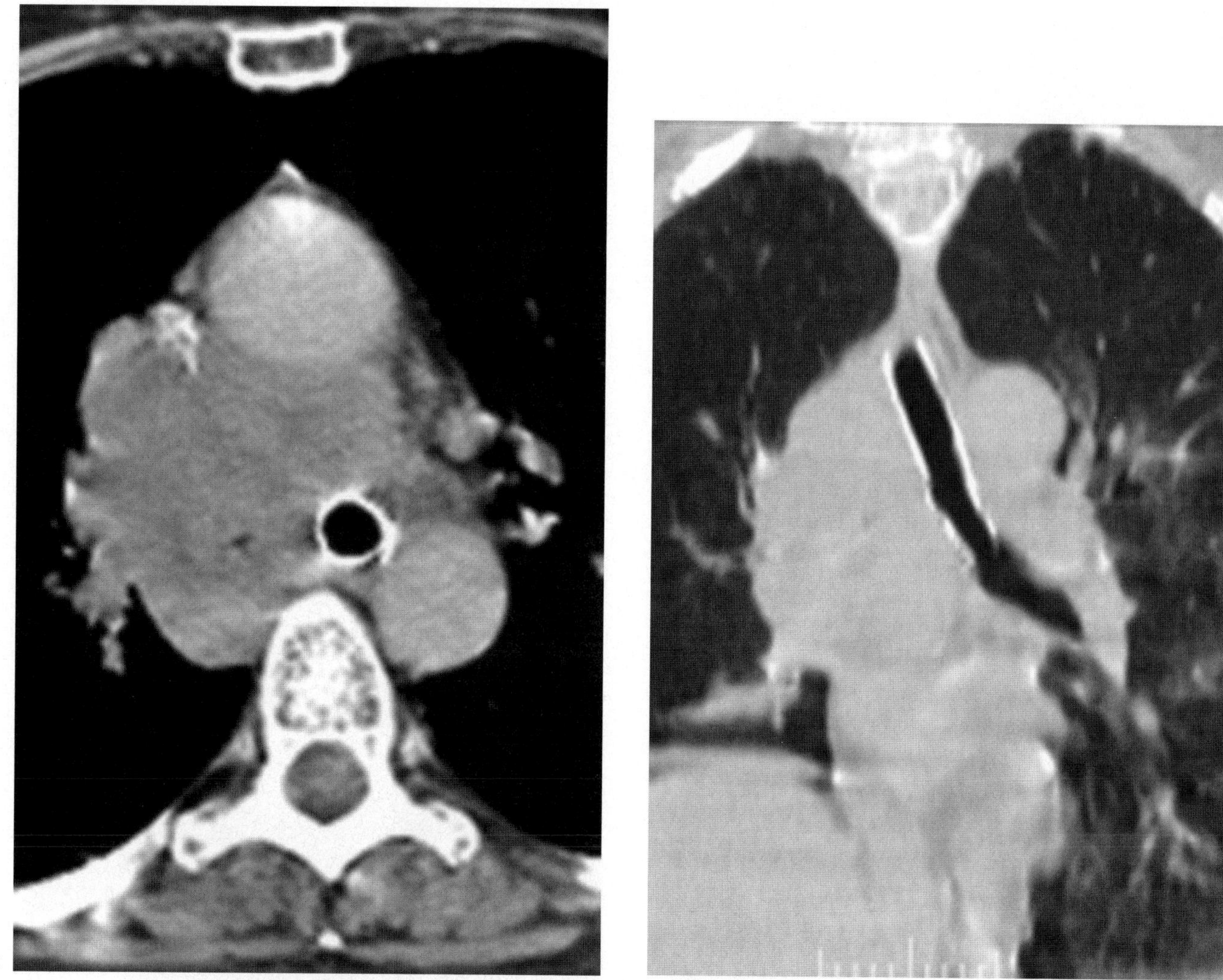

Figure 3-19 *(continued)* **C** and **D:** Axial and coronal images, respectively, following successful insertion of a stent in the distal trachea and left mainstem bronchus. In this nonsurgical case, palliation was best achieved by insuring patency of the left mainstem bronchus.

Infectious Tracheobronchitis

A number of infections, both acute and more often chronic, may affect the trachea and proximal bronchi, resulting in both focal and diffuse airway disease.

Acute Tracheitis

Typically seen in children, acute bacterial tracheitis may rarely be seen in an adult population. Most often characterized by acute upper airway obstruction resulting in stridor, endoscopically there may be evidence of purulent debris, mucosal ulcerations, and edema (69). Not surprisingly, acute bacterial infection most often occurs in patients with underlying malignancies or AIDS (70). Although CT reports are lacking, we recently encountered a patient with known lymphoma who rapidly developed diffuse tracheal wall thickening associated with diffuse mediastinal edema, who subsequently rapidly improved on antibiotic therapy (Fig. 3-21).

Tuberculosis of the Trachea and Mainstem Bronchi

Tuberculosis typically involves the distal trachea and proximal mainstem bronchi; isolated tracheal disease is rare (71,72). Clinically, patients often present with a barking cough that is unresponsive to antitussive medication and associated with variable amounts of sputum. Less commonly, patients present with localized wheezing or hemoptysis (73). Radiographically, there is usually evidence of either parenchymal consolidation or atelectasis consequent to bronchial obstruction; however, normal radiographs may occur in as many as 8% of patients (73). Bronchoscopic findings reflect the stage of disease. Early in the course of infection, hyperplastic changes are identified with congestion and edema causing luminal narrowing. Histologically there is evidence of lymphocytic infiltration of the bronchial mucosa with subsequent ulceration and caseous necrosis. Endoscopic examination at this time reveals luminal narrowing frequently accompanied by a whitish

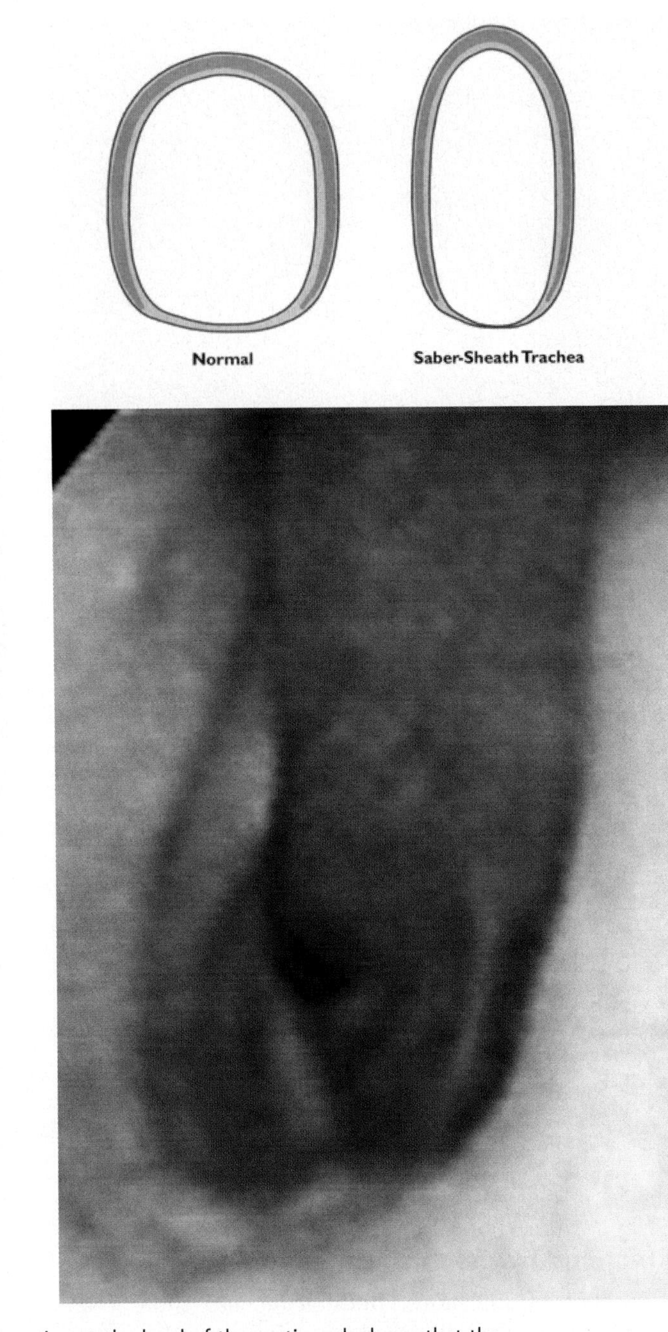

A

Figure 3-20 Saber-sheath trachea. **A:** Axial section at the level of the aortic arch shows that the sagittal length of the trachea is more than twice the width of the trachea—a finding characteristic of a saber-sheath trachea. **B:** Typical appearance of saber-sheath trachea compared with normal trachea. Cartilage appears as dark gray. Narrowing of the trachea is caused by deformity of tracheal cartilage. Mucosa and submucosa appear normal. **C:** Bronchoscopic image in the same patient shows similar appearance of marked narrowing of the width of the trachea. Note that, although the lumen of the trachea appears smooth on CT, accurate evaluation of the tracheal mucosa requires endoscopy. (**B:** From Webb EM, Elicker BM, Webb WR. Using CT to diagnose nonneoplastic tracheal abnormalities: appearance of the tracheal wall. *AJR Am J Roentgenol* 2000;174:1315–1321, with permission.)

pseudomembrane. Subsequent fibrosis of the lamina propria with healing of mucosal ulcerations leads to cicatricial stenosis. Surprisingly, despite active infection, prebronchoscopic sputum samples are often negative; in a study of 121 patients with documented endobronchial tuberculosis, Lee et al. (73) noted that only 17% of patients had smears positive for acid-fast bacilli (AFB). In this same series, the overall diagnostic yield from sputum evaluation was still only 79%. It should be noted that even endoscopic evaluation may not be diagnostic; in a study of 28 patients with endobronchial tuberculosis evaluated by Choe et al. (74), endobronchial biopsy proved nonspecific in 10.

The role of CT in evaluating patients with endobronchial tuberculosis has been extensively described

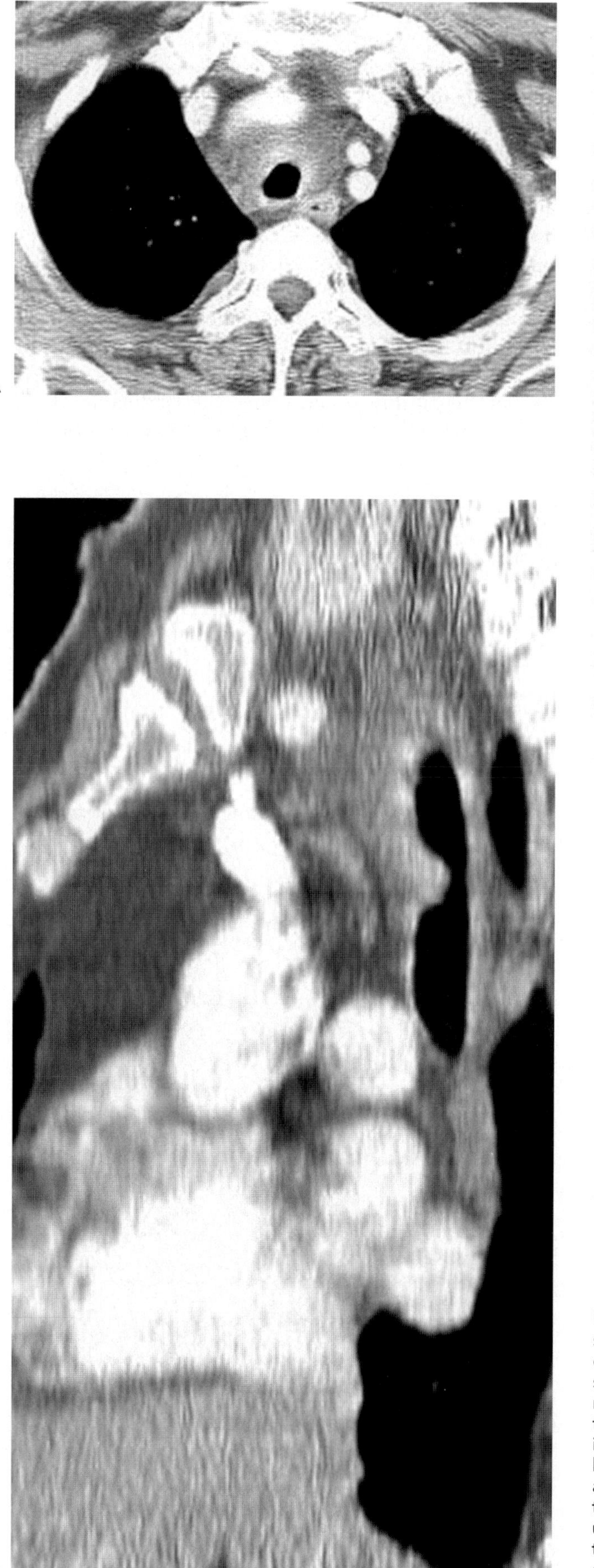

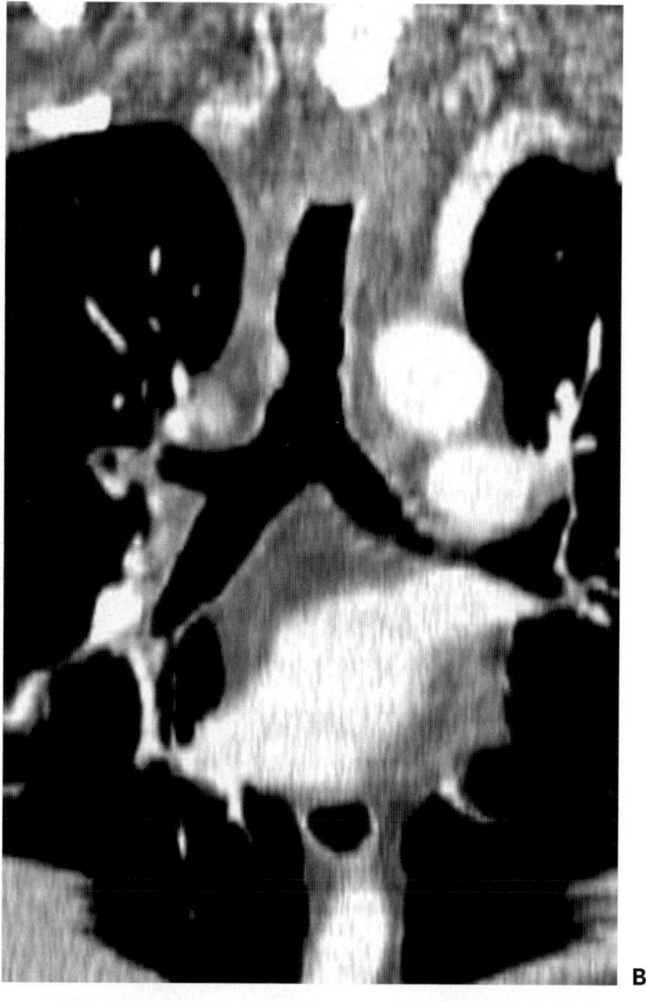

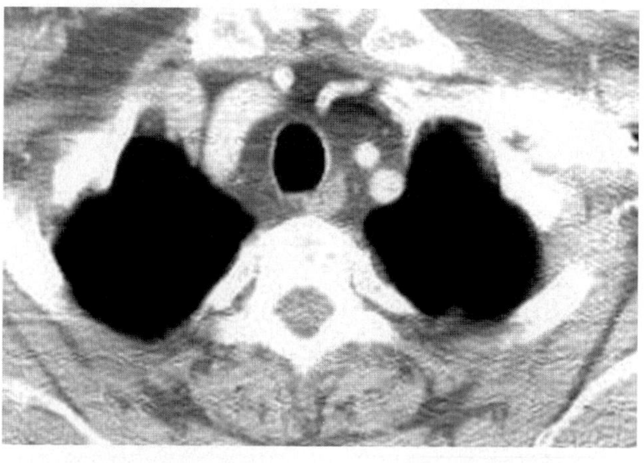

Figure 3-21 Acute bacterial tracheitis. **A** to **C:** Axial, coronal, and sagittal images through the trachea, respectively, show evidence of diffuse peritracheal edema with loss of visualization of the normally sharply defined tracheal wall, in this case owing to edematous mediastinal fat. The tracheal lumen appears narrowed. CT of the thorax several months before this study showed no evidence of intrathoracic pathology in this patient with a known nasopharyngeal lymphoma (not shown). Endoscopic biopsy performed several days after initiation of antibiotic therapy showed nonspecific inflammation only, without evidence of tumor. **D:** Axial image through the upper trachea shows complete resolution of mediastinal inflammation with a normal tracheal wall and tracheal lumen following a course of antibiotic therapy.

(71,72,74). Not surprisingly, CT findings tend to reflect the stage of disease. In patients with acute or subacute infection, the most common finding is loss of definition of the bronchial wall resulting from adjacent lymphadenopathy, usually accompanied by nonspecific bronchial narrowing or obstruction (Fig. 3-22). Distal tracheal and proximal mainstem bronchial involvement is the rule (74). Both enhancement of the tracheal wall and rim enhancement of adjacent tuberculous lymph nodes have been reported in patients with acute inflammation after the administration of intravenous contrast material (72,74). Rarely, tuberculous nodes may be observed to cavitate resulting in communication with the adjacent airway (Fig. 3-23). Acute infection may even lead to the expectoration of portions of tracheal cartilage (75). Clearly, in this stage, CT differentiation between infection and tumor may prove difficult.

In distinction, in patients with late-stage or fibrotic stenoses, CT typically shows evidence of concentric bronchial stenosis associated with either smooth or irregular bronchial wall thickening, typically involving a long—greater than 3 cm—airway segment (Fig. 3-24). Unlike active infection, which involves both mainstem bronchi equally, fibrotic tuberculosis has been reported to more often involve the left main bronchus, perhaps because of its greater length. Fibrotic stenosis may be subtle. In their study of 28 patients with tuberculous stenoses, Choe et al. (74) found that two patients had normal CT examinations, despite the acquisition of high-resolution 1.5-mm images.

A variety of theories have been proposed to account for endobronchial disease, including direct implantation of tubercle bacilli in bronchi; infiltration by adjacent medi-

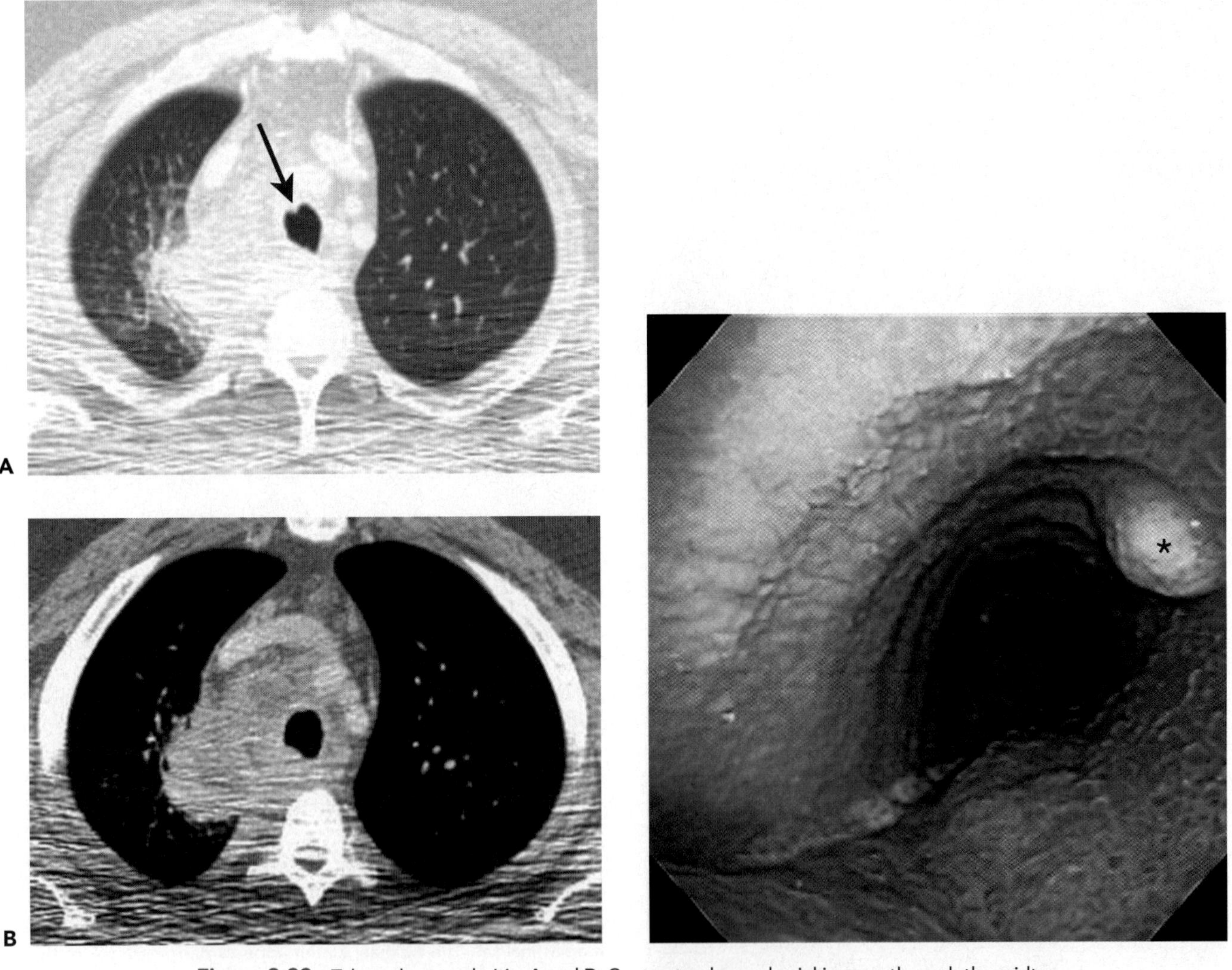

Figure 3-22 Tuberculous tracheitis. **A** and **B:** Contrast-enhanced axial images through the midtrachea, imaged with wide and narrow windows, respectively, show extensive low-density, rim-enhancing right paratracheal nodes causing eccentric narrowing of the posterolateral tracheal wall. Note apparent small nodule in the anterior tracheal wall in **A** *(arrow)*. **C:** Bronchoscopic image corresponding to the CT section in **A** shows extrinsic compression of the posterolateral tracheal wall on the right side *(asterisk)*, associated with diffuse, irregular nodularity of the trachea mucosa. Suspected polypoid lesion seen on CT is seen to better effect endoscopically. Endoscopically proved tuberculosis.

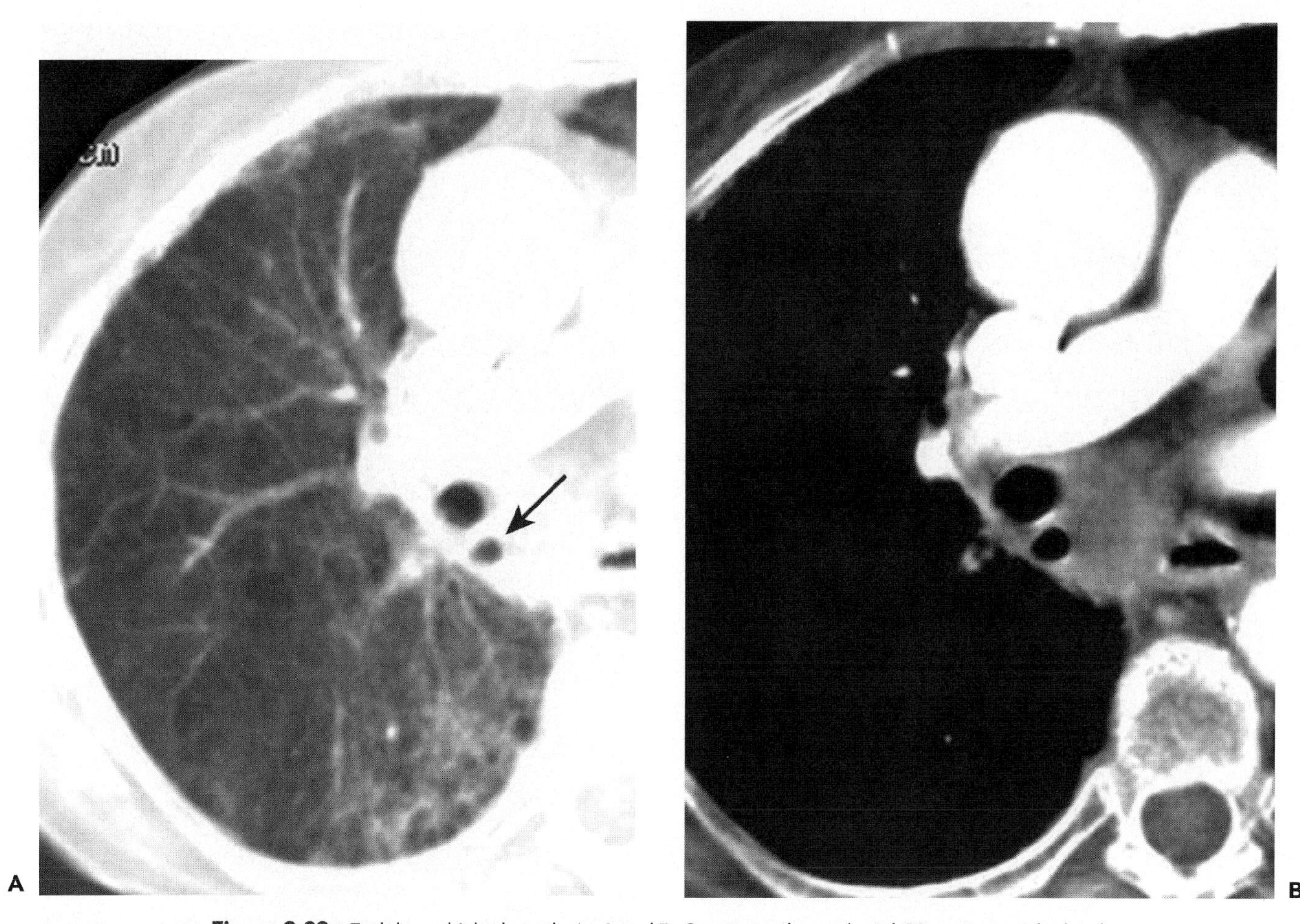

Figure 3-23 Endobronchial tuberculosis. **A** and **B:** Contrast-enhanced axial CT sections at the level of the bronchus intermedius, imaged with wide and narrow windows, respectively, show enlarged subcarinal nodes. A focal collection of air can be identified medial to the bronchus intermedius, separate from the air-filled esophageal lumen (*arrow* in **A**). At this stage, communication between the subcarinal nodes and adjacent bronchus was not prospectively identified. *(continued)*

astinal or hilar lymph nodes; and lymphohematogenous spread, in particular extension into the peribronchial region by lymphatic drainage from areas of active infection within the lungs (73). With appropriate antituberculous drugs and corticosteroid therapy, infection is usually, although not invariably, reversible. CT findings in patients with central airway tuberculosis are rarely specific. As noted by Moon et al. (72), findings that help to differentiate tuberculous disease from bronchogenic carcinoma include longer circumferential involvement and the absence of an intraluminal mass. Notwithstanding these distinctions, accurate diagnosis usually requires histologic evaluation.

Nontuberculous Granulomatous Tracheobronchitis/Rhinoscleroma

Rhinoscleroma (RS) is a slowly progressive granulomatous infection caused by *Klebsiella rhinoscleromatis,* a capsulated gram-negative bacterium (76–78). Typically involving the upper respiratory tract, in particular the nose, upper lip, hard palate, and maxillary sinuses, this organism may also involve the trachea and proximal bronchi in up to 10% of patients (78). RS is endemic in tropical and subtropical areas with more than 80% of cases reported from Central and South America, Africa, India, Indonesia, and Eastern and Central Europe (79). Although only sporadically seen in the United States, the prevalence of this disease is rising as a consequence of the ease of international travel. Clinically and pathologically the disease is usually divided into three stages. In the catarrhal-atrophic stage, there is evidence of profuse purulent inflammation. Histologically, there is evidence of squamous metaplasia associated with neutrophilic infiltration. In the granulomatous phase, nodules and masses are present, causing usually partial obstruction of the involved airways and leading to hoarseness and stridor when the larynx is involved. Histologically, this phase is typified by so-called pseudoepitheliomatous hyperplasia characterized by Mikulicz cells, large, vacuolated histiocytes, and Russell bodies, eosinophilic structures within the cytoplasm of plasma cells (79). In the final sclerotic stage, the airways appear deformed, with stenoses developing secondary to fibrosis. The diagnosis is generally established by either biopsy or positive culture, present in approximately 50% of patients. CT evaluation shows evidence of diffuse nodular

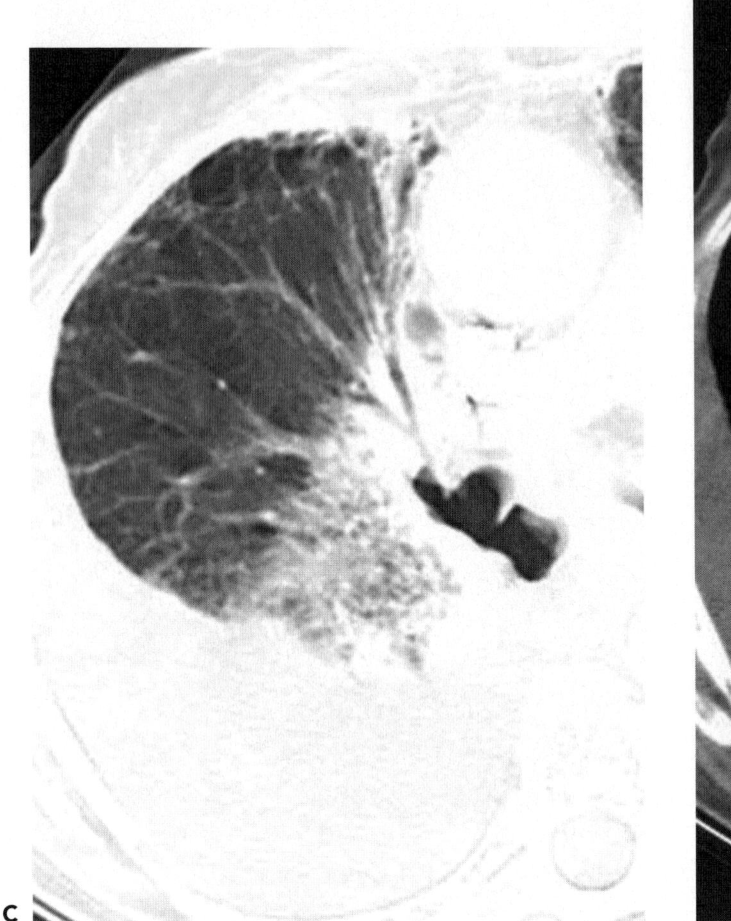

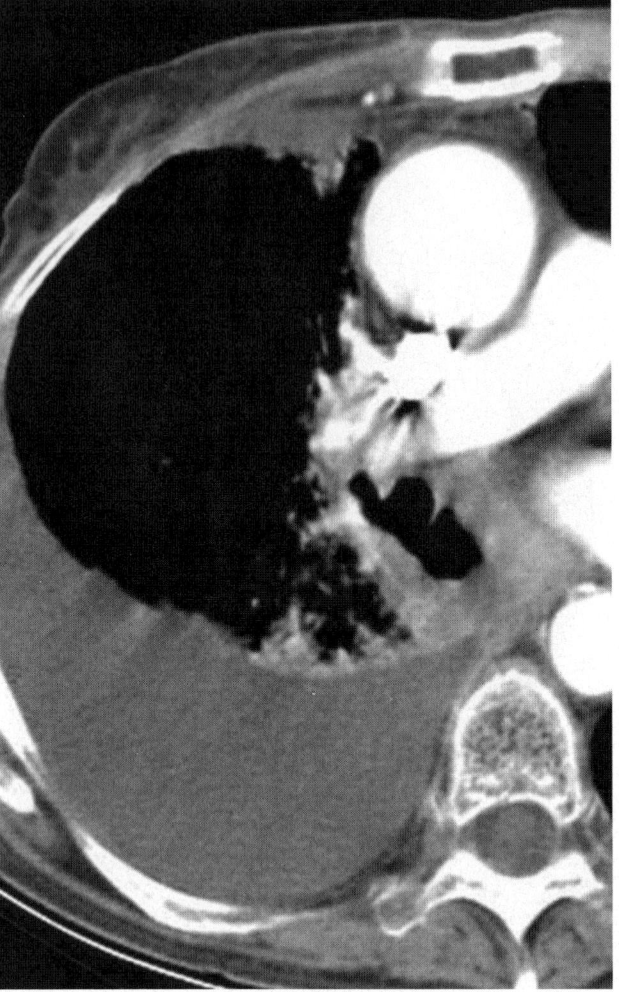

Figure 3-23 *(continued)* **C** and **D:** Follow-up CT sections obtained several days later following the development of a large right-sided effusion, show wide-open fistulization between the bronchus and adjacent necrotic lymph nodes. Endobronchial tuberculosis was subsequently verified endoscopically.

thickening of the trachea and proximal bronchi with associated narrowing of the airways (Fig. 3-25). There may also be evidence of mediastinal or hilar adenopathy. With airway obstruction, patchy parenchymal consolidation may also be identified. Although antibiotics generally result in immediate improvement, RS is difficult to eradicate, and the infection frequently relapses.

Fungal Tracheobronchitis/Aspergillosis

Aspergillosis infection is associated with a wide range of intrathoracic manifestations. Within the airways, aspergillosis takes many forms, including saprophytic colonization, tracheobronchitis, ulcerative tracheobronchitis with or without pseudomembrane formation, and necrotizing (invasive) aspergillosis (80). Necrotizing aspergillosis may be further subdivided into acute and chronic airway invasive forms (81). Acute tracheobronchitis is uncommon and is usually restricted to the central airways. It usually occurs in severely immunocompromised individuals, especially those with underlying malignancies or AIDS or following bone marrow, lung, or heart transplantation (82). Histologically there is evidence of respiratory epithelial ulceration and submucosal inflammation. CT examination reveals nonspecific multifocal or diffuse tracheobronchial wall thickening, resulting in either smooth or nodular luminal narrowing (80,81,83). To date, treatment with antifungal agents has generally proved unsuccessful in immunocompromised patients. Necrotizing tracheobronchitis in an immunocompromised patient resulting in acute obstruction of the right mainstem bronchus with subsequent bronchial wall necrosis and rupture of the adjacent pulmonary artery and leading to death has been reported (84).

Sarcoidosis

Involvement of the peripheral airways is common in sarcoidosis as a result of the presence of perilymphatic granulomas and accounts for the high diagnostic yield of transbronchial biopsies in most patients (85). Involvement of the larynx and subglottic space is still rarer, reported to occur in only 1% to 3% of patients (31). On high-resolution CT,

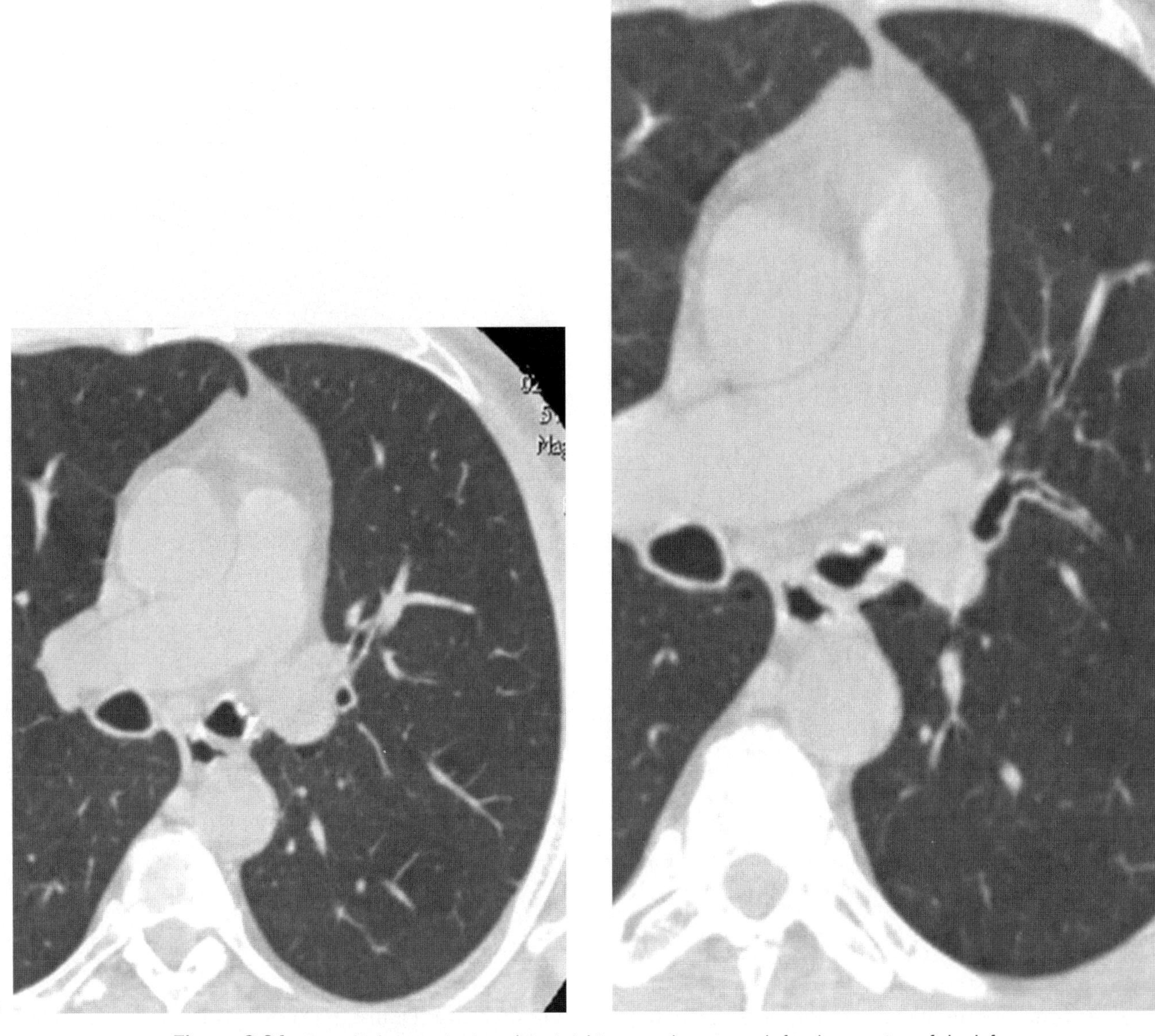

Figure 3-24 Bronchial stenosis. **A** and **B:** Axial images show smooth focal narrowing of the left mainstem bronchus in this patient with a history of tuberculosis treated earlier. Note the absence of mediastinal adenopathy, apparent even with wide windows. *(continued)*

focal nodular thickening of segmental and subsegmental bronchi is commonly seen. Although the trachea and mainstem bronchi may appear narrowed because of the presence of extensive mediastinal and hilar adenopathy, visualization of discrete endobronchial lesions is uncommon (Fig. 2-10) (68).

Relapsing Polychondritis

Relapsing polychondritis is a rare multisystem disorder that results in the inflammation and destruction of cartilaginous tissue throughout the body (31,43,53,69). Thought to be related to abnormal acid mucopolysaccharide metabolism, relapsing polychondritis also affects proteoglycan-rich structures including the cardiovascular system, eyes, skin, and internal organs (86). Involvement of medium- and large-sized blood vessels results in aneurysms, and in a small percentage of patients, valvular heart disease including aortic and mitral insufficiency may develop (79,87). The diagnosis is made on clinical grounds; there are no pathognomonic histologic or laboratory findings. As proposed by McAdam et al. (88), the diagnosis is considered conclusive when patients have at least three of the following six defined features of the disease: respiratory tract, bilateral auricular, or nasal chondritis; nonerosive seronegative inflammatory arthritis; ocular inflammation; or audiovestibular damage.

Clinically the disease is characterized by recurrent episodes of inflammation that most often affect the ears, joints, and respiratory tract. Respiratory tract symptoms represent the initial clinical findings in approximately 15% of patients, and involvement of the trachea and bronchi ultimately occurs in up to 50% of patients. Patients typically

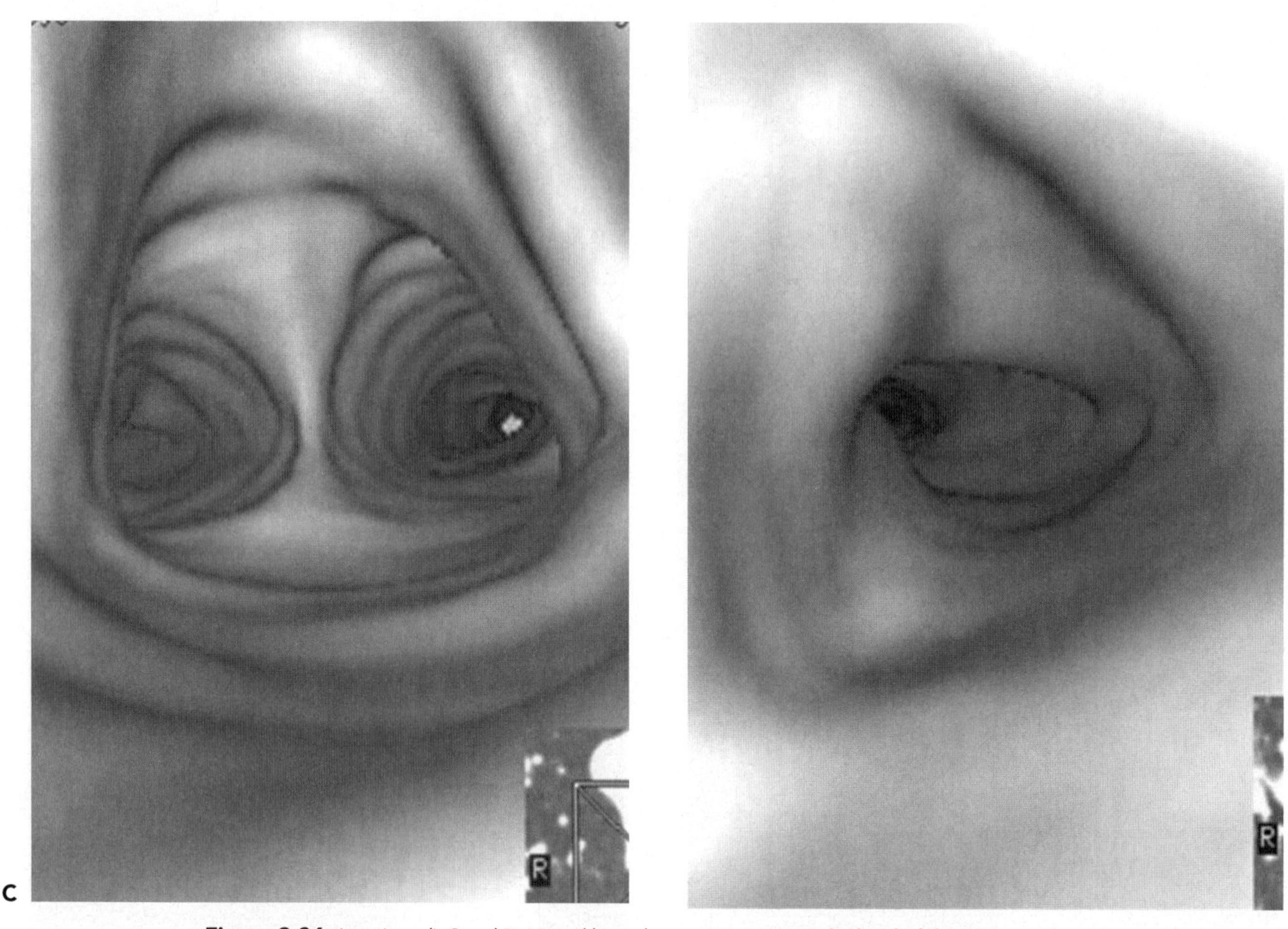

Figure 3-24 *(continued)* **C** and **D:** Virtual bronchoscopic images at the level of the carina and proximal left mainstem bronchus (in this case oriented in the same direction as the corresponding CT) also shows a focal bronchial stricture to good advantage.

present with nonspecific respiratory tract symptoms, including cough, dyspnea, and wheezing; hoarseness and aphonia are also frequently noted (86). Progressive laryngotracheal inflammation may lead eventually to severe tracheal stenosis from a combination of edema, granulation tissue, cartilage destruction, and fibrosis (86,87). With increasing severity, airway obstruction and recurrent episodes of atelectasis and pneumonia may result. Unfortunately, respiratory tract involvement is one of the most serious consequences of this disease, accounting for up to 50% of deaths (86).

Several early reports documented the CT findings in patients with relapsing polychondritis (31). Most commonly seen is a combination of increased airway wall attenuation in association with smooth tracheal and/or bronchial wall thickening that characteristically spares the posterior membranous portions of the trachea (Figs. 3-26 and 3-27) (89). As described by Behar et al. (90), the degree of increased attenuation may range from subtle to a finding of frank calcification (Fig. 3-27); the latter may be difficult to differentiate from calcifications owing to advanced age. Diffuse tracheal narrowing usually represents a later phase of disease, occurring in at least one series in only 33% of patients (90). Focal stenoses may also occur, although far less commonly (89). Unlike other diffuse tracheal diseases, relapsing polychondritis is rarely associated with either diffuse parenchymal lung disease or bronchiectasis.

No single therapy has yet proved universally effective. The disease may either remain indolent or prove rapidly fatal (91). Most patients with airway disease have been managed with a combination of medications, including nonsteroidal antiinflammatory drugs; corticosteroids and other immunosuppressive agents, including azathioprine, methotrexate, and cyclosporine, among others. Although these drugs may temporarily decrease the severity and intensity of recurrences, they fail to prevent disease progression. CT may be of particular value in documenting a response to therapy by demonstrating decreased tracheal wall thickening, potentially obviating more invasive follow-up procedures (87). In refractory cases, self-expandable metallic stents have been used to provide long-term palliation (91).

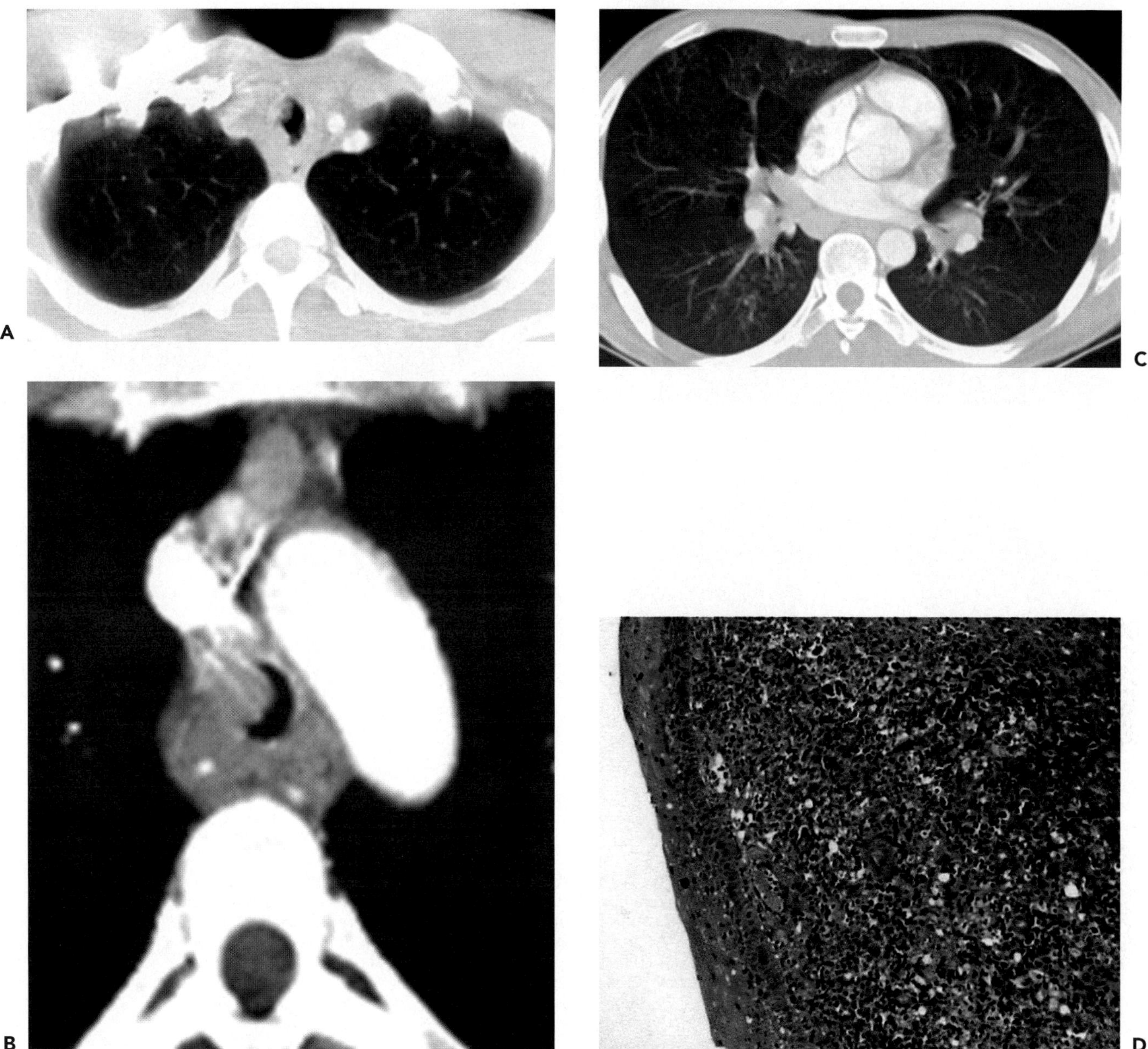

Figure 3-25 Rhinoscleroma. **A** to **C:** Axial CT sections at the level of the thoracic inlet, distal trachea, and proximal lower lobe bronchi, respectively, in a 26-year-old immigrant complaining of persistent cough and chest pain. These images show a combination of nodular thickening of the tracheal and bronchial walls, resulting in marked luminal narrowing associated with mediastinal and hilar adenopathy. **D:** Endoscopic biopsy of the tracheal wall shows squamous mucosa with acute inflammation, characterized by dense infiltration with plasma cells, lymphocytes, and histiocytes. Subsequent evaluation revealed intracellular bacilli consistent with rhinoscleroma.

Wegener's Granulomatosis (WG)

Wegener's granulomatosis is a disease of unknown etiology that is characterized by a necrotizing granulomatous vasculitis. Characteristically involving the upper and lower respiratory tract and kidneys, it is now recognized that the disease may involve any organ in the body, including the skin, joints, middle ear, eye, and nervous system (92). Formerly considered universally fatal, early diagnosis leading to successful treatment with immunosuppressive therapy has been facilitated by the recognition that in 90% of patients, highly specific serum antineutrophil cytoplasmic antibodies (cANCA)—characterized by a diffuse granular cytoplasmic immunofluorescent staining pattern—may be detected (92).

The lungs are the most commonly affected organ; disease restricted to the respiratory system, so-called limited Wegener's, is found in up to 10% of patients (93). Clinically, patients present with a wide spectrum of nonspecific symptoms including cough, dyspnea, and chest pain. Hemoptysis has been noted to occur in up to 40% of patients (93).

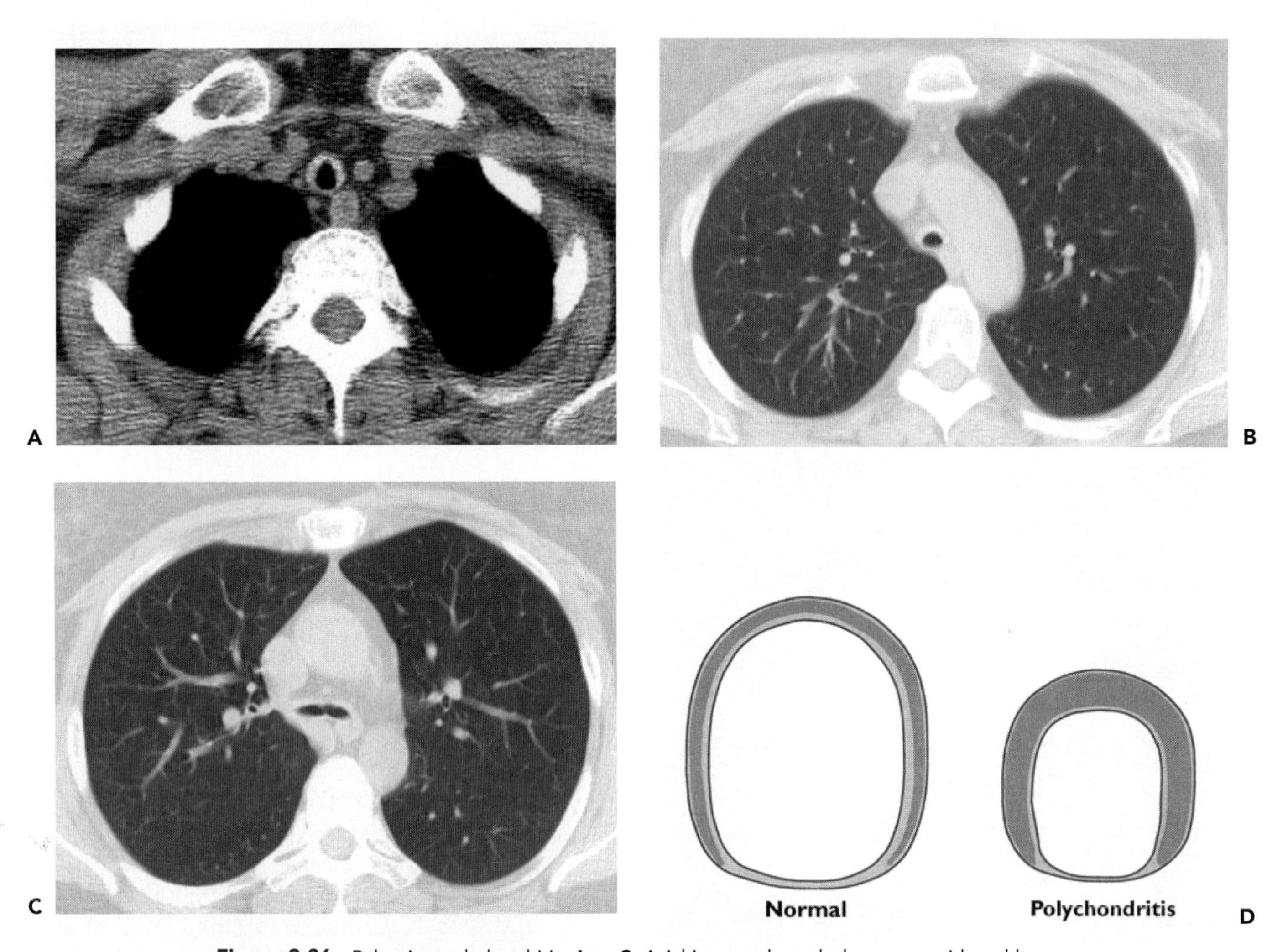

Figure 3-26 Relapsing polychondritis. **A** to **C:** Axial images through the upper, mid, and lower trachea/carina, respectively, show typical appearance of diffuse, uniform tracheal and mainstem bronchial wall thickening with sparing of the posterior membranous wall of the trachea. Note the absence of mediastinal adenopathy. **D:** Drawing shows typical appearance of polychondritis with thickened anterior and lateral tracheal walls resulting from thickened tracheal cartilage with sparing of the posterior membranous tracheal wall. (**C:** Webb EM, Elicker BM, Webb WR. Using CT to diagnose nonneoplastic tracheal abnormalities: appearance of the tracheal wall. *AJR Am J Roentgenol* 2000;174:1315–1321, with permission.)

Radiographically, Wegener's granulomatosis usually manifests as multiple, frequently cavitary parenchymal nodules or as areas of either diffuse or, more commonly, focal consolidation (93). These may be either bilateral or unilateral without an apparent predilection for any specific lung zone. Although most patients have radiographic evidence of lung disease, findings indicative of airway disease are only rarely observed.

CT findings have been extensively reported (93–103). In one study of 30 patients with documented Wegener's granulomatosis, 29 of 30 (97%) had abnormal CT studies at the time of presentation (98). Nodules and masses were most commonly observed and occurred in 90% of patients. Most often bilateral, these nodules characteristically proved to be either subpleural (simulating pulmonary infarction) or peribronchovascular in distribution (98). Interestingly, feeding vessels were a frequent observation, consistent with underlying vasculitis. Central cavitation, both irregular and thick walled and smooth and thin walled, was also common, typically occurring only in lesions larger than 2 cm. In this study, patchy foci of consolidation or ground-glass attenuation were less frequently noted, occurring in approximately 25% of patients (98).

Involvement of both central and peripheral airways is a common and important manifestation of Wegener's granulomatosis. Cordier et al. (93), in a study of 77 patients with documented disease, found that 55% in whom fiberoptic bronchoscopy was performed proved to have airway involvement, including inflammatory lesions with and without bronchial stenosis, ulcerations and pseudotumors, and isolated hemorrhagic foci. Similarly, Daum et al. (95), in their study of 51 patients who were all evaluated bronchoscopically, found endobronchial abnormalities in

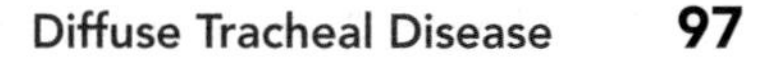

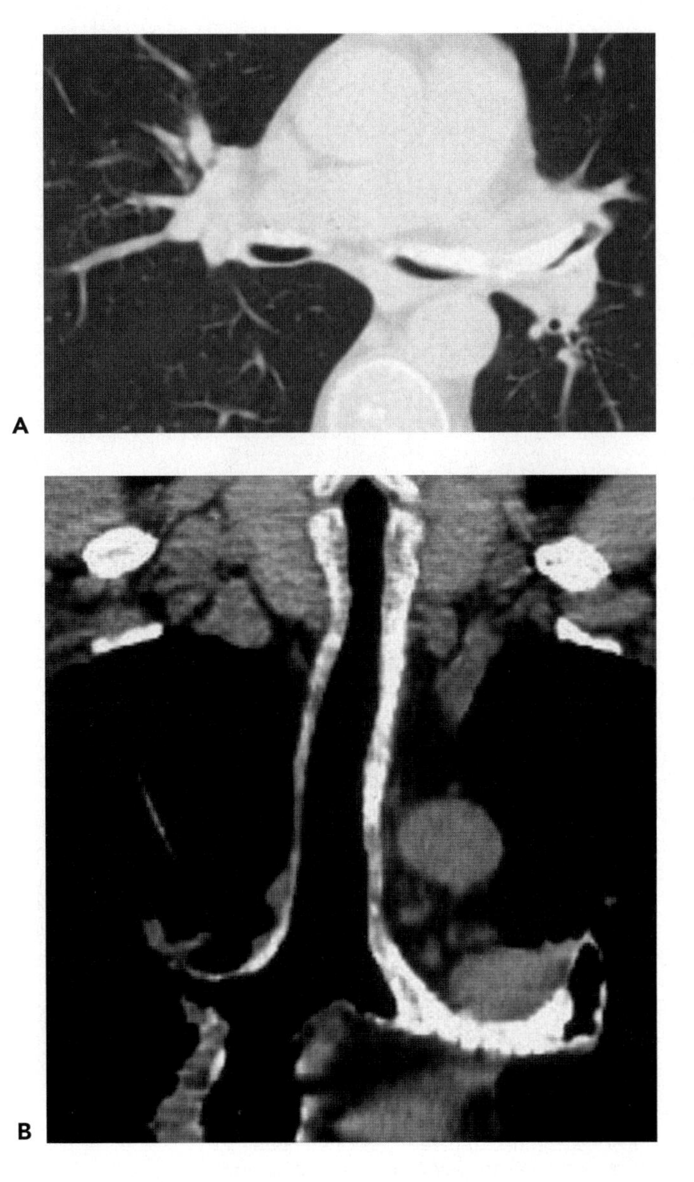

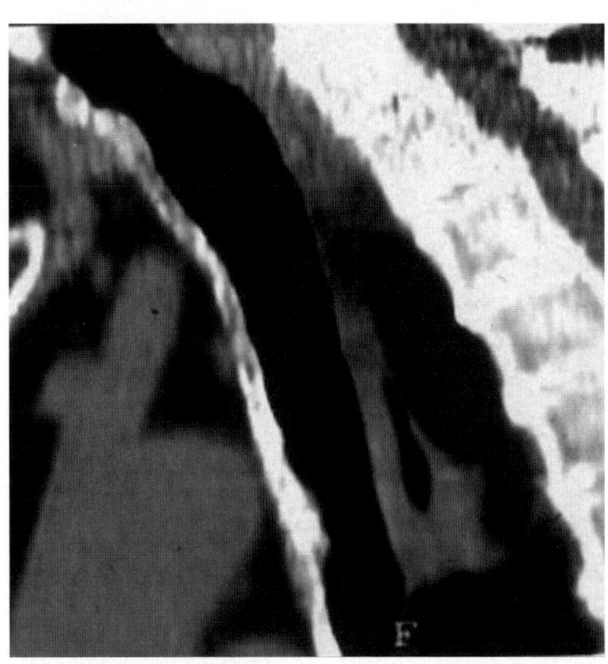

Figure 3-27 Relapsing polychondritis. **A:** Axial image through the subcarinal space shows marked narrowing/stenosis of the bronchus intermedius and especially of the left mainstem and upper lobe bronchi without evidence of adenopathy. Note sparing of the posterior wall of the bronchus intermedius. **B** and **C:** Coronal and sagittal reconstructions, respectively, show extensive tracheal and bronchial cartilage calcifications with marked diffuse narrowing. (From Grenier PA, et al. New frontiers in CT imaging of the airways. *Eur Radiol* 2002;12:1022–1044, with permission.)

59%, including subglottic stenosis in 17%, ulcerating tracheobronchitis in 60%, tracheal or bronchial stenoses in 13%, and hemorrhage without an identifiable source in another 4% of patients. Interestingly, in this same study, no correlation was noted between cANCA levels and the presence of tracheobronchial inflammation. Furthermore, a specific histologic diagnosis of Wegener's granulomatosis could be made bronchoscopically in only approximately 17% of patients.

Recent studies also have confirmed that airway lesions are common, seen on CT in up to 40% of patients (101–103). Lee et al. (98), for example, reported that central airway abnormalities could be identified in 30% of patients, while evidence of segmental and subsegmental bronchial wall thickening with and without luminal narrowing or obliteration was identifiable in 73% of patients (Figs. 3-28 to 3-30). Centrilobular nodules were also noted, presumably the result of peripheral bronchiolar inflammation. In this same study, bronchiectasis was diagnosed by CT in 13% of patients. Screaton et al. (97), in a study of 10 patients with known tracheal involvement, noted that 90% of lesions were subglottic and identifiable as short segments of circumferential mucosal thickening; the degree of luminal narrowing ranged from 23% to 100%. Two patients showed evidence of cartilaginous involvement resulting in deformed airways. Additional reported CT findings include marked airway narrowing on expiration, consistent with tracheobronchomalacia, as well as diffuse mediastinal adenopathy.

In addition to assessing the extent of disease initially, CT has proved of value in follow-up. Lee et al. (98) evaluated 20 follow-up CT studies; in 25% there was total resolution of previously identified parenchymal and airway abnormalities, whereas in 12 only partial resolution was noted. Evidence of recurrent disease was identified in only three patients. Airway lesions may occur in the course of therapy, possibly because of prolonged survival with use of cytotoxic agents. Aberele et al. (94), in their series of 19 patients, identified symptomatic airway lesions in 5 patients in the

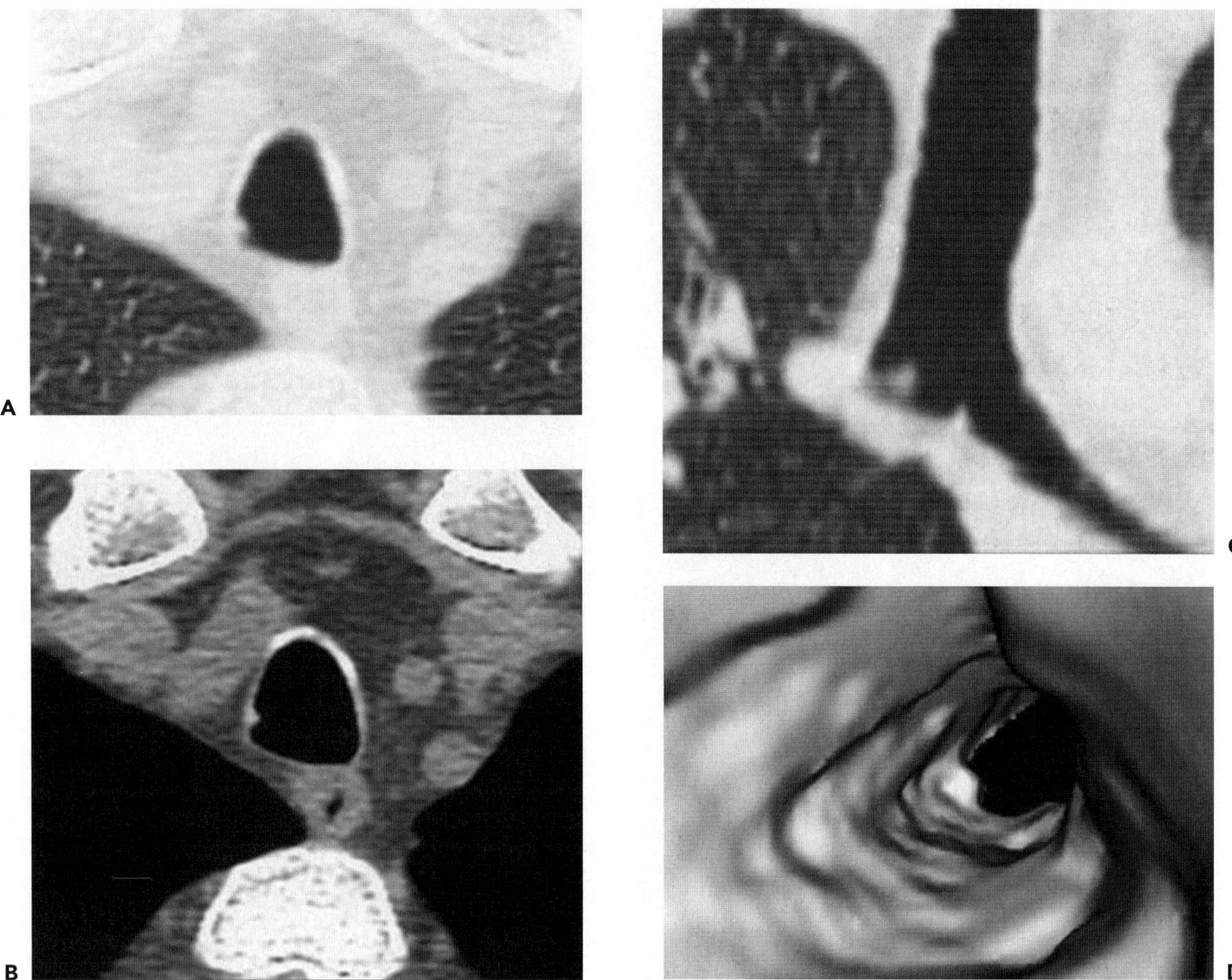

Figure 3-28 Wegener's granulomatosis. **A** and **B:** Axial section through the upper trachea imaged with wide and narrow windows, respectively, shows a tiny, well-defined apparently calcified nodule in the posterolateral wall of the trachea. **C:** Coronal reconstruction at the level of the proximal right mainstem bronchus shows an additional well-defined nodule. **D:** Virtual bronchoscopic image shows diffuse nodularity throughout the trachea, with the largest nodule corresponding to the nodule identified in **C.** In this case, the true extent of disease is best seen on the virtual endoscopic images. Findings subsequently confirmed bronchoscopically. (Grenier PA, et al. New frontiers in CT imaging of the airways. *Eur Radiol* 2002;12:1022–1044, with permission.)

course of eight relapses, manifested as hoarseness, cough, or stridor. More recently, in an attempt to distinguish active pulmonary disease from inactive cicatricial disease, Komocsi et al. (104) evaluated high-resolution CT findings in 28 patients before and after immunotherapy. Although CT disclosed evidence of substantial residual damage, including residual nodules, it could be distinguished from active disease by the small nodule size (<15 mm) and lack of cavitation. Residual reticular markings—both septal and nonseptal—were also frequently noted, some occurring after initiation of therapy. However, over a 2-year follow-up period, patients with residual nodules or reticular densities had no more relapses than patients in whom initial lesions completely resolved, suggesting that CT is of value in distinguishing active from inactive inflammation. Finally, in select patients, CT may prove invaluable by demonstrating optimal sites for tracheostomy as well as by defining the true extent of disease when bronchial narrowing precludes complete bronchoscopic evaluation. In this setting, virtual bronchoscopy has been advocated as a means for evaluating central airway stenoses (105).

Amyloidosis

Amyloidosis refers to a collection of disease entities characterized by the deposition of an autologous fibrillar protein and associated protein derivatives in extracellular tissues. Together these elements are arranged in a pleated sheet, secondary structure that can accumulate either in single organs or diffusely throughout the body, resulting in a wide range of clinical symptoms. Histochemically,

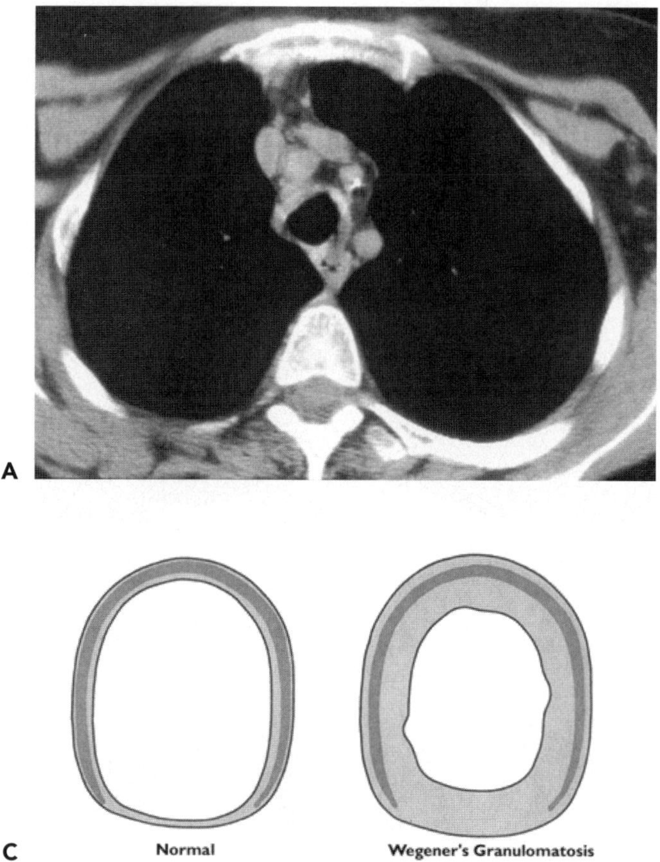

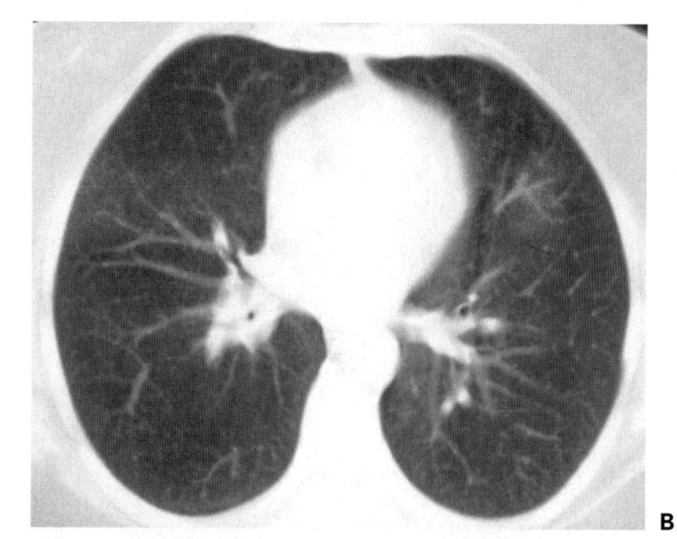

Figure 3-29 Wegener's granulomatosis. **A:** Axial image through the midtrachea showing irregular nodular thickening of the tracheal wall associated with increased soft tissue density in the right paratracheal space. **B:** Axial section shows marked narrowing of the origin of the middle lobe bronchus associated with hilar adenopathy. In this case, the lung parenchyma appeared normal. **C:** Drawing showing typical appearance of Wegener's granulomatosis with evidence of mucosal and submucosal inflammation resulting in concentric thickening of the tracheal wall with mucosal ulcerations identifiable in some patients. (**C:** Webb EM, Elicker BM, Webb WR. Using CT to diagnose nonneoplastic tracheal abnormalities: appearance of the tracheal wall. *AJR Am J Roentgenol* 2000;174:1315–1321, with permission.)

amyloid binds with Congo red, showing green birefringence in polarized light. Although amyloidosis is classically divided into two broad categories, primary and secondary, as defined by the World Health Organization, precise classification is dependent on recognition of the specific fibrillar protein that defines the type of amyloidosis (106). In primary amyloidosis, the defining protein is almost always a fragment of the variable immunoglobulin light chain (AL) and thus varies from person to person. In distinction, secondary amyloidosis involves the amino acid terminus of the acute phase protein serum amyloid A (SAA) and is identical in all patients. SAA is subsequently cleaved by macrophages to form amyloid A (AA) (107). As the name implies, secondary amyloidosis usually develops

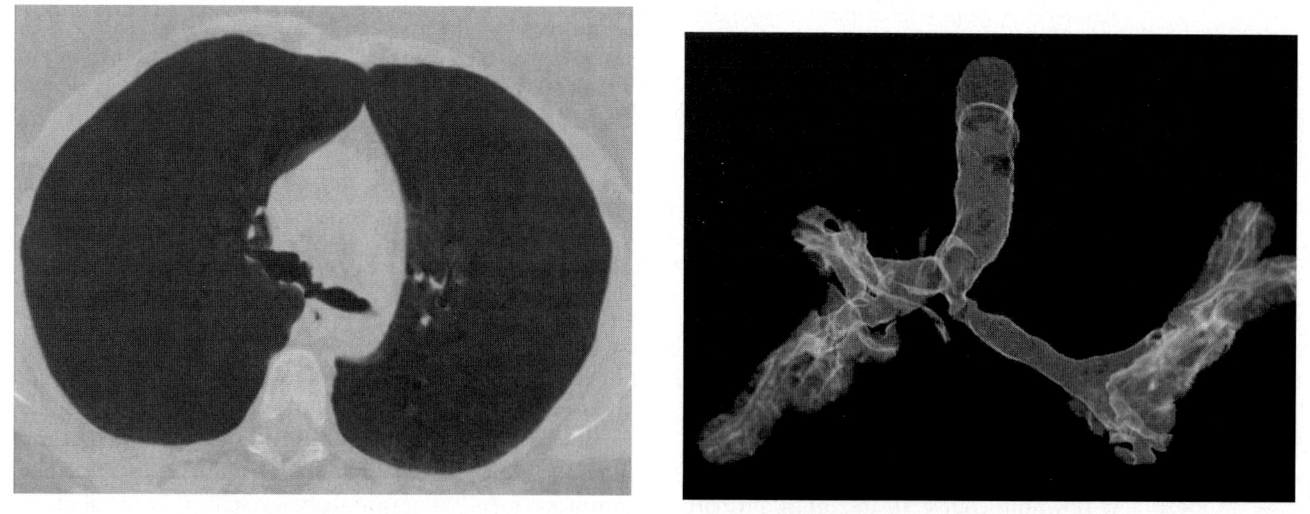

Figure 3-30 Wegener's granulomatosis. **A:** Axial minimum-intensity projection image shows irregular nodular thickening of the carina. **B:** 3D surface rendering of same patient showing to advantage focal stenosis at the origin of the left mainstem bronchus. As shown in Fig. 3-31, additional retrospective imaging may be of value in select cases to more accurately reflect airway abnormalities.

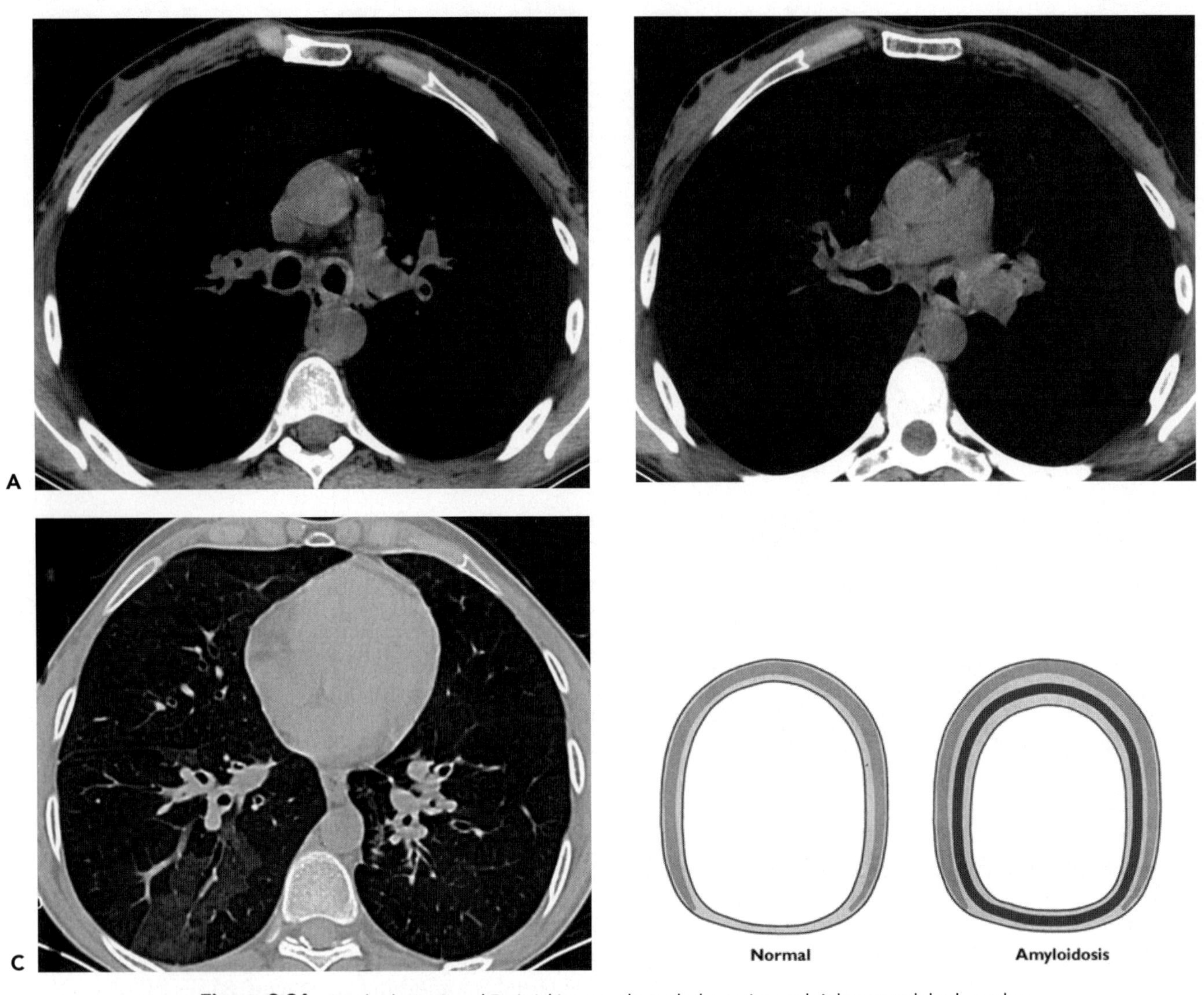

Figure 3-31 Amyloidosis. **A** and **B:** Axial images through the carina and right upper lobe bronchus, respectively, show diffuse bronchial wall thickening causing diffuse luminal narrowing, in this case in the absence of abnormal calcifications. **C:** Axial image through the lower lobes shows that bronchial wall thickening extends peripherally into the proximal basilar bronchi. Note the presence of mosaic attenuation consistent with air trapping, presumably the result of coexisting small-airway disease. **D:** Drawing shows typical appearance of tracheal amyloidosis. Submucosal deposits of amyloid result in concentric smooth or nodular thickening of the tracheal wall. Calcification (shown in black) is common and may also be concentric or nodular in appearance. (Case courtesy of Dr. Page McAdams, Chapel Hill, North Carolina; **D:** Webb EM, Elicker BM, Webb WR. Using CT to diagnose nonneoplastic tracheal abnormalities: appearance of the tracheal wall. *AJR Am J Roentgenol* 2000;174:1315–1321, with permission.)

as a response to a wide range of chronic inflammatory diseases, including cystic fibrosis, tuberculosis, and bronchiectasis, among others.

Primary systemic amyloidosis results from clonal expansion of plasma cells within the bone marrow and results in multiorgan accumulation of amyloid. It is this form of the disease that is frequently associated with either multiple myeloma or Waldenström's macroglobulinemia and tends to have an inexorable downhill course. In the lungs, primary systemic amyloidosis results in diffuse interstitial infiltration.

In distinction, localized amyloidosis typically involves a single organ. Although this form of the disease is also characterized by deposition of monoclonal immunoglobulin light chains, there is no evidence of marrow plasmacytosis, nor is there evidence of proteinuria as is usually seen in patients with primary systemic amyloidosis. Within the lung, three types of localized amyloidosis have been identified: tracheobronchial, nodular, and diffuse alveolar septal amyloidosis (108,109).

Although tracheobronchial amyloidosis is the most common form of respiratory system involvement in patients with localized amyloidosis, to date only several hundred cases have been reported (110). The disease is characterized by the presence of either multifocal or diffuse

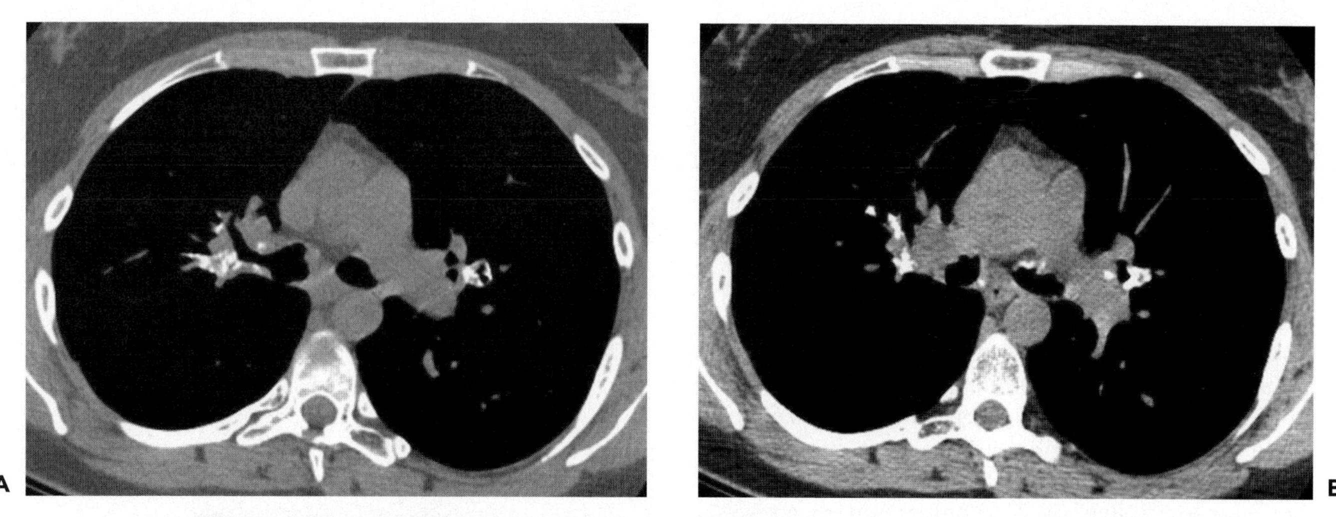

Figure 3-32 Amyloidosis. **A** and **B:** Axial images through the carina and subcarinal space, respectively, show extensive nodular calcifications throughout the bronchial tree associated with mild bronchial wall thickening. This appearance should not be confused with the cartilaginous calcifications typically seen in elderly individuals.

submucosal plaques or masses. Endobronchial biopsies are diagnostic. Clinical manifestations reflect the portion of the tracheobronchial tree affected (109). In patients with proximal subglottic or laryngeal involvement, patients typically present with hoarseness or stridor. In distinction, involvement of the distal trachea or mainstem, lobar, or proximal segmental bronchi results in cough, wheezing, dyspnea, or hemoptysis. In cases in which bronchial obstruction occurs, patients may present with fever secondary to obstructive pneumonitis (111). Nodular parenchymal amyloidosis is less commonly seen than is tracheobronchial amyloidosis and is usually characterized by multiple peripheral or subpleural nodules that vary from a few millimeters to several centimeters in size; calcifications are identified in up to 50% of lesions. Patients are rarely symptomatic (111). Diffuse parenchymal amyloidosis, although typically identified in patients with primary systemic amyloidosis, is the least common form of

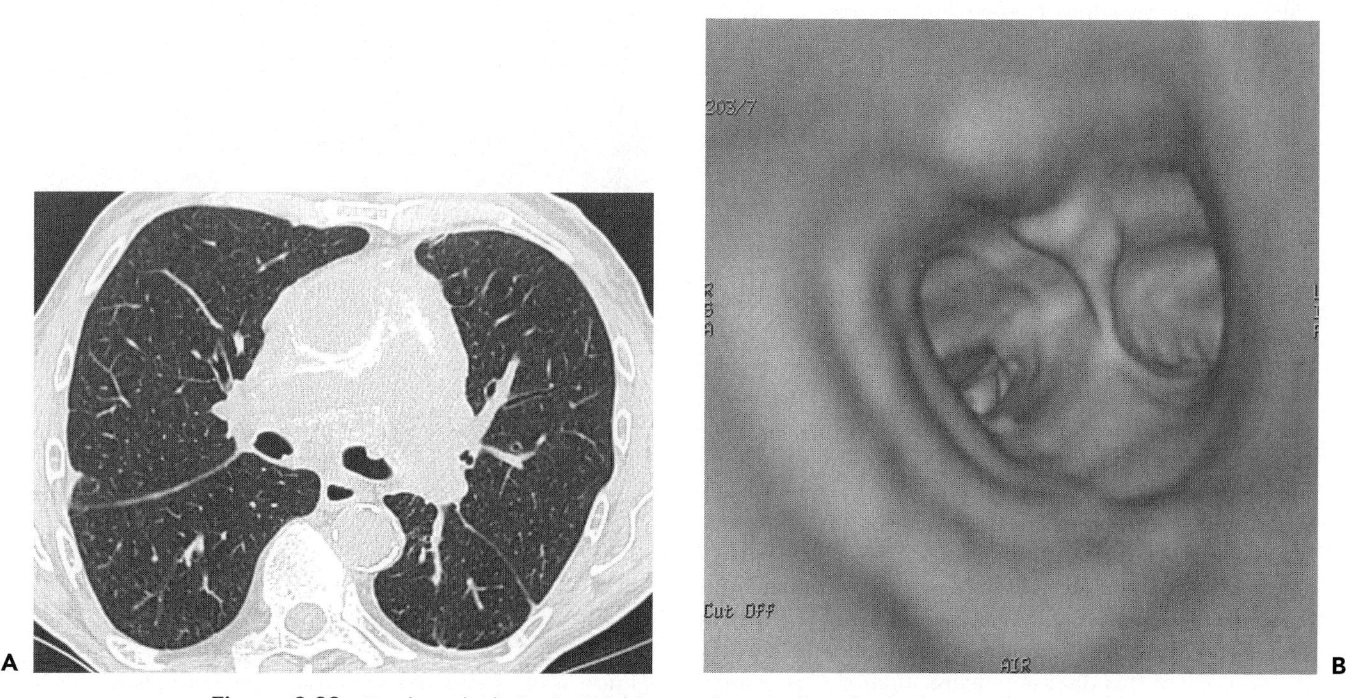

Figure 3-33 Focal amyloidosis. **A:** Axial image through the subcarinal space shows discrete nodules in the medial wall of the bronchus intermedius and the anterior wall of the left mainstem bronchus. **B:** Virtual bronchoscopic image showing additional nodules in the distal trachea and carina. Biopsy proved amyloidosis.

localized amyloidosis. It is characterized by diffuse reticulonodular opacities with prominent interlobular and intralobular septae (111).

CT findings in patients with tracheobronchial amyloid have been reported (99,107,109–114). Typically, amyloid results in circumferential tracheal or bronchial wall thickening because of the submucosal deposition of nodules or plaques, frequently resulting in luminal narrowing (Figs. 3-31 and 3-32). In its nodular form, amyloid appears as a focal mass partially or completely occluding airways and with infiltration of the adjacent paratracheal or bronchial tissues (Fig. 3-33). In this form, it may mimic the appearance of both benign and malignant tracheal neoplasms. Mural calcifications are prominent features, although calcifications are rarely identified bronchoscopically. It should be emphasized that calcifications are in themselves a nonspecific finding. In addition to the presence of calcified tracheal and bronchial rings in older populations or, more rarely, those occurring in association with warfarin therapy, care must also be taken to differentiate cartilaginous calcifications from calcified lymph nodes (115,116). In patients with recurrent infiltrates, bronchiectasis may also be identified. Differential diagnosis includes relapsing polychondritis, tracheobronchopathia osteochondroplastica (TPO), and granulomatous tracheitis. Interestingly, there have been rare reports of concurrent tracheobronchial amyloid and TPO (110). However, in the vast majority of cases, these entities prove pathologically distinct; specifically, although both result in heterotopic calcifications, in patients with TPO, Congo red stains are uniformly negative.

In patients with severe narrowing, therapy usually involves repeated attempts at debulking lesions using either forceps or Nd:YAG laser resection. Despite initial response, disease progression often necessitates repeated resections (110). In patients with subglottic involvement, tracheostomies may be required. In these patients, unfortunately, an association has been noted between proximal death and early death resulting from respiratory insufficiency (109).

Tracheobronchopathia Osteochondroplastica

TPO is a rare disorder characterized by multiple submucosal cartilaginous or osseous nodules or spicules that project into the tracheobronchial lumen. Histologically these have been shown to contain heterotopic bone, cartilage, and calcified acellular protein matrix as well as hemopoietic and fatty elements. The overlying bronchial mucosa is typically normal in appearance. Although any part of the tracheobronchial tree may be affected, in most series the distal trachea and proximal bronchi are most often involved. Because they arise from cartilaginous tracheal and bronchial rings, the membranous posterior wall of the trachea is characteristically spared. Although the etiology of this disease remains unknown, two theories have been proposed. In one, nodules have been attributed to enchondroses and exostoses arising from the perichondrium of cartilage rings; in the other, nodules have been attributed to cartilaginous or bony metaplasia (117). Other theories, including the possibility that TPO represents the end stage of tracheobronchial amyloidosis, have largely been discredited.

Most patients remain asymptomatic, with the diagnosis made clinically in less than 10% of patients (118). Tracheopathia osteochondrolytica has been reported to cause hemoptysis (119). Other symptoms include cough, dyspnea, hoarseness, and stridor. Recurrent lower respiratory tract infections may occur secondary to rare instances of bronchial obstruction.

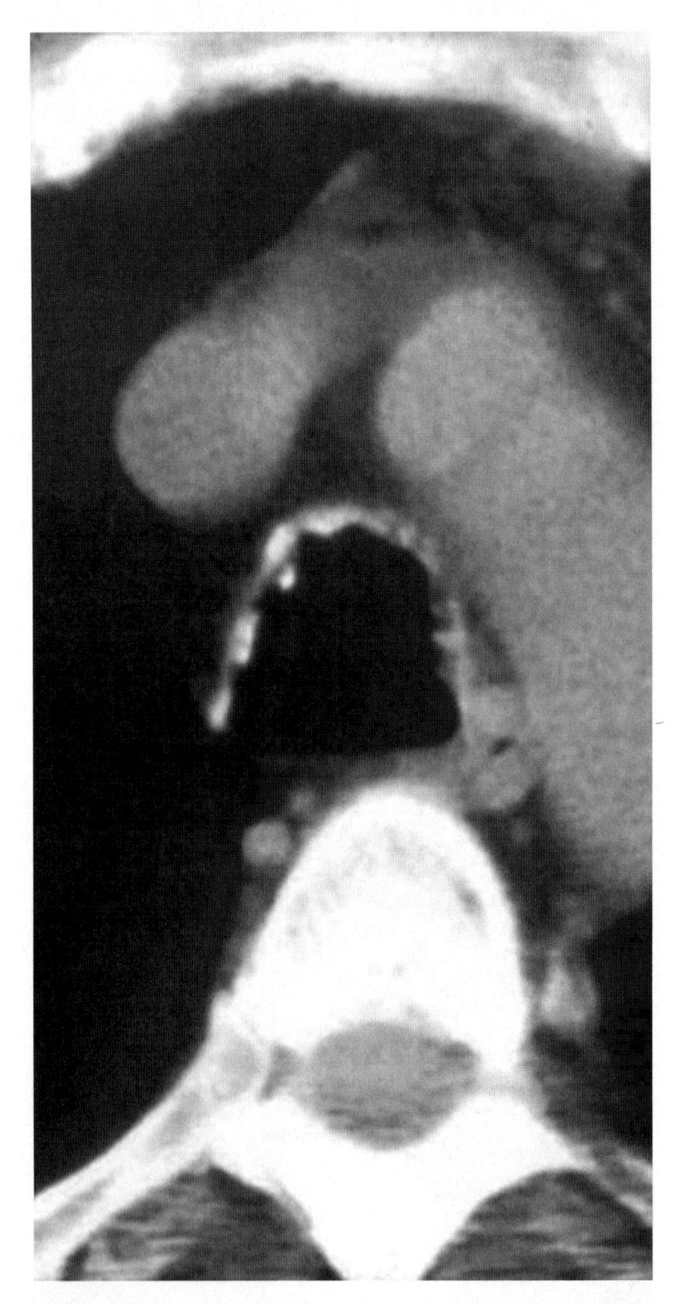

Figure 3-34 Tracheobronchopathia osteochondroplastica (TPO). Axial image through the midtrachea shows characteristic appearance of calcified nodules, in this case resulting in no appreciable luminal narrowing. Note the absence of involvement of the posterior membranous trachea wall (also see Fig. 2-6).

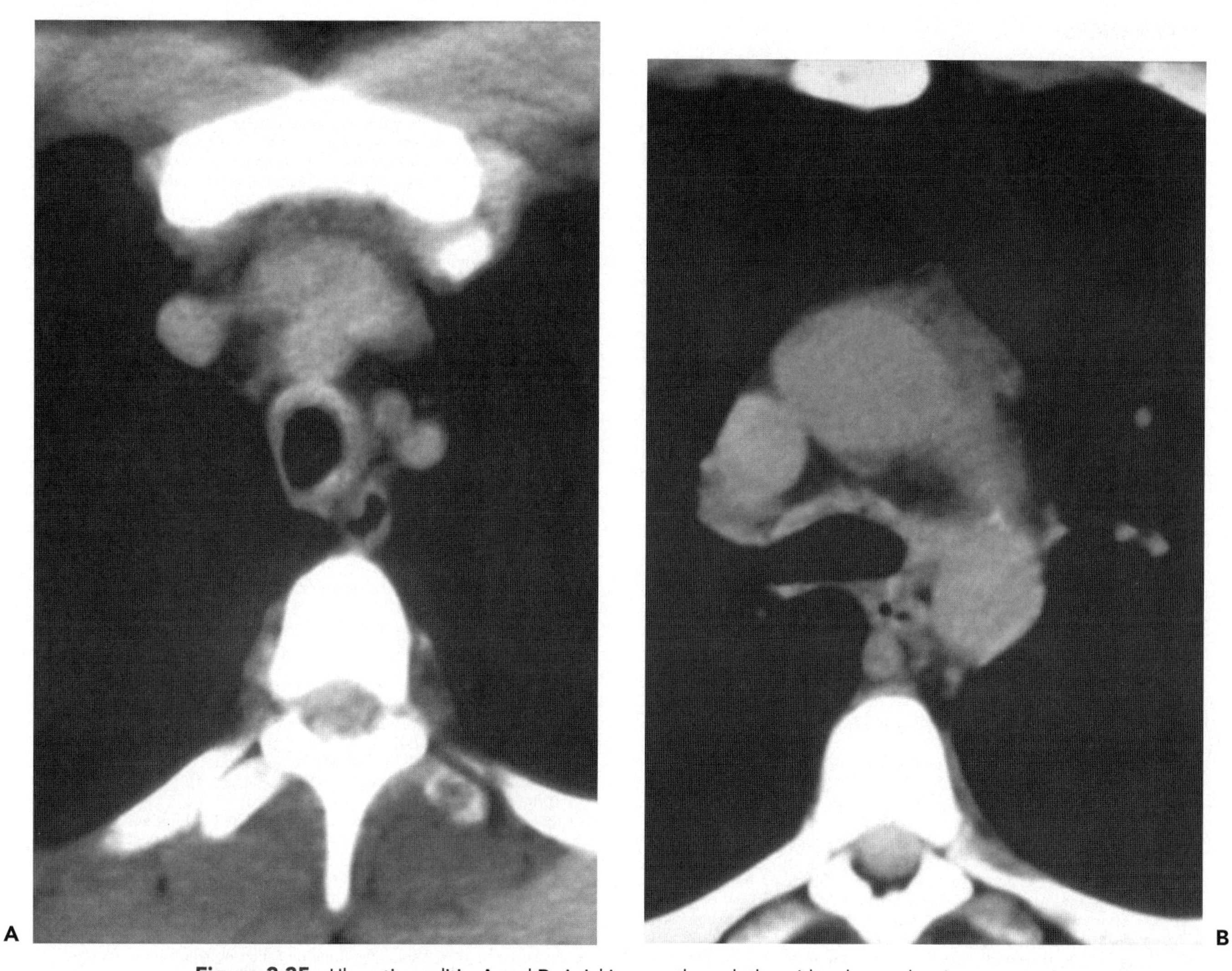

Figure 3-35 Ulcerative colitis. **A** and **B:** Axial images through the midtrachea and carina, respectively, show nonspecific, diffuse wall thickening typical of central airway involvement in patients with inflammatory bowel disease.

Bronchoscopically, lesions appear as multiple yellow-white, hard papillary nodules that may be difficult to biopsy because of their bony nature (Fig. 3-34; see also Fig. 2-6). The trachea is usually described as exceedingly rigid. Although chest radiographs are usually interpreted as normal, even in retrospect the diagnosis is easily established with CT (31,120–122). Findings include horseshoe-shaped thickening of the tracheal wall associated with multifocal calcific densities, the largest of which protrude into the tracheal lumen. The cartilaginous rings themselves may also appear deformed. As noted previously, the posterior membranous portion of the trachea is spared. In most patients, the disease progresses slowly, if at all. Therapy is requisite only when the tracheal or bronchial lumens become compromised.

Ulcerative Colitis

Ulcerative colitis is a known, albeit rare, cause of pulmonary disease. Abnormalities reported to date include pulmonary vasculitis as well as apical fibrosis. An association with chronic bronchitis and bronchiectasis has also been reported (123). Wilcox et al. (124) have also reported two patients with documented ulcerative colitis presenting with severe airflow obstruction. In one, findings similar to those found in patients with constrictive bronchiolitis were identified; however, histologic evaluation revealed an unusual pattern of sclerosing peribronchiolitis in the absence of inflammation or fibrosis predominantly involving terminal airways. The other patient showed evidence of marked compromise of the tracheal and proximal bronchial lumens secondary to a diffuse sclerosing tracheobronchitis without evidence of bronchiectasis (Fig. 3-35). These findings, although considerably varied, suggest that a spectrum of airway pathology exists in association with inflammatory bowel disease. To date, no apparent relationship has been established between disease activity within the colon and airway inflammation; in fact, airway disease may occur even years after colectomy (124).

REFERENCES

1. Berkmen YM. The trachea: the blind spot in the chest. *Radiol Clin North Am* 1984;22:539–562.
2. Karmy-Jones R, Jurkovich GJ. Blunt chest trauma. *Curr Prob Surg* 2004;41:223–380.
3. Baumgartner F, et al. Tracheal and main bronchial disruptions after blunt chest trauma: presentation and management. *Ann Thorac Surg* 1990;50:569–574.
4. Rossbach MM, et al. Management of major tracheobronchial injuries: a 28-year experience. *Ann Thorac Surg* 1998;65:182–186.
5. Kirsh MM, et al. Management of tracheobronchial disruption secondary to nonpenetrating trauma. *Ann Thorac Surg* 1976;22:93–101.
6. Carbognani P, et al. Management of postintubation membranous tracheal rupture. *Ann Thorac Surg* 2004;7:406–409.
7. Unger JM, et al. Tears of the trachea and main bronchi caused by blunt trauma: radiologic findings. *AJR Am J Roentgenol* 1989;153:1175–1180.
8. Chen J-D, et al. Using CT to diagnose tracheal rupture. *AJR Am J Roentgenol* 2001;176:1273–1280.
9. Rollins RJ, Tocino I. Early radiographic signs of tracheal rupture. *AJR Am J Roentgenol* 1987;148:695–698.
10. Palder SB, Shandling B, Manson D. Rupture of the thoracic trachea following blunt trauma: diagnosis by CAT scan. *J Pediatr Surg* 1991;26:1320–1322.
11. Lupetin AR. Computed tomographic evaluation of laryngotracheal trauma. *Curr Probl Diagn Radiol* 1997;26:185–206.
12. Wintermark M, Schnyder P, Wicky S. Blunt traumatic rupture of a mainstem bronchus: spiral CT demonstration of the "fallen lung" sign. *Eur Radiol* 2001;11:409–411.
13. Balci AE, et al. Surgical treatment of post-traumatic tracheobronchial injuries: 14-year experience. *Eur J Cardio Thorac Surg* 2002;22:984–989.
14. Tsunezuka Y, et al. Spontaneous tracheal rupture associated with acquired tracheobronchomalacia. *Ann Thorac Cardiovasc Surg* 2003; 9:394–396.
15. Stark P. Imaging of tracheobronchial injuries. *J Thorac Imaging* 1995;10:206–219.
16. Zwischenberger JB, Sankar AB. Surgery of the thoracic trachea. *J Thorac Imaging* 1995;10:199–205.
17. Devine N, et al. Bronchial anastomotic complications in lung transplantation: CT assessment. *J Radiol* 1996;77:477–481.
18. Fullerton DA, Campbell DN. Airway problems in lung transplantation. *Semin Respir Crit Care Med* 1996;17:187–196.
19. Herman S, et al. Single-lung transplantation: imaging features. *Radiology* 1989;170:89–93.
20. Murray JG, et al. Pictorial essay. Complications of lung transplantation: radiologic findings. *AJR Am J Roentgenol* 1996;166:1405–1411.
21. O'Donovan P. Imaging of complications of lung transplantation. *Radiographics* 1993;13:787–796.
22. Whyte RI, et al. Helical computed tomography for the evaluation of tracheal stenosis. *Ann Thorac Surg* 1995;60:27–31.
23. Ferretti GR, et al. Benign abnormalities and carcinoid tumors of the central airways: diagnostic impact of CT bronchography. *AJR Am J Roentgenol* 2000;174:1307–1313.
24. Hoppe H, et al. Grading airway stenosis down to the segmental level using virtual bronchoscopy. *Chest* 2004;125:704–711.
25. Rea F, et al, Benign tracheal and laryngotracheal stenosis: surgical treatment and results. *Eur J Cardio Thorac Surg* 2002;22:352–356.
26. Pearson FG, Todd TRJ, Cooper JD. Experience with primary neoplasms of the trachea. *J Thorac Cardiovasc Surg* 1984;88:511–516.
27. Grillo HC, Mathisen DJ. Primary tracheal tumors: treatment and results. *Ann Thorac Surg* 1990;49:69–77.
28. Grillo HC, Mathisen DJ, Wain JC. Management of tumors of the trachea. *Oncology* 1992;6:61–67.
29. Hazama K, et al. Clinicopathological investigation of 20 cases of primary tracheal cancer. *Eur J Cardio Thorac Surg* 2003;23:1–5.
30. McCarthy MJ, Rosado-de-Christenson ML. Tumors of the trachea. *J Thorac Imaging* 1995;10:180–198.
31. Kwong JS, Muller NL, Miller RR. Disease of the trachea and main-stem bronchi: correlation of CT with pathologic findings. *Radiographics* 1992;12:645–657.
32. Kwon JW, et al. Mucous gland adenoma of the bronchus: CT findings in two patients. *J Comput Assist Tomogr* 1999;23:758–760.
33. Kim TS, et al. Sialadenoid tumors of the respiratory tract: radiologic-pathologic correlation. *AJR Am J Roentgenol* 2001;177:1145–1150.
34. Maziak DE, et al. Adenoid cystic carcinoma of the airway: thirty-two-year experience. *J Thorac Cardiovasc Surg* 1996;112:1522–1531.
35. Kim TS, et al. Mucoepidermoid carcinoma of the tracheobronchial tree: radiographic and CT findings in 12 patients. *Radiology* 1999; 212:643–648.
36. Jeung M-Y, et al. Bronchial carcinoid tumors of the thorax: spectrum of radiologic findings. *Radiographics* 2002;22:351–365.
37. Rosado de Christenson ML, et al. Thoracic carcinoids: radiologic-pathologic correlation. *Radiographics* 1999;19:707–736.
38. Naidich DP. CT/MR correlation in the evaluation of tracheobronchial neoplasia. *Radiol Clin North Am* 1990;28:555–571.
39. Zwiebel BR, Austin JHM, Grines MM. Bronchial carcinoid tumors: assessment with CT of location and intratumoral calcification in 31 patients. *Radiology* 1991;179:483–486.
40. Barzo P, Molnar L, Minik K. Bronchial papillomas of various origins. *Chest* 1987;92:132–136.
41. Kramer SS, et al. Pulmonary manifestations of juvenile laryngotracheal papillomatosis. *AJR Am J Roentgenol* 1985;144:687–694.
42. Cosio BG, et al. Endobronchial hamartoma. *Chest* 2002;122:202–205.
43. Nguyen PT, Kvale PA. Endobronchial chondroid hamartoma. *J Bronchol* 1999;6:263–265.
44. Siegelman SS, Khouri NF, Scott WW. Pulmonary hamartoma: CT findings. *Radiology* 1986;160:313–317.
45. Reittner P, Muller NL. Tracheal hamartoma: CT findings in two patients. *J Comput Assist Tomogr* 1999;23:957–958.
46. Carlin BW, et al. Endobronchial metastases due to colorectal cancer. *Chest* 1989;96:1110–1114.
47. Wang J-C, et al. Tracheal invasion by thyroid carcinoma: prediction using MR imaging. *AJR Am J Roentgenol* 2001;177:929–936.
48. Nadrous HF, et al. Glomus tumor of the trachea: value of multidetector computed tomographic virtual bronchoscopy. *Mayo Clin Proc* 2004;79:237–240.
49. Muraoka M, et al. Endobronchial lipoma—review of 64 cases reported Japan. *Chest* 2003;123:293–296.
50. Allen MS. Malignant tracheal tumors. *Mayo Clin Proc* 1993;68:680–684.
51. Chan AL, et al. Advances in the management of endobronchial lung malignancies. *Curr Opin Pulm Med* 2003;9:301–308.
52. Webb EM, Elicker BM, Webb WR. Using CT to diagnose nonneoplastic tracheal abnormalities: appearance of the tracheal wall. *AJR Am J Roentgenol* 2000;174:1315–1321.
53. Choplin RH, Wehunt WD, Theros EG. Diffuse lesions of the trachea. *Semin Roentgenol* 1983;18:38–50.
54. Schwartz M, Rossoff L. Tracheobronchomegaly. *Chest* 1994;106:1589–1590.
55. Dunne MG, Reiner B. CT features of tracheobronchomegaly. *J Comput Assist Tomogr* 1988;12:388–391.
56. Roditi GH, Weir J. The association of tracheomegaly and bronchiectasis. *Clin Radiol* 1994;49:608–611.
57. Woodring JH, et al. Acquired tracheomegaly in adults as a complication of diffuse pulmonary fibrosis. *AJR Am J Roentgenol* 1989;152:743–747.
58. Shin MS, Jackson RM, Ho K-J. Case report. Tracheobronchomegaly (Mounier-Kuhn syndrome): CT diagnosis. *AJR Am J Roentgenol* 1988;150:777–779.
59. Stern EJ, et al. Normal trachea during forced expiration: dynamic CT measurements. *Radiology* 1993;187:27–31.
60. Aquino SL, et al. Acquired tracheomalacia: detection by expiratory CT scan. *J Comput Assist Tomogr* 2001;25:394–399.
61. Stern EJ, Webb WR. Dynamic imaging of lung morphology with ultrafast high-resolution computed tomography. *J Thorac Imaging* 1993;8:273–282.
62. Nishino M, et al. Value of volumetric data acquisition in expiratory high-resolution computed tomography of the lung. *J Comput Assist Tomogr* 2004;28:209–214.
63. Hein E, et al. Dynamic and quantitative assessment of tracheomalacia by electron beam tomography: correlation with clinical symptoms and bronchoscopy. *J Comput Assist Tomogr* 2000;24:247–252.
64. Marom EM, Goodman PC, McAdams HP. Pictorial essay—diffuse abnormalities of the trachea and main bronchi. *AJR Am J Roentgenol* 2001;176:713–717.
65. Greene R. "Saber sheath" trachea: relation to chronic obstructive pulmonary disease. *AJR Am J Roentgenol* 1978;130:441–445.
66. Gamsu G, Webb WR. Computed tomography of the trachea: normal and abnormal. *AJR Am J Roentgenol* 1982;139:3321–326.
67. Gamsu G, Webb WR. Computed tomography of the trachea and mainstem bronchi. *Semin Roentgenol* 1983;18:51–60.
68. Shepard JO, McLoud TC. Imaging the airways. *Clin Chest Med* 1991;12:151–168.
69. Kalender WA. Technical foundations of spiral CT. *Semin Ultrasound CT MRI* 1994;15:81–89.
70. Valor RR, et al. Bacterial tracheitis with upper airway obstruction in a patient with the acquired immunodeficiency syndrome. *Am Rev Respir Dis* 1992;146:1598–1599.
71. Kim Y, et al. Tuberculosis of the trachea and main bronchi: CT findings in 17 patients. *AJR Am J Roentgenol* 1997;168:1051–1056.
72. Moon WK, et al. Tuberculosis of the central airways: CT findings of active and fibrotic disease. *AJR Am J Roentgenol* 1997;169:649–653.
73. Lee JH, et al. Endobronchial tuberculosis: clinical and bronchoscopic features in 121 cases. *Chest* 1992;102:990–994.
74. Choe KO, Jeong HJ, Sohn HY. Tuberculous bronchial stenosis: CT findings in 28 cases. *AJR Am J Roentgenol* 1990;155:971–976.
75. Park MJ, et al. Endobronchial tuberculosis with expectoration of tracheal cartilages. *Eur Respir J* 2000;15:800–802.
76. Yigla M, et al. Laryngotracheobronchial involvement in a patient with nonendemic rhinoscleroma. *Chest* 2000;117:1795–1798.
77. Sedano HO, Carlos R, Koutlas IG. Respiratory scleroma: a clinicopathologic and ultrastructural study. *Oral Surg Oral Med Oral Pathol Oral Radiol Endod* 1996;81:665–671.

78. Amoils CP, Shindo ML. Laryngotracheal manifestations of rhinoscleroma. *Ann Otol Rhinol Laryngol* 1996;105:336–340.
79. Hart CA, Rao SK. Rhinoscleroma [Editorial]. *J Med Microbiol* 2000; 49:395–396.
80. Franquet T, et al. Necrotizing aspergillosis of large airways. CT findings in eight patients. *J Comput Assist Tomogr* 2002;26:342–345.
81. Buckingham SJ, Hansell DM. Aspergillus in the lung: diverse and coincident forms. *Eur Radiol* 2003;13:1786–1800.
82. Miller WTJ, et al. Pulmonary aspergillosis in patients with AIDS. Clinical and radiographic correlations. *Chest* 1994;105:37–44.
83. Franquet T, et al. Aspergillus infection of the airways computed tomography and pathologic findings. *J Comput Assist Tomogr* 2004;28:10–16.
84. Putnam JB, et al. Acute airway obstruction and necrotizing tracheobronchitis from invasive mycosis. *Chest* 1994;106:1265–1267.
85. Lenique F, et al. CT assessment of bronchi in sarcoidosis: endoscopic and pathologic correlations. *Radiology* 1995;194:419–423.
86. Trentham DE, Le CH. Relapsing polychondritis. *Ann Intern Med* 1998;129:114–122.
87. Im J-G, et al. CT manifestations of tracheobronchial involvement in relapsing polychondritis. *J Comput Assist Tomogr* 1988;12:792–793.
88. McAdam LP, et al. Relapsing polychondritis: prospective study of 23 patients and a review of the literature. *Medicine* 1976;55:193–215.
89. Tillie-Leblond I, et al. Respiratory involvement in relapsing polychondritis, clinical, functional, endoscopic, and radiographic evaluations. *Medicine* 1998;77:168–176.
90. Behar JV, et al. Relapsing polychondritis affecting the lower respiratory tract. *AJR Am J Roentgenol* 2002;178:173–177.
91. Sarodia BD, Dasgupta A, Mehta AC. Management of airway manifestations of relapsing polychondritis. Case reports and review of literature. *Chest* 1999;116:1669–1675.
92. Katzenstein A-LA. In: *Katzenstein and Askin's surgical pathology of non-neoplastic lung disease.* Philadelphia: WB Saunders, 1997.
93. Cordier JF, et al. Pulmonary Wegener's granulomatosis. A clinical and imaging study of 77 cases. *Chest* 1990;97:906–912.
94. Aberle DR, Gamsu G, Lynch D. Thoracic manifestations of Wegener granulomatosis: diagnosis and course. *Radiology* 1990;174:703–709.
95. Daum TE, et al. Tracheobronchial involvement in Wegener's granulomatosis. *Am J Respir Crit Care Med* 1995;151:522–526.
96. Deremee RA, Homburger HA, Specks U. Lesions of the respiratory tract associated with the finding of anti-neutrophil cytoplasmic autoantibodies with a perinuclear staining pattern. *Mayo Clin Proc* 1994; 69:819–824.
97. Screaton NJ, et al. Tracheal involvement in Wegener's granulomatosis: evaluation using spiral CT. *Clin Radiol* 1998;53:809–815.
98. Lee KS, et al. Thoracic manifestation of Wegener's granulomatosis: CT findings in 30 patients. *Eur Radiol* 2003;13:43–51.
99. Prince JS, et al. Nonneoplastic lesions of the tracheobronchial wall: radiologic findings with bronchoscopic correlation. *Radiographics* 2002; 22:S215–S230.
100. Kuhlman JE, Hruban RH, Fishman EK. Wegener granulomatosis: CT features of parenchymal lung disease. *J Comput Assist Tomogr* 1991; 15:948–952.
101. Foo SS, et al. Wegener granulomatosis presenting on CT with atypical bronchovasocentric distribution. *J Comput Assist Tomogr* 1990;14:1004–1006.
102. Maskell RG, Lockwood CM, Flower CDR. Computed tomography of the lung in Wegener's granulomatosis. *Clin Radiol* 1993;48:377–380.
103. Papiris SA, et al. Imaging of thoracic Wegener's granulomatosis: the computed tomographic appearance. *Am J Med* 1992;93:529–536.
104. Komocsi A, et al. Active disease and residual damage in treated Wegener's granulomatosis: an observational study using pulmonary high-resolution computed tomography. *Eur Radiol* 2003;13:36–42.
105. Summers RM, et al. CT virtual bronchoscopy of the central airways in patients with Wegener's granulomatosis. *Chest* 2002;121:242–250.
106. WHO–IUIS Nomenclature Sub-committee. Nomenclature of amyloid and amyloidosis. *Bull World Health Organ* 1993;71:105–112.
107. Georgiades CS, et al. Amyloidosis: review and CT manifestations. *Radiographics* 2004;24:405–416.
108. Utz JP, Patel AM, Edell ES. The role of transcarinal needle aspiration in the staging of bronchogenic carcinoma. *Chest* 1993;104:1012–1016.
109. O'Regan A, et al. Tracheobronchial amyloidosis. The Boston University experience from 1984 to 1999. *Medicine* 2000;79:69–79.
110. Mares DC, et al. Tracheobronchial amyloidosis: a review of clinical and radiographic characteristics, bronchoscopic diagnosis, and management. *J Bronchol* 1998;5:147–155.
111. Kim HY, et al. Localized amyloidosis of the respiratory system: CT features. *J Comput Assist Tomogr* 1999;23:627–631.
112. Urban BA, et al. CT evaluation of amyloidosis: spectrum of disease. *Radiographics* 1993;13:1295–1308.
113. Kirchner J, et al. CT findings in extensive tracheobronchial amyloidosis. *Eur Radiol* 1998;8:352–354.
114. Howard ME, Ireton J, Daniels F. Pulmonary presentations of amyloidosis. *Respirology* 2001;6:61–64.
115. Moncada RM, et al. Tracheal and bronchial cartilaginous rings: warfarin sodium-induced calcification. *Radiology* 1992;184:437–439.
116. Kim HY, et al. Bronchial anthracofibrosis (Inflammatory bronchial stenosis with anthracotic pigmentation): CT findings. *AJR Am J Roentgenol* 2000;174:523–527.
117. Briones-Gomez A, et al. Tracheopathia osteoplastica. *J Bronchol* 2000; 7:301–305.
118. Prakash UBS, et al. Tracheopathia osteoplastica: familial occurrence. *Mayo Clin Proc* 1989;64:1091–1096.
119. Martin CJ. Tracheopathia osteochondroplastica. Arch Otolaryngol 1974; 64:290–293.
120. Mariotta S, et al. Spiral CT and endoscopic findings in a case of tracheobronchopathia osteochondroplastica. *J Comput Assist Tomogr* 1997; 21:418–420.
121. Bottles K, et al. Case report. CT diagnosis of tracheobronchopathia osteochondroplastica. *J Comput Assist Tomogr* 1983;7:324–327.
122. Onitsuka H, et al. Computed tomography of tracheopathia osteoplastica. *AJR Am J Roentgenol* 1983;140:268–270.
123. Kraft SC, et al. Unexplained bronchopulmonary disease with inflammatory bowel disease. *Arch Intern Med* 1976;136:454–459.
124. Wilcox P, et al. Airway involvement in ulcerative colitis. *Chest* 1987; 92:18–22.
125. Grenier PA, et al. New frontiers in CT imaging of the airways. *Eur Radiol* 2002;12:1022–1044.

Bronchiectasis

4

Bronchiectasis is most simply defined as irreversible bronchial dilatation. It is usually associated with structural abnormalities of the bronchial wall, and chronic or recurrent infection is usually present. Bronchiectasis may occur as a result of various pathologic processes and thus may be a feature of a number of different lung and airway diseases (1–4).

Although chronic cough and expectoration of purulent sputum are common in patients with bronchiectasis, symptoms and physiologic abnormalities are usually nonspecific and a clinical diagnosis is often difficult to make. On the other hand, because bronchiectasis is defined by abnormal morphology, imaging provides an accurate diagnosis in most cases. Volumetric spiral computed tomography (SCT) with thin slices and high-resolution computed tomography (HRCT) are both highly accurate in the diagnosis of bronchiectasis and are routinely used in clinical practice.

PATHOLOGY OF BRONCHIECTASIS

Regardless of its cause, bronchiectasis is usually associated with (a) bronchial wall inflammation and infiltration by inflammatory cells; (b) destruction of the elastic, muscular, and cartilaginous elements of the bronchial wall; (c) bronchial wall fibrosis; (d) irregularity of the bronchial lumen; (e) chronic infection; (f) mucous plugging; and (g) replacement of the ciliated epithelium by squamous or columnar epithelium in some cases. The surrounding lung parenchyma often shows evidence of fibrosis, inflammation, atelectasis, and sometimes pneumonia. Bronchioles often demonstrate abnormalities similar to those affecting the larger airways, and constrictive bronchiolitis (bronchiolitis obliterans) may be present (1–4).

PATHOGENESIS

Several mechanisms are involved in the development of bronchiectasis. These include bronchial infection, inflammation, peribronchial fibrosis, and bronchial obstruction (Table 4-1). Underlying structural abnormalities of the bronchial wall, either congenital or acquired, may also be present in some patients. In many patients with bronchiectasis, several mechanisms acting in concert contribute to the development of airway abnormalities. Infection is almost always present.

Infection

The most common cause of bronchiectasis is acute, chronic, or recurrent infection. In otherwise healthy individuals, acute infection by organisms capable of causing tissue necrosis may lead to bronchial wall destruction and bronchiectasis. Such infections include tuberculosis (TB), pertussis, staphylococcus, and viral diseases. In such cases, a single childhood illness may result in eventual bronchiectasis.

In other patients, underlying conditions that predispose them to chronic airway infection may lead to bronchiectasis. Such conditions include (a) congenital or acquired immune deficiency and (b) abnormal bronchial mucociliary clearance related to ciliary abnormalities (e.g., dyskinetic cilia syndrome), abnormal mucus (e.g., cystic fibrosis), bronchial obstruction (e.g., neoplasm), or structural bronchial abnormalities (e.g., tracheobronchomegaly) (1,5–7). In patients with chronic infection, cytokines released by macrophages and airway epithelial cells result in neutrophil recruitment and subsequent release of elastase, collagenase, and other active substances; these lead to airway wall inflammation and destruction. Common organisms found on sputum culture of patients with chronic bronchiectasis include *Haemophilus influenzae* (29% to 42% of patients), *Pseudomonas aeruginosa* (13% to 31%), *Streptococcus pneumoniae* (6% to 13%), *Branhamella catarrhalis,* and *Staphylococcus aureus,* in approximate order of frequency (1).

It is crucial to recognize that the presence of bronchial dilatation itself (i.e., bronchiectasis) results in abnormal mucociliary clearance, which in turn predisposes a patient to chronic bronchial infection. To make matters worse, infection may contribute to abnormal mucociliary clearance through release of toxins from the infecting organisms;

TABLE 4-1
CAUSES OF BRONCHIECTASIS AND POSSIBLE MECHANISMS

Condition	Mechanisms
Infection (bacteria, mycobacteria, fungus, virus)	Impaired mucociliary clearance, disruption of respiratory epithelium, microbial toxins, host-mediated inflammation, fibrosis, bronchostenosis
Immunodeficiency	Genetic or acquired predisposition to recurrent infection
Bronchial obstruction (tumor, foreign body, congenital abnormalities)	Impaired mucociliary clearance, recurrent infection, mucous plugging
Cystic fibrosis	Abnormal airway epithelial chloride transport, impaired mucous clearance, recurrent infection
Asthma	Airway inflammation, mucous plugging
Allergic bronchopulmonary aspergillosis (ABPA)	Type I and Type III immune responses to fungus in airway lumen, mucous plugging
Dyskinetic cilia syndrome (Kartagener's syndrome)	Genetic defect, absent or dyskinetic cilia, impaired mucous clearance, recurrent infection
Young's syndrome (obstructive azoospermia)	Abnormal mucociliary clearance
Yellow nails and lymphedema syndrome	Unknown, lymphatic hypoplasia and sometimes immune deficiency, predisposition to recurrent infection
Alpha$_1$-antitrypsin deficiency	Proteinase–antiproteinase imbalance
Tracheobronchomegaly (Mounier-Kuhn syndrome)	Congenital deficiency of membranous and cartilaginous parts of tracheal and bronchial walls, impaired mucous clearance, recurrent infection
Williams-Campbell syndrome	Congenital deficiency of bronchial cartilage, obstruction, impaired mucous clearance, recurrent infection
Systemic diseases (e.g., collagen vascular diseases, inflammatory bowel disease)	Various, including inflammation, infection, fibrosis
Chronic fibrosis	Traction bronchiectasis
Bronchiolitis obliterans (postinfectious, lung transplant, etc.)	Bronchial wall inflammation, epithelial damage, recurrent infection in some cases
Aspiration, toxic fume inhalation	Inflammation

Modified from Davis AL, Salzman SH, eds. *Bronchiectasis*. Philadelphia: WB Saunders, 1991.

these may cause abnormalities of ciliary function. In this manner, a vicious circle is created: bronchiectasis and infection lead to abnormal airway clearance, which predisposes the airway to infection, which results in further airway wall inflammation and destruction.

Inflammation

Bronchiectasis may also result from bronchial inflammation without obvious infection in patients with collagen vascular diseases, inflammatory bowel disease, bronchiolitis obliterans, or allergic bronchopulmonary aspergillosis or in those who inhale toxic fumes or aspirate corrosive liquids.

Fibrosis

Peribronchial fibrosis, occurring in conjunction with bronchial and peribronchial infection (i.e., in patients with bronchiectasis) or fibrotic lung disease (e.g., TB, sarcoidosis, usual interstitial pneumonia) may result in or contribute to bronchial dilatation. In patients with bronchiectasis resulting from chronic infection, peribronchial fibrosis undoubtedly contributes to bronchial dilatation and luminal irregularity. In patients with fibrotic lung disease, fibrous tissue results in traction on the bronchial wall and causes them to dilate. Bronchiectasis related to fibrotic lung diseases is termed "traction bronchiectasis" (8). It is not a primary airway disease and is not characteristically associated with airway infection or typical symptoms of bronchiectasis. Traction bronchiectasis is best thought of as a sign of lung fibrosis and not an airway disease.

Bronchial Obstruction

Bronchial narrowing or obstruction with accumulation of mucus distal to the obstruction and chronic infection may lead to bronchiectasis. Bronchial obstruction may occur because of endobronchial neoplasm, foreign body, postinflammatory stricture, or congenital bronchial abnormality (e.g., bronchial atresia) or as a result of external compression.

Structural Bronchial Abnormalities

In patients with bronchiectasis occurring because of other causes, chronic infection and inflammation result in destruction of the elastic, muscular, and cartilaginous elements of the bronchial wall, leading to bronchial dilatation. Uncommonly, bronchiectasis results from an inherent structural abnormality of the bronchial wall that predisposes the bronchi to dilatation. Examples include Williams-Campbell syndrome and tracheobronchomegaly, in which cartilaginous, elastic, or muscular elements of the bronchial wall are deficient.

CLINICAL PRESENTATION

The presentation of patients with bronchiectasis is often nonspecific. In general, a clinical diagnosis of bronchiectasis is possible only in the most severely affected patients, and even in this setting, differentiation from chronic bronchitis or other airway diseases may be difficult (9).

Patients with bronchiectasis may have symptoms related to both airway infection and underlying or associated conditions, such as chronic bronchitis, emphysema, asthma, or bronchiolitis obliterans. Nearly all patients with bronchiectasis have chronic cough with purulent sputum production and recurrent pulmonary infections (1,2,4–6,10). Other symptoms may include fever, wheezing, chest pain, and weight loss. Hemoptysis also is frequent, occurring in up to 50% of patients, and may be the only clinical finding; it usually reflects the presence of bronchial artery enlargement associated with chronic inflammation (6,11,12).

Pulmonary function test (PFT) findings vary with the underlying cause of the bronchiectasis. However, most patients have some degree of airflow obstruction; mild restriction and hypoxemia also may be present (1,4,13). The presence of obstructive abnormalities on PFTs may partially reflect the collapse of abnormal bronchi with expiration but is more likely related to associated small airway abnormalities, such as bronchiolitis obliterans, infectious bronchiolitis, and asthma or associated emphysema. Mild restrictive abnormalities are sometimes present on PFTs, usually in patients with diseases resulting in lung fibrosis or reduced lung volume. Low diffusing capacity may be present in some patients with bronchiectasis, perhaps resulting from ventilation–perfusion mismatch.

RADIOGRAPHIC FINDINGS

The radiographic manifestations of bronchiectasis have been well described (14). These include (a) a loss of definition of vascular markings in affected lung segments, presumably resulting from peribronchial fibrosis and volume loss, (b) evidence of bronchial wall thickening with "tram tracks," (c) obvious bronchial dilatation, manifested in severely affected patients by discrete tubular or cystic lesions, and (d) mucus- or fluid-filled bronchi (Fig. 4-1).

It has been suggested that the radiographic diagnosis of bronchiectasis may be made more sensitive and accurate by the use of specific anatomic criteria (15). The most important of these is assessment of bronchial dilatation, either by comparing the diameters of end-on bronchi in normal and abnormal areas of the lung or by the measurement of bronchoarterial ratios.

Although radiographs are abnormal in 80% to 90% of patients with bronchiectasis, findings are often nonspecific and a definitive diagnosis is usually difficult to make except in advanced cases (9). Overall, the correct diagnosis may be made on chest radiographs in only about 40% of patients.

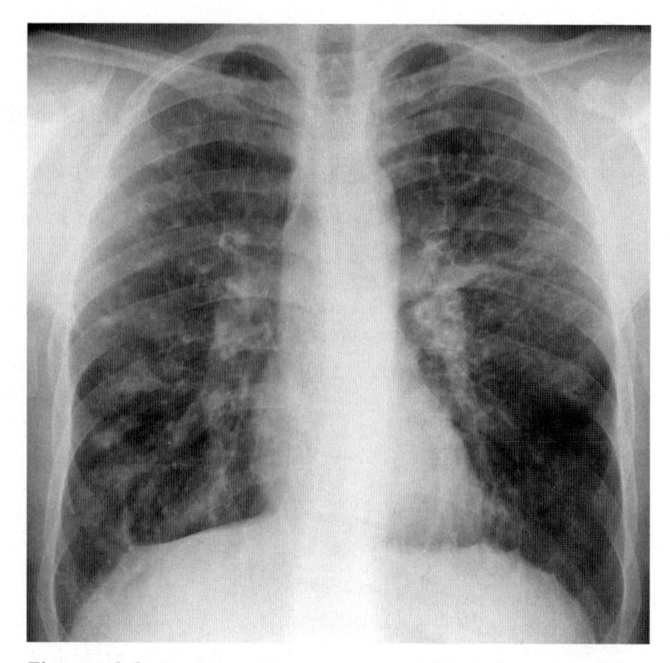

Figure 4-1 Radiographic appearance of bronchiectasis. Chest radiograph in a patient with severe bronchiectasis associated with cystic fibrosis shows tram tracks and ring shadows resulting from dilated and thick-walled bronchi. Ill-defined nodular opacities represent mucous plugs.

BRONCHOGRAPHIC FINDINGS

Bronchography is rarely used in clinical practice to diagnose bronchiectasis. Nonetheless, the bronchographic findings of patients with bronchiectasis have been described in detail, and knowledge of the typical bronchographic findings is helpful in understanding CT diagnosis of this disease.

Bronchographic findings indicative of bronchiectasis include (a) proximal and/or distal bronchial dilatation, (b) lack of normal tapering of peripheral airways (i.e., cylindrical bronchiectasis), (c) bronchial contour abnormalities (i.e., varicose and cystic bronchiectasis), (d) pruning (reduction in the number) of bronchial branches, (e) luminal occlusion, and (f) luminal filling defects resulting from mucoid or purulent secretions.

CT FINDINGS OF BRONCHIECTASIS

Direct findings of bronchiectasis include bronchial dilatation, bronchial contour abnormalities, lack of normal bronchial tapering, and visibility of airways in the lung periphery (Table 4-2) (2–4,16,17). Indirect findings of bronchiectasis (i.e., those not directly related to bronchial dilatation) include bronchial wall thickening and irregularity and mucoid impaction of the bronchial lumen. Small airway abnormalities are also often associated with bronchiectasis, with HRCT showing bronchiolectasis, centrilobular nodules, and "tree-in-bud." A combination of

TABLE 4-2
HRCT FINDINGS IN BRONCHIECTASIS

DIRECT SIGNS	INDIRECT SIGNS
1. Bronchial dilatation Increased bronchoarterial ratio Signet-ring sign (vertically oriented bronchi) Contour abnormalities Cylindrical, varicose, or cystic bronchiectasis	1. Bronchial wall thickening >0.5 times the diameter of an adjacent pulmonary artery (vertically oriented bronchi)
2. Lack of tapering >2 cm distal to bifurcation	2. Mucoid impaction or fluid-filled bronchi Tubular or Y-shaped structures Branching or rounded opacities in cross section Air-fluid levels
3. Visibility of peripheral airways within 1 cm of the costal pleura	3. Centrilobular nodules or tree-in-bud
	4. Mosaic perfusion
	5. Air trapping on expiratory scan
	6. Bronchial artery hypertrophy
	7. Atelectasis or emphysema

these findings enables an accurate diagnosis in a large percentage of patients.

Additional CT findings that may be seen in some patients with bronchiectasis include mosaic perfusion visible on inspiratory scans, focal air trapping identifiable on expiration scans, tracheomegaly, bronchial artery enlargement, atelectasis, and emphysema.

Bronchial Dilatation

Because bronchiectasis is defined by the presence of bronchial dilatation, recognition of increased bronchial diameter is key to the CT diagnosis of this abnormality. Various methods for measuring airway dimensions have been proposed. These include the use of digital image analysis programs requiring operator-dependent definition of a "seed point" at the lumen–wall interface to obtain isocontour lines of the bronchial lumen (18) and automated thresholding to detect the airway lumen area (19). Although these approaches may allow precise quantitative assessment of airways, and may prove particularly valuable in physiologic studies, subjective visual criteria for establishing the presence of bronchial dilatation are most often used in the interpretation of clinical scans (20–25).

For the purposes of CT interpretation, bronchial dilatation may be diagnosed (a) by comparing the bronchial diameter to that of the adjacent pulmonary artery branch (i.e., determining the bronchoarterial ratio), (b) by detecting a lack of bronchial tapering, and (c) by identifying airways in the peripheral lung.

Bronchoarterial Ratio

In most normal subjects, the diameters of bronchi and adjacent pulmonary arteries are nearly the same. Their diameters may be compared by using the *bronchoarterial ratio (B/A ratio)*, defined as the internal diameter (i.e., luminal diameter) of the bronchus divided by the diameter of the adjacent pulmonary artery (Fig. 4-2). To avoid the exaggeration of diameters caused by obliquity of the bronchus and artery relative to the scan plane, the least diameter of the bronchus and artery are used for measurement. The B/A ratio in normal subjects generally averages 0.65 to 0.70 (Fig. 4-3) (26,27).

The definition of an abnormal or increased B/A ratio varies widely among authors (16,20,22,24,25,27,28). In most cases, bronchiectasis is considered to be present when the internal diameter of a bronchus is greater than the diameter of the adjacent pulmonary artery branch, that is, when the B/A ratio is greater than 1 (16). The accuracy of this finding in diagnosing bronchiectasis has been validated in a number of studies comparing CT with bronchography in patients with bronchiectasis (29–32). A B/A ratio of more than 1 is recognizable on HRCT in 95% of patients with bronchiectasis (21).

However, in patients with bronchiectasis, the bronchial diameter is often much larger than the pulmonary artery diameter (i.e., the B/A ratio is >1.5), a finding that reflects not only the presence of bronchial dilatation but also some reduction in pulmonary artery size as a consequence of

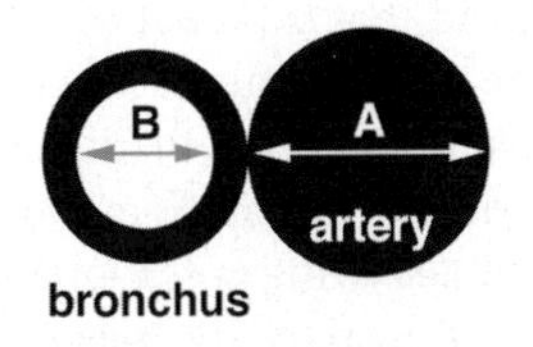

Figure 4-2 Bronchoarterial ratio (B/A ratio). The B/A ratio is calculated by dividing the internal diameter (i.e., luminal diameter) of the bronchus (B) by the diameter of the adjacent pulmonary artery (A).

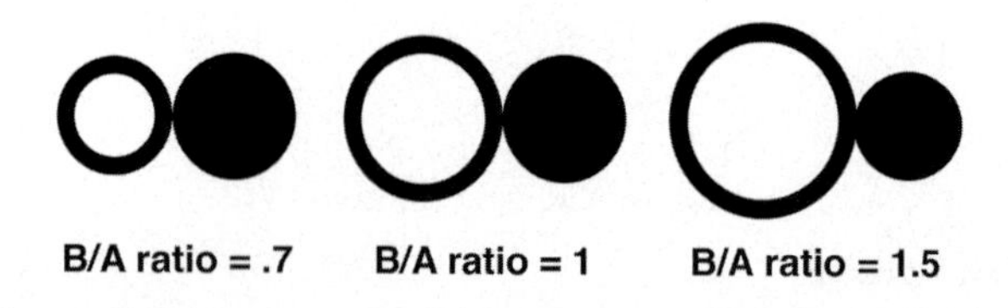

Figure 4-3 Normal and abnormal bronchoarterial (B/A) ratios. A normal B/A ratio averages 0.65 to 0.7 in young or middle-aged patients. A B/A ratio of 1 or more may be seen in some normals older than 65 years or in patients living at high altitude. A B/A ratio of 1.5 is typical of bronchiectasis and usually reflects increased bronchial diameter and decrease in size of the artery. This appearance mimics a signet ring and is termed the *signet-ring sign*.

decreased lung perfusion in affected lung regions (i.e., mosaic perfusion) (21). The association of a dilated bronchus with a much smaller adjacent pulmonary artery branch has been termed the *signet-ring sign* (Fig. 4-4) (33). This classic sign is very useful in recognizing bronchiectasis and in distinguishing dilated airways from other cystic lung diseases, which tend not to be associated with this finding.

Although an abnormal B/A ratio is typical of bronchiectasis, a B/A ratio slightly exceeding 1 may be seen in some normal subjects. For example, in an HRCT evaluation of 14 normal subjects (27), although the B/A ratio averaged 0.65 ± 0.16, 7% of scan interpretations were felt to show some evidence of bronchial dilatation.

The presence of a B/A ratio >1 in normal subjects has been associated with increasing age. In a study by Matsuoka et al. (26), B/A ratios were measured at the segmental and subsegmental levels in the apical and posterior basal segments in 85 normal subjects. A significant correlation was found between the B/A ratio and age ($r = 0.768$, $p < .0001$). When the subjects were considered in three age groups, the mean B/A ratios were 0.609 ± 0.05 in subjects 21 to 40 years old, 0.699 ± 0.067 in subjects 41 to 64 years old, and 0.782 ± 0.078 in subjects 65 years and older ($p < .0001$). At least one bronchus with a B/A ratio >1 was seen in 41% of patients older than 65 years, and in this group, 19% of measured bronchi had a B/A ratio >1. Seven percent of subjects 41 to 64 years of age had at least one bronchus (5% of measured bronchi) with a B/A ratio greater than 1. None of the subjects 21 to 40 years of age showed this finding.

An increase in normal B/A ratio may also be seen in subjects living at high altitude (21,23,24). It has been suggested that this results from mild hypoxemia with bronchial dilatation and vasoconstriction; the same mechanism may result in an increased B/A ratio in older patients. Kim et al. (21) found that 9 (53%) of 17 normal subjects living at an altitude of 1,600 meters had evidence of at least one bronchus equal to or greater in diameter than the adjacent pulmonary artery; these authors found that only 2 of 16 (12.5%) individuals living at sea level similarly showed a similar finding. In this study, the mean B/A ratio was 0.76 at an altitude of 1,600 meters, greater than that seen in subjects living at sea level. Similarly, Lynch et al. (23) compared the internal diameters of lobar, segmental,

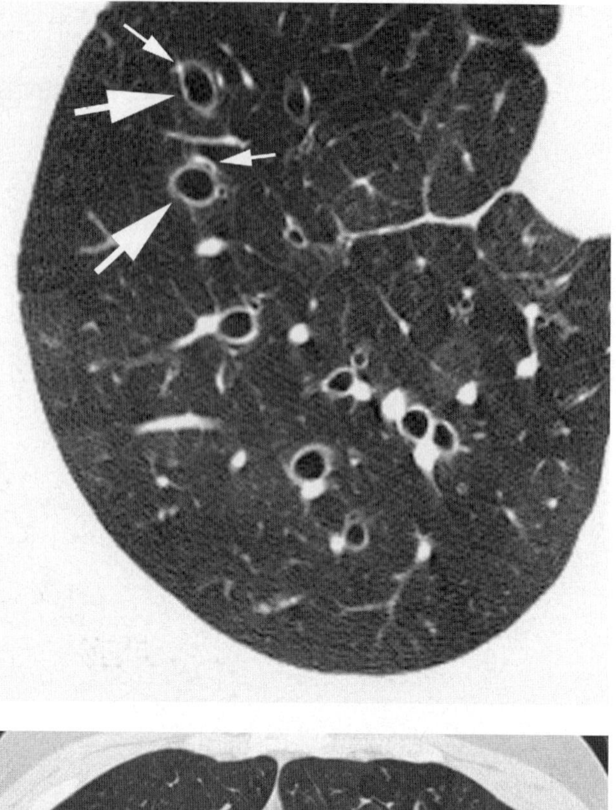

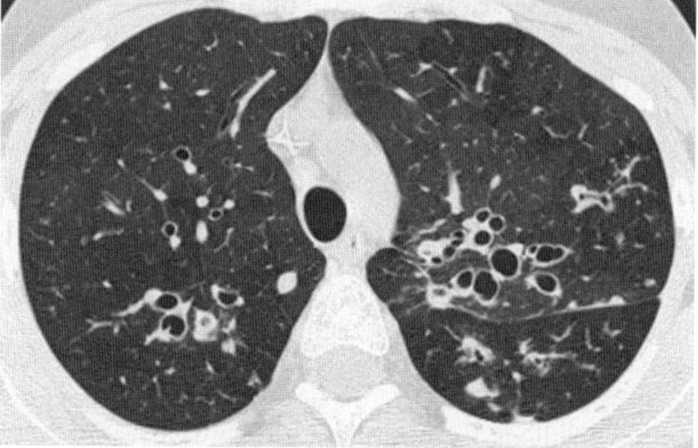

Figure 4-4 Bronchiectasis in two patients with increased B/A ratio. **A:** Bronchiectasis is visible in the right lower lobe, with increase in the B/A ratio. This is the result of both increase in bronchial diameter *(large arrows)* and a decrease in size of the accompanying artery *(small arrows)*. This appearance is termed the signet-ring sign. **B:** Increased B/A ratio in a patient with bilateral upper lobe bronchiectasis. This finding is easiest to recognize when the bronchus and artery are imaged in cross section.

subsegmental, and smaller bronchi with those of adjacent pulmonary artery branches in 27 normal subjects living in Denver at an altitude of about 1 mile. The authors found that 37 (26%) of 142 bronchi evaluated, and 59% of individuals, had increased B/A ratios.

A convincing relationship has not been shown between the B/A ratio and the location of the bronchi being evaluated. Evaluation of the distribution of bronchi with a B/A ratio >1 has generally failed to reveal any relationship to lobe or anteroposterior location within the lungs (21,25).

It must be emphasized that bronchiectasis should not be diagnosed on the basis of an increased B/A ratio alone, unless the B/A ratio is significantly greater than 1 (e.g., 1.5).

Bronchial wall thickening is almost always seen in association with bronchial dilatation in patients with bronchiectasis, as are irregularities in bronchial diameter or lack of bronchial tapering. In the normal subjects studied by Lynch et al. (23) who demonstrated an increased B/A ratio, bronchial wall thickening was relatively uncommon, and it is unlikely that any of the subjects in this study would have been diagnosed on clinical HRCT studies as having true bronchiectasis.

Bronchial diameter may be reliably measured using CT, and although objective measurements may be valuable in some cases, visual inspection with a subjective determination of B/A ratio usually suffices for clinical diagnosis (22,34,35). Desai et al. (34) evaluated both interobserver and intraobserver variability in CT measurements of bronchial wall circumference in 61 subsegmental bronchi and found the reproducibility of these measurements to be sufficient for clinical usefulness. Using visual inspection only, Diederich et al. (22) found close agreement among three readers in both the detection ($\kappa = 0.78$) and assessment of the severity ($\kappa = 0.68$) of bronchiectasis. It should also be pointed out, however, that visual inspection alone may lead to an overestimation of B/A ratio because of an optical illusion in which the diameter of empty circles appears larger than that of solid circles despite their being identical in diameter (21).

A potential limitation of the use of B/A ratios is the necessity of identifying both airways and accompanying arteries. This may not always be possible in patients with coexisting parenchymal consolidation (24). Kang et al. (24), in a study of 47 resected lobes with documented bronchiectasis, were unable to determine the B/A ratios in three patients owing to the presence of parenchymal consolidation.

Lack of Bronchial Tapering

Lack of bronchial tapering has come to be recognized as an important finding in the diagnosis of bronchiectasis and, in particular, subtle cylindrical bronchiectasis. It has been suggested that, for this finding to be present, the diameter of the airway should remain unchanged for at least 2 cm distal to a branching point (Fig. 4-5) (21). First emphasized by Lynch et al. (23) as a necessary finding for diagnosis, lack of bronchial tapering has been reported by some to be the most sensitive means for diagnosing bronchiectasis. Kang et al. (24), for example, in an assessment of 47 lobes with pathologically proved bronchiectasis found lack of tapering of bronchial lumina in 37 cases (79%) as compared with increased B/A ratios seen in only 28 (60%). In another study (36), lack of tapering of bronchi was seen in 10% of HRCT interpretations in healthy subjects compared with 95% of reviews in patients with bronchiectasis. It should be emphasized that the accurate detection of this finding is difficult in the absence of contiguous HRCT sections or thin-collimation SCT, especially for vertically or obliquely oriented airways. The value of this sign is doubtful when HRCT scans are obtained in spaced intervals in a noncontiguous fashion.

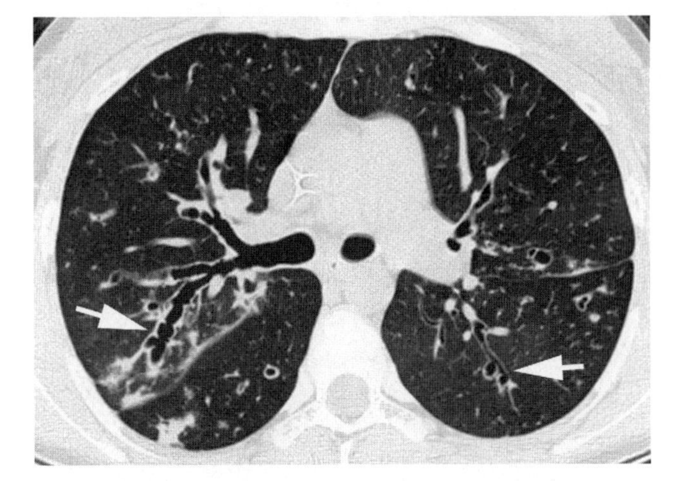

Figure 4-5 Lack of bronchial tapering in bronchiectasis. Two upper lobe bronchi *(arrows)* show a lack of bronchial tapering distal to a branch point. This is easiest to recognize when the bronchi lie in the plane of the scan.

Visibility of Peripheral Airways

Another finding valuable in the diagnosis of bronchiectasis is visibility of airways in the peripheral 1 cm of lung (Fig. 4-6) (24,36). The smallest airways normally visible using HRCT or thin-collimation SCT techniques have a diameter of approximately 2 mm and a wall thickness of about 0.2 to 0.3 mm (37); in normal subjects, airways in the peripheral 2 cm of lung are uncommonly seen because their walls are too thin (38).

Peribronchial fibrosis and bronchial wall thickening in patients with bronchiectasis, in combination with dilatation of the bronchial lumen, allow small airways in the lung periphery to be seen on HRCT or thin-slice SCT. In a study by Kang et al. (24), bronchi visualized within 1 cm of pleura were seen in 21 of 47 (45%) bronchiectatic lobes.

Kim et al. (36) further assessed the value of this sign in the diagnosis of bronchiectasis. The authors emphasized that although normal bronchi are not visible within 1 cm of the costal pleural surfaces, they may be seen within 1 cm of the mediastinal pleural surfaces. In their study, bronchi were visible within 1 cm of the mediastinal pleura in 40% of normal subjects (36). Bronchi within 1 cm of the costal pleural surface or bronchi touching the mediastinal pleural surfaces were visible in 81% and 53%, respectively, of HRCT interpretations in patients with clinical or pathologic evidence of cylindrical bronchiectasis.

Bronchial Wall Thickening

Although bronchial wall thickening is a nonspecific finding seen in various airway diseases, it is usually present in patients with bronchiectasis (Fig. 4-6).

Anatomically, the normal thickness of an airway wall is related to its diameter. Second- to fourth-generation (lobar to segmental) bronchi have a wall thickness of approximately 1.5 mm and a mean diameter between 5 and 8 mm (i.e., the bronchial wall thickness is about 20% to 30% of

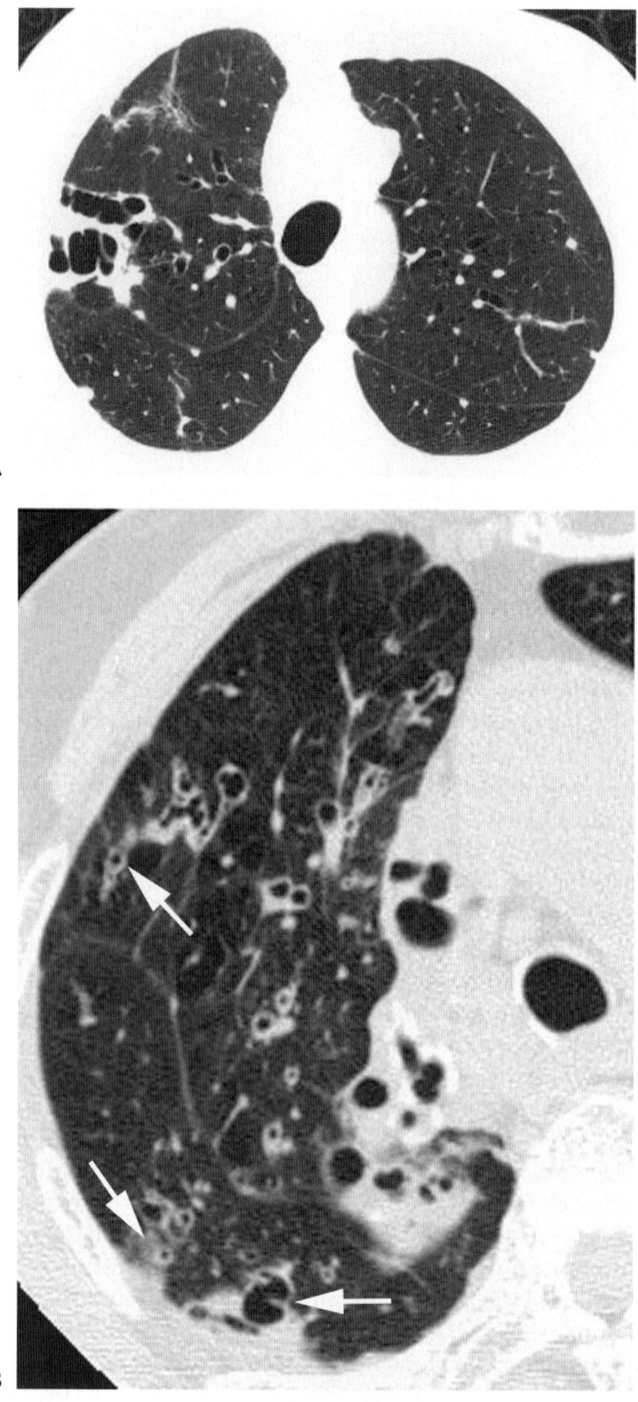

Figure 4-6 Visible bronchi in the peripheral 1 cm of lung in two patients with bronchiectasis. **A:** Dilated bronchi are seen extending to the pleural surface in the right upper lobe. The bronchial walls are abnormally thickened, and the bronchi are markedly dilated (i.e., cystic bronchiectasis). **B:** Dilated bronchi are visible about 1 cm from the pleural surface.

the bronchial diameter), sixth- to eighth-generation (subsegmental) airways have a wall approximately 0.3 mm thick and a mean diameter between 1.5 and 3 mm (the airway wall is 10% to 20% of its diameter), and eleventh- to thirteenth-generation airways have a diameter measuring 0.7 to 1 mm with walls of 0.1 to 0.15 mm (the airway wall is about 15% of its diameter) (39,40).

This relationship between bronchial wall thickness and diameter may be expressed by using the thickness-to-diameter (T/D) ratio, defined as wall thickness (T) divided by the total diameter of the bronchus (D) (Fig. 4-7). This ratio may be measured using CT and averages about 20% for segmental and subsegmental bronchi, similar to the anatomic measurements described previously. In one study (26), HRCT was performed in 85 subjects without cardiopulmonary disease. The T/D ratio was measured at the segmental and subsegmental levels of the apical and posterior basal segments. The images were viewed at a window level of −450 H and a window width of 1500 H, thought best for accurate bronchial measurements (41,42). Overall, the T/D ratio measured 0.200 ± 0.015 (range 0.171 to 0.227). No significant correlation was seen between the T/D ratio and age. Although no significant differences in T/D ratio were seen between smokers and nonsmokers in the entire group studies, the T/D ratio was found to be significantly higher in smokers than in nonsmokers when patients 65 years or older were considered as a separate group ($p = .021$). In another study, the T/D ratio measured 0.23 (±0.04) in 14 normal subjects (43).

The relationship between bronchial wall thickness and bronchial diameter may also be assessed by using the bronchial lumen ratio (BLR), defined as the inner diameter of the bronchus divided by its outer diameter (25). In essence, the BLR represents $1 - (2 \times T/D)$. At the subsegmental level, the BLR in normal subjects averaged 0.66 ± 0.06, with a range of 0.51 to 0.86 (25).

There is no widespread agreement as to what constitutes bronchial wall thickening or how it should be measured using CT, although various methods have been proposed (22,26,28,44,45). Identification of thickened bronchial walls for the purpose of interpretation of clinical scans remains largely subjective (24,46).

Simply determining the T/D ratio or BLR is problematic in the diagnosis of bronchial wall thickening, because bronchiectasis increases the bronchial diameter at the same time the wall becomes thick (Fig. 4-8A). Comparing the bronchial wall thickness with the diameter of the adjacent pulmonary artery is useful as an objective measurement, and bronchial wall thickening is diagnosed if the airway wall is at least 0.5 times the width of an adjacent vertically oriented pulmonary artery (Fig. 4-8A and B) (28,44,47).

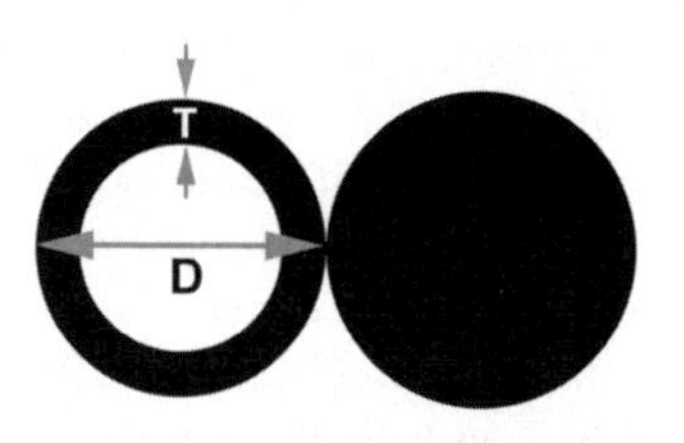

Figure 4-7 Measurement of bronchial wall thickness using the T/D ratio. This ratio is defined as wall thickness (T) divided by the total diameter of the bronchus (D). In normals, it averages about 0.2 or 20%.

Because bronchiectasis and bronchial wall thickening are often multifocal rather than diffuse and uniform, a comparison of bronchi in one lung region with those in another can be helpful in making this diagnosis (Fig. 4-8C). Remy-Jardin et al. (45) considered bronchial wall thickening to be present if a bronchial wall measured twice the thickness of the wall of a similar but normal bronchus.

The quantitative measurement of bronchial wall thickness is tedious and uncommonly performed in clinical practice. Fortunately, it has been shown that visual assessment of wall thickening may be reliable. Using visual estimation, Diederich et al. (22) found acceptable levels of agreement among three readers regarding the presence or absence of bronchial wall thickening (κ = 0.64), although the validity of this diagnosis was not assessed. On the other hand, Bankier et al. (48) found relatively low sensitivity in the diagnosis of abnormally thick-walled segmental and subsegmental bronchi, evaluated by three independent observers, on two occasions. Sensitivity in detecting abnormal bronchi averaged 45% with a specificity of 72% (48), although it should be emphasized that the airway abnormalities evaluated in this study were subtle with abnormal segmental and subsegmental wall thickness measuring 1.77 mm and 0.95 mm, respectively, as compared with normal segmental and subsegmental airways measuring 1.14 and 0.46 mm, respectively.

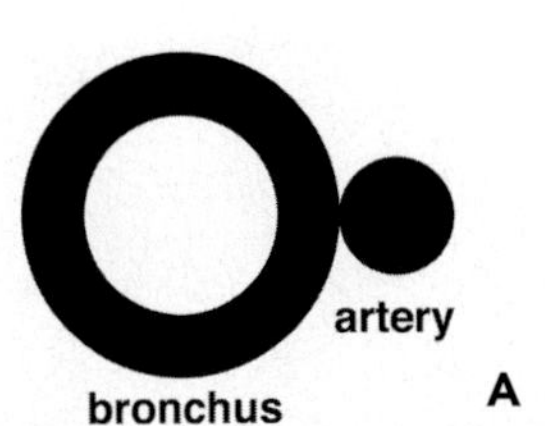

Figure 4-8 Increased wall thickness in bronchiectasis. **A:** Diagram of bronchial wall thickening in bronchiectasis. The bronchus is thick walled, but the T/D ratio is normal (i.e., about 0.2) because the bronchus is dilated. Note that the bronchial wall is more than half the diameter of the adjacent artery. This finding may be valuable in the diagnosis of wall thickening in the presence of bronchiectasis. **B:** Bronchial wall thickening in bronchiectasis as a result of CF. **C:** Bronchial wall thickening in bronchiectasis may not be uniform, and thick-walled bronchi *(large arrows)* can be contrasted with normal bronchi seen in other locations *(small arrows)*.

Mucoid Impaction

The presence of mucus- or fluid-filled bronchi may be helpful in confirming a diagnosis of bronchiectasis. The HRCT appearance of fluid or mucus-filled airways is dependent on both their size and orientation relative to the scan plane (Fig. 4-9). Larger mucus-filled airways result in abnormal lobular or branching structures when they lie in the same plane as the CT scan. Although they may be confused with abnormally dilated vessels, in most cases the recognition of dilated, fluid-filled airways is simplified by the identification of other areas of bronchiectasis in which the bronchi are air filled; these are usually revealed with careful examination. In problematic cases, distinction between larger fluid-filled bronchi and dilated blood vessels is easily made by rescanning patients following the bolus injection of intravenous contrast agent. Alternatively, with the introduction of newer generation scanners, it is possible to obtain high-quality multiplanar and maximum-intensity projection images in a variety of imaging planes as a means for further evaluation.

Although commonly associated with bronchiectasis and infection, dilated mucus-filled airways in the central lung can also result from congenital bronchial abnormalities, such as bronchopulmonary sequestration or bronchial atresia (49–54). It should also be emphasized that the presence of dilated mucus-filled airways, especially when central or predominantly segmental or lobar in distribution, should alert one to the possibility of central endobronchial obstruction, resulting from either tumor or foreign body aspiration.

Small Airway Abnormalities

Most patients with bronchiectasis also have pathologic or HRCT evidence of small airway disease or bronchiolitis

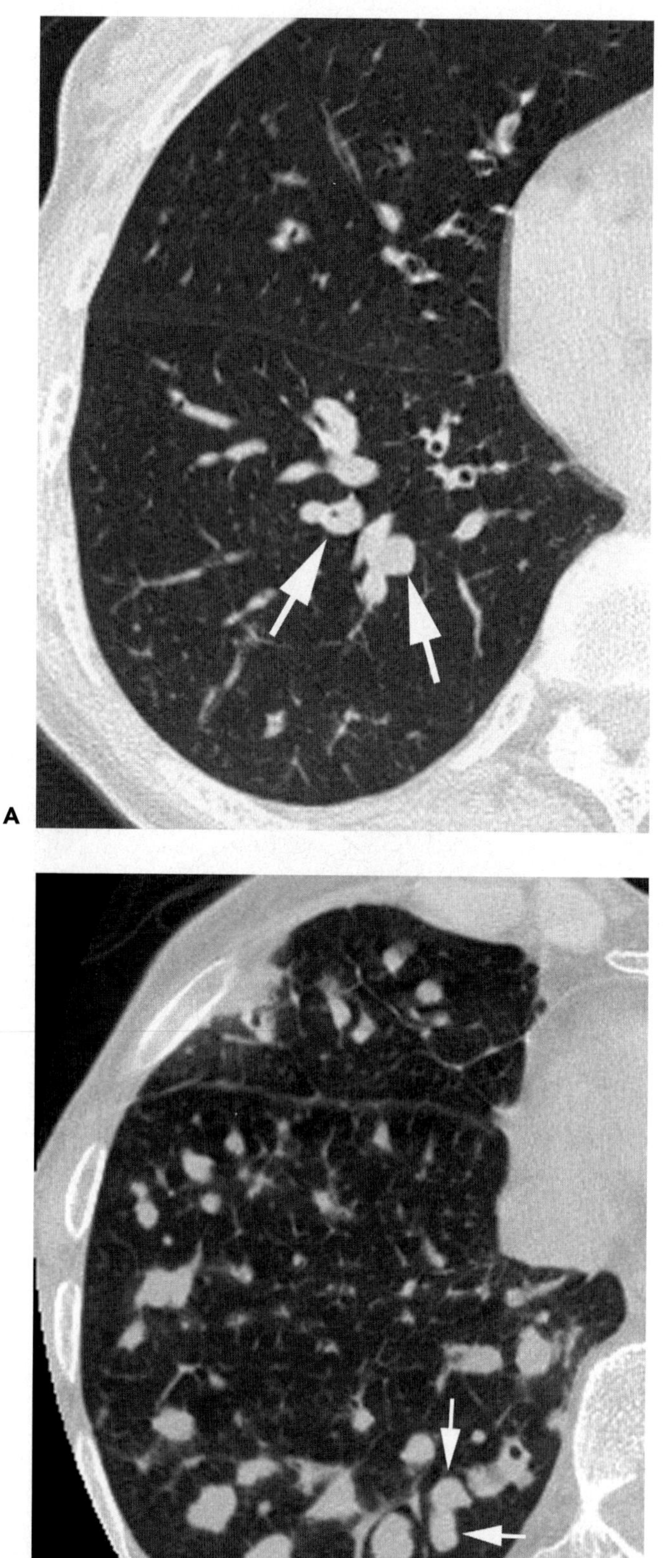

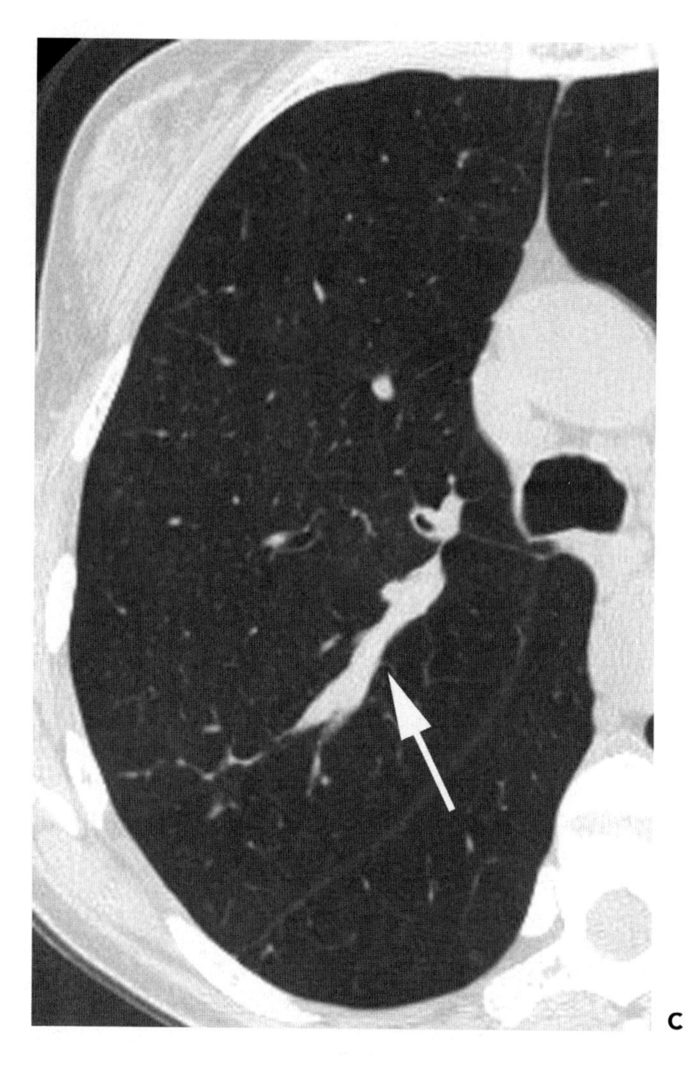

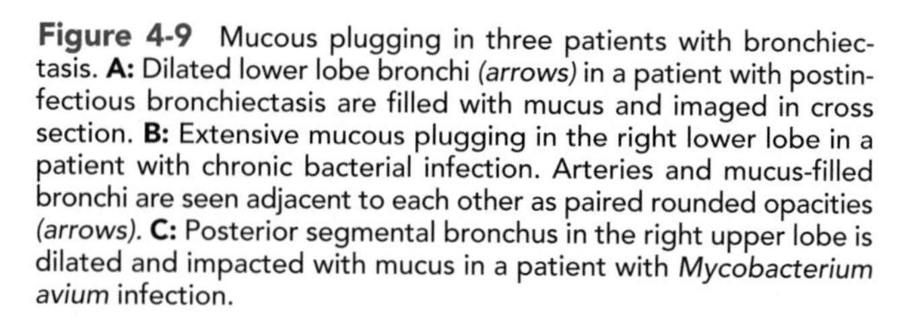

Figure 4-9 Mucous plugging in three patients with bronchiectasis. **A:** Dilated lower lobe bronchi *(arrows)* in a patient with postinfectious bronchiectasis are filled with mucus and imaged in cross section. **B:** Extensive mucous plugging in the right lower lobe in a patient with chronic bacterial infection. Arteries and mucus-filled bronchi are seen adjacent to each other as paired rounded opacities *(arrows)*. **C:** Posterior segmental bronchus in the right upper lobe is dilated and impacted with mucus in a patient with *Mycobacterium avium* infection.

(Figs. 4-10 and 4-11). For example, Kang et al. (24) found pathologic evidence of bronchiolitis in 85% of 47 resected lobes in patients with bronchiectasis. These included 18 lobes with inflammatory or suppurative bronchiolitis, 16 lobes with both inflammatory and obliterative bronchiolitis, and 6 lobes with obliterative bronchiolitis. HRCT findings consistent with bronchiolitis were identified in 30 (75%) of the 47 lobes, including a pattern of mosaic perfusion (n = 21), bronchiolectasis (n = 17), and centrilobular nodular and/or branching opacities (i.e., tree-in-bud) (n = 10) (24).

Bronchiolitis in patients with bronchiectasis may be recognized on HRCT by the presence of (a) bronchiolectasis (dilatation of small peripheral or centrilobular airways), (b) tree-in-bud (dilatation and mucoid impaction of centrilobular bronchioles), (c) centrilobular nodules, or (d) mosaic perfusion and air trapping. The HRCT findings of bronchiolitis are also described in Chapter 5.

Bronchiolectasis, Tree-in-bud, and Centrilobular Nodules

Dilated air-filled bronchioles may be recognized on HRCT in a centrilobular location in some patients with bronchiectasis, but more often the finding termed tree-in-bud is visible.

Tree-in-bud is very important in the diagnosis of infectious or cellular bronchiolitis and reflects the presence of dilated centrilobular bronchioles, their lumina impacted with mucus, fluid, or pus and often associated with peribronchiolar inflammation (Fig. 4-10) (55–59). On HRCT, the finding of tree-in-bud is usually easy to recognize. It may be associated with a typical centrilobular branching appearance, with the most peripheral branches being several millimeters from the pleural surface. Abnormal bronchioles that produce a tree-in-bud pattern can usually be distinguished from normal centrilobular vessels by their more irregular appearance, a lack of tapering, and a knobby or bulbous appearance at the tips of small branches. Normal centrilobular arteries are considerably thinner than the branching bronchioles seen in patients with this finding and are much less conspicuous. Furthermore, because tree-in-bud is often patchy in distribution, it is easy to contrast its appearance with that of adjacent normal lung regions.

Tree-in-bud is commonly associated with bronchiectasis. In a study by Aquino et al. (56), 26 of 27 (96%) patients showing tree-in-bud on HRCT also showed bronchiectasis or bronchial wall thickening on HRCT. Furthermore, 25% of patients with bronchiectasis and 18% of patients with infectious bronchitis reviewed in this study showed tree-in-bud, but this finding was not visible in patients with other diseases involving the airways, such as respiratory bronchiolitis, bronchiolitis obliterans, bronchiolitis obliterans organizing pneumonia, and hypersensitivity pneumonitis (56).

Ill-defined centrilobular nodules representing areas of peribronchiolar inflammation or bronchopneumonia may also be seen in patients with bronchiectasis and airway disease (58). They may be associated with bronchiolectasis or tree-in-bud and are commonly present in patients with bronchiectasis associated with active infection.

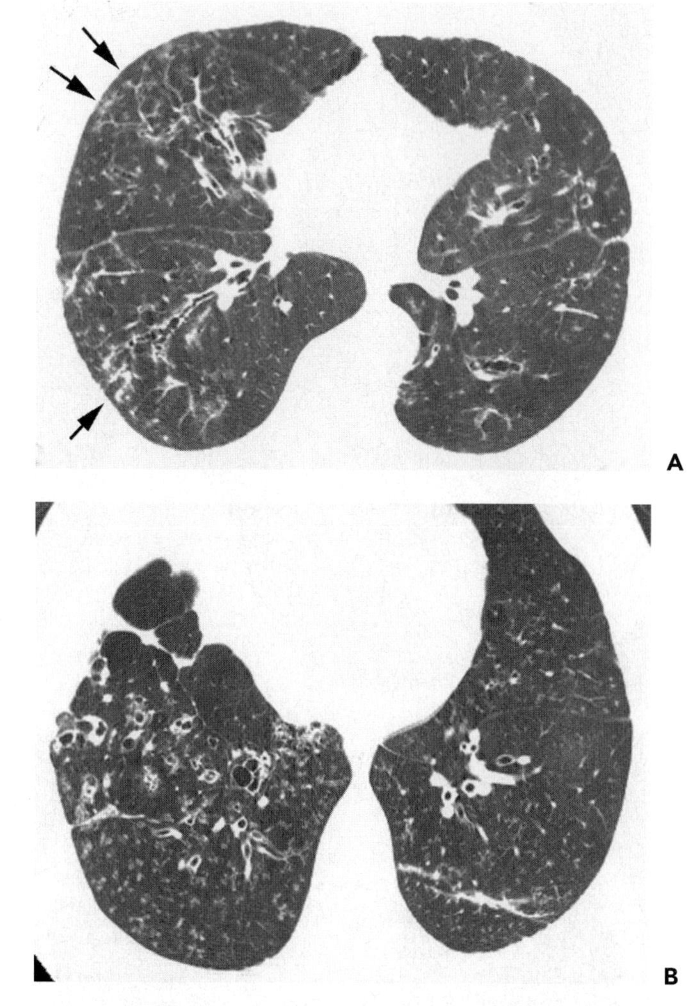

Figure 4-10 Small-airway abnormalities in bronchiectasis with tree-in-bud. **A:** In a patient with CF, branching opacities in the lung periphery are typical of tree-in-bud (*arrows*) and represent small airways impacted by pus. Central bronchiectasis is also visible. **B:** Extensive tree-in-bud in the right lower lobe in a patient with bronchiectasis and small-airway infection.

Mosaic Perfusion and Air Trapping

HRCT findings of mosaic perfusion on inspiratory scans and focal air trapping on expiratory scans are useful in the diagnosis of bronchiolitis associated with bronchiectasis (Fig. 4-11). In a study of 70 patients with HRCT evidence of bronchiectasis in 52% of lobes evaluated, areas of decreased attenuation (i.e., mosaic perfusion) were visible on inspiratory scans in 20% of lobes and on expiration (air trapping) in 34% (60). Although areas of decreased attenuation on expiratory scans were more prevalent in lobes with severe bronchiectasis (59% of cases) or localized bronchiectasis (28% of cases), air trapping was identified in the absence of associated bronchiectasis in 17% of lobes. In this same study, the presence of decreased attenuation on expiratory scans was also associated with mucoid impaction. Air trap-

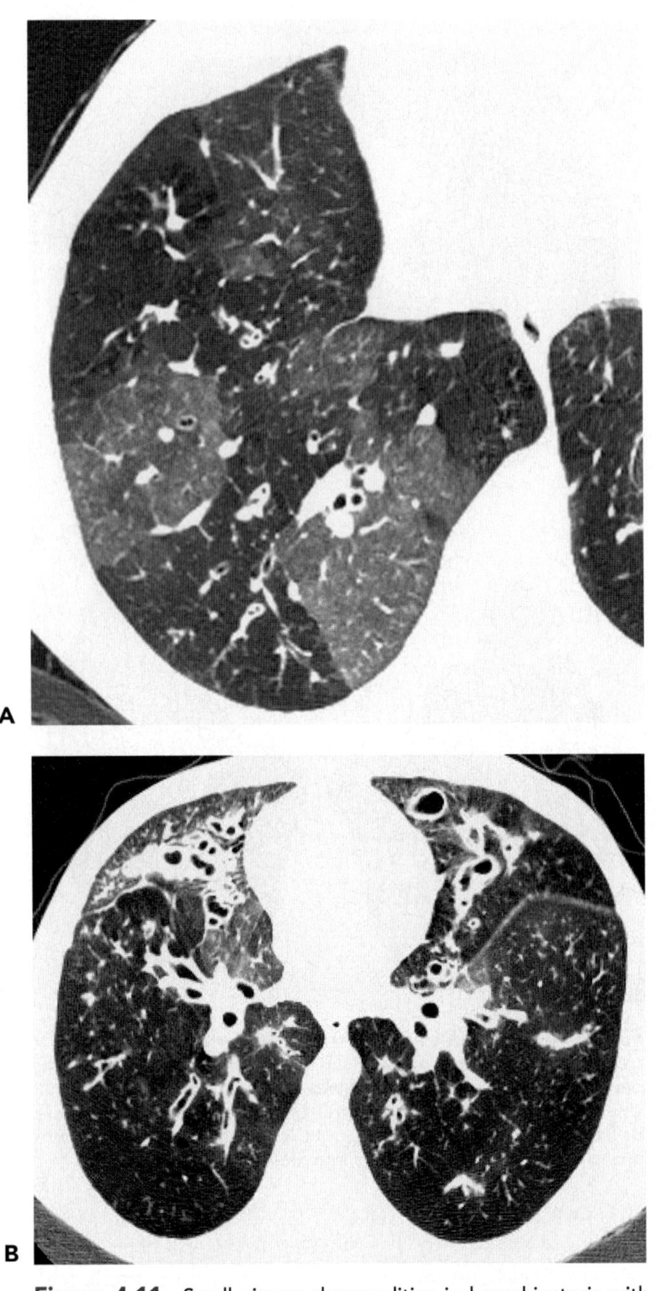

Figure 4-11 Small airway abnormalities in bronchiectasis with mosaic perfusion. **A:** Patchy mosaic perfusion in CF. Geographic regions of decreased lung attenuation in the right lower lobe are the result of small airway obstruction, poor ventilation, and reflex vasoconstriction. Lucent lung regions contain smaller vessels than dense lung regions. This is diagnostic of mosaic perfusion. Bronchial wall thickening is also visible. **B:** Mosaic perfusion in CF. Extensive bronchiectasis is visible. Heterogeneous lung attenuation results from mosaic perfusion.

ping was seen in 73% of lobes with large mucus plugs and in 58% of those with centrilobular mucus plugs. These same authors noted a correlation ($r = 0.40$, $p < .001$) between the total extent and severity of bronchiectasis and the extent of decreased attenuation shown on expiratory CT. Furthermore, in the 55 patients who had pulmonary function tests, the extent of expiratory attenuation abnormalities was inversely related to measures of airway obstruction such as forced expiratory volume in 1 second (FEV_1) and FEV_1/forced vital capacity (FVC) (60).

Bronchial Artery Hypertrophy

Bronchial arteries extend from the hila, along the central airways, to a level a few bronchial generations proximal to the terminal bronchioles; they represent the primary bronchial blood supply (61). Arising directly from the proximal descending thoracic aorta, these typically measure <2 mm in size. Enlarged bronchial arteries are identified pathologically in most cases of bronchiectasis, accounting for the common occurrence of hemoptysis in these patients. With thin-slice SCT obtained during contrast infusion, it has proved possible to identify both normal and abnormal bronchial arteries; this is more difficult to do with unenhanced HRCT (62,63).

Song et al. (64) were able to demonstrate good correlation between non–contrast-enhanced HRCT images and corresponding CT angiograms for demonstrating hypertrophied bronchial arteries in patients with bronchiectasis. Specifically, these authors showed that the finding of tubular or nodular areas of soft tissue attenuation, distinct from blood vessels within the mediastinum and adjacent to the central airways, correctly predicted bronchial artery hypertrophy in 88% and 53% of patients, respectively. Although the diagnosis of bronchiectasis rarely is dependent on demonstrating bronchial artery hypertrophy, identification of focal bronchial wall abnormalities resulting from enlarged bronchial arteries is important before attempting bronchoscopy because inadvertent biopsy may lead to significant hemorrhage (64).

In patients with bronchiectasis and massive hemorrhage, CT can be valuable in determining the cause and localizing the site of bleeding (Fig. 4-12). In a comparison of CT to bronchoscopy in patients with massive hemoptysis, most of whom had bronchiectasis (65), CT was more accurate in identifying the cause of bleeding (77% vs. 8%, respectively; $p < .001$), whereas the two methods were comparable for identifying the site of bleeding (70% vs. 73%, respectively).

MORPHOLOGIC CLASSIFICATION OF BRONCHIECTASIS

Bronchiectasis traditionally has been classified into three types based on the severity of bronchial dilatation and the degree of luminal irregularity. These three types are *cylindrical, varicose,* and *cystic* (66). Although a distinction among these three types of bronchiectasis is sometimes helpful in diagnosis and correlates with the severity of both the anatomic and functional abnormality (28), their differentiation is generally less important clinically than a determination of the extent and distribution of the airway disease.

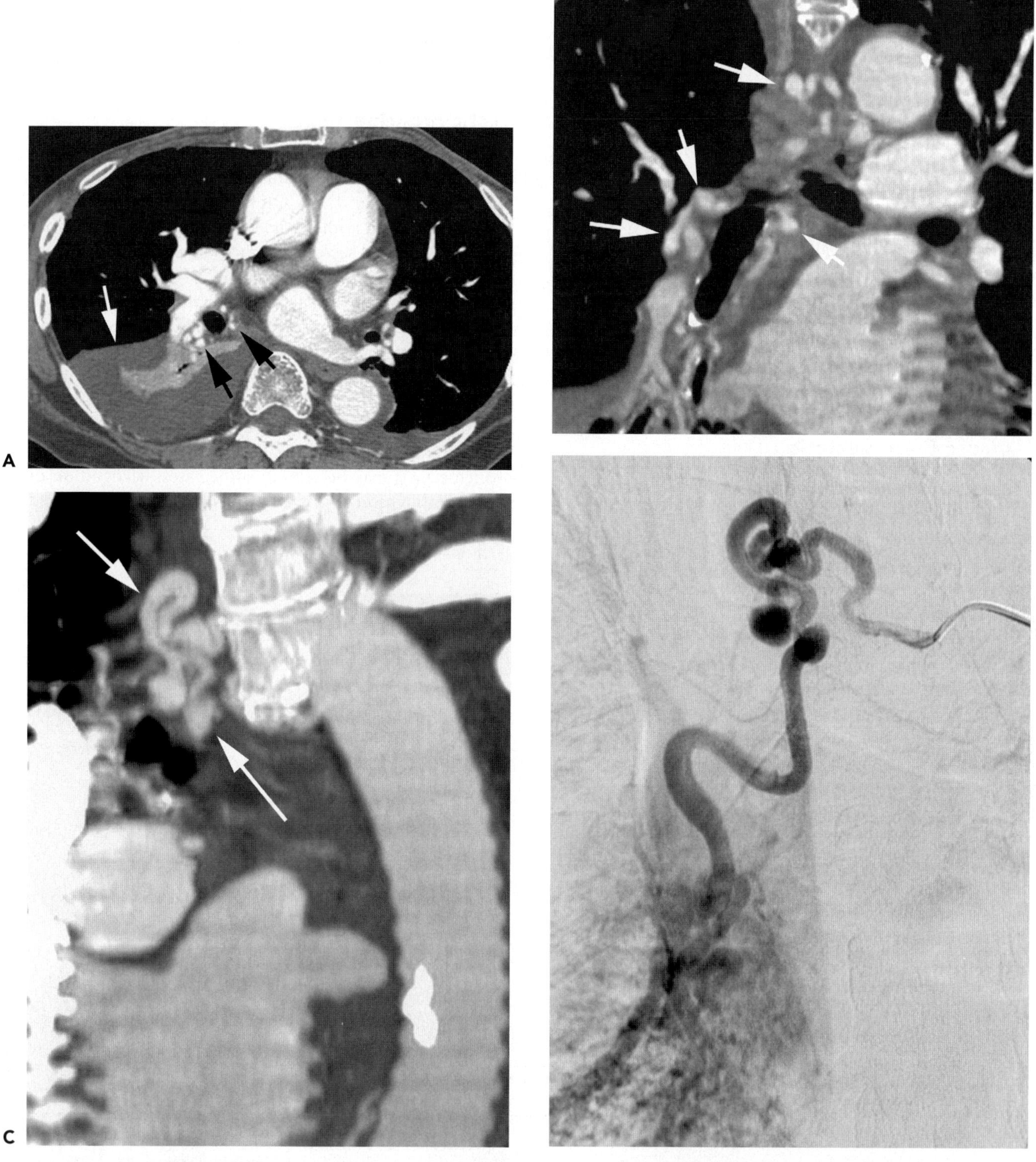

Figure 4-12 Bronchial artery enlargement in bronchiectasis. **A:** Multidetector CT (1.25-mm slice thickness) during contrast infusion in a patient with hemoptysis. Right lower lobe collapse and consolidation *(white arrow)* is the result of bronchiectasis. There is marked enlargement of bronchial arteries in the hilum *(black arrows)*. **B:** Reconstruction in the coronal plane shows enlargement of bronchial arteries in the hilum and mediastinum *(arrows)*. **C:** Oblique reconstruction shows the enlarged mediastinal bronchial artery *(arrows)*. **D:** Arteriogram in the same plane as (**C**) shows bronchial artery enlargement. The bronchial artery was embolized for treatment of the patient's hemoptysis.

Cylindrical Bronchiectasis

Mild, or cylindrical, bronchiectasis is diagnosed if the dilated bronchi are of relatively uniform caliber and have roughly parallel walls (Fig. 4-13). The appearance of cylindrical bronchiectasis varies depending on whether the abnormal bronchi have a horizontal or a vertical course relative to the scan plane. When horizontal, bronchi are visualized along their length and are recognizable as branching "tram tracks" that fail to taper as they extend peripherally and are visible more peripherally than is normal. When cylindrically dilated bronchi are oriented vertically, they are scanned in cross section and appear as thick-walled, circular lucencies. In most cases, dilated bronchi seen in cross section can be easily distinguished from emphysema or other causes of lung cysts by identifying the signet-ring sign and the continuity of the dilated bronchus on adjacent scans.

Varicose Bronchiectasis

With increasingly severe abnormalities of the bronchial wall, bronchi may assume a beaded configuration, referred to as varicose bronchiectasis (Fig. 4-14). This diagnosis may be difficult to make unless the involved bronchi course horizontally in the plane of the scan. Varicose bronchiectasis is much less frequent than cylindrical bronchiectasis.

Cystic Bronchiectasis

With severe, or cystic, bronchiectasis, involved airways are cystic or saccular in appearance and may extend to the pleural surface (Fig. 4-15). On HRCT, cystic bronchiectasis may be associated with the presence of (a) air–fluid levels, caused by retained secretions in the dependent portions of the dilated bronchi; (b) a string of cysts, caused by sectioning irregularly dilated bronchi along their length; or (c) a cluster of cysts, caused by multiple dilated bronchi lying adjacent to each other. Clusters of cysts are most frequently seen in atelectatic lobes, presumably as a result of chronic infection.

In general, the dilated airways in patients with cystic bronchiectasis are thick walled, but thin-walled cystic bronchiectasis may be seen in some cases. Recognition of some combination of dilated bronchi, air–fluid levels, and

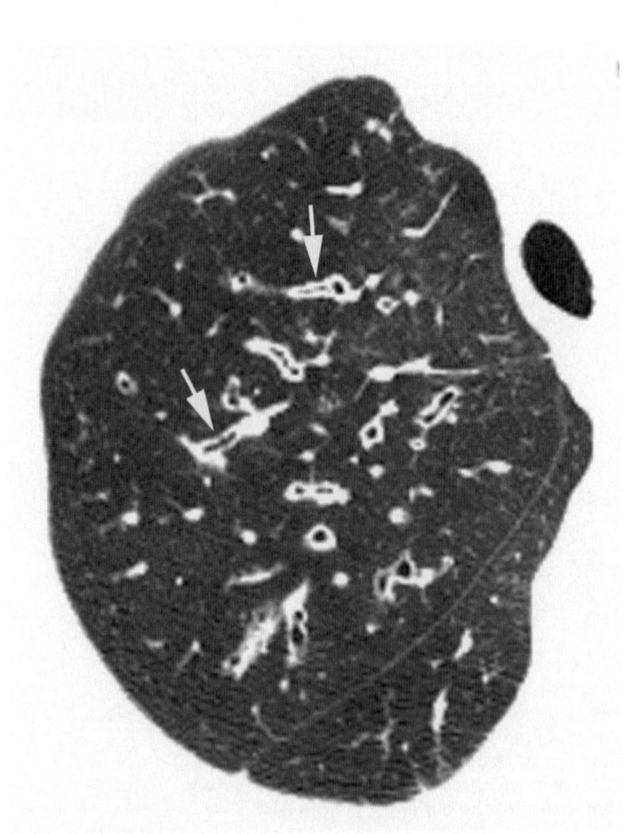

Figure 4-13 Cylindrical bronchiectasis in CF. Bronchi are mildly dilated and thick walled. Bronchi seen along their axis have roughly parallel walls *(arrows)*. Bronchi in cross section show the signet-ring sign.

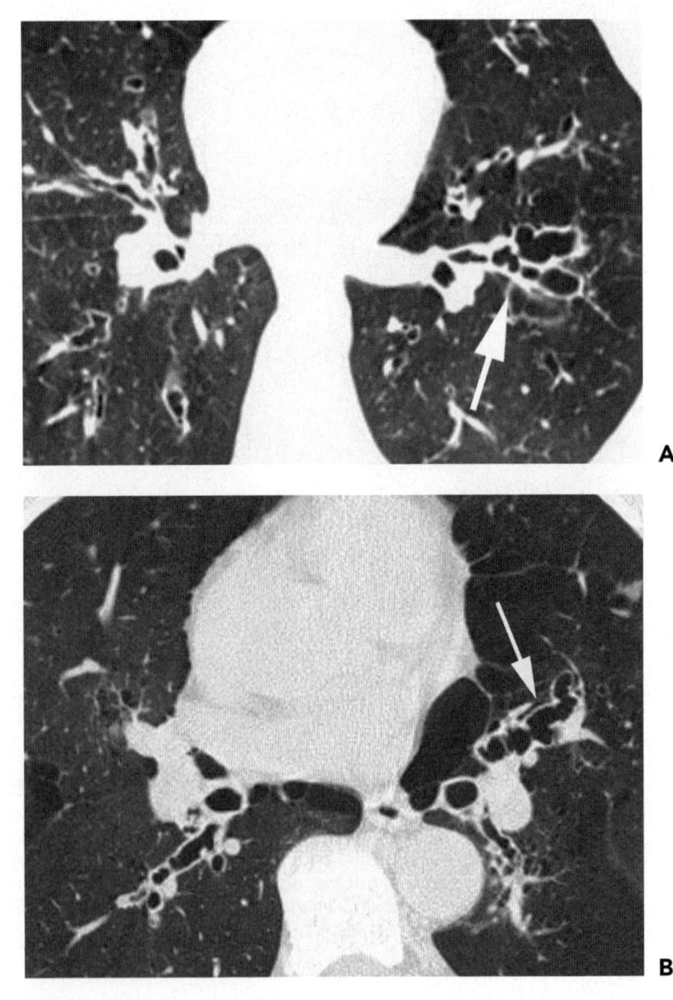

Figure 4-14 Varicose bronchiectasis in ABPA. **A** and **B:** Irregular bronchial dilatation *(arrow)* is visible.

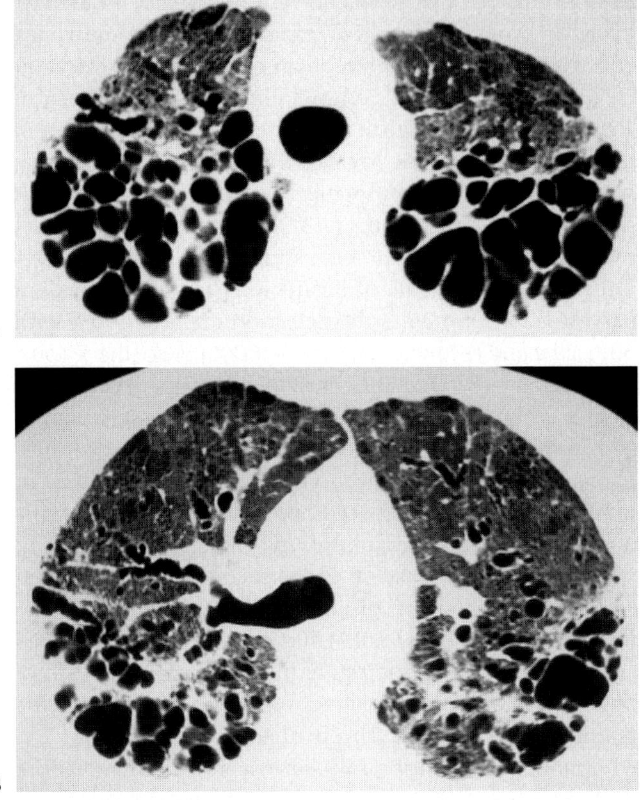

Figure 4-15 Cystic bronchiectasis. **A** and **B:** Cystic lucencies in both upper lobes represent bronchiectasis. Several dilated bronchi have a branching appearance.

strings or clusters of cysts should be considered diagnostic of cystic bronchiectasis (67).

Cystic bronchiectasis may be associated with a greater incidence of infection and greater functional impairment than milder forms of disease. In a study of patients with symptomatic bronchiectasis shown on CT (13), patients with cystic bronchiectasis were significantly more likely to grow *Pseudomonas* from their sputum and to have purulent sputum than were patients with cylindrical or varicose bronchiectasis. Also, patients with cystic bronchiectasis had significantly lower FEV^1 and FVC values than did patients with cylindrical or varicose bronchiectasis (13).

ACCURACY OF CT FOR THE DIAGNOSIS OF BRONCHIECTASIS

In our experience, most patients studied using HRCT have clinically suspected disease and subtle abnormalities identified on chest radiographs. Symptomatic patients with entirely normal radiographs are the exception. In a prospective study comparing chest radiographs and HRCT (68), a normal chest radiograph was found to exclude significant bronchiectasis with a high degree of accuracy. In this study, 37 patients had a normal radiograph, and 32 of these had a normal HRCT. The other 5 had mild cylindrical bronchiectasis. In the 47 patients with an abnormal radiograph, 36 had signs of bronchiectasis at HRCT and 11 had a normal HRCT. Thus, in this study, the sensitivity of chest radiography for detecting bronchiectasis diagnosed by HRCT was 88%, with a specificity of 74%.

CT obtained using 10-mm slice thickness is inadequate for the diagnosis of bronchiectasis, with a sensitivity of only 60% to 80% (29–31,69–72). The use of HRCT or thin-slice SCT results in significant improvement in sensitivity and accuracy.

Grenier et al. (73), using 1.5-mm-thick sections obtained every 10 mm, retrospectively compared CT and bronchography in 44 lungs in 36 patients and found that CT confirmed the diagnosis of bronchiectasis with a sensitivity of 97% and a specificity of 93%. Young et al. (32) also assessed the reliability of HRCT in the assessment of bronchiectasis, as compared with bronchography, in 259 segmental bronchi from 70 lobes of 27 lungs. HRCT was positive in 87 of 89 segmental bronchi shown to have bronchiectasis (sensitivity 98%). HRCT was negative in 169 of 170 segmental bronchi without bronchiectasis at bronchography (specificity 99%). Similar results have been reported by Giron et al. (74).

It should be emphasized that, despite the excellent sensitivity of HRCT, bronchiectasis may be focal and exceedingly subtle on HRCT scans. Cylindrical bronchiectasis, in particular, can be missed on HRCT, especially if care is not taken to obtain images in deep inspiration (73–75). Giron et al. (74), in a study of 54 patients with bronchographic evidence of bronchiectasis, found that they missed three patients, all with mild cylindrical bronchiectasis, using 1-mm slices obtained every 10 mm.

The introduction of SCT has led to a reconsideration of optimal scan protocols in patients with suspected bronchiectasis. In a study by Lucidarme et al. (76) of 50 consecutive patients with suspected bronchiectasis, 1.5-mm HRCT sections obtained at 10-mm intervals were compared with a volumetric acquisition using 3-mm collimation. These authors found volumetric data acquisition to be more accurate than routine HRCT for the identification of bronchiectasis. Specifically, bronchiectasis was noted in 77 segments (22 patients) on thin-section CT scans compared with 90 segments (26 patients) on helical CT scans. Interobserver agreement was significantly better ($p < .05$) in identification of segments that were positive for bronchiectasis on helical CT scans ($\kappa = 0.87$) than on thin-section CT scans ($\kappa = 0.71$). Although helical CT failed to identify bronchiectasis in seven segments in which the disease was diagnosed with HRCT, in four cases a diagnosis of subsegmental cylindrical bronchiectasis was made only with helical CT. In comparison, there were no patients in whom a diagnosis of bronchiectasis was established by HRCT alone.

SCT shows greatest promise in the diagnosis of subtle cylindrical bronchiectasis. The absence of bronchial tapering is often difficult to diagnose using noncontiguous 1-mm sections.

TECHNICAL CONSIDERATIONS IN THE CT DIAGNOSIS OF BRONCHIECTASIS

Most important for accurate evaluation of bronchiectasis is the use of appropriate window level and mean, especially in those cases for which quantitative information is desired. As first shown by Webb et al. (41) using phantoms composed of Lucite cylinders, an optimal window level for assessing the airway lumen and walls is −450 HU. A similar conclusion was reached by McNamara et al. also using a reference phantom (42,77). In distinction, others have suggested that window width is as important as or more important than window level in airway measurements. Bankier et al. (78), using inflation-fixed lungs to evaluate the effect of window width and levels on bronchial wall thickness confirmed by planimetry, concluded that an optimal window width should vary between 1,000 and 1,400 HU and that window levels could vary as much as −250 to −700 HU. In our experience, for practical purposes, these windows and levels are adequate for routine visual assessment.

Standard CT protocols for the assessment of suspected airway disease and bronchiectasis have generally involved the use of HRCT obtained at spaced intervals (e.g., 10 mm) (32,73,74). Such HRCT protocols have proved highly accurate. However, the development and evolution of multidetector SCT scanners are changing our approach to the diagnosis of this disease. Using multidetector SCT, the entire thorax may be imaged volumetrically, with scans being viewed using varying slice thicknesses and in different planes after completion of the study (79,80).

SCT with a slice thickness of 3 mm or less has proved comparable to or superior to spaced HRCT images in making the diagnosis of bronchiectasis and determining its extent. It is most advantageous for the diagnosis of subtle cylindrical bronchiectasis. For example, as reviewed in the preceding section, Lucidarme et al. (76) found that a volumetric spiral acquisition using 3-mm collimation was more accurate than routine HRCT (1.5-mm HRCT sections obtained at 10-mm intervals) in the identification of bronchiectasis. Although SCT failed to identify bronchiectasis in seven segments in which the disease was diagnosed with HRCT, in four cases a diagnosis of subsegmental cylindrical bronchiectasis was made only with helical CT. In comparison, in no patients was a diagnosis of bronchiectasis established by HRCT alone.

Similarly, in a study using multidetector SCT, both 3-mm-thick and 1-mm-thick slices were reconstructed in 40 patients suspected of having bronchiectasis (4 × 1-mm detectors, 120 kV, 0.5 sec/rotation, 80 mA/slice, pitch of 1.75) (81). No significant differences were found between 3-mm-thick and 1-mm-thick slices in the detection of bronchiectasis, the evaluation of bronchiectasis extent, or the characterization of bronchiectasis type (81).

With multidetector SCT, the entire thorax may be scanned in a single breath hold using a 1- to 1.25-mm detector width. This enables reformation of the scan data in any plane, with similar spatial resolution. Viewing the scan data in multiple planes may be advantageous in the diagnosis of bronchiectasis. For example, in one study, the effectiveness of coronal reconstructions of multidetector CT (120 kVp, 70 mA, 2.5-mm collimation, table speed of 15 mm/sec, table rotation time 1 sec) (82) was assessed in the diagnosis of bronchiectasis. In 110 patients who were suspected of having bronchiectasis, both axial (2.5-mm slice thickness) and coronal (1.3- to 2.0-mm slice thickness) reformatted images were reconstructed. With axial images only, the detection rate of bronchiectasis on a per-patient basis was 97%, whereas the detection rate was 100% with both axial and coronal images ($p = .0001$). Also, the readers' confidence as to the distribution of bronchiectasis was greater when both axial and coronal images were viewed ($p = .008$) (82). In another study (83), the use of multiplanar reconstruction of 1-mm multidetector CT resulted in improved agreement between observers as to the diagnosis of bronchiectasis (kappa improved from 0.29 to 0.54) (83).

Furthermore, the use of reconstruction techniques such as maximum-intensity projection (MIP) and minimum-intensity projection (MinIP) images and precise internal and external volumetric renderings of the airways are of potential value in the diagnosis of bronchiectasis, as is the possibility of creating CT bronchograms (84,85).

Although volumetric CT results in a greater radiation dose than does spaced HRCT scanning, low-dose volumetric CT may be used with a significant reduction in radiation but without loss of diagnostic information (86). In one study, 52 patients with suspected airway disease were studied using both spaced HRCT (120 kVp, 170 mA, 1-mm collimation, and 10-mm intervals) and low-dose volumetric SCT (120 kVp, 40-mA, 3-mm collimation, pitch of 2, and reconstruction interval of 2 mm). Eighty-six percent and 90% of patients were diagnosed with bronchiectasis at HRCT and low-dose helical CT, respectively. Of 928 segments evaluated by five observers, bronchiectasis was seen in 152.5 segments on HRCT and in 193.5 segments on helical CT. The radiation dose of the 40-mA helical technique averaged 3.21 mGy as compared with 2.17 mGy for HRCT (86). In another study (87), the image quality of multidetector CT scans (120 kVp, a 2.5-mm collimation, pitch of 6, 2.5-mm reconstruction interval) obtained in patients with suspected bronchiectasis was assessed with six different mA settings (170, 100, 70, 40, 20, 10 mA). Independently, two chest radiologists assessed and compared the quality of the images obtained at the six mA exposures. The mean image quality at exposures of 170, 100, and 70 mA were similar, and images obtained at 70 mA were rated significantly better than those obtained at 40 mA or less ($p < .01$). The mean radiation doses at 170, 100, 70, 40, 20, and 10 mA were 23.72, 14.39, 10.54, 5.41, 2.74, and 1.50 mGy, respectively (87).

The use of low-dose HRCT techniques for performing routine follow-up scans in patients with severe chronic disease has also been suggested (44,88). Bhalla et al. (44), evaluating scans obtained using both 70 and 20 mA showed that high-quality HRCT images of bronchiectatic airways could be obtained in patients with cystic fibrosis.

Given these options, it is apparent that choice of scan technique depends on the type of scanner available as well as available postprocessing capabilities. It is also likely that specific protocols will continue to evolve with continued clinical experience.

HRCT or multidetector SCT may also be used to evaluate the presence of air trapping in patients with suspected bronchiectasis (60,89–93). This may be accomplished either by repeatedly acquiring scans at one preselected level during a forced expiration or as two separate acquisitions, first in deep inspiration followed by scans obtained through the same region in expiration (18,60,79,91,94–98). This technique of paired inspiratory and expiratory images may be obtained using HRCT or spiral, volumetric techniques. It should be emphasized that although a variety of protocols for acquiring expiratory scans have been proposed, including volumetric expiratory imaging, 1-mm images obtained at three levels (aortic arch, tracheal carina, and above the diaphragm) are usually sufficient to identify significant air trapping, even when inspiratory scans are normal (91).

ASSESSMENT OF BRONCHIECTASIS EXTENT AND SEVERITY

Systems for grading the severity and extent of bronchiectasis by using CT findings have been proposed by various authors and have been used primarily in the assessment of patients with cystic fibrosis (CF). Bhalla et al. (44), in the first description of such a system, used nine separate variables, including the extent of mucus plugging, peribronchial thickening, generations of bronchial divisions involved, number of bullae, and the presence of emphysema, to calculate a global CT score. Based on this approach, CT was found to be a valuable tool for objectively evaluating the extent and severity of bronchiectasis in patients with CF (44).

Subsequent modifications of this system have been proposed by a number of authors (20,28,47,99–102), including differences in the definition of bronchial dilatation, bronchial wall thickening, and the extent of bronchiectasis. For example, although Bhalla et al. (44) assessed segments in their scoring system, Smith et al. (20) and others have assessed bronchiectasis extent by lobes, using a five-point scale based on the visual assessment of the number of abnormal bronchi (<25%, 25% to 49%, 50% to 74%, or >75%).

Other differences among scoring systems include the methods of describing the axial extent of disease. Some investigators assess the number of generations of airways involved (44,101,102), whereas others localize abnormal airways either in the peripheral half or one third of the lung (28,47,99) or describe the overall extent of disease as assessed regionally by lobe and zone (100). More recent scoring systems have also emphasized the inclusion of centrilobular nodules and mosaic perfusion as additional signs of airway disease (47,99,101,102).

Despite these differences, most reports have shown good correlation between the HRCT assessment of bronchiectasis extent and severity when compared with more traditional radiographic, clinical, or functional criteria for assessing CF patients (20,44,47,101,102). For example, Shah et al. (47), found that HRCT severity scores in symptomatic and asymptomatic patients correlated with FVC ($r = 0.44, p = .01$) and FEV_1 ($r = 0.34, p = .04$), and severity of bronchiectasis correlated with FVC ($r = 0.50, p = .004$) and FEV_1 ($r = 0.40, p = .02$). In symptomatic patients, improvement in HRCT score correlated with changes in FEV_1/FVC ($r = 0.39, p = .049$).

A relationship between the severity and extent of bronchiectasis and lung function also has been shown in patients who have other causes of airway diseases. Although largely assessing the same parameters, different investigators have tended to use slightly different criteria for determining the severity and extent of bronchiectasis and relating these findings to lung function or symptoms. Despite these differences, similar conclusions have been reached in several studies. The degree of bronchial wall thickening and the severity and extent of bronchiectasis correlate with PFT findings of obstruction (13,93,103,104) as do the extent of mosaic perfusion or air trapping (103,104). On multivariate analysis, bronchial wall thickness has proved to be the strongest independent determinant of airflow obstruction (93,103). In one study (103), the severity of symptoms tended to correlate with either bronchial wall thickening or the presence of small airway abnormalities.

For example, Lynch et al. (13) studied 261 patients with symptomatic bronchiectasis, excluding patients with CF, allergic bronchopulmonary aspergillosis, and fungal or mycobacterial infections. There was a weak but significant correlation between the degree of morphologic abnormality on CT and the extent of physiologic impairment. Scores for the severity and extent of bronchiectasis correlated with the FEV_1 ($r = -0.362, p = .0001$) and the FVC ($r = -0.362, p = .0001$). Scores for bronchial wall thickening correlated with the FEV_1 ($r = -0.367, p = .0001$) and FVC ($r = -0.239, p = .001$).

Similarly, in a study by Roberts et al. (93) of 100 patients with bronchiectasis, the extent and severity of bronchiectasis and the severity of bronchial wall thickening correlated strongly with the severity of airflow obstruction; the closest relationship found was between decreased FEV_1 and the extent of decreased attenuation on the expiratory scan ($r = -0.55, p < .00005$). On multivariate analysis bronchial wall thickness and decreased attenuation were the strongest independent determinants of airflow obstruction. The severity of bronchial dilatation was negatively associated with airflow obstruction.

In another study, the severity of bronchial wall thickening and the extent of bronchiectasis, small airway abnormalities (i.e., centrilobular nodules, tree-in-bud, and bronchiolectasis), and mosaic perfusion were evaluated in 60 patients with bronchiectasis and associated with clinical and functional parameters (103). The frequency of clinical exacerbations was associated with the degree of bronchial wall thickening ($r = 0.29$, $p = .04$) and the 24-hour sputum volume correlated with bronchial wall thickening and small airway abnormalities ($r = 0.30$, $p = .03$ and $r = 0.39$, $p = .004$, respectively). The extent of bronchiectasis, bronchial wall thickening, and mosaic perfusion, respectively, were related to FEV_1 ($r = -0.43$ to -0.60, $p < .001$), forced expiratory flow, midexpiratory phase ($FEF_{25\%-75\%}$) ($r = -0.38$ to -0.57, $p < .001$), FVC ($r = -0.36$ to -0.46, $p < .01$), and FEV_1/FVC ratio ($r = -0.31$ to -0.49, $p < .01$). After multiple regression analyses, bronchial wall thickening remained a significant determinant of airflow obstruction, whereas small airway abnormalities remained associated with 24-hour sputum volume (103).

Edwards et al. (104) reviewed bronchiectasis in children that was unrelated to CF. Comparisons between HRCT scan and lung function parameters showed that the strongest relationships were between the extent of bronchiectasis, bronchial wall thickening, and air trapping with FEV_1 and $FEF_{25\%-75\%}$. No relationship was demonstrated between chronic sputum infection and CT score.

Bronchial wall thickening also correlates with functional deterioration over time in patients with bronchiectasis. In one study (105), the relationships between pulmonary function indices and CT scan findings were evaluated at baseline and at follow-up at a median interval of 28 months (range 6 to 74 months) in 48 adult patients with bronchiectasis. Greater severity of mucous plugging, bronchiectasis, and bronchial wall thickness on the baseline CT were predictive of significant declines in pulmonary function over time; severe bronchial wall thickness was the most adverse prognostic determinant (105).

PITFALLS IN THE DIAGNOSIS OF BRONCHIECTASIS

A variety of pitfalls in the diagnosis of bronchiectasis have been reported (106). For the most part, they can be avoided.

Most frequent among the pitfalls are artifacts that result from cardiac and respiratory motion. Transmitted cardiac motion (pulsation) artifacts frequently obscure detail in the lingula and left lower lobe (107). With pulsation artifacts, thin streaks radiate from the edges of vessels and resemble stars and small areas of apparent lucency may be seen between these streaks. These lucent areas, if not recognized as artifactual, may be mistaken for dilated bronchi (107).

Respiratory motion or cardiac pulsation can cause ghosting artifacts that very closely mimic the appearance of tram tracks (Fig. 4-16). Such an artifact results when a linear structure, such as a fissure or vessel, is in slightly different positions (because of breathing or pulsation) when scanned from opposite directions. The structure is seen as double because of its motion during the scan, which can mimic the appearance of a bronchus with thick parallel walls (108,109). Recognizing that other structures such as

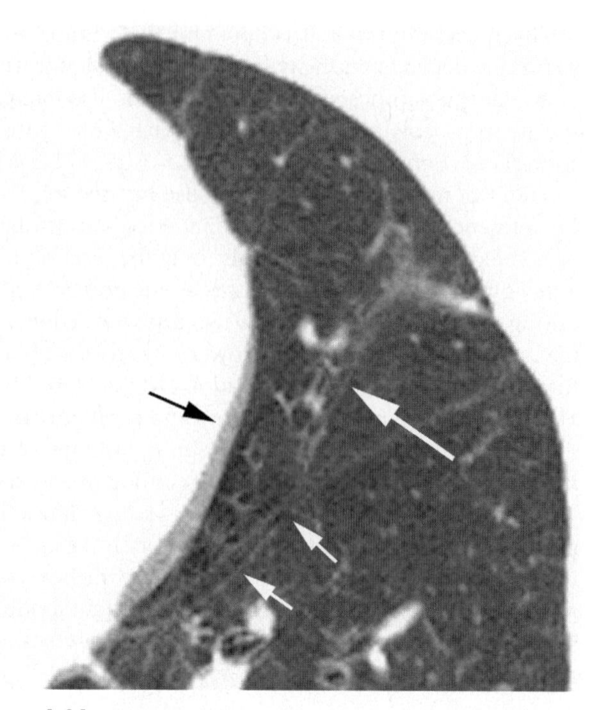

Figure 4-16 Motion artifact simulating bronchiectasis. Motion during the scan causes a ghosting artifact *(large arrow)* that mimics tram tracks. Note that the major fissure is also seen as two parallel lines *(small white arrows)* and the left heart border *(black arrow)* is seen as a double shadow.

the heart border or fissure appear double is helpful in making the correct interpretation.

The appearance of bronchial wall thickening is dependent on the use of appropriate window widths and levels (78). Using an inappropriate window can make a bronchus appear thick walled. Furthermore, on expiratory scans, bronchi can appear thicker walled and narrower than on inspiratory scans.

Bronchiectasis is difficult to diagnose in patients with concurrent parenchymal consolidation or atelectasis. In such patients, dilated peripheral airways seen on CT may revert to normal following resolution of the lung disease. This is so-called reversible bronchiectasis (Fig. 4-17) (110). Follow-up scans are recommended in patients with lung disease and apparent bronchiectasis.

Cystic lung diseases may be difficult to differentiate from bronchiectasis in some cases. In patients with Langerhans cell histiocytosis, bizarre-shaped cysts are often seen, especially in the upper lobes. Because these may seem to branch, their appearance may be suggestive of bronchiectasis. Pathologically, some of these cystic abnormalities do indeed represent abnormally dilated bronchi, presumably the result of peribronchiolar inflammation. Cystic lesions in other diseases (e.g., in patients with *Pneumocystis carinii* pneumonia) may superficially simulate bronchiectasis. The presence of the signet-ring sign can be helpful in distinguishing true bronchiectasis from cystic lung disease.

Bronchi may become dilated in association with lung fibrosis, so-called traction bronchiectasis (Fig. 4-18). Traction

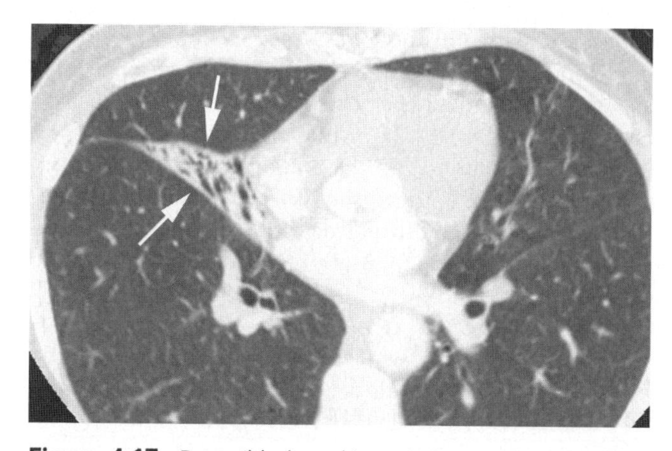

Figure 4-17 Reversible bronchiectasis in a patient with right middle lobe atelectasis. The collapsed middle lobe *(arrows)* outlines dilated and air-filled bronchi. In patients with atelectasis, apparent bronchial dilatation disappears following re-expansion.

bronchiectasis may be accurately diagnosed in most cases. Dilated bronchi appear irregularly thick walled or corkscrewed and are invariably found in association with either diffuse reticular changes or honeycombing (8). Mucoid impaction or fluid within bronchi is not present. Traction bronchiectasis does not represent primary airway disease and is unassociated with symptoms (8).

Thickening of the peribronchovascular interstitium (i.e., peribronchial cuffing), as may occur in patients with pulmonary edema, fibrosis, or infiltrative lung diseases, mimics bronchial wall thickening. Both the overall bronchial diameter and bronchial wall thickness will be increased, but the bronchial lumen is unaffected. The diameter of the adjacent pulmonary artery also will appear increased because of thickening of the surrounding interstitium, and the B/A ratio will remain normal.

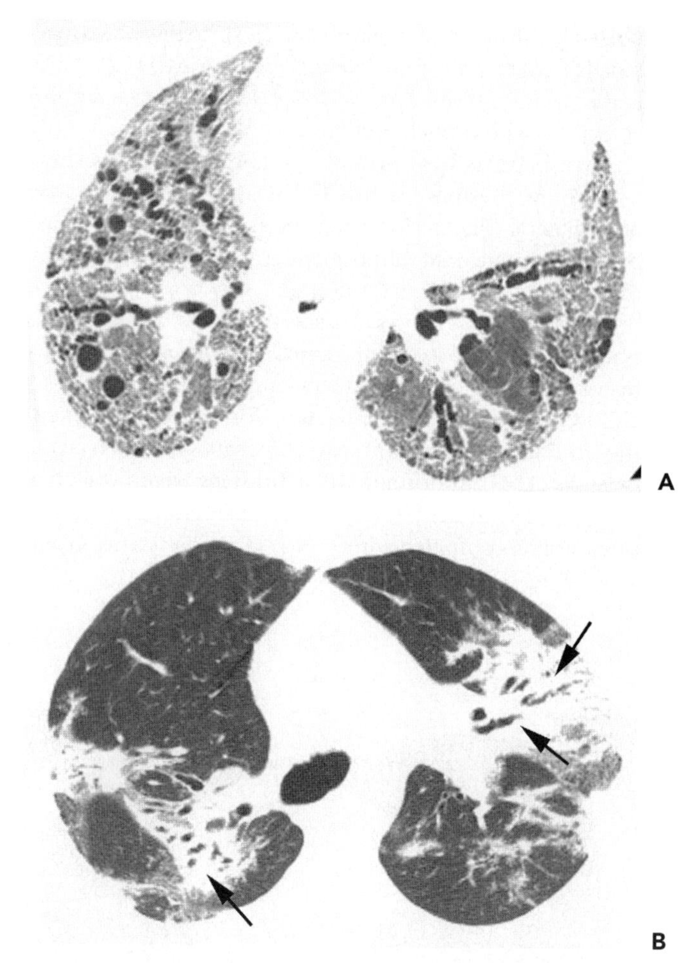

Figure 4-18 Traction bronchiectasis in patients with pulmonary fibrosis. **A:** A patient with idiopathic pulmonary fibrosis shows extensive lung fibrosis with reticulation. Multiple irregularly dilated bronchi are visible. **B:** End-stage sarcoidosis with perihilar fibrosis and associated traction bronchiectasis *(arrows)*.

SPECIFIC CAUSES OF BRONCHIECTASIS

Bronchiectasis has been associated with a wide variety of causes, the most frequent of which is acute, chronic, or recurrent infection (Table 4-1) (5–7). In a recent review of 123 patients with documented bronchiectasis, an antecedent potentially causative event, usually pneumonia, could be identified in 70% of patients (10). In another study of 150 patients with bronchiectasis (111), a cause could be identified in only 47%; in 29%, the cause was early childhood pneumonia, pertussis, or measles.

Bronchiectasis may occur in patients with a variety of genetic abnormalities, especially those with abnormal mucociliary clearance, immune deficiency, or structural abnormalities of the bronchus or bronchial wall (17). In addition to CF, causes of bronchiectasis having a genetic basis include alpha$_1$-antitrypsin deficiency; dyskinetic cilia syndrome; Young's syndrome; Williams-Campbell syndrome (congenital deficiency of the bronchial cartilage); Mounier-Kuhn syndrome (congenital tracheobronchomegaly); immunodeficiency syndromes, including Bruton's hypogammaglobulinemia, IgA, and combined IgA-IgG subclass deficiencies; and the yellow nail syndrome (yellow nails, lymphedema, and pleural effusions). Chronic or recurrent infection is common in these conditions.

Noninfectious diseases that result in airway inflammation and mucous plugging can result in bronchiectasis. These include ABPA and, to a lesser extent, asthma (23,46,112). Bronchiectasis may also occur in patients with bronchiolitis obliterans regardless of its cause, but including chronic rejection following heart-lung or lung transplantation (113–119) or bone marrow transplantation, most often as a result of rejection or chronic graft-versus-host disease (GVHD) (120).

POSTINFECTIOUS BRONCHIECTASIS

Bronchiectasis often results from chronic or severe bacterial infection, especially by those organisms associated with tissue necrosis, such as *Staphylococcus, Klebsiella,* or *Bordetella pertussis* (7). Granulomatous infections, including those caused by *Mycobacterium tuberculosis* (55), atypical mycobacteria (*Mycobacterium avium-intracellulare* or MAC) (121–123), and fungal organisms such as *Histoplasma capsulatum* are also associated with bronchiectasis.

Most patients with postinfectious bronchiectasis show nonspecific findings on HRCT. Airway abnormalities may be unilateral (Fig. 4-19) or may be seen in multiple lobes. A predominance of abnormalities in the lower lobes, middle lobe, and lingula is typical.

Bronchiectasis may be associated with bronchiolitis obliterans or the Swyer-James syndrome in patients with a history of viral or mycoplasma pneumonia. For example, 38 children requiring hospitalization for *Mycoplasma* pneumonia had HRCT from 1.0 to 2.2 years after their acute episode (124). Abnormal HRCT findings were present in 37% (14/38) of the patients with a history of *Mycoplasma* pneumonia, compared with 12% (2/17) of a control group of children with a history of *Mycoplasma* upper respiratory infection. The HRCT abnormalities in the group with a history of pneumonia, included mosaic perfusion ($n = 12$), bronchiectasis ($n = 8$), bronchial wall thickening ($n = 4$), decreased vascularity ($n = 1$), and air trapping on expiratory scan (9 of 29). The area affected by these abnormalities, usually involving two or more lobes, corresponded to the location of radiographic abnormalities occurring at the time of pneumonia.

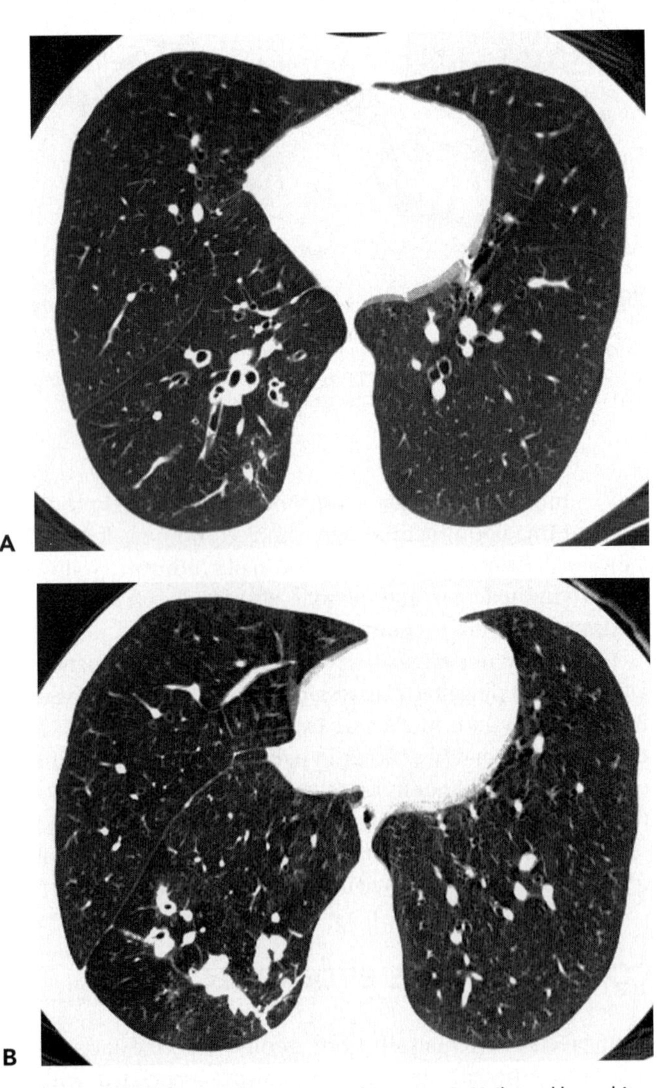

Figure 4-19 Postinfectious bronchiectasis. **A:** Unilateral bronchiectasis is visible in the right lower lobe. **B:** At a lower level, mucous plugging is visible in the right lower lobe.

NONTUBERCULOUS (ATYPICAL) MYCOBACTERIAL INFECTION

Nontuberculous, or atypical, mycobacteria (NTMB) are ubiquitous in the environment, being found in soil, lakes, streams, various food sources, and domestic animals (125,126). A number of species of NTMB have been identified, but pulmonary disease is usually the result of *Mycobacterium kansasii* or organisms classified as belonging to MAC (125–128). Because NTMB cultured from the sputum can be a contaminant rather than a pathogen, or can reflect the presence of inconsequential airway colonization in patients with morphologic abnormalities such as bronchiectasis, emphysema, or pneumoconiosis, criteria for the diagnosis of NTMB lung disease have been established by the American Thoracic Society (ATS) (129) and were updated in 1997 (130). These criteria apply only to symptomatic patients with radiographic evidence of infiltrative, nodular, or cavitary lung disease or HRCT showing multifocal bronchiectasis and/or multiple small nodules. In general terms, the ATS criteria for NTMB infection require (a) three positive cultures or two positive cultures and one positive smear for acid-fast bacilli (AFB) from three sputum samples or bronchial washings obtained in the preceding 12 months, (b) a positive bronchial washing with a 2+ to 4+ AFB smear or 2+ to 4+ growth on solid media, or (c) a transbronchial or open lung biopsy yielding NTMB or showing histopathologic features of mycobacterial infection (granulomatous inflammation and/or AFB) and one or more positive sputum or bronchial washing samples for an NTMB, even in low numbers (130). It cannot be overemphasized that definite diagnosis is a prerequisite for good patient management because treatment usually requires a prolonged course of multidrug therapy.

NTMB infection can be associated with a variety of clinical and radiographic presentations, but two common patterns are seen in immunocompetent individuals (125,126). The first of these, so-called classical NTMB infection, closely resembles TB; the second form of infection, which has been termed the "nonclassical" form of NTMB, has distinct radiographic and clinical features (125).

Classical NTMB infection is seen predominantly in men, most commonly in their fifties, sixties, and seventies, and many patients have an underlying lung disease, such as chronic obstructive pulmonary disease (COPD) or emphysema or other risk factors such as smoking, alcohol abuse, diabetes, or nonpulmonary malignancies (125,131,132). Symptoms are often insidious and include cough, hemoptysis, and weight loss; fever is present in a minority of patients. Radiographs typically show apical opacities that are nodular or consolidative and are associated with scarring and volume loss (125,126,131,133,134). As seen on chest radiographs, cavitation occurs in the large majority (90%) of patients and is frequently associated with pleural thickening (40%) or endobronchial spread of infection (60%) (131,133). Pleural effusion and lymph node enlargement are less common. Disseminated infection with an appearance mimicking that of miliary TB is uncommon, being seen in only a few percent of patients (126). Traction bronchiectasis may be seen in patients with chronic disease and fibrosis.

The second form occurs in 20% to 30% of immunocompetent patients with NTMB and is typically produced by infection with MAC (125). Patients generally lack predisposing conditions. Women constitute about 80% of patients, and many are in their seventies (121–123,125, 135,136). The onset of disease is insidious, with chronic cough and hemoptysis being the most common symptoms. Fever is uncommon (125). Typical pathologic findings include bronchiectasis, extensive granuloma formation throughout the airways, bronchiolitis, centrilobular lesions, consolidation, and cavitation (137). It is thought that the bronchiectasis commonly seen in patients with MAC represents the result of infection rather than a preexisting and predisposing condition.

Typical radiographic findings include multiple bilateral, poorly defined nodules that involve the lung in a patchy fashion and lack the upper lobe predominance seen in patients with classical disease. Patchy bronchiectasis is commonly visible radiographically, being most common in the middle lobe and lingula (138).

HRCT Findings

The HRCT appearance of pulmonary NTMB infection varies with the form of disease (121–123,125,135,136,139,140). As would be expected, the CT appearance of classical NTMB mimics that seen in patients with TB. Findings include apical opacities, cavities that may be smooth or irregular in appearance, bronchiectasis in regions of severe lung damage, pleural thickening adjacent to abnormal lung regions, and small nodules (0.5 to 2.0 cm) in areas of lung distant to the dominant focus of infection (125), probably representing endobronchial spread of infection.

In patients with nonclassical NTMB infection caused by MAC (121–123), CT typically shows a variable combination of bronchiectasis, small nodules, and tree-in-bud (Figs. 4-20 to 4-22) (121,123,135). These abnormalities tend to predominate in the right middle lobe and lingula and at the lung bases (138), although extensive lung involvement may be present in some (Figs. 4-20 to 4-22). Other findings may include atelectasis, consolidation, cavities, mediastinal lymph node enlargement, and pleural disease (138).

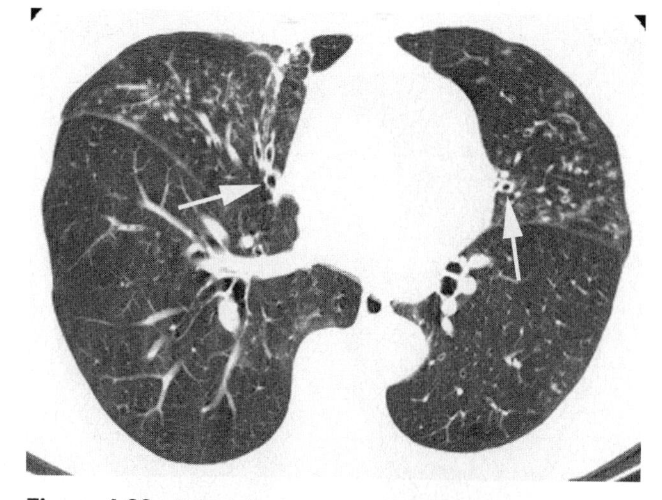

Figure 4-20 MAC infection in an elderly woman. HRCT shows bronchial wall thickening and bronchiectasis in the middle lobe and lingula *(arrows)* with small centrilobular nodules and tree-in-bud.

Similar abnormalities may be seen in patients infected with several different species of NTMB, but the severity of bronchiectasis and prevalence of nodules seen on HRCT are highest in patients with MAC infection (141).

In a study by Hartman et al. (121), CT scans were reviewed in 62 patients with positive MAC cultures. Of these, 60 had pulmonary opacities, which were nodular in 39, and 40 had bronchiectasis. Most significant, all 35 patients with small nodular infiltrates also had bronchiectasis. None of these 35 patients were immunocompromised, and 29 (83%) of them were women, with a mean age of 66 years. Of the 27 patients without small nodular infiltrates and bronchiectasis, 25 had underlying malignancy or immunocompromise. Findings of bronchiectasis, tree-in-bud, and nodules are most common in the middle lobe and lingula. The presence of reduced lung attenuation as a result of air trapping and mosaic perfusion has also been stressed as an important finding in MAC, occurring with or without bronchiectasis or small nodules in 41% of lung zones assessed in one study (142).

Moore (123) reviewed the CT and HRCT findings in 40 patients with cultures that were positive for atypical mycobacteria. Common findings included bronchiectasis (80%), consolidation or ground-glass opacity (73%), nodules (70%), and evidence of scarring and/or volume loss (28%). Less commonly observed were cavities, lymphadenopathy, and pleural disease. Both small (<1 cm), well-defined nodules and large, ill-defined nodules were seen; some small nodules were centrilobular and associated with a tree-in-bud appearance. In some patients, bronchiectasis was seen to develop in previously normal lung regions, suggesting that this finding results from the mycobacterial infection and does not represent a preexisting or predisposing condition; this has been confirmed by others (137,143). Moore concluded that some combination of bronchiectasis, consolidation, and nodules on CT scans should raise the possibility of atypical mycobacterial infec-

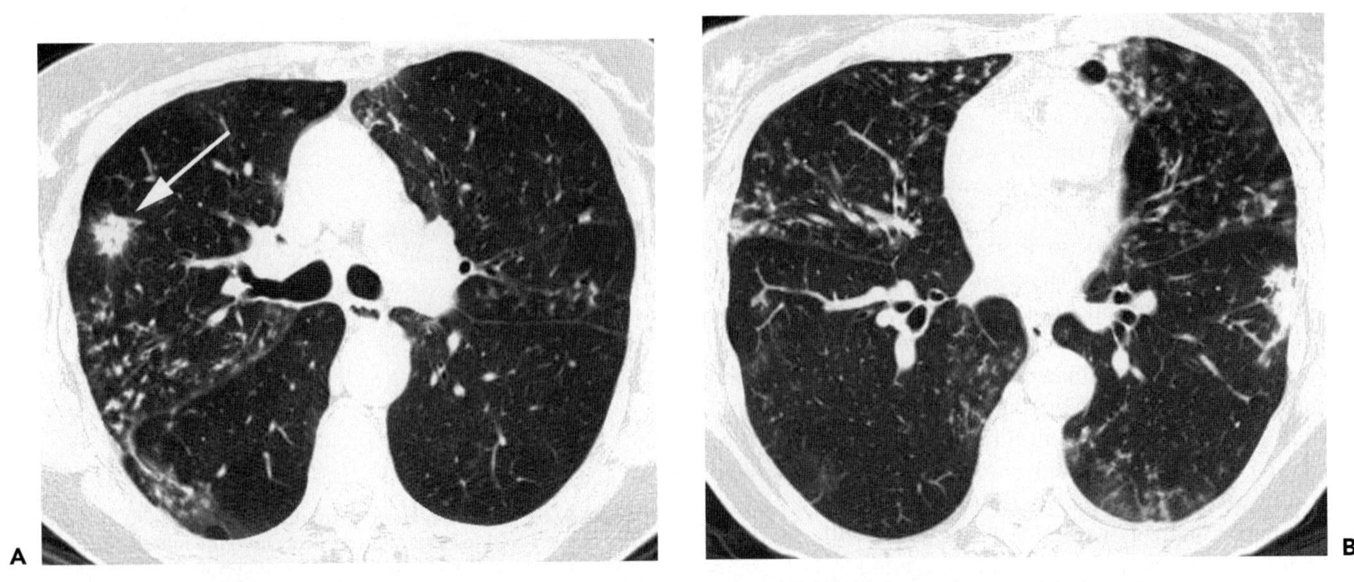

Figure 4-21 MAC infection in a 69-year-old woman. **A** and **B:** HRCT shows a large nodule *(arrow)*, small centrilobular nodules, and tree-in-bud. Abnormalities are diffuse but predominate in the middle lobe and lingula.

tion; 30 of the 40 patients showed two or three of these findings. Similar results were reported in a study of 70 patients with MAC. CT findings included bronchiectasis (97%), small nodules (89%), parenchymal distortion (60%), bronchial wall thickening (56%), consolidation (50%), and cavity formation (49%) (144).

Swensen et al. (122) tested the hypothesis that bronchiectasis and multiple small lung nodules seen on chest CT are indicative of MAC infection or colonization by reviewing the CT scans of 100 patients with a CT diagnosis of bronchiectasis; 24 of these 100 patients also had multiple pulmonary nodules visible on CT. Mycobacterial cultures were performed in 15 of the 24 patients with lung nodules seen in combination with bronchiectasis and 48 of the 76 patients who had bronchiectasis without lung nodules. Of the 15 patients with bronchiectasis and lung nodules, 8 (53%) had cultures positive for MAC, as did 2 of the 48 (4%) patients with no CT evidence of lung nodules. Thus, the authors found that CT findings of small lung nodules in association with bronchiectasis had a sensitivity of 80%, a specificity of 87%, and an accuracy of 86% in predicting positive cultures for MAC. Similar findings were documented by Tanaka et al. (145) in a prospective study of 26 patients evaluated over a 4-year period with findings on CT suggestive of MAC pulmonary disease, including clusters of small nodules in the lung periphery and bronchiectasis. Thirteen of these patients

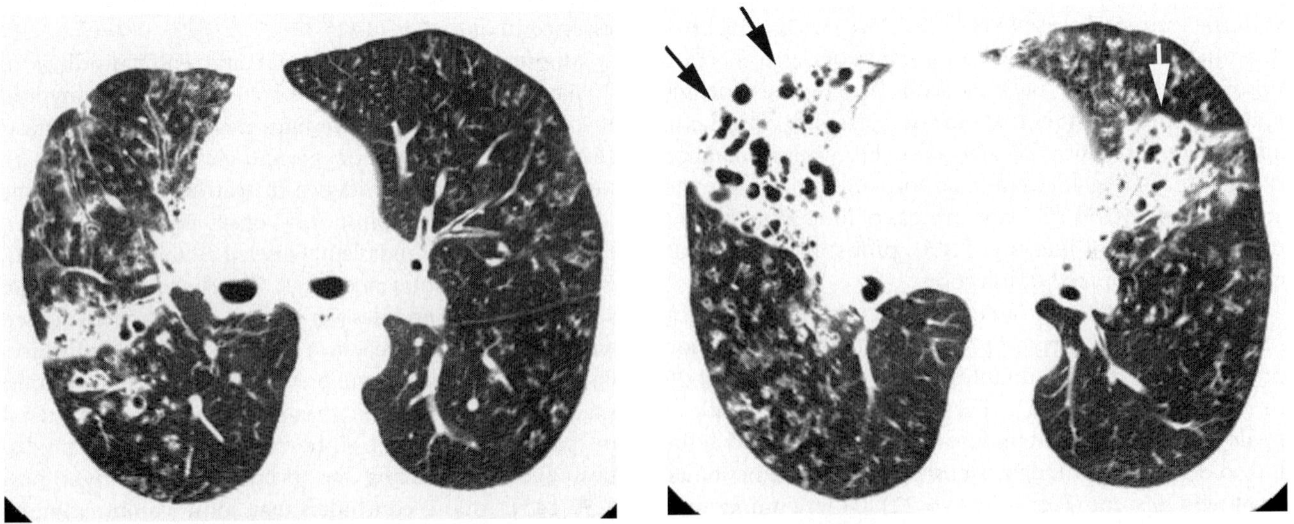

Figure 4-22 MAC infection in a 65-year-old woman. **A** and **B:** HRCT shows bronchiectasis in the right middle lobe and lingula *(arrows)*, small centrilobular nodules, and tree-in-bud.

(50%) proved to have positive MAC cultures from bronchial washings (145), and epithelioid granulomas were demonstrated in 8 of the 13 on biopsy.

CT findings of MAC may progress, improve, or remain stable on follow-up studies (143). In a study of 18 women and 7 men with a median age of 66 years who had a diagnosis of MAC, the initial chest CT examination showed findings typical of MAC, including bronchiectasis (visible in 53% of lung regions examined), centrilobular nodules (69%), nodules (32%), air-space disease (12%), and cavities (4%). The middle lobe and lingula were most frequently involved. Bronchiectasis scores were significantly higher on CT studies obtained an average of 28 months after the initial examination; bronchiectasis progressed in 15 patients and improved in 4 patients. Centrilobular nodules progressed in 9 patients and improved in 7 during follow-up. Similarly, in another study, CT scans before and during follow-up were reviewed (142). Pretreatment CT scans showed small nodules in 47% of the lung zones studied, reduced lung attenuation in 41%, and bronchiectasis in 27%. In patients without treatment, or with noncurative treatment, bronchiectasis developed or worsened in 46% of lung zones. In contrast, after curative treatment, small nodules disappeared completely in 48% of lung zones.

TUBERCULOSIS

The CT and HRCT findings seen in association with TB are numerous and varied and reflect the protean manifestations of this disease (55,135,146–155). HRCT findings of airway abnormalities associated with endobronchial spread of infection are common in patients with newly diagnosed active TB or recent reactivation of disease. Of 29 patients with newly diagnosed active TB (55), 28 (97%) had HRCT findings of endobronchial spread of infection, with centrilobular nodules or centrilobular branching structures (97%), a tree-in-bud appearance (72%), and bronchial wall thickening (79%) with or without bronchiectasis. These findings typically indicate active airway inflammation.

Bronchiectasis and bronchial wall thickening may be seen in patients with reactivation TB, both before and after treatment (156,157). They largely reflect the presence of lung fibrosis and volume loss (i.e., traction bronchiectasis) (Fig. 4-23) (55) but may also be the result of primary airway infection or secondary bronchial obstruction occurring as a result of bronchial stricture (Fig. 4-24). In 12 patients with reactivation TB reported by Im et al. (55), HRCT findings included distortion of bronchovascular structures (58%), bronchiectasis (58%), emphysema (50%), and fibrotic bands (50%). Similarly, Hatipoglu et al. (158) compared the HRCT findings in 32 patients with newly diagnosed active pulmonary TB and 34 patients with inactive disease. Active TB was associated with HRCT findings of infectious bronchiolitis such as centrilobular nodules and/or branching linear opacities present (91% of patients) and tree-in-bud (71%), whereas patients with inactive disease showed findings of

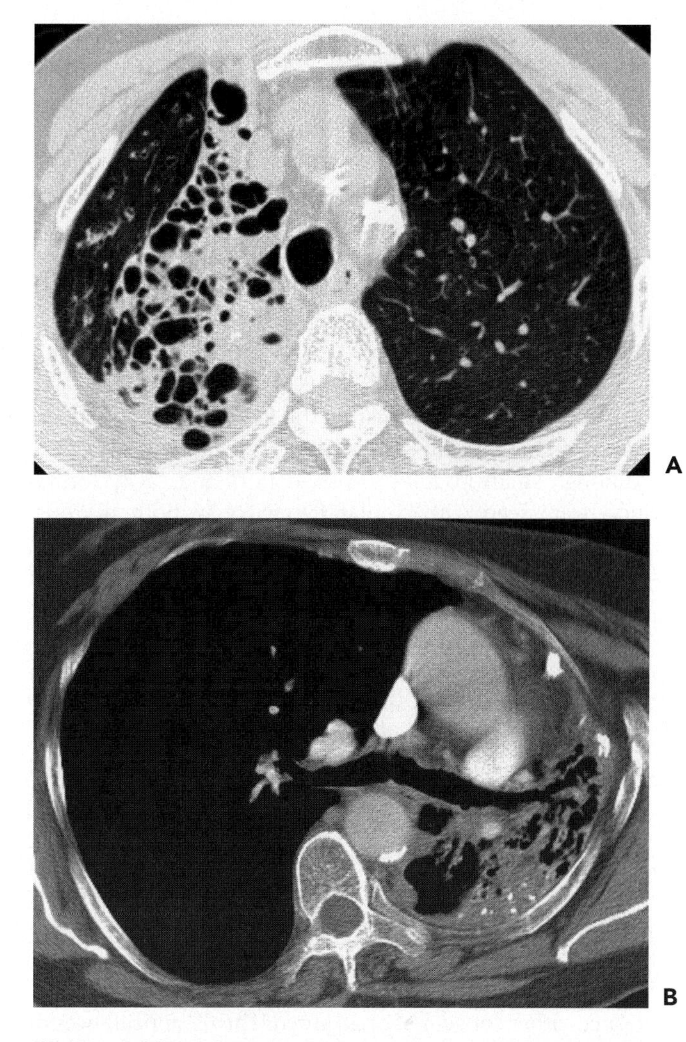

Figure 4-23 Tuberculosis with traction bronchiectasis in two patients. **A:** Right upper volume loss with traction bronchiectasis. **B:** Extensive left lung atelectasis with mediastinal shift. Traction bronchiectasis is visible within the left lung. Calcified granulomas are also visible within consolidated lung.

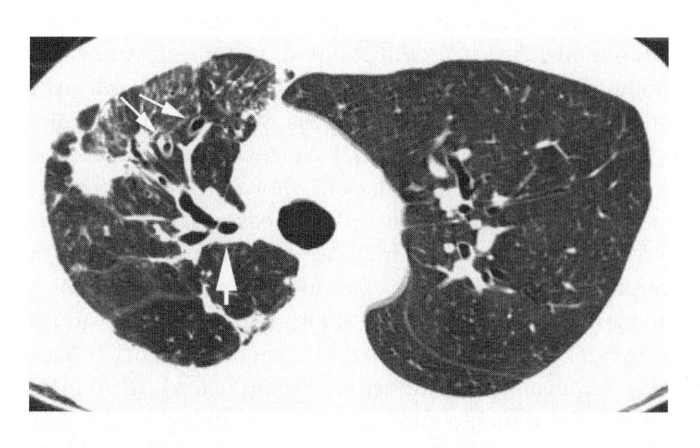

Figure 4-24 Tuberculosis with bronchial stricture and bronchiectasis. Narrowing of the right upper lobe bronchus is the result of a tuberculous stricture *(large arrow)*. Areas of bronchiectasis *(small arrows)* are visible in the right upper lobe, associated with volume loss, a large nodule, and small centrilobular nodules. The stricture was treated with placement of a stent.

fibrosis (100%), including distortion of bronchovascular structures (94%) and bronchiectasis (71%) (158). Other airway abnormalities occurring as sequelae of TB include tracheobronchial stenosis and broncholithiasis (159).

Because reactivation TB often occurs in the upper lobes and may be unilateral or asymmetrical, bronchiectasis seen in patients with TB may be unilateral and may have an upper lobe predominance. This distribution is less common in other causes of bronchiectasis. In one study assessing the accuracy of CT in diagnosing the cause of bronchiectasis, a correct diagnosis of TB as a cause was made in 16 of 24 patients (67%) (100).

In a study (135) comparing the frequency of bronchiectasis in patients with TB to that seen with MAC infection, although small nodules, consolidation, and cavity formation were seen with similar frequency in both diseases, bronchiectasis was found to be significantly more common in patients with MAC (94% vs. 27% for patients with TB). Similar results were reported by Lynch et al. (136) in a study of 15 subjects with TB and 55 subjects with MAC. Bronchiectasis involving four or more lobes (often associated with centrilobular nodules) and the combination of right middle lobe and lingular bronchiectasis were seen only in MAC. Kasahara et al. (144) found bronchiectasis and parenchymal distortion to be significantly more common in patients with MAC as compared with those with TB.

IMMUNE DEFICIENCY

Bronchiectasis is common in patients with immune deficiency, either congenital or acquired. The CT appearances of bronchiectasis in these conditions are largely nonspecific and typical of patients with bronchiectasis occurring because of severe or chronic infection (160).

Hypogammaglobulinemia

The radiographic and HRCT study of 22 patients with primary hypogammaglobulinemia (18 with common variable immunodeficiency, 4 with X-linked agammaglobulinemia) showed pulmonary abnormalities in most, despite adequate immunoglobulin replacement therapy (161). HRCT revealed pulmonary abnormalities in 21 patients, and bronchiectasis was present in 16 patients. PFT showed obstruction in 5 patients. In a 3-year follow-up of 14 patients, progression of bronchiectasis occurred in 5, all of whom were receiving appropriate intravenous immunoglobulin replacement therapy (161). Similarly, in a study of 19 patients (mean age 33 years) with common variable immunodeficiency (CVID) and hypogammaglobulinemia, being treated with intravenous immunoglobulin replacement, bronchiectasis was diagnosed using HRCT in 11 patients (58%), and in 8 patients (42%) abnormalities were multilobar (162). All patients also underwent complete PFTs. Chronic airflow limitation (CAL) was present in 10 patients (53%), and 11 patients (58%) had a decrease in single-breath carbon monoxide diffusing capacity (DLCO) (162).

HIV- and AIDS-Related Airway Disease and Bronchiectasis

A number of reports have shown an increased prevalence of airway-related infections in HIV-positive and AIDS patients (163–168). Bacterial pneumonia and bronchitis have superseded *Pneumocystis* pneumonia as the most common pulmonary infection in AIDS patients (169–171). Wallace et al. (171), for example, in a study of more than 1,000 HIV-positive patients without an AIDS-defining illness found a significantly higher incidence of acute bronchitis compared with HIV-negative subjects (171). Airway infection most commonly results from organisms such as *H. influenzae, P. aeruginosa, Streptococcus viridans,* or *S. pneumoniae,* although both mycobacterial and fungal organisms may also be involved (164).

An accelerated form of bronchiectasis occurs in HIV-positive patients with airway infection (163,167,172). Although the etiology is unclear, it is likely that bronchiectasis results from recurrent bacterial infections affecting airways, possibly made more susceptible because of the direct effects of HIV infection on the pulmonary immune system. Recently, a correlation has been shown between airway dilatation identified by CT and the presence of elevated levels of neutrophils on bronchoalveolar lavage (BAL). In a study comparing BAL findings in 50 HIV-positive subjects with those of 11 HIV-negative individuals, King et al. (165) showed that patients with bronchial dilatation on CT had significantly higher BAL neutrophil counts ($p = .014$) as well as significantly lower diffusing capacity ($p = .003$). As noted by these authors, neutrophils are an important mediator of pulmonary damage, possibly because of the action of human neutrophil elastase.

Bronchiectasis is commonly identified in patients with HIV infection or AIDS (163). King et al. (165) have shown that bronchial dilatation is common in HIV-positive patients, being seen in 36% of them. Because various manifestations of airway infection and bronchiectasis may be present, this condition is often called AIDS-related airway disease.

AIDS-related airway disease is manifested by a variety of HRCT abnormalities, a fact that reflects the different organisms that may be involved. Findings include bronchial wall thickening, bronchiectasis, bronchial or bronchiolar impaction with tree-in-bud, endoluminal masses or nodules, and consolidation (164). A lower lobe predominance is typical, and abnormalities are often bilateral and symmetrical (Fig. 4-25). The common HRCT finding of air trapping in HIV-positive patients suggests that small airway disease may be a significant contributor to pulmonary function decline and may precede more obvious findings of airway disease (173). Gelman et al. (173) evaluated the HRCT scans of 59 subjects using inspiratory and expiratory HRCT, 48 of whom were HIV positive and 11 of whom were

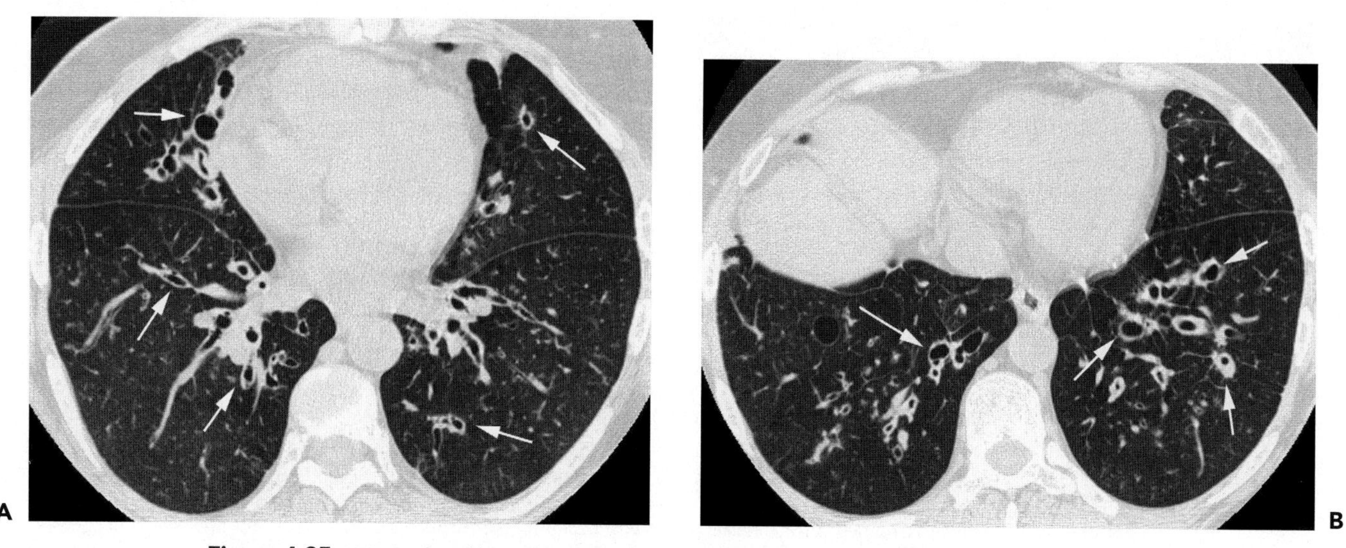

Figure 4-25 AIDS-related bronchiectasis. **A** and **B:** HRCT shows multifocal bronchiectasis *(arrows)* involving the middle lobe, lingula, and both lower lobes.

HIV negative. Expiratory CT revealed focal air trapping in 33 subjects, 30 of whom were HIV positive and 3 of whom were HIV negative ($p = .0338$). The mean values of FEV_1, forced midexpiratory flow, and diffusion capacity were significantly lower for subjects with focal air trapping than for those with normal findings on CT ($p = .001$, $p = .021$, and $p = .003$, respectively).

It should also be noted that, although less common than bacterial or viral infections, the airways may be infected by fungal organisms; *Aspergillus* is most common. Typically occurring late in the course of HIV infection, and usually in association with other risk factors, including corticosteroid use and granulocytopenia, approximately 10% of all reported cases of aspergillosis in AIDS patients affect the airways (164). Several distinct subtypes of airway aspergillosis have been described, including necrotizing tracheobronchitis, obstructing bronchopulmonary aspergillosis, and chronic cavitary parenchymal aspergillosis (174–176).

Obstructing bronchial aspergillosis represents a stage before frank tissue invasion. It typically presents acutely with fever, dyspnea, and progressive cough associated with the expectoration of fungal casts and is characterized on CT by the presence of mucoid impaction typically involving the lower lobe airways (176). It has been suggested that this form of disease is unique to AIDS patients.

Rarely, aspergillosis primarily affects the small airways in the absence of bronchial inflammation. This form of infection has been termed chronic cavitary parenchymal aspergillosis and results in necrotic debris and fungi filling respiratory bronchioles with extension into adjacent alveolar spaces (177).

Necrotizing tracheobronchial aspergillosis (also referred to as diffuse, ulcerative, and pseudomembranous tracheobronchitis) is associated with frank tissue invasion resulting in a range of abnormalities on CT from subtle focal irregularity and nodularity of airway walls to airway obstruction with or without accompanying parenchymal infiltrates.

BRONCHIAL OBSTRUCTION

Bronchial narrowing or obstruction may result in bronchiectasis because of chronic infection, mucous plugging, and chronic atelectasis with fibrosis. Obstruction may be associated with an aspirated foreign body, postinflammatory stricture, congenital bronchial abnormality, or bronchial neoplasm or as a result of external compression by a mass or enlarged lymph nodes.

Focal bronchiectasis associated with volume loss in the affected lung region and bronchial impaction are typically present (Fig. 4-26). Dilated and mucus-filled bronchi may be visible as mucous bronchograms within consolidated lung. Bronchial abnormalities may also be seen after the cause of obstruction has been relieved and the bronchi are air filled. In patients with atelectasis, distinction of postobstructive bronchiectasis from reversible atelectasis is difficult (Figs. 4-17 and 4-26B).

CYSTIC FIBROSIS

CF is the most common cause of pulmonary insufficiency in the first three decades of life (178,179). It results from an autosomal recessive genetic defect in the structure of the cystic fibrosis transmembrane regulator protein, which leads to abnormal chloride transport across epithelial membranes. The mechanisms by which this abnormality leads to lung disease are not entirely understood, but an abnormally low

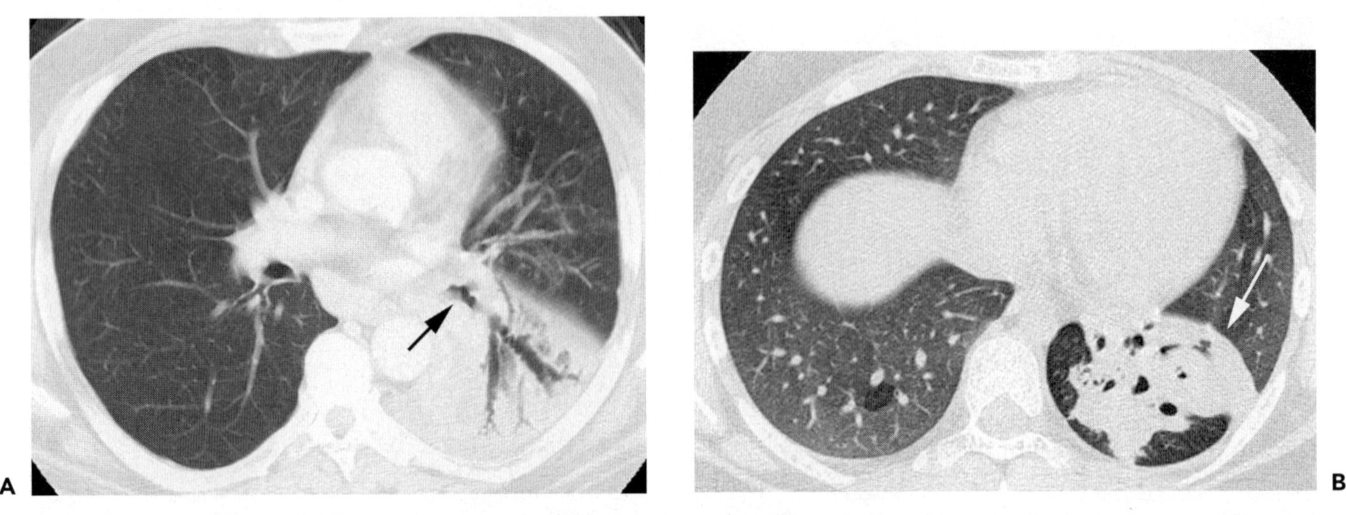

Figure 4-26 Postobstructive bronchiectasis in two patients. **A:** Bronchiectasis distal to an obstructing carcinoma. The proximal left lower lobe bronchus is narrowed (arrow). Left lower lobe atelectasis and irregular bronchiectasis are present. **B:** Left lower lobe atelectasis *(arrow)* resulting from bronchial obstruction is associated with bronchiectasis. This appearance is difficult to distinguish from reversible bronchiectasis.

water content of airway mucus is at least partially responsible, resulting in decreased mucous clearance, mucous plugging of airways, and an increased incidence of bacterial airway infection. Bronchial wall inflammation progressing to secondary bronchiectasis is universal in patients with longstanding disease and is commonly visible on chest radiographs (180).

Plain radiographs can be diagnostic in patients with CF, showing increased lung volumes, accentuated linear opacities in the central or upper lung regions resulting from bronchial wall thickening or bronchiectasis, central bronchiectasis, and mucoid impaction (180). However, plain film findings in patients with early or mild disease may be quite subtle. Hyperinflation, which can represent an early finding, reflects the presence of obstruction of small airways by mucus; thickening of the wall of the right upper lobe bronchus, best seen on the lateral radiograph, can also be an early sign of disease (181). In adult patients with CF and patients with chronic disease, abnormalities can include cystic regions in the upper lobes, representing cystic bronchiectasis, healed abscess cavities, or bullae; atelectasis; findings of pulmonary hypertension or cor pulmonale; pneumothorax; and pleural effusion (182). In the large majority of patients with an established diagnosis of CF, clinical findings and chest radiographs are sufficient for clinical management. On the other hand, it should be recognized that the symptoms of patients with CF can be significantly exacerbated with little visible radiographic change (183).

HRCT Findings

HRCT findings in patients with CF have been well described (44,47,99,101,102,179,184–186). Bronchiectasis is present in all patients with advanced CF (44,47,99,101,102,179, 184,185). Proximal or parahilar bronchi are always involved when bronchiectasis is present, and bronchiectasis is limited to these central bronchi in about a third of patients, a finding that is referred to as "central bronchiectasis." Both

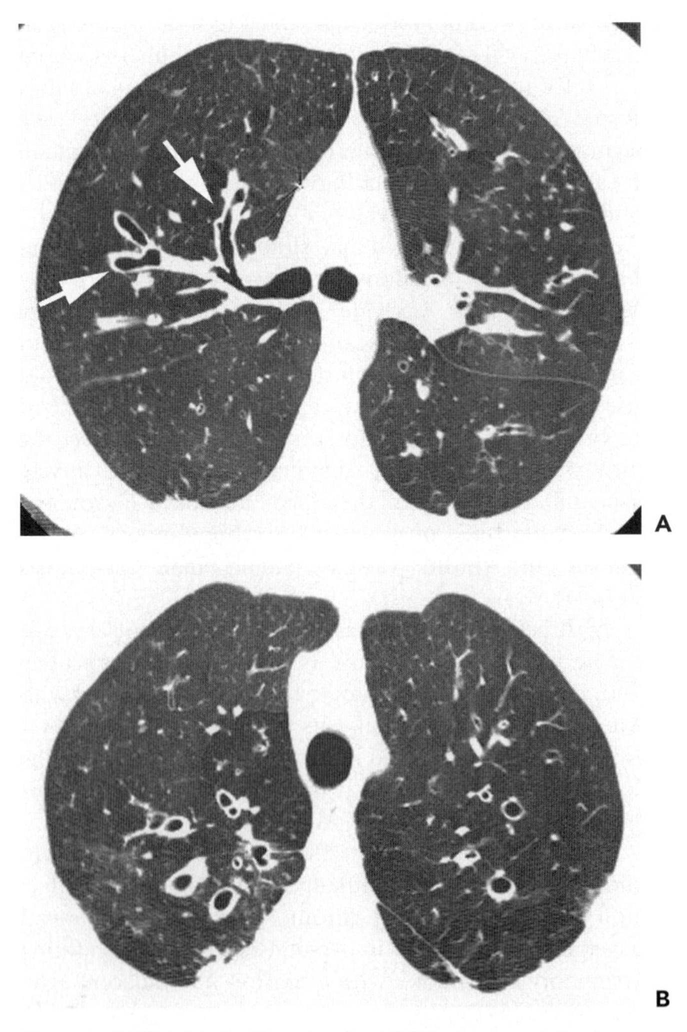

Figure 4-27 Cystic fibrosis. **A:** HRCT shows predominant involvement of the right upper lobe bronchi *(arrows)* with bronchial wall thickening and bronchiectasis. Central bronchial involvement is typical. **B:** Central bronchial wall thickening and bronchiectasis are visible in both upper lobes.

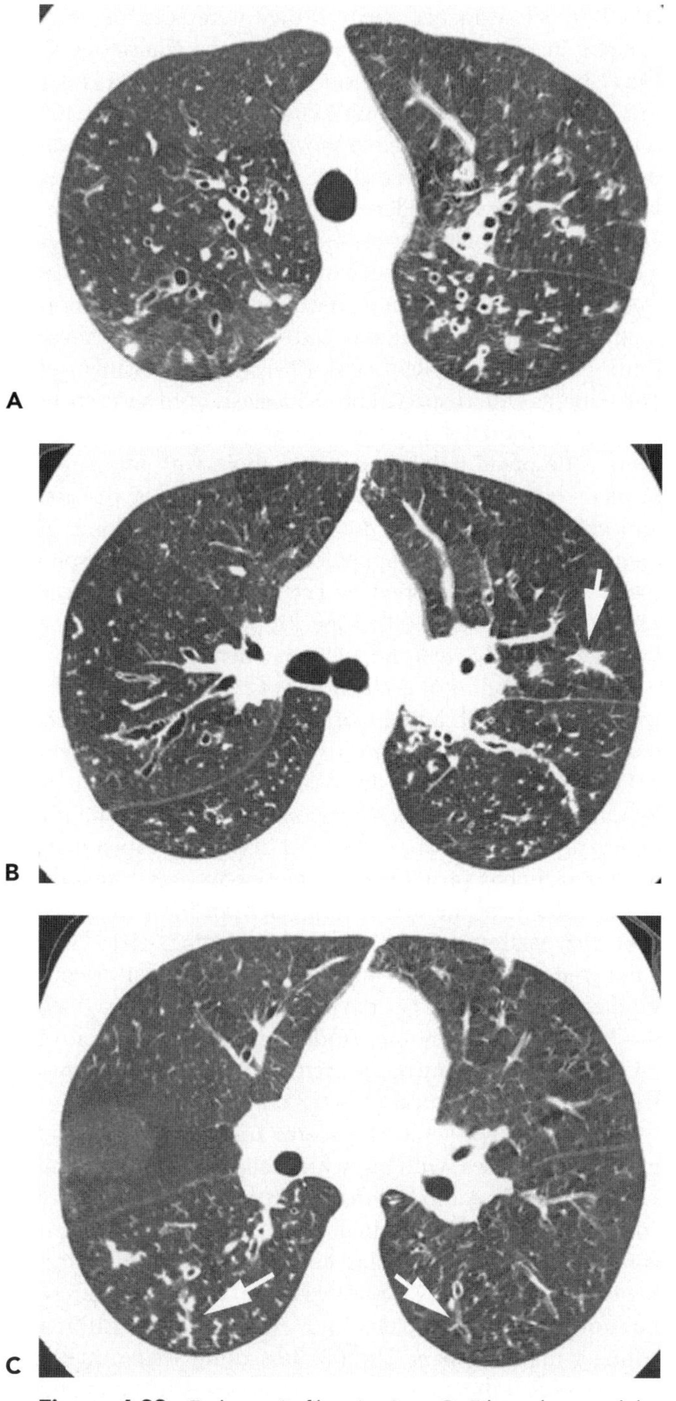

Figure 4-28 Early cystic fibrosis. **A** to **C:** Bilateral upper lobe bronchiectasis is visible. The most abnormal bronchi are central in location. Nodule opacity (*arrow*, **B**) represents a mucous plug. Tree-in-bud is also visible (*arrows*, **C**).

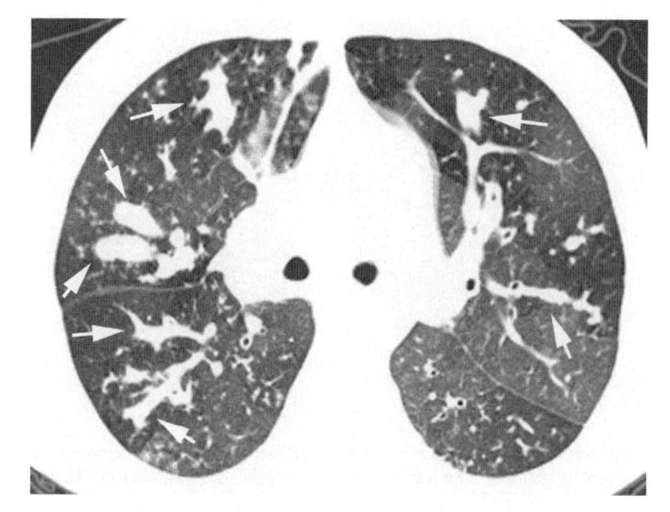

Figure 4-29 Mucous plugging in cystic fibrosis. A 9-year-old child shows extensive mucous plugging in the upper lobes *(arrows)*. As with bronchiectasis in CF, the mucous plugging is centrally located.

the central and peripheral bronchi are abnormal in about two thirds of patients (Figs. 4-27 and 4-28) (44,184).

All lobes are typically involved, although early in the disease abnormalities are often predominantly distributed in the upper lobe, and a right upper-lobe predominance may be present in some patients (Figs. 4-27 and 4-28) (44,47,99,101,102,179,184–186). It has also been pointed out, however, that in children, bronchiectasis may be primarily present in the lower lobe. In a study of HRCT in 16 children younger than 12 years, Marchant et al. (187) found that the lower lobes were universally involved but that 5 of the 16 children did not have any upper lobe disease. Cylindrical bronchiectasis is the most frequent pattern seen and was visible in 94% of lobes in one study of patients with severe disease (184); 34% of lobes in this study showed cystic bronchiectasis, and varicose bronchiectasis was seen in 11%. In another report, cystic lesions representing cystic bronchiectasis or abscess cavities were present in 8 of 14 (57%) patients (44).

Bronchial wall and/or peribronchial interstitial thickening is also common in patients with CF (Figs. 4-27 to 4-29) (99,101,102,188). It is generally more evident than bronchial dilatation in patients who have early disease and may be seen independent of bronchiectasis (44,186). Thickening of the wall of proximal right upper lobe bronchi was the earliest abnormal feature visible on HRCT in studies of patients with mild CF (44,186).

Mucous plugging is also common, reported in between one quarter and one half of patients (Figs. 4-28B and 4-29) (99,101,102), and may be visible in all lobes (44,185). Collapse or consolidation can be seen in as many as 80% of patients (Fig. 4-30) (44,99,188). Volume loss was visible in 20% of lobes in patients with advanced disease (184).

Branching or nodular centrilobular opacities (i.e., tree-in-bud), which reflect the presence of bronchiolar dilatation with associated mucous impaction, infection, or peribronchiolar inflammation, can be an early sign of disease (Fig. 4-28) (185). Focal areas of decreased lung opacity, representing air trapping or mosaic perfusion, are common (Fig. 4-11). These can be seen to correspond to pulmonary lobules or subsegments and may appear to surround dilated, thick-walled, or mucus-plugged bronchi (185) in as

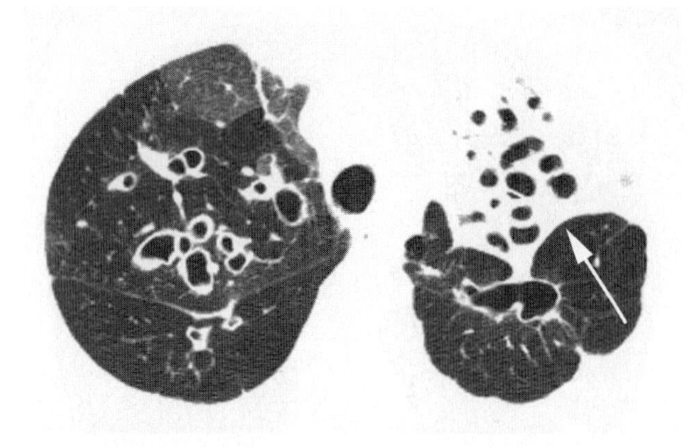

Figure 4-30 Atelectasis in CF. Upper lobe bronchiectasis is present bilaterally. The left upper lobe *(arrow)* is collapsed. Air bronchograms are visible within the collapsed lobe.

many as two thirds of patients (101). Air trapping can often be seen on expiratory scans (184).

Lung volumes may appear increased on CT, although this diagnosis is rather subjective and may be better assessed on chest radiographs (184). Cystic or bullous lung lesions can also be visible and typically predominate in the subpleural regions of the upper lobes (Fig. 4-31) (44,184). Hilar or mediastinal lymph node enlargement and pleural abnormalities can also be seen, largely reflecting chronic infection. Pulmonary artery dilatation resulting from pulmonary hypertension can also be seen in patients with longstanding disease.

HRCT Correlation with Clinical Measures in CF

HRCT can demonstrate morphologic abnormalities in patients with early CF who are asymptomatic, have normal pulmonary function, or have normal chest radiographs. In a study of 38 patients with mild CF who had normal pulmonary function (186), chest radiographs were normal in 17 (45%), showed mild bronchial wall thickening in 17, and revealed mild bronchiectasis in 4 (10%). On HRCT in this group, features of bronchiectasis were present in 77% of all patients and in 65% of those with normal chest radiographs; only 3 patients had a normal HRCT (186). In another study of HRCT findings in 12 largely asymptomatic pediatric patients with early CF, chest radiographs were normal in 7, but HRCT was normal in only 2. HRCT findings not visible on radiographs included bronchial wall thickening, bronchiectasis, centrilobular small airway abnormalities, and lobular or segmental inhomogeneity representing mosaic perfusion or air trapping (185).

In patients with more advanced disease, HRCT can also show abnormalities not visible on chest radiographs. In a study of 14 patients with CF (44), HRCT was found to be superior to chest radiographs in detecting bronchiectasis and mucous plugging. Of a total of 162 segments assessed, bronchiectasis was detected in 124 segments using HRCT, whereas only 71 segments were considered to show this finding on chest radiographs. Mucous plugs were detected on HRCT in 38 segments, whereas they were seen on radiographs in only 4 segments. In a study by Hansell et al. (184), bronchiectasis was considered to be present on HRCT in 124 of 126 lobes; on chest radiographs, only 84 of 102 lung zones were considered to show this finding. Chest radiographs also failed to reveal the extent of bronchiectasis. Bronchiectasis was considered to be both central and peripheral in only 31% of lung zones on chest radiographs, whereas a diffuse distribution was seen in 59% of lobes using HRCT.

Despite numerous reports detailing the range of abnormalities identified in patients with CF, few if any of these findings are specific. Reiff et al. (28), in an assessment of 168 patients with suspected bronchiectasis from a variety of etiologies, found that patients with adult CF tended to have more widespread involvement than those with idiopathic bronchiectasis ($p < .01$). In patients with early disease, abnormalities are often predominantly upper lobe in distribution, with a right upper lobe predominance. Despite these findings, as reported by Lee et al. (189) and more recently Cartier et al. (100), a specific diagnosis of adult CF was made in only 38% and 68% of patients, respectively.

The routine clinical evaluation of CF makes use of clinical and radiograph-based scoring systems. Several authors have also suggested the use of an HRCT scoring system (44,99,190); these were described in detail earlier. It is hypothesized that such a scoring system may facilitate the objective evaluation of existing and newly developed therapeutic regimens (44). One scoring system (44), based on an assessment of the degree and extent of bronchiectasis, bronchial wall thickening, mucous plugging, atelectasis, emphysema, and other findings, showed a statistically significant correlation to the percent ratios of FEV_1/FVC ($r = 0.69$, $p = .006$) (44). In another study based on assessment of bronchiectasis and mucous plugging (190), CT scores correlated highly with clinical ($r = 0.88$, $p < .0001$) and radiographic ($r = 0.93$, $p < .0001$) scores and several PFTs. The best correlation was with bronchiectasis. Two of the scoring systems (Bhalla and Nathanson) have been directly compared in young children, that is, the age group in which other objective markers of disease are scarce. Marchant et al. (187) reviewed the clinical findings, pulmonary function data, and HRCT of 16 children younger than 12 years. The Bhalla scoring system had a better correlation with FEV_1 ($r = -0.65$, $p = .012$) than did the Nathanson score ($r = 0.53$, $p = 0.05$).

CT offers a reliable alternative to routine radiographic and clinical methods for monitoring disease status and progression as well as for assessing response to treatment (44,102,190,191). These studies consistently document close correlation between HRCT findings and both clinical and pulmonary functional evaluation of these patients.

HRCT may be used to closely monitor potentially reversible morphologic changes as a means for monitoring both disease progression and treatment therapy. Shah et al. (47), using a modification of the scoring system proposed by Bhalla et al. (44), reported findings in 19 symptomatic patients with adult CF evaluated initially and

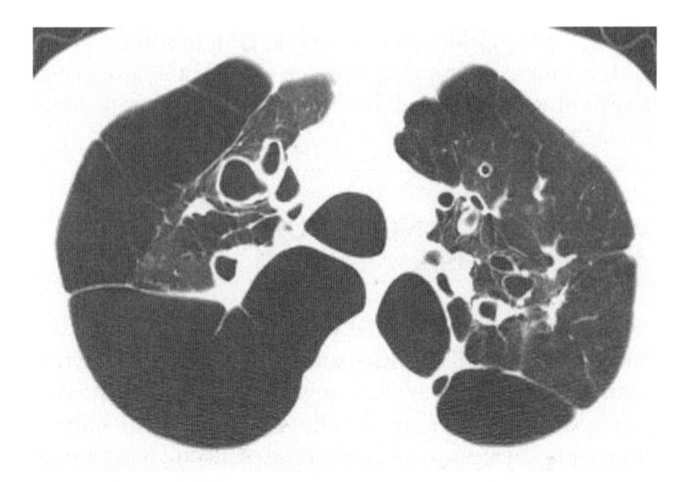

Figure 4-31 Bullae in CF. Upper lobe bronchiectasis is associated with large bullae in the peripheral lung.

following 2 weeks of therapy compared with a control group of 8 asymptomatic CF patients. Reversible findings included air–fluid levels in bronchiectatic cavities, centrilobular nodules, mucous plugging, and peribronchial thickening. Significantly, although severity of bronchiectasis was found to correlate with FVC ($p = .004$) and FEV_1 ($p = .02$), no correlation was identified between PFT parameters and either mucous plugging or centrilobular nodules, suggesting that PFTs were an insensitive means for identifying potentially reversible and hence treatable disease (47).

In a related study, Helbich et al. (102) evaluated serial CT studies obtained at various time intervals up to 48 months in 107 patients to determine both the evolution of findings as well as optimal time intervals for sequential CT evaluation. These authors found that 6- to 18-month follow-up was valuable for identifying potentially reversible morphologic changes and, in particular, the presence of mucous plugging. In distinction, progression of bronchiectasis and mosaic perfusion progressed at a significantly slower rate, rendering them less useful as a means for monitoring therapeutic interventions. Of particular interest was the finding that, although CT correlated significantly with PFTs and clinical scores, these same parameters by comparison with CT were relatively insensitive means for identifying either improvement or disease progression (102). Although mucous plugging could be identified in 25% of patients reexamined by CT within 18 months, for example, only minor changes could be identified through pulmonary function testing.

These findings support the contention that HRCT should be added to the follow-up regimens of patients with CF. In distinction, it has been reported that CT may play only a limited role in the preoperative assessment of patients with CF before lung transplantation (192). In a recent retrospective review of 26 patients with CF who subsequently underwent bilateral lung transplantation, in no case was an unsuspected malignancy identified (192). Of particular surgical interest, CT proved of little value in predicting the presence of pleural adhesions, a potential concern before transplantation.

ASTHMA

Asthma is characterized by hyperreactivity of the airways to various stimuli, airway inflammation, and largely reversible airway obstruction (193,194). Pathologically, patients with asthma show bronchial wall thickening caused by inflammation and edema and excess mucus production that can result in mucous plugging (195). Bronchiectasis may be seen in some patients with longstanding asthma.

Radiographic findings associated with asthma include increased lung volume, increased lung lucency, mild bronchial wall thickening, and mild prominence of hilar vasculature resulting from transient pulmonary hypertension (196–199). Bronchial wall thickening is visible in about half of patients (23,199). Bronchiectasis is not usually recognized, but small mucous plugs can sometimes be seen. Associated complications of asthma, although uncommon, include pneumonia, atelectasis, pneumomediastinum, and pneumothorax (198). Radiographic abnormalities are generally more common and more severe in children with asthma (197,198).

Plain radiographs are uncommonly used to make a diagnosis of asthma (193,197). The usefulness of radiography in patients with an established diagnosis of asthma who suffer an acute attack is also limited. Correlation between the severity of radiographic findings and the severity and reversibility of an asthma attack is generally poor (196–198), and radiographs provide significant information that alters treatment in only 5% or less of patients with acute asthma (200,201). Although it is difficult to generalize regarding the role of radiographs in both adults and children with acute asthma, chest films are often used to exclude the presence of associated pneumonia or other complications when significant symptoms and/or appropriate clinical or laboratory findings are suggestive (196–198,200).

HRCT Findings

HRCT is uncommonly indicated in the routine assessment of patients with asthma. However, it is sometimes used when complications of asthma, such as ABPA, are suspected (46) or in documenting the presence of emphysema in smokers with asthma (202,203). ABPA is associated with more severe bronchiectasis than that typically seen in patients with uncomplicated asthma.

Bronchial dilatation, bronchial wall thickening, mucoid impaction, centrilobular bronchiolar abnormalities such as tree-in-bud, patchy areas of mosaic perfusion, and regional air trapping on expiratory scans may be identified on HRCT in patients with uncomplicated asthma. On the whole, the severity of these abnormalities correlates with the severity of asthma measured by pulmonary function. In one study, FEV_1 values were inversely correlated with bronchial wall thickening, hyperlucency, mucoid impaction, linear shadows, centrilobular prominence, and bronchiectasis (204).

Mild bronchial dilatation has been reported in 15% to 77% of patients with uncomplicated asthma (23,27,46,199, 205). In a study by Lynch et al. (23), 77% of asthmatic patients and 153 (36%) of 429 bronchi assessed in asthmatic patients were associated with a B/A ratio exceeding 1. In a study by Grenier et al. (205), bronchial dilatation was found in 28.5% of the asthmatic subjects, primarily involving subsegmental and distal bronchi. Apparent bronchial dilatation in asthmatic patients may partially reflect reduction in pulmonary artery diameter, resulting from changes in blood volume or local hypoxia, or may be physiologic (23,193); Lynch (193) suggests caution in diagnosing mild bronchiectasis in this patient population.

On the other hand, bronchial diameter may decrease significantly during an asthma attack. In experimental studies in dogs (18) and asthmatic subjects (206–208), bronchial luminal diameter was measured using HRCT before and during a histamine- or methacholine-induced bronchospasm. These studies found a significant reduction in the luminal diameter of small bronchi in association with acute asthma. Also, a significant decrease in lung attenuation as a result of air trapping was seen in association with induced bronchospasm in these subjects (207).

Bronchial wall thickening has been reported in 16% to 92% of patients (23,27,199,205), and there is a tendency for the degree of bronchial wall thickening to correlate with the severity of disease (27,43,209). For example, Awadh et al. (43) measured the ratio of airway wall thickness to the outer airway diameter (i.e., T/D ratio) in normal subjects and in asthmatic patients with varying severity of disease (43). The mean T/D was significantly higher (0.27) in patients with an episode of near-fatal asthma, as compared to those with mild asthma (0.25) or normals (0.23).

Mucoid impaction has been reported in as many as 21% of patients (199); this abnormality may clear following treatment. Branching or nodular centrilobular opacities have been reported to be present in as many as 10% to 21% of patients, sometimes manifested as tree-in-bud. These likely reflect bronchiolar wall thickening or inflammation, with or without mucoid impaction. However, this finding is absent or tends to be inconspicuous in most patients with asthma.

Focal or diffuse hyperlucency has been observed on inspiratory scans in 18% to 31% of patients (23,205, 210,211), undoubtedly owing to small airway obstruction, air trapping, and mosaic perfusion. A significant positive correlation has been found between PFT findings of small airway obstruction and the HRCT mosaic perfusion score ($p = .05$) (211).

Expiratory CT can show evidence of patchy air trapping in asthmatic patients (212). In a study by Park et al. (27), air trapping involving more than a segment was seen in 50% of asthmatic patients. Furthermore, in a study of 22 patients classified as having moderate asthma and 12 healthy volunteer nonsmokers (211), air-trapping scores were significantly higher in the asthmatic patients than in the normal controls ($p = .003$). In addition, both FEV_1 and reversibility of small airway obstruction values correlated with air-trapping score ($p = .03$ and $p = .007$, respectively) (211). In some patients with asthma, air trapping may be seen in the absence of morphologic abnormalities visible on inspiratory scans (92,213).

ALLERGIC BRONCHOPULMONARY ASPERGILLOSIS

ABPA reflects a hypersensitivity reaction to *Aspergillus* species and is characteristically associated with eosinophilia, symptoms of asthma such as wheezing, and findings of central or proximal bronchiectasis, usually associated with mucoid impaction, atelectasis, and sometimes consolidation similar to that seen in patients with eosinophilic pneumonia.

ABPA is associated with asthma; in one recent study, the prevalence of ABPA in asthma patients was shown to be 16% (214). ABPA has also been noted to occur in 2% to 10% of patients with CF (215,216).

ABPA results from both type I and type III (IgE and IgG) immunologic responses to the endobronchial growth of *Aspergillus*. The immune reactions result in symptoms of asthma (type I) and central bronchiectasis (type III), which is usually varicose or cystic in appearance, and the formation of mucous plugs that contain fungus and inflammatory cells. A type IV reaction may also be involved.

It has been suggested that disease progression be divided into five separate phases. These include (1) an acute phase; (2) usually leading to resolution, during which time pulmonary infiltrates clear and serum IgE declines; (3) followed by remission; (4) evolving to a phase of dependence on corticosteroids, and finally leading in some cases (5) to diffuse pulmonary fibrosis (215). ABPA may vary greatly in severity (217).

HRCT Findings

Central bronchiectasis is characteristic of patients with ABPA (Figs. 4-14, 4-32 to 4-34) (28,46,100,112,189,193, 218–224). For example, in a study of 23 patients with ABPA, central bronchiectasis could be identified in 85% of lobes and 52% of lung segments (223). The degree of bronchial dilatation may be severe and is considerably more extensive than that seen in asthmatic patients. For example, HRCT was evaluated in 19 patients with documented ABPA and 18 asthmatic controls (225). Seventeen patients (89%) with ABPA had central cystic or varicoid bronchiectasis in at least one lobe, and the majority had diffuse disease, manifested by bronchiectasis in four or five lobes. Only three asthmatic patients (17%) had findings of cylindrical bronchiectasis (225).

Mucous plugs are commonly seen in patients with ABPA, within the ectatic airways. High-attenuation mucoid impaction is common and suggests this diagnosis (Figs. 4-33 to 4-35) (226,227). High-density mucous plugs presumably represent the presence of calcium concentrated by the fungus. This finding has been seen in as many as 28% of

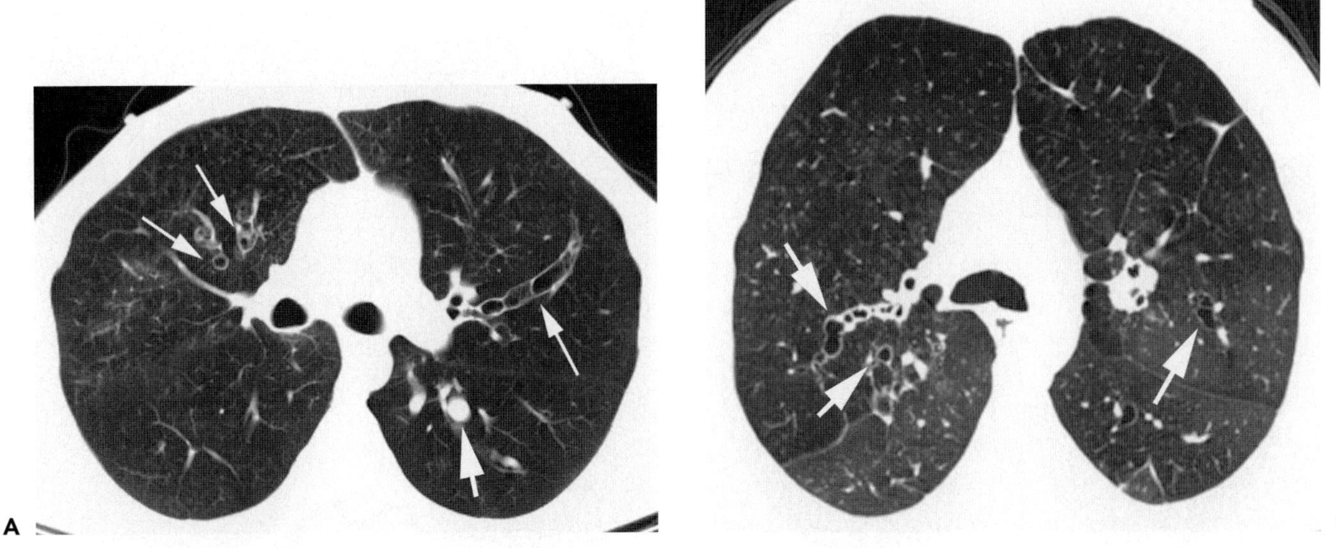

Figure 4-32 ABPA with central bronchiectasis in two patients. **A:** Bronchiectasis is visible in central lung regions *(small arrows)*. A mucous plug is visible within a dilated bronchus in the left lower lobe. **B:** Central varicose bronchiectasis is visible *(arrows)*.

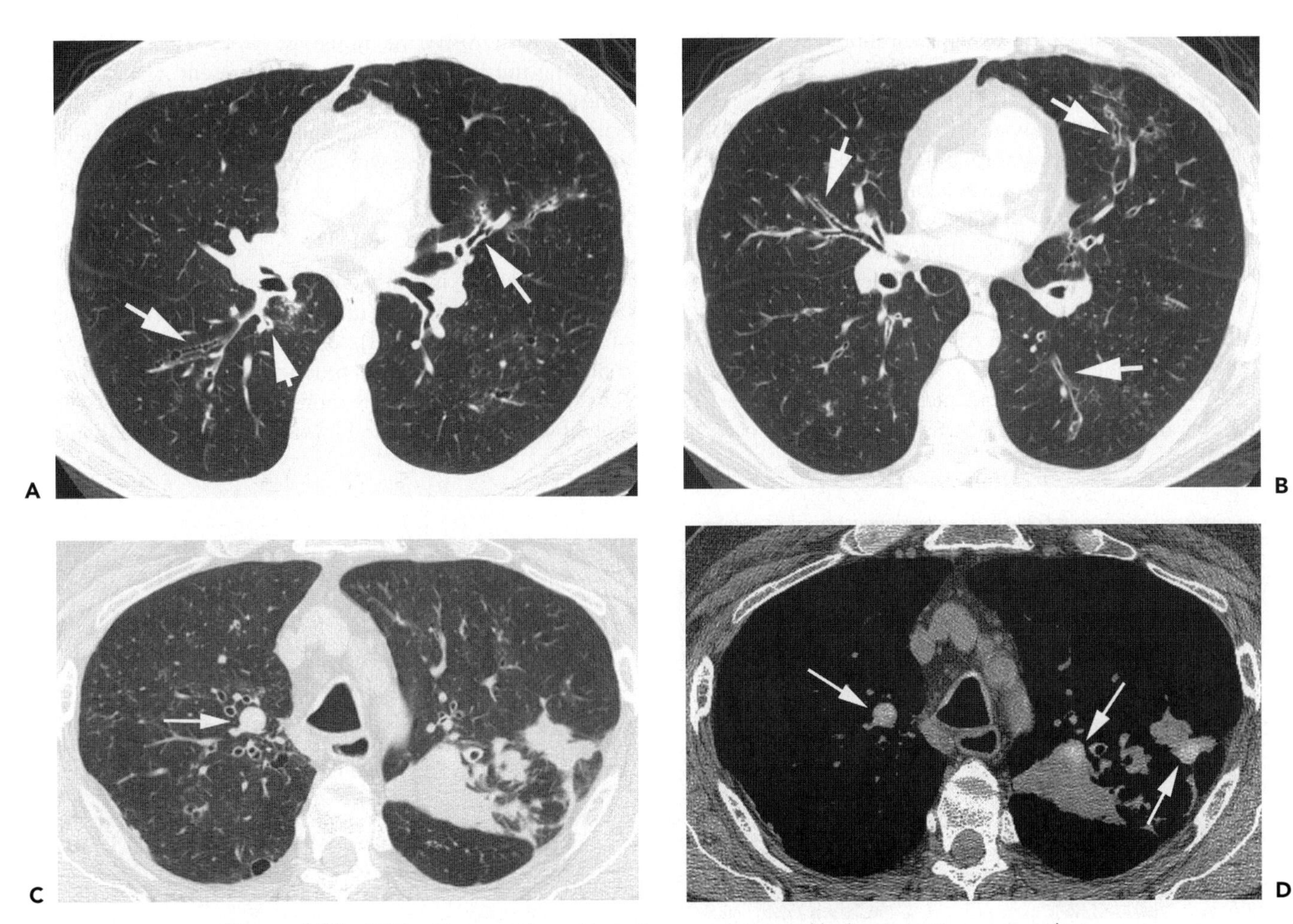

Figure 4-33 ABPA with central bronchiectasis, progression, and high-attenuation mucous plugs. **A** and **B:** HRCT in a patient with asthma shows central bronchiectasis and bronchial wall thickening. **C:** HRCT six years later shows mucous plugging in the right upper lobe *(arrow)* with patchy left upper lobe atelectasis. **D:** Soft tissue window image at the same level as **(C)** shows high-attenuation mucous plugs in both upper lobes *(arrows)*.

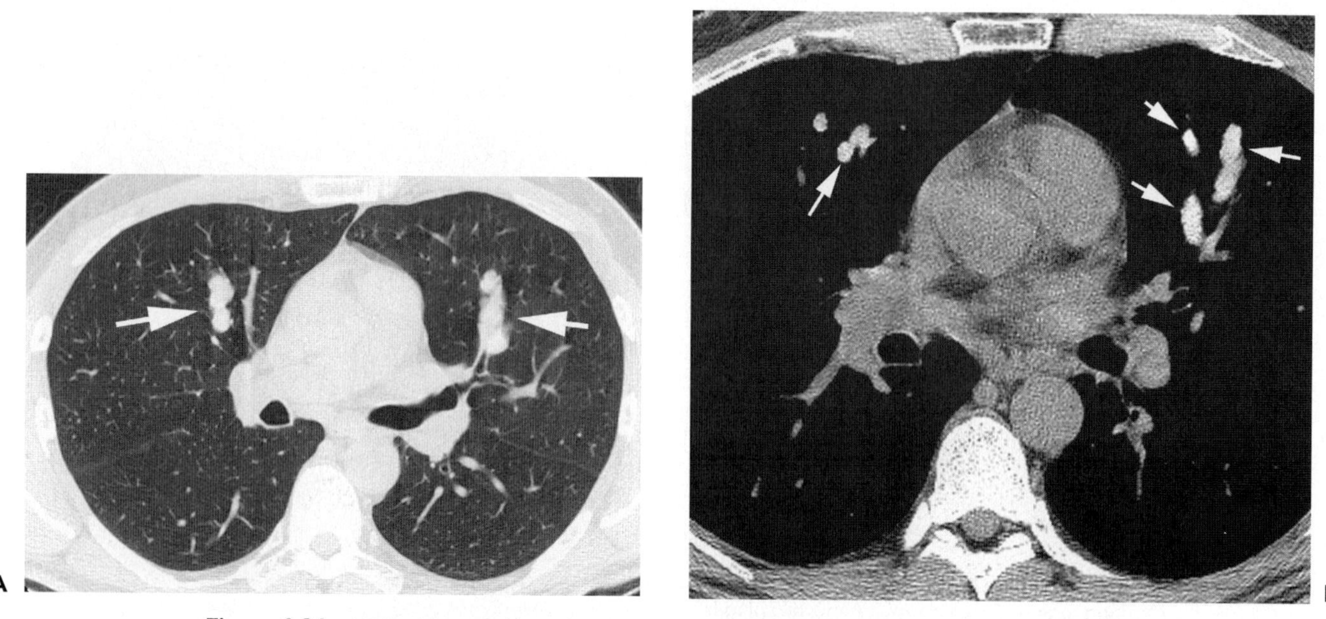

Figure 4-34 ABPA with central bronchiectasis and high-attenuation mucous plugs. **A:** Lung window scan shows bilateral upper lobe bronchiectasis with mucoid impaction *(arrows)*. **B:** Soft tissue window setting CT shows high-attenuation mucous plugs *(arrows)*.

patients with ABPA and when present should be considered highly suggestive of the diagnosis (227).

The finding of aspergillomas in ectatic airways in patients with ABPA has also been reported (228). Additional parenchymal abnormalities, including consolidation, collapse (Fig. 4-35), cavitation, and bullae, may be identified especially in the upper lobes in as many as 43% of patients (223). An identical percentage of patients also had evidence of pleural abnormalities, especially focal pleural thickening. Mass-like foci of eosinophilic pneumonia also may be seen in ABPA patients with acute exacerbations (229,230).

In addition to widespread and central bronchiectasis, a number of ancillary findings have been reported to occur in patients with ABPA. As noted by Webb (213), disease involving the small airways is often present, resulting in either a tree-in-bud appearance resulting from mucus-filled bronchioles or mosaic perfusion and air trapping owing to bronchiolar obstruction with resulting air trapping.

Use of HRCT

Although ABPA is classically associated with central bronchiectasis, this finding in itself is nonspecific and insensitive (189). Reiff et al. (28), for example, in a study of 168 patients with chronic sputum production, found that patients with ABPA were significantly more likely than patients with other diseases to have central bronchiectasis ($p < .005$), and

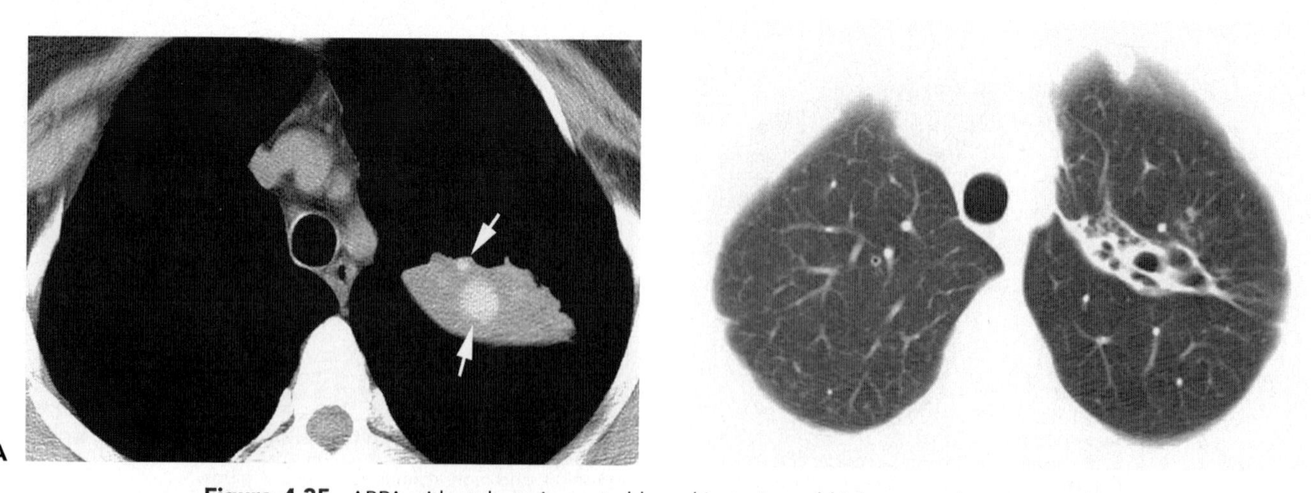

Figure 4-35 ABPA with atelectasis, central bronchiectasis, and high-attenuation mucous plugs. **A:** Soft tissue window scan shows focal left upper-lobe atelectasis containing high-attenuation mucous plugs *(arrows)*. **B:** Several months later, the atelectasis and mucous plugging have cleared. Focal left upper lobe bronchiectasis is visible.

bronchiectasis was more likely to be varicose or cylindrical morphologically ($p < .01$); however, the sensitivity of central bronchiectasis in this same study proved to only be 37% in diagnosing ABPA. Similarly, in a retrospective study of 82 consecutive patients with bronchiectasis with known etiologies, Cartier et al. (100) found that in only five of nine patients (56%) was a diagnosis of ABPA specifically suggested.

HRCT may be valuable in the early identification of lung damage in patients with ABPA and thus help in planning treatment (218,219). HRCT is more sensitive than plain radiographs in detecting abnormalities associated with ABPA (220). In one study, narrow-section (3 mm) CT and plain chest radiography were compared in 10 patients with ABPA (218). Bronchiectasis was reported in 31 of 60 lobes on CT scans but was visible in only 15 lobes on plain chest radiographs; CT was also more sensitive in detecting central bronchiectasis. In another study, CT with 8-mm collimation was compared with bronchography in two pediatric patients with ABPA (219); CT was able to identify 24 of 27 segments that showed central bronchiectasis.

ABPA may be difficult to diagnose on clinical grounds alone in a patient with asthma; many of the features of asthma and ABPA overlap. In addition to the finding of bronchiectasis, these include serum precipitants to *A. fumigatus* in up to 10% of asthmatics, a positive skin test to *Aspergillus* in up to 25% asthmatics, and elevated IgE levels and eosinophilia. In a study by Neeld et al. (46), the HRCT findings in patients with ABPA were compared with those in patients with uncomplicated asthma. Bronchial dilatation was seen in 41% of lobes in the patients with ABPA, as compared with 15% in the patients with asthma.

In the most extensive evaluation to date, Ward et al. (224) retrospectively assessed the accuracy of CT in the diagnosis of ABPA in asthmatic patients. Comparing the CT findings in 44 patients with documented ABPA with those in 36 asthmatic controls, these authors noted a clear distinction in the frequency of a number of CT findings in patients with ABPA, including: bronchiectasis in 95% of patients versus 29% of asthmatics; centrilobular nodules in 93% of patients versus 28% of asthmatics; and mucoid impaction in 67% versus 4% of asthmatics. Furthermore, as noted by others, patients with ABPA consistently had more severe and extensive disease compared with asthmatics, especially when present in three or more lobes (224). It should be noted that the prevalence of bronchiectasis in this study far exceeds that reported in most other studies. In comparison to patients with CF, who often have diffuse cylindrical bronchiectasis, those with ABPA more typically show bronchiectasis that is cystic in appearance (184).

DYSKINETIC CILIA SYNDROME AND KARTAGENER'S SYNDROME

Dyskinetic cilia syndrome (DCS; primary ciliary dyskinesia) is characterized by abnormal ciliary structure and function, resulting in reduced mucociliary clearance and chronic airway infection (231,232). Bronchiectasis and sinusitis are common manifestations. About half of patients with DCS also have situs inversus. The combination of bronchiectasis, sinusitis, and situs inversus is termed Kartagener's syndrome (Fig. 4-36).

DCS results from a genetic abnormality having autosomal recessive transmission and an incidence of about 1 in 20,000 births. Men and women are equally affected. A variety of ultrastructural abnormalities of ciliary microtubules have been reported in association with this syndrome, although in some cases, the cilia appear normal. In men, the syndrome may be associated with immotile spermatozoa and infertility; the fertility of women is not affected. Other congenital abnormalities may also be present. In patients with chronic infections and situs inversus, the diagnosis is not difficult. In the absence of situs inversus, criteria for attributing chronic infection to DCS may include immotile spermatozoa (in men), a family history of DCS, or abnormal cilia on biopsy.

Symptoms of recurrent bronchitis, pneumonia, and sinusitis often date from childhood. Radiographs and CT typically show bilateral bronchiectasis with a basal (lower or middle lobe) predominance, similar to that seen in patients with other causes of postinfectious bronchiectasis (Fig. 4-36). Cylindrical bronchiectasis is most common. Appropriate antibiotic treatment is associated with a normal life expectancy.

As is common in many patients with bronchiectasis, a diffuse bronchiolitis may be present in patients with DCS or

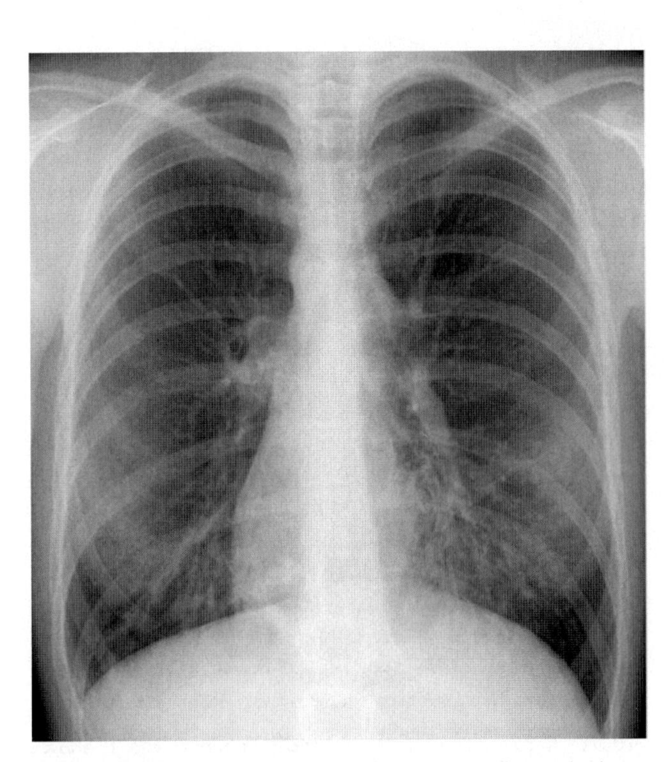

Figure 4-36 Kartagener's syndrome. Chest radiograph shows situs inversus and basal bronchiectasis.

Kartagener's syndrome. For example, in a study of eight patients with Kartagener's syndrome, CT showed diffuse small centrilobular nodules in six, and histopathologic examination of lung specimens showed obliterative thickening of the walls of the membranous bronchioles with infiltration by lymphocytes, plasma cells, and neutrophils. PFTs revealed marked obstructive impairment in all patients (FEV_1 = 57.0%) (233).

YOUNG'S SYNDROME

Young's syndrome, also referred to as obstructive azoospermia, is characterized by male infertility caused by obstruction of the epididymis, bronchiectasis, and sinusitis (234). It may resemble DCS clinically, but ciliary abnormalities are absent. The cause is unknown. The radiographic appearance of the bronchiectasis is nonspecific.

YELLOW NAILS AND LYMPHEDEMA

This syndrome is characterized by (a) slowly growing nails that are thickened, curved, and yellow-green in color; (b) lymphedema, usually of the lower extremities resulting from lymphatic hypoplasia, and (c) exudative pleural effusions associated with pleural lymphatic dilatation (235). Not all three manifestations need be present; pleural effusion is least common. Chronic sinusitis, airway infection, and bronchiectasis are present in about one half of patients (Fig. 4-37). Although their etiology is unclear, these manifestations may be related to abnormal lymphatic drainage, immunologic abnormalities, or ciliary dysfunction. Presentation is typically in adulthood.

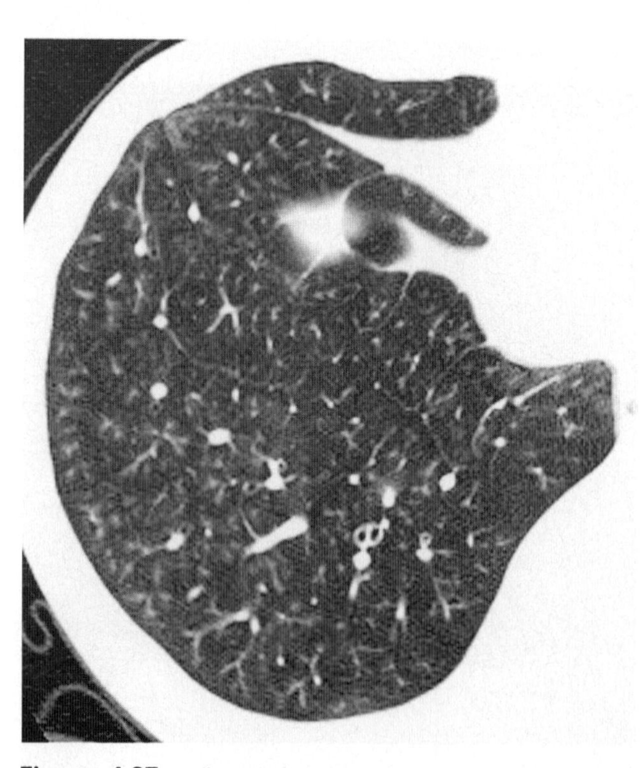

Figure 4-37 Yellow nails and lymphedema. HRCT shows bronchial wall thickening in the right lower lobe and bronchiolitis manifested by tree-in-bud.

ALPHA$_1$-ANTITRYPSIN DEFICIENCY

In addition to emphysema, bronchiectasis is also frequently identified in patients with α_1-antitrypsin deficiency. In a study of 14 patients with α_1-antitrypsin deficiency, King et al. (236) found evidence of bronchiectasis in 6 (43%). Approximately 50% of patients with α_1-antitrypsin deficiency have symptoms of airway disease, in particular chronic sputum production.

It is thought that bronchiectasis occurs by mechanisms similar to those resulting in emphysema in patients with this deficiency. In the presence of airway infection, neutrophils release elastases and other proteolytic enzymes. These elastases have the ability to cleave a variety of proteins, including collagen and elastin. The bronchi are normally protected from excessive elastase-induced damage by α_1-protease inhibitor (α_1-antiprotease or antitrypsin and other circulating antiproteinases.

TRACHEOBRONCHOMEGALY

The term *tracheobronchomegaly,* also known as Mounier-Kuhn syndrome, is used to describe marked dilatation of the trachea and mainstem bronchi, with or without central bronchiectasis, in otherwise heterogeneous patients (237–239). Histologic examination of the trachea shows deficient smooth muscle and elastic fibers and absence of the myenteric plexus. A cartilage abnormality is undoubtedly present as well, although this may be acquired. This syndrome can be associated with recurrent lower respiratory tract infection. Tracheobronchomegaly most often is diagnosed in men in their third and fourth decades (240,241).

The etiology of tracheobronchomegaly is uncertain and may be multifactorial. The presence of structural abnormalities of the tracheal wall and the association of this condition with congenital connective tissue disorders (including Marfan's syndrome, CF, Ehlers-Danlos syndrome, and cutis laxa in children) suggest that genetic abnormalities are at least partially responsible in some patients (240,241). An association between tracheomegaly and diffuse pulmonary fibrosis has also been reported; in such patients, tracheal dilatation is presumably the result of increased traction on the tracheal wall resulting from increased pulmonary elastic recoil (240,241).

Tracheobronchomegaly may be diagnosed if the trachea measures more than 3 cm in diameter at a level 2 cm above the aortic arch and the right and left main bronchi measure more than 2.4 and 2.3 cm, respectively (Fig. 4-38)

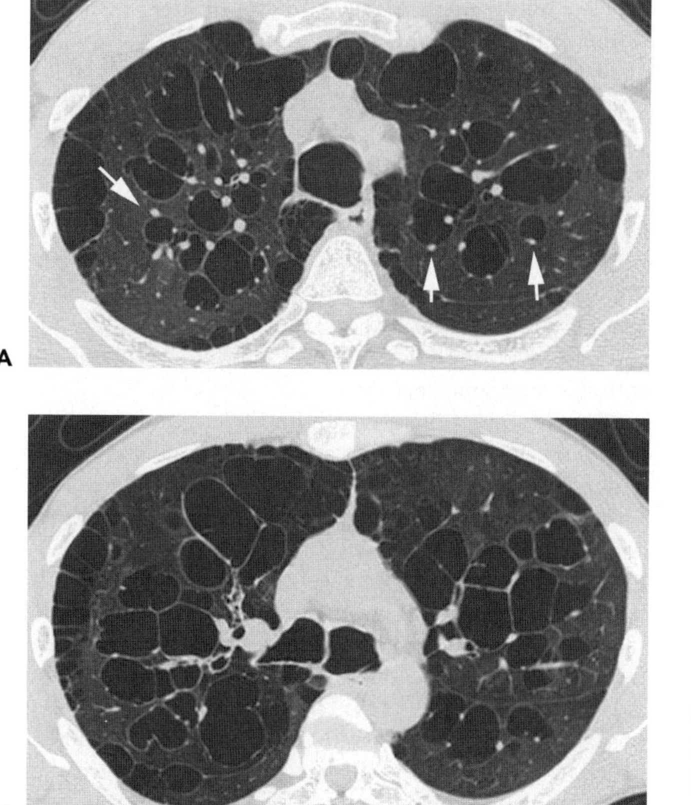

Figure 4-38 Tracheobronchomegaly. **A:** CT shows tracheal dilatation and central cystic bronchiectasis. Note the presence of the signet-ring sign *(arrows)* in relation to cystic lesions, indicating that they represent bronchiectasis. Peripheral bullae are also present. **B:** Cystic bronchiectasis is also visible at a lower level. (Courtesy of Harold Litt, MD.)

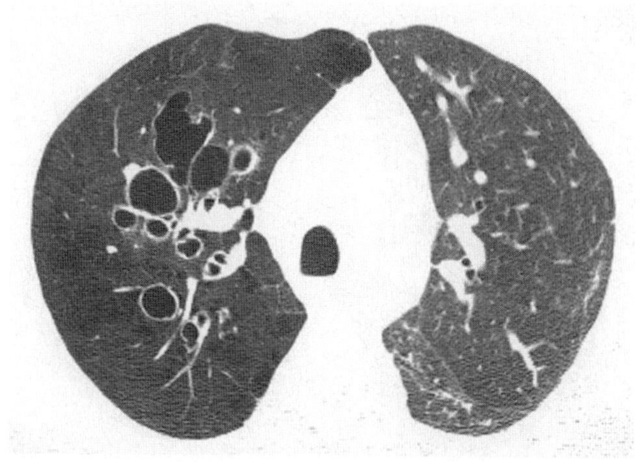

Figure 4-39 Williams-Campbell syndrome with left lung transplantation. Cystic bronchiectasis is visible in the central right lung. The peripheral right lung appears lucent because of bronchiolitis and air trapping.

(242). Additional findings include tracheal scalloping and/or diverticula, the latter especially common along the posterior tracheal wall (242–244). Tracheomalacia is also common, with a marked decrease in the tracheal diameter on expiration.

Central bronchiectasis having a cystic appearance may be seen in some patients with tracheobronchomegaly. The presence of this type of bronchiectasis is likely related to abnormalities of the bronchial wall similar to those seen in the trachea (Fig. 4-38). However, the presence of tracheal abnormalities may also contribute to bronchiectasis by predisposing to chronic infection. In a study of 75 consecutive patients referred for CT evaluation of possible bronchiectasis, Roditi and Weir (240) found that 12% of patients had tracheal dilatation, including 7 of 42 patients (17%) with CT evidence of bronchiectasis and 3 of 32 (6%) without.

WILLIAMS-CAMPBELL SYNDROME

Williams-Campbell syndrome is rare and results in central cystic bronchiectasis owing to deficiency of cartilage in the fourth- to sixth-order bronchi (245,246). It typically presents in children with chronic cough, fever, sputum production, and failure to thrive. HRCT can show areas of central cystic bronchiectasis (Fig. 4-39) with distal regions of abnormal lucency, probably related to air trapping or bronchiolitis (247). Ballooning of central bronchi on inspiration and collapse on expiration have also been reported (248).

BRONCHIECTASIS ASSOCIATED WITH SYSTEMIC DISEASES

Bronchiectasis may seen in a number of major systemic diseases. Of particular interest is the association between bronchiectasis and both collagen vascular diseases and inflammatory bowel disease.

Rheumatoid Arthritis

Rheumatoid arthritis (RA) may be associated with a variety of pulmonary abnormalities, including interstitial pneumonia, organizing pneumonia, respiratory tract infections, and necrobiotic nodules. Airway diseases, including both bronchiectasis and bronchiolectasis, are also common (249).

Based on studies of HRCT, it has been estimated that bronchiectasis occurs in up to 35% of patients with RA (Fig. 4-40) (250–253). For example, McDonagh et al. (251) evaluated 20 patients with clinical and radiologic evidence of RA and found that bronchiectasis could be identified in 6 patients, including 2 previously thought to have diffuse interstitial lung disease on the basis of chest radiographs. In this same study, bronchiectasis was also identified in 4 of 20 asymptomatic control patients with RA and normal chest radiographs. A study of 38 patients with RA reported by Rémy-Jardin et al. (250) revealed

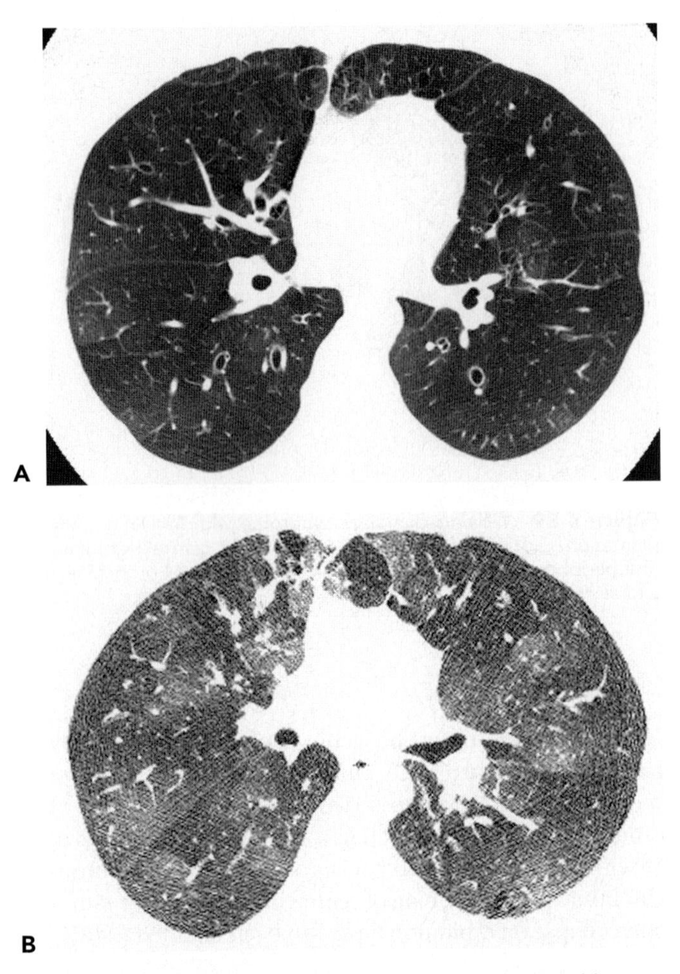

Figure 4-40 RA with bronchiectasis and bronchiolitis obliterans. **A:** HRCT shows bilateral bronchiectasis. The lung appears heterogeneous in attenuation because of mosaic perfusion. **B:** Dynamic, low-dose expiratory HRCT shows patchy air trapping as a result of bronchiolitis obliterans.

evidence of either bronchiectasis or bronchiolectasis in 23 (30%), including 8% of asymptomatic patients, with additional features suggestive of small airway disease in another 6 patients. These findings included linear and/or branching centrilobular opacities thought by these authors to represent bronchiolitis obliterans (250). Although this group included 7 patients with traction bronchiectasis in areas of honeycombing, in the remaining 16 patients bronchiectasis was seen in the absence of CT evidence of lung fibrosis.

More recently, it has been shown that in RA patients with normal radiographs, the prevalence of airway disease may be considerably higher than previously thought. In a study of 50 RA patients without radiographic evidence of lung disease, Perez et al. (253) reported findings of bronchial and/or bronchiolar disease in 35 (70%), including air trapping on expiratory scans in 32%, cylindrical bronchiectasis in 30%, mosaic attenuation on inspiratory scans in 20%, and centrilobular nodules in 6%. Importantly, HRCT depicted features of small airway disease in 20 of 33 patients with normal PFTs.

In a study of 46 patients with RA who underwent HRCT, bronchiectasis or bronchiolectasis was found in 23 patients (50%). Eighteen of the 23 patients had not been diagnosed with bronchiectasis before the study, and 13 were free of respiratory symptoms. No significant differences were found between the 23 patients with and the 23 patients without bronchiectasis for age at onset or duration of the RA, extra-articular involvement, positive rheumatoid factors, bony erosions, use of corticosteroids or immunosuppressives, respiratory manifestations, smoking, or spirometry parameters (254).

Bronchiolitis obliterans with findings of bronchiectasis, mosaic perfusion, and air trapping may also be seen in patients with RA but is uncommon (Fig. 4-40) (250,255).

It has long been observed that airway obstruction is common in patients with RA (256), leading to speculation that bronchiectasis may predispose to the development of RA. For example, it has been suggested that chronic bacterial infections may trigger an immune reaction in genetically predisposed individuals, leading to development of an autoimmune disease (249). In this regard, it has been observed that bronchiectasis may precede the development of RA by several decades. It has also been suggested that steroid therapy or related treatment, especially with immunosuppressive therapy, itself may lead to an increased incidence of respiratory infections in RA patients. It has further been suggested that the association between RA and bronchiectasis may reflect a shared genetic predisposition, although this remains controversial (252).

Regardless of the precise role played by bronchiectasis in the development of RA, it has been shown that patients with bronchiectasis appear to have decreased survival. As shown by Swinson et al. (257), in a study comparing the 5-year survival of 32 RA patients with both arthritis and bronchiectasis matched for age, sex, and disease duration with 32 patients having arthritis alone and an additional 31 patients with bronchiectasis alone, these authors found that patients with both RA and bronchiectasis were 7.3 times more likely to die than the general population, 5 times more likely to die than patients with RA alone, and 2.4 times more likely to die than patients with bronchiectasis alone.

Systemic Lupus Erythematosus

Bronchiectasis may be identified in up to 20% of patients with systemic lupus erythematosus (SLE) (258). Bankier et al. (259), in a prospective study of 45 patients with SLE and normal radiographs, found abnormal CT findings in 38%, including bronchial wall thickening in 20% and bronchiectasis in another 18%.

Sjögren's Syndrome

A high prevalence of airway pathology has been noted in patients with primary Sjögren's syndrome (260). In a study of 60 patients with primary Sjögren's syndrome, HRCT showed bronchiectasis in 38% (261). Small airway abnormalities may also be seen.

Inflammatory Bowel Disease

Pulmonary involvement is common in patients with inflammatory bowel disease and includes a wide range of abnormalities, such as interstitial pneumonia, bronchiectasis, air trapping, and fibrosis (262). In a study of 23 patients with ulcerative colitis and 13 patients with Crohn's disease, HRCT revealed abnormalities in 19; 42% of the patients with a HRCT abnormality were free of respiratory symptoms (262). Airway abnormalities are present in about half of patients with lung disease and include chronic bronchitis or bronchiolitis, bronchiectasis, or chronic infection (Fig. 4-41). Histologic examination of the bronchi shows abnormalities similar to those of the bowel, including mucosal ulceration and cellular infiltration.

Generally, lung abnormalities are most common with ulcerative colitis. In patients with ulcerative colitis, airway abnormalities may include subglottic stenosis, chronic bronchitis, and chronic suppurative inflammation of both large and small airways (249). Similar to what is seen in patients with RA, chronic suppurative airway disease may precede, coexist with, or follow the development of inflammatory bowel disease. Of particular interest is that, unlike other causes of bronchiectasis, chronic airway disease associated with ulcerative colitis frequently responds to treatment with inhaled steroids (249).

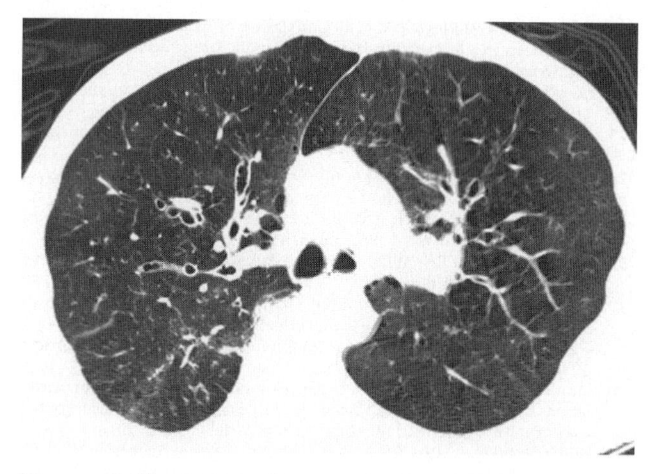

Figure 4-41 Crohn's disease with bronchiectasis. Bilateral bronchial wall thickening and bronchiectasis are present.

CT DIFFERENTIATION OF CAUSES OF BRONCHIECTASIS

The reliability of CT for distinguishing among the causes of bronchiectasis is somewhat controversial (28,100,189). Reiff et al. (28) evaluated the HRCT scans of 168 patients with chronic purulent sputum production suspected of having bronchiectasis. With the exception of a predominant lower lobe distribution in patients with syndromes of impaired mucociliary clearance, these authors found no significant difference in lobar distribution between cases of idiopathic bronchiectasis and those with a known etiology. Although central bronchiectasis was more common in patients with ABPA, the sensitivity of this finding as a diagnostic feature proved to be only 37% (28). Similarly, although the extent and severity of disease was more pronounced in patients with both ABPA and CF, these features were of only limited value in individual cases (28).

Lee et al. (189), in a similar study of CT scans in 108 patients with bronchiectasis from a variety of causes, found that a correct first-choice diagnosis was made by three experienced observers in only 45% of cases; more problematic still, a high confidence level was reached in only 9%, and of these a correct diagnosis was made in only 35%. Furthermore, interobserver agreement was poor (mean $\kappa = 0.20$) leading these investigators to conclude that CT was of little value in diagnosing specific etiologies of bronchiectasis. It should be emphasized that CT scans were interpreted in the absence of clinical data (189).

More recently, Cartier et al. (100) reported better results in a retrospective study of 82 consecutive patients with bronchiectasis having a known cause. These authors noted that a correct diagnosis was reached by two independent observers in 61% of cases, including a correct diagnosis in 68% of patients with CF, 67% of patients with TB, and 56% of patients with ABPA (100). Specifically, in this study a bilateral upper lobe distribution was most commonly seen in patients with CF and ABPA, unilateral upper lobe distribution was most common in patients with TB, and a lower lobe distribution was most often seen in patients after childhood viral infections.

REFERENCES

1. Barker AF. Bronchiectasis. *N Engl J Med* 2002;346:1383–1393.
2. Kumar NA, Nguyen B, Maki D. Bronchiectasis: current clinical and imaging concepts. *Semin Roentgenol* 2001;36:41–50.
3. McGuinness G, Naidich DP. CT of airways disease and bronchiectasis. *Radiol Clin North Am* 2002;40:1–19.
4. Hansell D. Bronchiectasis. *Radiol Clin North Am* 1998;36:107–128.
5. Barker AF, Bardana EJ. Bronchiectasis: update on an orphan disease. *Am Rev Respir Dis* 1988;137:969–978.
6. Stanford W, Galvin JR. The diagnosis of bronchiectasis. *Clin Chest Med* 1988;9:691–699.
7. Davis AL, Salzman SH, eds. *Bronchiectasis.* Philadelphia: WB Saunders, 1991.
8. Westcott JL, Cole SR. Traction bronchiectasis in end-stage pulmonary fibrosis. *Radiology* 1986;161:665–669.
9. Currie DC, Cooke JC, Morgan AD, et al. Interpretation of bronchograms and chest radiographs in patients with chronic sputum production. *Thorax* 1987;42:278–284.
10. Nicotra MB, Rivera M, Dale AM, et al. Clinical, pathophysiologic, and microbiologic characterization of bronchiectasis in an aging cohort [see comments]. *Chest* 1995;108:955–961.
11. Millar A, Boothroyd A, Edwards D, Hetzel M. The role of computed tomography (CT) in the investigation of unexplained hemoptysis. *Respir Med* 1992;86:39–44.
12. Naidich DP, Funt S, Ettenger NA, Arranda C. Hemoptysis: CT-bronchoscopic correlations in 58 cases. *Radiology* 1990;177:357–362.

13. Lynch DA, Newell J, Hale V, et al. Correlation of CT findings with clinical evaluations in 261 patients with symptomatic bronchiectasis. *AJR Am J Roentgenol* 1999;173:53–58.
14. Gudjberg CE. Roentgenologic diagnosis of bronchiectasis: an analysis of 112 cases. *Acta Radiol (Stockh)* 1955;43:209–226.
15. Woodring JH. Improved plain film criteria for the diagnosis of bronchiectasis. *J Ky Med Assoc* 1994;92:8–13.
16. Naidich DP, McCauley DI, Khouri NF, et al. Computed tomography of bronchiectasis. *J Comput Assist Tomogr* 1982; 6:437–444.
17. McGuinness G, Naidich DP. Bronchiectasis: CT/clinical correlations. *Semin Ultrasound CT MR* 1995;16:395–419.
18. Herold CJ, Brown RH, Mitzner W, et al. Assessment of pulmonary airway reactivity with high-resolution CT. *Radiology* 1991;181:369–374.
19. McNitt-Gray MF, Goldin JG, Johnson TD, et al. Development and testing of image-processing methods for the quantitative assessment of airway hyperresponsiveness from high-resolution CT images. *J Comput Assist Tomogr* 1997;21:939–947.
20. Smith IE, Jurriaans E, Diederich S, et al. Chronic sputum production: correlations between clinical features and findings on high resolution computed tomographic scanning of the chest. *Thorax* 1996;51:914–918.
21. Kim JS, Müller NL, Park CS, et al. Bronchoarterial ratio on thin section CT: comparison between high altitude and sea level. *J Comput Assist Tomogr* 1997;21:306–311.
22. Diederich S, Jurriaans E, Flower CD. Interobserver variation in the diagnosis of bronchiectasis on high-resolution computed tomography. *Eur Radiol* 1996;6:801–806.
23. Lynch DA, Newell JD, Tschomper BA, et al. Uncomplicated asthma in adults: comparison of CT appearance of the lungs in asthmatic and healthy subjects. *Radiology* 1993;188:829–833.
24. Kang EY, Miller RR, Müller NL. Bronchiectasis: comparison of preoperative thin-section CT and pathologic findings in resected specimens. *Radiology* 1995;195:649–654.
25. Kim SJ, Im JG, Kim IO, et al. Normal bronchial and pulmonary arterial diameters measured by thin section CT. *J Comput Assist Tomogr* 1995;19:365–369.
26. Matsuoka S, Uchiyama K, Shima H, et al. Bronchoarterial ratio and bronchial wall thickness on high-resolution CT in asymptomatic subjects: correlation with age and smoking. *AJR Am J Roentgenol* 2003;180:513–518.
27. Park CS, Müller NL, Worthy SA, et al. Airway obstruction in asthmatic and healthy individuals: inspiratory and expiratory thin-section CT findings. *Radiology* 1997;203:361–367.
28. Reiff DB, Wells AU, Carr DH, et al. CT findings in bronchiectasis: limited value in distinguishing between idiopathic and specific types. *AJR Am J Roentgenol* 1995;165:261–267.
29. Joharjy IA, Bashi SA, Abdullah AK. Value of medium-thickness CT in the diagnosis of bronchiectasis. *AJR Am J Roentgenol* 1987;149:1133–1137.
30. Cooke JC, Currie DC, Morgan AD, et al. Role of computed tomography in diagnosis of bronchiectasis. *Thorax* 1987;42:272–277.
31. Silverman PM, Godwin JD. CT/bronchographic correlations in bronchiectasis. *J Comput Assist Tomogr* 1987;11:52–56.
32. Young K, Aspestrand F, Kolbenstvedt A. High resolution CT and bronchography in the assessment of bronchiectasis. *Acta Radiol* 1991;32:439–441.
33. Ouellette H. The signet ring sign. *Radiology* 1999;212:67–68.
34. Desai SR, Wells AU, Cheah FK, et al. The reproducibility of bronchial circumference measurements using CT. *Br J Radiol* 1994;67:257–262.
35. Seneterre E, Paganin F, Bruel JM, et al. Measurement of the internal size of bronchi using high resolution computed tomography (HRCT). *Eur Respir J* 1994;7:596–600.
36. Kim JS, Müller NL, Park CS, et al. Cylindrical bronchiectasis: diagnostic findings on thin-section CT. *AJR Am J Roentgenol* 1997;168:751–754.
37. Murata K, Itoh H, Todo G, et al. Centrilobular lesions of the lung: demonstration by high-resolution CT and pathologic correlation. *Radiology* 1986;161:641–645.
38. Webb WR, Stein MG, Finkbeiner WE, et al. Normal and diseased isolated lungs: high-resolution CT. *Radiology* 1988;166:81–87.
39. Weibel ER. High resolution computed tomography of the pulmonary parenchyma: anatomical background. Presented at the The Fleischner Society Symposium on Chest Disease, Scottsdale, Arizona, 1990.
40. Weibel ER, Taylor CR. Design and structure of the human lung. In: Fishman AP, ed. *Pulmonary diseases and disorders,* 2nd ed. New York: McGraw-Hill, 1988:11–60.
41. Webb WR, Gamsu G, Wall SD, et al. CT of a bronchial phantom: factors affecting appearance and size measurements. *Invest Radiol* 1984;19:394–398.
42. McNamara AE, Muller NL, Okazawa M, et al. Airway narrowing in excised canine lungs measured by high-resolution computed tomography. *J Appl Physiol* 1992;73:307–316.
43. Awadh N, Müller NL, Park CS, et al. Airway wall thickness in patients with near fatal asthma and control groups: assessment with high resolution computed tomographic scanning. Thorax 1998;53:248–253.
44. Bhalla M, Turcios N, Aponte V, et al. Cystic fibrosis: scoring system with thin-section CT. *Radiology* 1991;179:783–788.
45. Remy-Jardin M, Remy J, Boulenguez C, et al. Morphologic effects of cigarette smoking on airways and pulmonary parenchyma in healthy adult volunteers: CT evaluation and correlation with pulmonary function tests. *Radiology* 1993;186:107–115.
46. Neeld DA, Goodman LR, Gurney JW, et al. Computerized tomography in the evaluation of allergic bronchopulmonary aspergillosis. *Am Rev Respir Dis* 1990;142:1200–1206.
47. Shah RM, Sexauer W, Ostrum BJ, et al. High-resolution CT in the acute exacerbation of cystic fibrosis: evaluation of acute findings, reversibility of those findings, and clinical correlation. *AJR Am J Roentgenol* 1997;169:375–380.
48. Bankier AA, Fleischmann D, De Maertelaer V, et al. Subjective differentiation of normal and pathological bronchi on thin-section CT: impact of observer training. *Eur Respir J* 1999;13:781–786.
49. Naidich DP, Rumancik WM, Ettenger NA, et al. Congenital anomalies of the lungs in adults: MR diagnosis. *AJR Am J Roentgenol* 1988;151:13–19.
50. Pugatch RD, Gale ME. Obscure pulmonary masses: bronchial impaction revealed by CT. *AJR Am J Roentgenol* 1983;141:909–914.
51. Rappaport DC, Herman SJ, Weisbrod GL. Congenital bronchopulmonary diseases in adults: CT findings. *AJR Am J Roentgenol* 1994;162:1295–1299.
52. Ikezoe J, Murayama S, Godwin JD, et al. Bronchopulmonary sequestration: CT assessment. *Radiology* 1990;176:375–379.
53. Finck S, Milne ENC. A case report of segmental bronchial atresia: radiologic evaluation including computed tomography and magnetic resonance. *J Thorac Imaging* 1988;3:53–58.
54. Ward S, Morcos SK. Congenital bronchial atresia—presentation of three cases and a pictorial review. *Clin Radiol* 1999;54:144–148.
55. Im JG, Itoh H, Shim YS, et al. Pulmonary tuberculosis: CT findings—early active disease and sequential change with antituberculous therapy. *Radiology* 1993;186:653–660.
56. Aquino SL, Gamsu G, Webb WR, Kee SL. Tree-in-bud pattern: frequency and significance on thin section CT. *J Comput Assist Tomogr* 1996;20:594–599.
57. Gruden JF, Webb WR. Identification and evaluation of centrilobular opacities on high-resolution CT. *Semin Ultrasound CT MR* 1995;16:435–449.
58. Gruden JF, Webb WR, Warnock M. Centrilobular opacities in the lung on high-resolution CT: diagnostic considerations and pathologic correlation. *AJR Am J Roentgenol* 1994;162:569–574.
59. Collins J, Blankenbaker D, Stern EJ. CT patterns of bronchiolar disease: what is "tree-in-bud"? *AJR Am J Roentgenol* 1998;171:365–370.
60. Hansell DM, Wells AU, Rubens MB, Cole PJ. Bronchiectasis: functional significance of areas of decreased attenuation at expiratory CT. *Radiology* 1994;193:369–374.
61. Jeffery PK. The development of large and small airways. *Am J Respir Crit Care Med* 1998;157:S174–S180.
62. Furuse M, Saito K, Kunieda E, et al. Bronchial arteries: CT demonstration with arteriographic correlation. *Radiology* 1987;162:393–398.
63. Murayama S, Hashiguchi N, Murakami J, et al. Helical CT imaging of bronchial arteries with curved reformation technique in comparison with selective bronchial arteriography: preliminary report. *J Comput Assist Tomogr* 1996;20:749–755.
64. Song JW, Im JG, Shim YS, et al. Hypertrophied bronchial artery at thin-section CT in patients with bronchiectasis: correlation with CT angiographic findings. *Radiology* 1998;208:187–191.
65. Revel MP, Fournier LS, Hennebicque AS, et al. Can CT replace bronchoscopy in the detection of the site and cause of bleeding in patients with large or massive hemoptysis? *AJR Am J Roentgenol* 2002;179: 1217–1224.
66. Reid LM. Reduction in bronchial subdivision in bronchiectasis. *Thorax* 1950;5:233–236.
67. Naidich DP. High-resolution computed tomography of cystic lung disease. *Semin Roentgenol* 1991;26:151–174.
68. van der Bruggen-Bogaarts BA, van der Bruggen HM, van Waes PF, Lammers JW. Screening for bronchiectasis. A comparative study between chest radiography and high-resolution CT. *Chest* 1996;109:608–611.
69. Müller NL, Bergin CJ, Ostrow DN, Nichols DM. Role of computed tomography in the recognition of bronchiectasis. *AJR Am J Roentgenol* 1984;143:971–976.
70. Mootoosamy IM, Reznek RH, Osman J. Assessment of bronchiectasis by computed tomography. *Thorax* 1985; 40:920–924.
71. Phillips MS, Williams MP, Flower CDR. How useful is computed tomography in the diagnosis and assessment of bronchiectasis? *Clin Radiol* 1986;37:321–325.
72. Munro NC, Cooke JC, Currie DC, et al. Comparison of thin section computed tomography with bronchography for identifying bronchiectatic segments in patients with chronic sputum production. *Thorax* 1990;45:135–139.
73. Grenier P, Maurice F, Musset D, et al. Bronchiectasis: assessment by thin-section CT. *Radiology* 1986;161:95–99.
74. Giron J, Skaff F, Maubon A, et al. [The value of thin-section CT scans in the diagnosis and staging of bronchiectasis: comparison with bronchography in a series of fifty-four patients]. *Ann Radiol* 1988;31:25–33.
75. Grenier P, Lenoir S, Brauner M. Computed tomographic assessment of bronchiectasis. *Semin Ultrasound CT MR* 1990;11:430–441.
76. Lucidarme O, Grenier P, Coche E, et al. Bronchiectasis: comparative assessment with thin-section CT and helical CT. *Radiology* 1996;200:673–679.
77. King GG, Müller NL, Pare PD. Evaluation of airways in obstructive pulmonary disease using high-resolution computed tomography. *Am J Respir Crit Care Med* 1999;159:992–1004.

78. Bankier AA, Fleischmann D, Mallek R, et al. Bronchial wall thickness: appropriate window settings for thin-section CT and radiologic-anatomic correlation. *Radiology* 1996;199:831–836.
79. Naidich DP, Gruden JF, McGuinness G, et al. Volumetric (helical/spiral) CT (VCT) of the airways. *J Thorac Imaging* 1997;12:11–28.
80. Grenier PA, Beigelman-Aubry C, Fetita C, et al. New frontiers in CT imaging of airway disease. *Eur Radiol* 2002;12:1022–1044.
81. Remy-Jardin M, Amara A, Campistron P, et al. Diagnosis of bronchiectasis with multislice spiral CT: accuracy of 3-mm-thick structured sections. *Eur Radiol* 2003;13:1165–1171.
82. Sung YM, Lee KS, Yi CA, et al. Additional coronal images using low-milliamperage multidetector-row computed tomography: effectiveness in the diagnosis of bronchiectasis. *J Comput Assist Tomogr* 2003;27:490–495.
83. Chooi WK, Matthews S, Bull MJ, Morcos SK. Multislice helical CT: the value of multiplanar image reconstruction in assessment of the bronchi and small airways disease. *Br J Radiol* 2003;76:536–540.
84. Remy-Jardin M, Remy J, Artaud D, et al. Volume rendering of the tracheobronchial tree: clinical evaluation of bronchographic images. *Radiology* 1998;208:761–770.
85. Remy-Jardin M, Remy J, Artaud D, et al. Tracheobronchial tree: assessment with volume rendering—technical aspects. *Radiology* 1998;208:393–398.
86. Jung KJ, Lee KS, Kim SY, et al. Low-dose, volumetric helical CT: image quality, radiation dose, and usefulness for evaluation of bronchiectasis. *Invest Radiol* 2000;35:557–563.
87. Yi CA, Lee KS, Kim TS, et al. Multidetector CT of bronchiectasis: effect of radiation dose on image quality. *AJR Am J Roentgenol* 2003;181: 501–505.
88. Zwirewich CV, Mayo JR, Müller NL. Low-dose high-resolution CT of lung parenchyma. *Radiology* 1991;180:413–417.
89. Stern EJ, Webb WR, Gamsu G. Dynamic quantitative computed tomography: a predictor of pulmonary function in obstructive lung diseases. *Invest Radiol* 1994;29:564–569.
90. Lucidarme O, Coche E, Cluzel P, et al. Expiratory CT scans for chronic airway disease: correlation with pulmonary function test results. *AJR Am J Roentgenol* 1998;170:301–307.
91. Arakawa H, Webb WR. Expiratory high-resolution CT scan. *Radiol Clin North Am* 1998;36:189–209.
92. Arakawa H, Webb WR. Air trapping on expiratory high-resolution CT scans in the absence of inspiratory scan abnormalities: correlation with pulmonary function tests and differential diagnosis. *AJR Am J Roentgenol* 1998;170:1349–1353.
93. Roberts HR, Wells AU, Milne DG, et al. Airflow obstruction in bronchiectasis: correlation between computed tomography features and pulmonary function tests. *Thorax* 2000;55:198–204.
94. Stern EJ, Graham CM, Webb WR, Gamsu G. Normal trachea during forced expiration: dynamic CT measurements. *Radiology* 1993;187:27–31.
95. Stern EJ, Webb WR. Dynamic imaging of lung morphology with ultrafast high-resolution computed tomography. *J Thorac Imaging* 1993;8: 273–282.
96. Webb WR, Stern EJ, Kanth N, Gamsu G. Dynamic pulmonary CT: findings in normal adult men. *Radiology* 1993;186:117–124.
97. Gotway MB, Lee ES, Reddy GP, et al. Low-dose, dynamic, expiratory thin-section CT of the lungs using a spiral CT scanner. *J Thorac Imaging* 2000;15:168–172.
98. Lucidarme O, Grenier PA, Cadi M, et al. Evaluation of air trapping at CT: comparison of continuous-versus suspended-expiration CT techniques. *Radiology* 2000;216:768–772.
99. Maffessanti M, Candusso M, Brizzi F, Piovesana F. Cystic fibrosis in children: HRCT findings and distribution of disease. *J Thorac Imaging* 1996;11:27–38.
100. Cartier Y, Kavanagh PV, Johkoh T, et al. Bronchiectasis: accuracy of high-resolution CT in the differentiation of specific diseases. *AJR Am J Roentgenol* 1999;173:47–52.
101. Helbich TH, Heinz-Peer G, Eichler I, et al. Cystic fibrosis: CT assessment of lung involvement in children and adults. *Radiology* 1999;213:537–544.
102. Helbich TH, Heinz-Peer G, Fleischmann D, et al. Evolution of CT findings in patients with cystic fibrosis. *AJR Am J Roentgenol* 1999;173:81–88.
103. Ooi GC, Khong PL, Chan-Yeung M, et al. High-resolution CT quantification of bronchiectasis: clinical and functional correlation. *Radiology* 2002;225:663–672.
104. Edwards EA, Metcalfe R, Milne DG, et al. Retrospective review of children presenting with non cystic fibrosis bronchiectasis: HRCT features and clinical relationships. *Pediatr Pulmonol* 2003;36:87–93.
105. Sheehan RE, Wells AU, Copley SJ, et al. A comparison of serial computed tomography and functional change in bronchiectasis. *Eur Respir J* 2002;20:581–587.
106. McGuinness G, Naidich DP, Leitman BS, McCauley DI. Bronchiectasis: CT evaluation. *AJR Am J Roentgenol* 1993;160:253–259.
107. Tarver RD, Conces DJ, Godwin JD. Motion artifacts on CT simulate bronchiectasis. *AJR Am J Roentgenol* 1988;151:1117–1119.
108. Mayo JR, Müller NL, Henkelman RM. The double-fissure sign: a motion artifact on thin-section CT scans. *Radiology* 1987;165:580–581.
109. Primack SL, Remy-Jardin M, Remy J, Müller NL. High-resolution CT of the lung: pitfalls in the diagnosis of infiltrative lung disease. *AJR Am J Roentgenol* 1996;167:413–418.
110. Mansour Y, Beck R, Danino J, Bentur L. Resolution of severe bronchiectasis after removal of long-standing retained foreign body. *Pediatr Pulmonol* 1998;25:130–132.
111. Pasteur MC, Helliwell SM, Houghton SJ, et al. An investigation into causative factors in patients with bronchiectasis. *Am J Respir Crit Care Med* 2000;162:1277–1284.
112. Kullnig P, Pongratz M, Kopp W, Ranner G. [Computerized tomography in the diagnosis of allergic bronchopulmonary aspergillosis]. *Radiologe* 1989;29:228–231.
113. Skeens JL, Fuhrman CR, Yousem SA. Bronchiolitis obliterans in heart-lung transplantation patients: radiologic findings in 11 patients. *AJR Am J Roentgenol* 1989;153:253–256.
114. O'Donovan P. Imaging of complications of lung transplantation. *Radiographics* 1993;13:787–796.
115. Morrish WF, Herman SJ, Weisbrod GL, Chamberlain DW. Bronchiolitis obliterans after lung transplantation: findings at chest radiography and high-resolution CT. *Radiology* 1991;179:487–490.
116. Lentz D, Bergin CJ, Berry GJ, et al. Diagnosis of bronchiolitis obliterans in heart-lung transplantation patients: importance of bronchial dilatation on CT. *AJR Am J Roentgenol* 1992;159:463–467.
117. Hruban RH, Ren H, Kuhlman JE, et al. Inflation-fixed lungs: pathologic-radiologic (CT) correlation of lung transplantation. *J Comput Assist Tomogr* 1990;14:329–335.
118. Herman S, Rappaport D, Weisbrod G, et al. Single-lung transplantation: imaging features. *Radiology* 1989;170:89–93.
119. Graham NJ, Müller NL, Miller RR, Shepherd JD. Intrathoracic complications following allogeneic bone marrow transplantation: CT findings. *Radiology* 1991;181:153–156.
120. Crawford SW, Clark JG. Bronchiolitis associated with bone marrow transplantation. *Clin Chest Med* 1993;14:741–749.
121. Hartman TE, Swensen SJ, Williams DE. Mycobacterium avium-intracellulare complex: evaluation with CT. *Radiology* 1993;187:23–26.
122. Swensen SJ, Hartman TE, Williams DE. Computed tomography in diagnosis of *Mycobacterium avium-intracellulare complex* in patients with bronchiectasis. *Chest* 1994;105:49–52.
123. Moore EH. Atypical mycobacterial infection in the lung: CT appearance. *Radiology* 1993;187:777–782.
124. Kim CK, Chung CY, Kim JS, et al. Late abnormal findings on high-resolution computed tomography after *Mycoplasma pneumonia*. *Pediatrics* 2000;105: 372–378.
125. Miller WT Jr. Spectrum of pulmonary nontuberculous mycobacterial infection. *Radiology* 1994;191:343–350.
126. Woodring JH, Vandiviere HM. Pulmonary disease caused by nontuberculous mycobacteria. *J Thorac Imaging* 1990;5:64–76.
127. Haque AK. The pathology and pathophysiology of mycobacterial infections. *J Thorac Imaging* 1990;5:8–16.
128. Patz EF Jr, Swensen SJ, Erasmus J. Pulmonary manifestations of nontuberculous *Mycobacterium*. *Radiol Clin North Am* 1995;33:719–729.
129. American Thoracic Society. Diagnosis and treatment of disease caused by nontuberculous mycobacteria. *Am Rev Respir Dis* 1990;142:940–953.
130. Diagnosis and treatment of disease caused by nontuberculous mycobacteria. This official statement of the American Thoracic Society was approved by the Board of Directors, March 1997. Medical Section of the American Lung Association. *Am J Respir Crit Care Med* 1997;156:S1–25.
131. Christensen EE, Dietz GW, Ahn CH, et al. Pulmonary manifestations of *Mycobacterium intracellularis*. *AJR Am J Roentgenol* 1979;59–66.
132. Rubin SA. Tuberculosis and atypical mycobacterial infections in the 1990s. *Radiographics* 1997;17:1051–1059.
133. Christensen EE, Dietz GW, Ahn CH, et al. Radiographic manifestations of pulmonary *Mycobacterium kansasii* infections. *AJR Am J Roentgenol* 1978;131:985–993.
134. Albelda SM, Kern JA, Marinelli DL, Miller WT. Expanding spectrum of pulmonary disease caused by nontuberculous mycobacteria. *Radiology* 1985;157:289–296.
135. Primack SL, Logan PM, Hartman TE, et al. Pulmonary tuberculosis and *Mycobacterium avium-intracellulare*: a comparison of CT findings. *Radiology* 1995;194:413–417.
136. Lynch DA, Simone PM, Fox MA, et al. CT features of pulmonary *Mycobacterium avium* complex infection. *J Comput Assist Tomogr* 1995;19:353–360.
137. Fujita J, Ohtsuki Y, Suemitsu I, et al. Pathological and radiological changes in resected lung specimens in *Mycobacterium avium-intracellulare* complex disease. *Eur Respir J* 1999;13:535–540.
138. Wittram C, Weisbrod GL. *Mycobacterium avium* complex lung disease in immunocompetent patients: radiography-CT correlation. *Br J Radiol* 2002;75:340–344.
139. Levin DL. Radiology of pulmonary *Mycobacterium avium-intracellulare* complex. *Clin Chest Med* 2002;23:603–612.
140. McKlendin K, Stark P. *Mycobacterium avium intracellulare* complex as a cause of bronchiectasis. *Semin Respir Infect* 2001;16:85–87.
141. Hollings NP, Wells AU, Wilson R, Hansell DM. Comparative appearances of non-tuberculous mycobacteria species: a CT study. *Eur Radiol* 2002;12:2211–2217.
142. Maycher B, O'Connor R, Long R. Computed tomographic abnormalities in *Mycobacterium avium* complex lung disease include the mosaic pattern of reduced lung attenuation. *Can Assoc Radiol J* 2000;51:93–102.

143. Obayashi Y, Fujita J, Suemitsu I, et al. Successive follow-up of chest computed tomography in patients with *Mycobacterium avium-intracellulare* complex. *Respir Med* 1999;93:11–15.
144. Kasahara T, Nakajima Y, Niimi H, et al. [HRCT findings of pulmonary *Mycobacterium avium* complex: a comparison with tuberculosis]. *Nihon Kokyuki Gakkai Zasshi* 1998;36:122–127.
145. Tanaka E, Amitani R, Niimi A, et al. Yield of computed tomography and bronchoscopy for the diagnosis of *Mycobacterium avium* complex pulmonary disease. *Am J Respir Crit Care Med* 1997;155:2041–2046.
146. Lee KS, Song KS, Lim TH, et al. Adult-onset pulmonary tuberculosis: findings on chest radiographs and CT scans. *AJR Am J Roentgenol* 1993;160:753–758.
147. Lee KS, Kim YH, Kim WS, et al. Endobronchial tuberculosis: CT features. *J Comput Assist Tomogr* 1991;15:424–428.
148. Im J-G, Webb WR, Han MC, Park JH. Apical opacity associated with pulmonary tuberculosis: high-resolution CT findings. *Radiology* 1991; 178:727–731.
149. McGuinness G, Naidich DP, Jagirdar J, et al. High resolution CT findings in miliary lung disease. *J Comput Assist Tomogr* 1992;16:384–390.
150. Ikezoe J, Takeuchi N, Johkoh T, et al. CT appearance of pulmonary tuberculosis in diabetic and immunocompromised patients: comparison with patients who had no underlying disease. *AJR Am J Roentgenol* 1992;159:1175–1179.
151. Leung AN. Pulmonary tuberculosis: the essentials. *Radiology* 1999;210: 307–322.
152. Lee KS, Im JG. CT in adults with tuberculosis of the chest: characteristic findings and role in management. *AJR Am J Roentgenol* 1995; 164:1361–1367.
153. Choi D, Lee KS, Suh GY, et al. Pulmonary tuberculosis presenting as acute respiratory failure: radiologic findings. *J Comput Assist Tomogr* 1999;23:107–113.
154. Kim WS, Moon WK, Kim IO, et al. Pulmonary tuberculosis in children: evaluation with CT. *AJR Am J Roentgenol* 1997;168:1005–1009.
155. Oh YW, Kim YH, Lee NJ, et al. High-resolution CT appearance of miliary tuberculosis. *J Comput Assist Tomogr* 1994;18:862–866.
156. Im JG, Itoh H, Han MC. CT of pulmonary tuberculosis. *Semin Ultrasound CT MR* 1995;16:420–434.
157. Poey C, Verhaegen F, Giron J, et al. High resolution chest CT in tuberculosis: evolutive patterns and signs of activity. *J Comput Assist Tomogr* 1997;21:601–607.
158. Hatipoglu ON, Osma E, Manisali M, et al. High resolution computed tomographic findings in pulmonary tuberculosis. *Thorax* 1996;51:397–402.
159. Kim HY, Song KS, Goo JM, et al. Thoracic sequelae and complications of tuberculosis. *Radiographics* 2001;21:839–858.
160. Curtin JJ, Webster AD, Farrant J, Katz D. Bronchiectasis in hypogammaglobulinaemia—a computed tomography assessment. *Clin Radiol* 1991;44:82–84.
161. Kainulainen L, Varpula M, Liippo K, et al. Pulmonary abnormalities in patients with primary hypogammaglobulinemia. *J Allergy Clin Immunol* 1999;104:1031–1036.
162. Martinez Garcia MA, de Rojas MD, Nauffal Manzur MD, et al. Respiratory disorders in common variable immunodeficiency. *Respir Med* 2001;95:191–195.
163. McGuinness G, Naidich DP, Garay SM, et al. AIDS associated bronchiectasis: CT features. *J Comput Assist Tomogr* 1993;17:260–266.
164. McGuinness G, Gruden JF, Bhalla M, et al. AIDS-related airway disease. *AJR Am J Roentgenol* 1997;168:67–77.
165. King MA, Neal DE, St John R, et al. Bronchial dilatation in patients with HIV infection: CT assessment and correlation with pulmonary function tests and findings at bronchoalveolar lavage. *AJR Am J Roentgenol* 1997;168:1535–1540.
166. Verghese A, al-Samman M, Nabhan D, et al. Bacterial bronchitis and bronchiectasis in human immunodeficiency virus infection. *Arch Intern Med* 1994;154:2086–2091.
167. Holmes AH, Trotman-Dickenson B, Edwards A, et al. Bronchiectasis in HIV disease. *Q J Med* 1992;85:875–882.
168. Moskovic E, Miller R, Pearson M. High resolution computed tomography of *Pneumocystis carinii* pneumonia in AIDS. *Clin Radiol* 1990;42:239–243.
169. Hirschtick RE, Glassroth J, Jordan MC, et al. Bacterial pneumonia in persons infected with the human immunodeficiency virus. Pulmonary Complications of HIV Infection Study Group [see comments]. *N Engl J Med* 1995;333:845–851.
170. Markowitz GS, Concepcion L, Factor SM, Borczuk AC. Autopsy patterns of disease among subgroups of an inner-city Bronx AIDS population. *J Acquir Immune Defic Syndr Hum Retrovirol* 1996;13:48–54.
171. Wallace JM, Hansen NI, Lavange L, et al. Respiratory disease trends in the Pulmonary Complications of HIV Infection Study cohort. Pulmonary Complications of HIV Infection Study Group. *Am J Respir Crit Care Med* 1997;155:72–80.
172. McGuinness G, Scholes JV, Jagirdar JS, et al. Unusual lymphoproliferative disorders in nine adults with HIV or AIDS: CT and pathologic findings. *Radiology* 1995;197:59–65.
173. Gelman M, King MA, Neal DE, et al. Focal air trapping in patients with HIV infection: CT evaluation and correlation with pulmonary function test results. *AJR Am J Roentgenol* 1999;172:1033–1038.
174. Klapholz A, Salomon N, Perlman DC, Talavera W. Aspergillosis in the acquired immunodeficiency syndrome. *Chest* 1991;100:1614–1618.
175. Denning DW. Aspergillus tracheobronchitis [letter; comment]. *Clin Infect Dis* 1994;19:1176–1177.
176. Staples CA, Kang EY, Wright JL, et al. Invasive pulmonary aspergillosis in AIDS: radiographic, CT, and pathologic findings. *Radiology* 1995;196: 409–414.
177. Wright JL, Lawson L, Chan N, Filipenko D. An unusual form of pulmonary aspergillosis in two patients with the acquired immunodeficiency syndrome. *Am J Clin Pathol* 1993;100:57–59.
178. Wood BP. Cystic fibrosis: 1997. *Radiology* 1997;204:1–10.
179. Stern RC. The diagnosis of cystic fibrosis. *N Engl J Med* 1997;336:487–491.
180. Friedman PJ. Chest radiographic findings in the adult with cystic fibrosis. *Semin Roentgenol* 1987;22:114–124.
181. Reinig JW, Sanchez FW, Thomason DM, Gobien RP. The distinctly visible right upper lobe bronchus on the lateral chest: a clue to adolescent cystic fibrosis. *Pediatr Radiol* 1985;15:222–224.
182. Schwartz EE, Holsclaw DS. Pulmonary involvement in adults with cystic fibrosis. *AJR Am J Roentgenol* 1974;122:708–718.
183. Greene KE, Takasugi JE, Godwin JD, et al. Radiographic changes in acute exacerbations of cystic fibrosis in adults: a pilot study. *AJR Am J Roentgenol* 1994;163:557–562.
184. Hansell DM, Strickland B. High-resolution computed tomography in pulmonary cystic fibrosis. *Br J Radiol* 1989;62:1–5.
185. Lynch DA, Brasch RC, Hardy KA, Webb WR. Pediatric pulmonary disease: assessment with high-resolution ultrafast CT. *Radiology* 1990;176:243–248.
186. Santis G, Hodson ME, Strickland B. High resolution computed tomography in adult cystic fibrosis patients with mild lung disease. *Clin Radiol* 1991;44:20–22.
187. Marchant JM, Masel JP, Dickinson FL, et al. Application of chest high-resolution computer tomography in young children with cystic fibrosis. *Pediatr Pulmonol* 2001;31:24–29.
188. Taccone A, Romano L, Marzoli A, Girosi D. [Computerized tomography in pulmonary cystic fibrosis]. *Radiol Med (Torino)* 1991;82:79–83.
189. Lee PH, Carr DH, Rubens MB, et al. Accuracy of CT in predicting the cause of bronchiectasis. *Clin Radiol* 1995;50:839–841.
190. Nathanson I, Conboy K, Murphy S, et al. Ultrafast computerized tomography of the chest in cystic fibrosis: a new scoring system. *Pediatr Pulmonol* 1991;11:81–86.
191. Shah RM, Friedman AC, Ostrum BJ, et al. Pulmonary complications of cystic fibrosis in adults. *Crit Rev Diagn Imaging* 1995;36:441–477.
192. Marom EM, McAdams HP, Palmer SM, et al. Cystic fibrosis: usefulness of thoracic CT in the examination of patients before lung transplantation. *Radiology* 1999;213:283–288.
193. Lynch DA. Imaging of asthma and allergic bronchopulmonary mycosis. *Radiol Clin North Am* 1998;36:129–142.
194. American Thoracic Society. Standards for the diagnosis and care of patients with chronic obstructive pulmonary disease (COPD) and asthma. *Am Rev Respir Dis* 1987;136:225–243.
195. Jeffery PK. Comparative morphology of the airways in asthma and chronic obstructive pulmonary disease. *Am J Respir Crit Care Med* 1994;150:S6–13.
196. Hodson ME, Simon G, Batten JC. Radiology of uncomplicated asthma. *Thorax* 1974;29:296–303.
197. Zieverink SA, Harper AP, Holden RW, et al. Emergency room radiology in asthma: an efficacy study. *Radiology* 1982;145:27–29.
198. Blair DN, Coppage L, Shaw C. Medical imaging in asthma. *J Thorac Imaging* 1986;1:23–35.
199. Paganin F, Trussard V, Seneterre E, et al. Chest radiography and high resolution computed tomography of the lungs in asthma. *Am Rev Respir Dis* 1992;146:1084–1087.
200. Sherman S, Skoney JA, Ravikrishnan KP. Routine chest radiographs in exacerbations of chronic obstructive pulmonary disease. Diagnostic value. *Arch Intern Med* 1989;149:2493–2496.
201. Gershel JC, Goldman HS, Stein REK, et al. The usefulness of chest radiographs in first asthma attacks. *N Engl J Med* 1983;309:336–339.
202. Kinsella M, Müller NL, Staples C, et al. Hyperinflation in asthma and emphysema: assessment by pulmonary function testing and computed tomography. *Chest* 1988;94:286–289.
203. Kondoh Y, Taniguchi H, Yokoyama S, et al. Emphysematous change in chronic asthma in relation to cigarette smoking: assessment by computed tomography. *Chest* 1990;97:845–849.
204. Harmanci E, Kebapci M, Metintas M, Ozkan R. High-resolution computed tomography findings are correlated with disease severity in asthma. *Respiration* 2002;69:420–426.
205. Grenier P, Mourey-Gerosa I, Benali K, et al. Abnormalities of the airways and lung parenchyma in asthmatics: CT observations in 50 patients and inter- and intraobserver variability. *Eur Radiol* 1996;6:199–206.
206. Kee ST, Fahy JV, Chen DR, Gamsu G. High-resolution computed tomography of airway changes after induced bronchoconstriction and bronchodilation in asthmatic volunteers. *Acad Radiol* 1996;3:389–394.
207. Goldin JG, McNitt-Gray MF, Sorenson SM, et al. Airway hyperreactivity: assessment with helical thin-section CT. *Radiology* 1998;208:321–329.
208. Beigelman-Aubry C, Capderou A, Grenier PA, et al. Mild intermittent asthma: CT assessment of bronchial cross-sectional area and lung attenuation at controlled lung volume. *Radiology* 2002;223:181–187.

209. Little SA, Sproule MW, Cowan MD, et al. High resolution computed tomographic assessment of airway wall thickness in chronic asthma: reproducibility and relationship with lung function and severity. *Thorax* 2002;57:247–253.
210. Park JW, Hong YK, Kim CW, et al. High-resolution computed tomography in patients with bronchial asthma: correlation with clinical features, pulmonary functions and bronchial hyperresponsiveness. *J Investig Allergol Clin Immunol* 1997;7:186–192.
211. Laurent F, Latrabe V, Raherison C, et al. Functional significance of air trapping detected in moderate asthma. *Eur Radiol* 2000;10:1404–1410.
212. Newman KB, Lynch DA, Newman LS, et al. Quantitative computed tomography detects air trapping due to asthma. *Chest* 1994;106:105–109.
213. Webb WR. High-resolution computed tomography of obstructive lung disease. *Radiol Clin North Am* 1994;32:745–757.
214. Kumar R, Gaur SN. Prevalence of allergic bronchopulmonary aspergillosis in patients with bronchial asthma. *Asian Pac J Allergy Immunol* 2000;18: 181–185.
215. Zhaoming W, Lockey RF. A review of allergic bronchopulmonary aspergillosis. *J Investig Allergol Clin Immunol* 1996;6:144–151.
216. Geller DE, Kaplowitz H, Light MJ, Colin AA. Allergic bronchopulmonary aspergillosis in cystic fibrosis: reported prevalence, regional distribution, and patient characteristics. Scientific Advisory Group, Investigators, and Coordinators of the Epidemiologic Study of Cystic Fibrosis. *Chest* 1999;116:639–646.
217. Kumar R. Mild, moderate, and severe forms of allergic bronchopulmonary aspergillosis: a clinical and serologic evaluation. *Chest* 2003;124:890–892.
218. Currie DC, Goldman JM, Cole PJ, Strickland B. Comparison of narrow section computed tomography and plain chest radiography in chronic allergic bronchopulmonary aspergillosis. *Clin Radiol* 1987;38:593–96.
219. Shah A, Pant CS, Bhagat R, Panchal N. CT in childhood allergic bronchopulmonary aspergillosis. *Pediatr Radiol* 1992;22:227–228.
220. Sandhu M, Mukhopadhyay S, Sharma SK. Allergic bronchopulmonary aspergillosis: a comparative evaluation of computed tomography with plain chest radiography. *Australas Radiol* 1994;38:288–293.
221. Angus RM, Davies ML, Cowan MD, et al. Computed tomographic scanning of the lung in patients with allergic bronchopulmonary aspergillosis and in asthmatic patients with a positive skin test to *Aspergillus fumigatus*. *Thorax* 1994;49:586–589.
222. Panchal N, Pant C, Bhagat R, Shah A. Central bronchiectasis in allergic bronchopulmonary aspergillosis: comparative evaluation of computed tomography with bronchography. *Eur Respir J* 1994;7:1290–1293.
223. Panchal N, Bhagat R, Pant C, Shah A. Allergic bronchopulmonary aspergillosis: the spectrum of computed tomography appearances. *Respir Med* 1997;91:213–219.
224. Ward S, Heyneman L, Lee MJ, et al. Accuracy of CT in the diagnosis of allergic bronchopulmonary aspergillosis in asthmatic patients. *AJR Am J Roentgenol* 1999;173:937–942.
225. Mitchell TA, Hamilos DL, Lynch DA, Newell JD. Distribution and severity of bronchiectasis in allergic bronchopulmonary aspergillosis (ABPA). *J Asthma* 2000;37:65–72.
226. Goyal R, White CS, Templeton PA, et al. High attenuation mucous plugs in allergic bronchopulmonary aspergillosis: CT appearance. *J Comput Assist Tomogr* 1992;16:649–650.
227. Logan PM, Müller NL. High-attenuation mucous plugging in allergic bronchopulmonary aspergillosis. *Can Assoc Radiol J* 1996;47:374–377.
228. Roberts CM, Citron KM, Strickland B. Intrathoracic aspergilloma: role of CT in diagnosis and treatment. *Radiology* 1987;165:123–128.
229. Logan PM, Muller NL. CT manifestations of pulmonary aspergillosis. *Crit Rev Diagn Imaging* 1996;37:1–37.
230. Logan PM, Müller NL. High-resolution computed tomography and pathologic findings in pulmonary aspergillosis: a pictorial essay. *Can Assoc Radiol J* 1996;47:444–452.
231. Rayner CF, Rutman A, Dewar A, et al. Ciliary disorientation alone as a cause of primary ciliary dyskinesia syndrome. *Am J Respir Crit Care Med* 1996;153:1123–1129.
232. de Iongh RU, Rutland J. Ciliary defects in healthy subjects, bronchiectasis, and primary ciliary dyskinesia. *Am J Respir Crit Care Med* 1995;151:1559–1567.
233. Homma S, Kawabata M, Kishi K, et al. Bronchiolitis in Kartagener's syndrome. *Eur Respir J* 1999;14:1332–1339.
234. Neville E, Brewis R, Yeates WK, Burridge A. Respiratory tract disease and obstructive azoospermia. *Thorax* 1983;38:929–933.
235. Wiggins J, Strickland B, Chung KF. Detection of bronchiectasis by high-resolution computed tomography in the yellow nail syndrome. *Clin Radiol* 1991;43:377–379.
236. King MA, Stone JA, Diaz PT, et al. Alpha 1-antitrypsin deficiency: evaluation of bronchiectasis with CT. *Radiology* 1996;199:137–141.
237. Choplin RH, Wehunt WD, Theros EG. Diffuse lesions of the trachea. *Semin Roentgenol* 1983;18:38–50.
238. Schwartz M, Rossoff L. Tracheobronchomegaly. *Chest* 1994;106:1589–1590.
239. Dunne MG, Reiner B. CT features of tracheobronchomegaly. *J Comput Assist Tomogr* 1988;12:388–391.
240. Roditi GH, Weir J. The association of tracheomegaly and bronchiectasis. *Clin Radiol* 1994;49:608–611.
241. Woodring JH, Barrett PA, Rehm SR, Nurenberg P. Acquired tracheomegaly in adults as a complication of diffuse pulmonary fibrosis. *AJR Am J Roentgenol* 1989;152:743–747.
242. Shin MS, Jackson RM, Ho KJ. Tracheobronchomegaly (Mounier-Kuhn syndrome): CT diagnosis. *AJR Am J Roentgenol* 1988;150:777–779.
243. Kwong JS, Müller NL, Miller RR. Diseases of the trachea and main-stem bronchi: correlation of CT with pathologic findings. *Radiographics* 1992;12:647–657.
244. Webb EM, Elicker BM, Webb WR. Using CT to diagnose nonneoplastic tracheal abnormalities: appearance of the tracheal wall. *AJR Am J Roentgenol* 2000;174:1315–1321.
245. Mitchell RE, Bury RG. Congenital bronchiectasis due to deficiency of bronchial cartilage (Williams-Campbell syndrome): a case report. *J Pediatr* 1975; 87:230–234.
246. Wayne KS, Taussig LM. Probable familial congenital bronchiectasis due to cartilage deficiency (Williams-Campbell syndrome). *Am Rev Respir Dis* 1976;114:15–22.
247. Kaneko K, Kudo S, Tashiro M, et al. Computed tomography findings in Williams-Campbell syndrome. *J Thorac Imaging* 1991;6:11–13.
248. Watanabe Y, Nishiyama Y, Kanayama H, et al. Congenital bronchiectasis due to cartilage deficiency: CT demonstration. *J Comput Assist Tomogr* 1987;11:701–703.
249. Cohen M, Sahn SA. Bronchiectasis in systemic diseases. *Chest* 1999;116: 1063–1074.
250. Remy-Jardin M, Remy J, Cortet B, et al. Lung changes in rheumatoid arthritis: CT findings. *Radiology* 1994;193:375–382.
251. McDonagh J, Greaves M, Wright AR, et al. High resolution computed tomography of the lungs in patients with rheumatoid arthritis and interstitial lung disease. *Br J Rheumatol* 1994;33:118–122.
252. Hassan WU, Keaney NP, Holland CD, Kelly CA. High resolution computed tomography of the lung in lifelong non-smoking patients with rheumatoid arthritis. *Ann Rheum Dis* 1995;54:308–310.
253. Perez T, Remy-Jardin M, Cortet B. Airways involvement in rheumatoid arthritis: clinical, functional, and HRCT findings. *Am J Respir Crit Care Med* 1998;157:1658–1665.
254. Despaux J, Manzoni P, Toussirot E, et al. Prospective study of the prevalence of bronchiectasis in rheumatoid arthritis using high-resolution computed tomography. *Rev Rhum Engl Ed* 1998;65:453–461.
255. Aquino SL, Webb WR, Golden J. Bronchiolitis obliterans associated with rheumatoid arthritis: findings on HRCT and dynamic expiratory CT. *J Comput Assist Tomogr* 1994;18:555–558.
256. Geddes DM, Webley M, Emerson PA. Airways obstruction in rheumatoid arthritis. *Ann Rheum Dis* 1979;38:222–225.
257. Swinson DR, Symmons D, Suresh U, et al. Decreased survival in patients with co-existent rheumatoid arthritis and bronchiectasis. *Br J Rheumatol* 1997;36:689–691.
258. Fenlon HM, Doran M, Sant SM, Breatnach E. High-resolution chest CT in systemic lupus erythematosus. *AJR Am J Roentgenol* 1996;166:301–307.
259. Bankier AA, Kiener HP, Wiesmayr MN, et al. Discrete lung involvement in systemic lupus erythematosus: CT assessment. *Radiology* 1995;196:835–840.
260. Franquet T, Giménez A, Monill JM, et al. Primary Sjögren's syndrome and associated lung disease: CT findings in 50 patients. *AJR Am J Roentgenol* 1997;169:655–658.
261. Koyama M, Johkoh T, Honda O, et al. Pulmonary involvement in primary Sjogren's syndrome: spectrum of pulmonary abnormalities and computed tomography findings in 60 patients. *J Thorac Imaging* 2001;16:290–296.
262. Songur N, Songur Y, Tuzun M, et al. Pulmonary function tests and high-resolution CT in the detection of pulmonary involvement in inflammatory bowel disease. *J Clin Gastroenterol* 2003;37:292–298.

Small Airway Diseases

Small airway disease is defined as a pathologic condition in which the small conducting airways are affected either primarily or in addition to alveolar or interstitial lung changes. For the pathologist, small airway disease has the same meaning as bronchiolitis, a nonspecific term used to describe inflammation of the membranous and respiratory bronchioles. Bronchiolitis can be classified according to its proved or its presumed etiology, the pulmonary or systemic diseases with which it is often associated, or its histologic features. The diagnosis of small airway disease is challenging for the clinician, because it has no pathognomonic clinical or functional features. The chest radiograph is normal or may show nonspecific findings. The highly variable radiographic abnormalities include hyperinflation and peripheral attenuation of vascular markings, peribronchial wall thickness, perihilar linear opacities, atelectasis, and airspace consolidation. However, there is considerable interobserver and intraobserver variability in interpretation of the radiographs and there is no real correlation between the clinical severity of the disease and the degree of radiographic changes. Thin-section computed tomography (CT) has become the best imaging technique for the assessment of the small airways and is clearly the radiologic method of choice for investigating a patient suspected on clinical, functional, or radiographic features of having bronchiolitis. CT findings are frequently suggestive of the diagnosis of small airway disease and are frequently the first indication of the presence of small airway pathology. In addition, CT provides the most reliable assessment of both the extent and the severity of disease. It is a reliable and easily repeatable technique for assessing response to therapy, avoiding the need for successive histologic evaluations. Nowadays the use of multidetector CT technique allows one to combine volumetric acquisition over the entire length during a single breath hold with the use of thin collimation. In addition, postprocessing techniques may contribute to improving the visualization of the characteristic findings of small airway disease and to assessing the extent of the lesions.

ANATOMY OF THE SMALL AIRWAYS

Small airways are those that do not contain cartilage and glands. They are called bronchioles (1). The bronchioles include two categories, membranous (lobular and terminal) bronchioles and respiratory bronchioles. The secondary pulmonary lobule, described by Miller (2) as the smallest portion of the lung that is surrounded by connective tissue septa (interlobular septa), is ventilated by a lobular bronchiole measuring approximately 1 mm in diameter and 0.15 mm in wall thickness (Fig. 5-1). The lobular bronchiole enters the core of the lobule accompanied by its homologous pulmonary artery and divides into 3 to 12 terminal bronchioles, according to the size of the lobule, at approximately 2-mm intervals (Fig. 5-2). The terminal bronchioles are found between the sixth and twenty-third generations of branching (3) and have an internal diameter of approximately 0.6 mm; their length varies from 0.8 to 2.5 mm (Fig. 5-3) (4,5). The walls of membranous bronchioles contain three compartments: (1) an inner wall consisting of epithelium, basement membrane, lamina propria, and submucosa, (2) a smooth muscle layer, and (3) an outer wall consisting of the connective tissue between the muscle layer and the surrounding parenchyma (6). The wall thickness varies between 0.05 and 0.1 mm. This is below the ability of CT to image, and as a result, normal airways with a diameter of less than approximately 1.5 mm cannot be identified on thin-section CT.

The terminal bronchioles and their accompanying homologous centrilobular pulmonary arterial branches and lymphatic vessels are "core structures," being clustered near

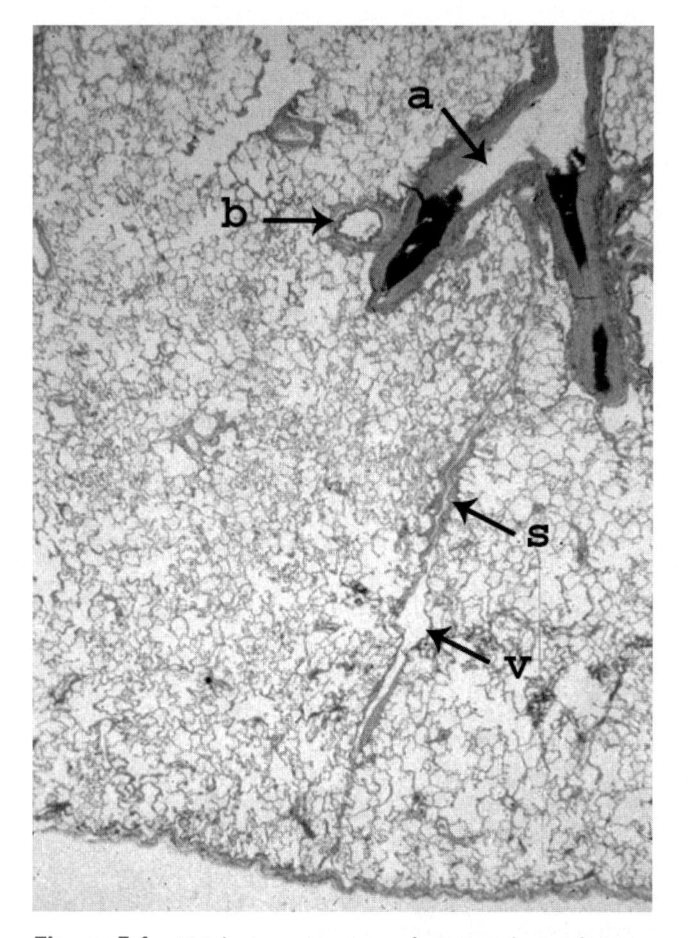

Figure 5-1 Histologic appearance of a secondary pulmonary lobule. The lobular bronchiole (b) is accompanied by its homologous pulmonary artery filled with a clot (a). The interlobular septum (s) contains the interlobular vein (v).

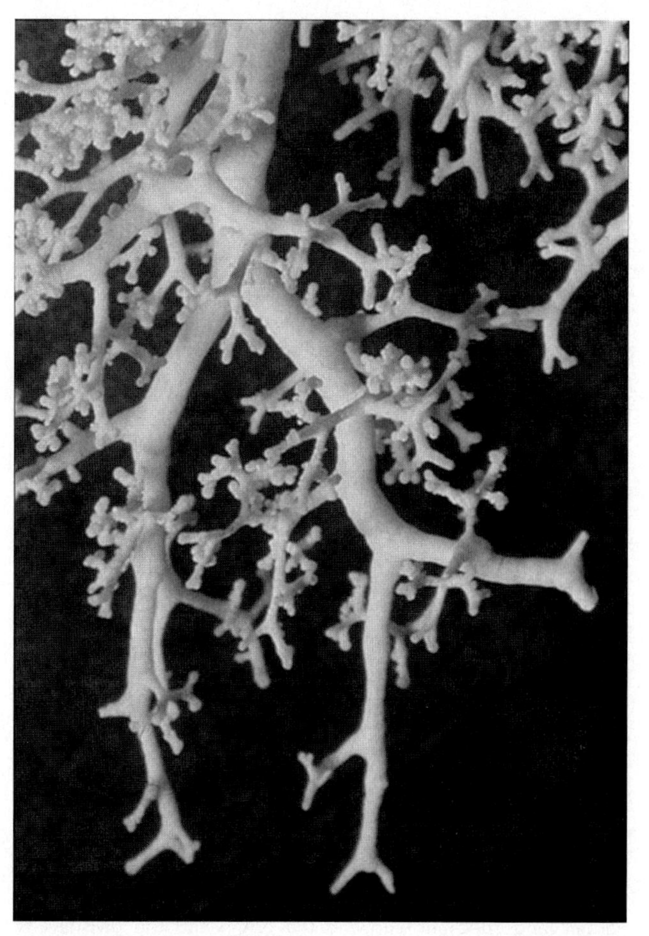

Figure 5-3 Bronchial cast from a human lung specimen showing the origin and divisions of several terminal bronchioles. (Courtesy of Ewald Weibel.)

the center of the secondary pulmonary lobule. Between these core structures and the interlobular septa, numerous alveolar spaces, capillaries, and respiratory bronchioles are present. This accounts for the characteristic centrilobular distribution of bronchiolar abnormalities detected on thin-section CT scans (7–9).

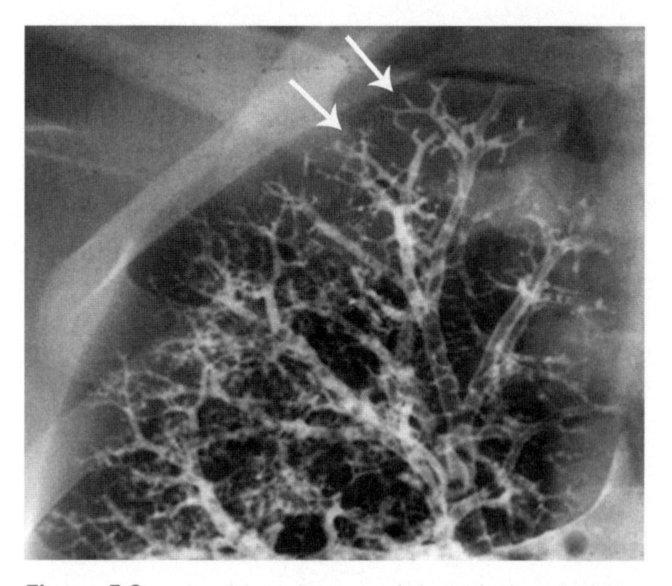

Figure 5-2 Normal bronchogram of the right bronchial tree targeted on the right upper lobe. The arrows show the normal appearance of lobular and terminal bronchioles.

The terminal bronchioles are purely conducting airways, and no alveoli arise directly from them. Each of the terminal bronchioles divides into several generations of respiratory bronchioles. Conversely, respiratory bronchioles have gas-exchanging alveoli arising from their walls. They communicate through alveolar ducts within numerous alveolar sacs (Fig. 5-4) (3).

PATHOLOGY

Initially bronchiolitis is an inflammatory disorder involving the bronchiolar wall, occurring as a reaction to an injury (10). The injury can be focal or multifocal or may affect all the bronchioles in both lungs. The injury can have a known cause or may be the result of an unknown trigger. The different causes of bronchiolitis are listed in Table 5-1. Although an etiologic classification may be useful when bronchiolitis is suspected, the simplest scheme for classifying bronchiolar disease is based on the histologic pattern, which shows a better

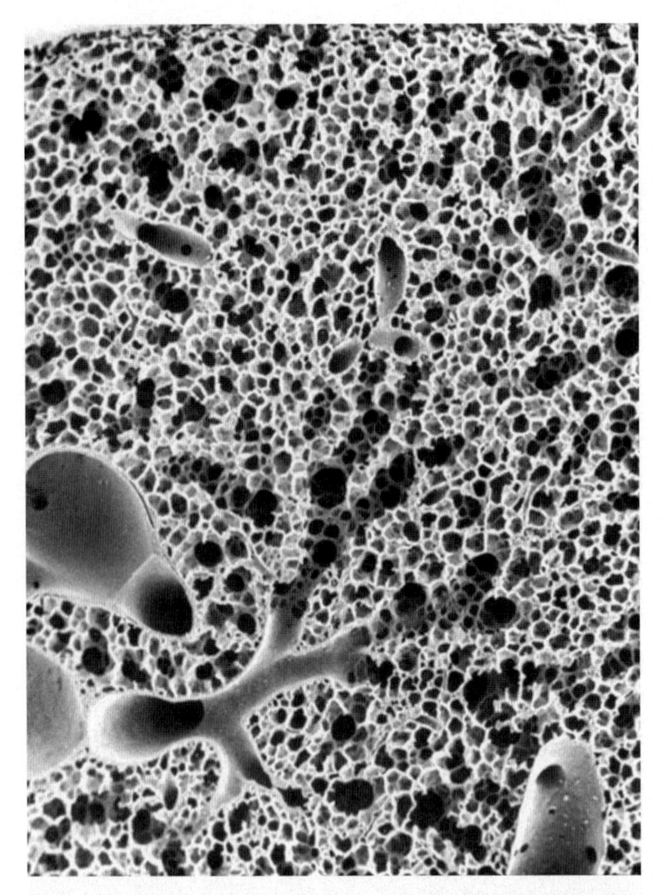

Figure 5-4 Low-power scanning electron microscopy of a normal lung specimen showing the origin and the divisions of terminal and respiratory bronchioles down to the alveolar ducts and sacs. (Courtesy of Ewald Weibel.)

correlation with the clinical and radiologic manifestations of disease. The histologic classification also shows better correlation with the natural history of the disease and its response to therapy.

Bronchiolitis can be subdivided into acute and chronic forms. Acute bronchiolitis usually results from processes that cause bronchiolar injury over a short period of time, such as viral infection or the inhalation of toxic gases. The lesions involve mainly the epithelium; necrosis and desquamation are followed by exudation, fibrin, inflammatory cell infiltration, and granuloma formation and subsequently by resorption and scarring. Chronic bronchiolitis is typically associated with prolonged injury and is characterized by bronchiolar infiltration by mononuclear cells typically followed by the development of a fibrotic process.

The current pathologic classification of bronchiolitis is based on three main histologic patterns: cellular bronchiolitis, bronchiolitis obliterans with intraluminal polyps, and obliterative bronchiolitis (10–14). Although two or three types of bronchiolitis may coexist in an individual, one pattern usually predominates in a given condition.

Besides bronchiolitis, the small airways may be involved indirectly. Changes adjacent to the bronchioles, such as lung fibrosis, and abnormalities in the bronchiolar wall, such as granulomas, can also cause distortion of the bronchiole and narrowing of the lumen (15). This phenomenon is particularly well illustrated in sarcoidosis.

TABLE 5-1
ETIOLOGIES AND CLINICAL CONDITIONS ASSOCIATED WITH BRONCHIOLITIS

Inhalation of gases, fumes, and dusts
Infection (e.g., viruses, *Mycoplasma pneumoniae, Chlamydia* species, *Aspergillus fumigatus*)
Irradiation
Aspiration
Drugs and chemicals
Organ transplantation
Bone marrow
Heart-lung
Lung
Connective tissue disease
Rheumatoid disease
Sjögren's syndrome
Systemic lupus erythematosus
Dermatomyosis
Progressive systemic sclerosis
Others
Hypersensitivity pneumonitis
Autoimmune diseases
Chronic eosinophilic pneumonia
Neoplasia (carcinoid tumor, neuroendocrine cell hyperplasia)

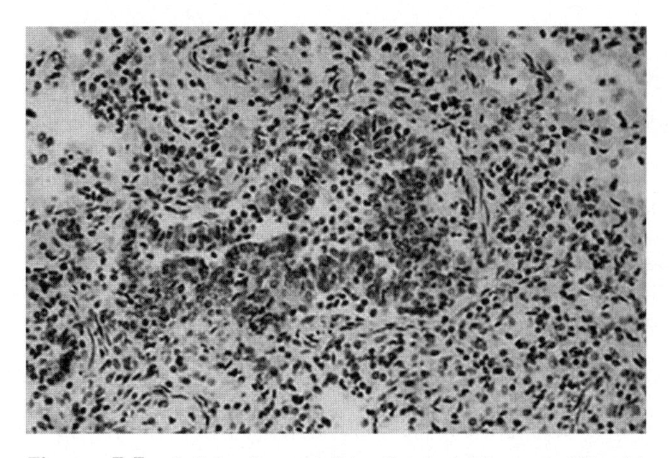

Figure 5-5 Cellular bronchiolitis. Surgical biopsy (×20) with immunohistochemical labeling. Inflammatory bronchiolitis caused by respiratory syncytial virus infection.

Cellular Bronchiolitis

The histologic pattern of cellular bronchiolitis is characterized by inflammatory cellular infiltrates involving both the bronchiolar lumen and walls with some degree of fibrosis. According to the predominant cell type and the clinical presentation, acute or chronic, the classification most commonly includes infectious bronchiolitis (Fig. 5-5), respiratory bronchiolitis, follicular bronchiolitis, panbronchiolitis, aspiration bronchiolitis, bronchiolitis associated with hypersensitivity pneumonitis, and asthma. The pattern of cellular bronchiolitis may regress under specific or anti-inflammatory treatment or may be followed by bronchiolitis obliterans or obliterative brochiolitis. (16).

Bronchiolitis Obliterans with Intraluminal Polyps

The histologic pattern of bronchiolitis obliterans with intraluminal polyps is characterized by the presence of granulation tissue polyps or plugs of fibroblastic tissue extending from the areas of epithelium damage into the lumens of respiratory bronchioles, resulting in partial, or occasionally complete, obstruction. Although the pattern may be the only abnormality present in the lungs, in most patients it is associated with similar epithelial injury and fibroblastic reaction in the more distal airspaces (Fig. 5-6). Mild interstitial chronic inflammation may be present and lung architecture is preserved. In such cases, bronchiolitis occurs in association with pneumonitis, and as a result the term bronchiolitis obliterans with organizing pneumonia (BOOP) is frequently used (17). Idiopathic BOOP is currently classified among the idiopathic interstitial pneumonias and is called cryptogenic organizing pneumonia (COP). Secondary BOOP is still regarded as an airway disease related to different types of injury (infection, drug toxicity, aspiration, irradiation, toxic fume inhalation) or associated with different conditions (collagen tissue disease, Wegener's granulomatosis, Behçet's disease, hypersensitivity pneumonitis, organ transplantation, tumors, infarction) (18–32). BOOP is responsive to steroids, with regression of the abnormalities in most patients.

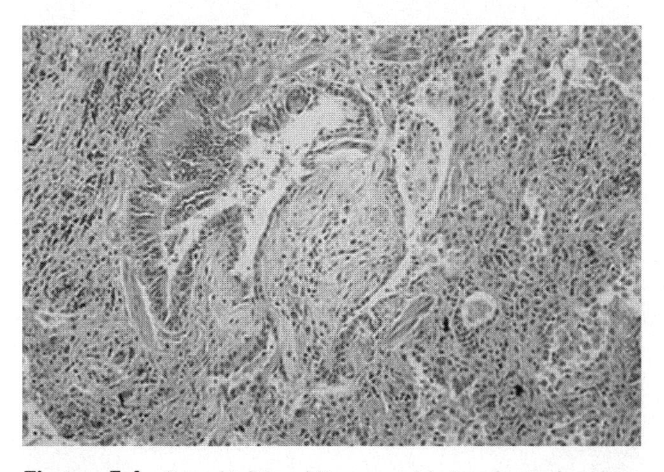

Figure 5-6 Bronchiolitis obliterans with intraluminal polyps. Surgical biopsy (×20, hematoxylin and eosin) obliteration of the lumen of a respiratory bronchiole by a fibroblastic plug floating in the lumen. The same type of fibroblastic reaction is also present in more distal airspaces (organizing pneumonia).

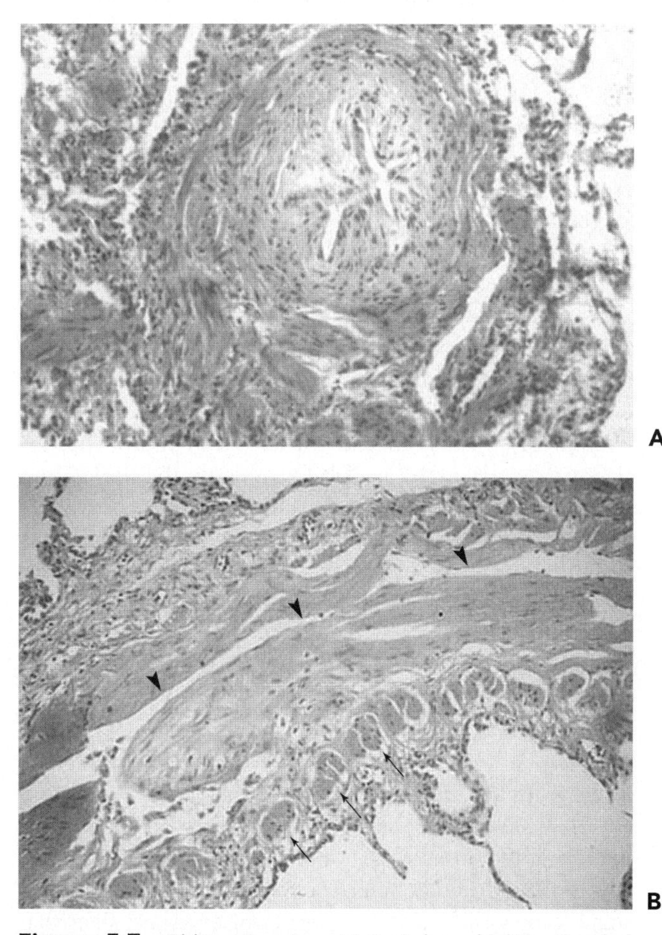

Figure 5-7 Obliterative (constrictive) bronchiolitis. Surgical biopsy (×20, HE). **A:** Section perpendicular to a terminal bronchiole showing a concentric narrowing of the bronchiolar lumen by subepithelial fibrosis. **B:** Section along the long axis of another terminal bronchiole showing the longitudinal extent of the subepithelial fibrosis. Arrows show the section of the smooth muscle fibers in the bronchiolar wall. Arrowheads show the narrowed bronchiolar lumen.

TABLE 5-2
CONDITIONS ASSOCIATED WITH OBLITERATIVE BRONCHIOLITIS

Infection (Table 5-3)
  Childhood viral infection (e.g., adenovirus, respiratory syncytial virus)
  Infection in adults and children (e.g., *Mycoplasma pneumoniae, Pneumocystis carinii* in AIDS patients, endobronchial spread of tuberculosis, bacterial bronchiolar infection)
Toxic fume inhalation (e.g., nitrogen dioxide, sulfur dioxide) (Table 5-4)
Connective tissue disease, particularly rheumatoid disease, and Sjögren's syndrome
Drug therapy (e.g., penicillamine, gold salts)
Chronic rejection following lung and heart-lung transplantation
Chronic graft-versus-host disease following bone marrow transplantation
Neuroendocrine cell hyperplasia
Inflammatory bowel disease
Idiopathic

Obliterative (or Constrictive) Bronchiolitis

The pattern of obliterative bronchiolitis is characterized by the development of an irreversible circumferential submucosal fibrosis, resulting in bronchiolar narrowing or obliteration of bronchioles in the absence of intraluminal granulation tissue polyps or surrounding parenchymal inflammation (Fig. 5-7) (10,33). Proliferation of fibrosis extends predominantly between the epithelium and the muscular mucosae and along the long axis of the airway, impairing collateral ventilation, and leading to airflow obstruction (Fig. 5-7B). The epithelium overlying the abnormal fibrosis tissue may be flattened or metaplastic and is usually intact without any ulceration. In some instances, the accompanying pulmonary artery is also obliterated by the same fibrotic process.

Although the histologic characterization of bronchiolitis clearly depends on the availability of tissue, the clinical and radiologic features associated with specific histologic patterns are often sufficiently characteristic to permit a strong, presumptive diagnosis. The various causes of obliterative bronchiolitis are shown in Table 5-2.

CT FINDINGS

Although the visualization of normal bronchioles is impaired by the spatial resolution limits of the thin-section CT, these airways may become directly visible when inflammation of the bronchiolar wall and accompanying exudate develop. On the other hand, bronchiolar changes can be too small to be visible directly but can cause indirect signs that suggest small airway involvement. Obstruction of the bronchioles may induce regional underventilation, leading to reflex vasoconstriction and expiratory air trapping, both of which may be visible on CT images. Five different CT patterns can express small airway pathology. The first two are direct signs, and the other three represent indirect manifestations.

Tree-in-Bud Sign

The tree-in-bud pattern comprises focal or multifocal areas of small centrilobular nodular and branching linear opacities. It reflects the abnormal bronchiolar wall thickening and dilatation of the bronchiolar lumen filled with liquid, mucus, or pus that is often associated with peribronchiolar inflammation (7). The branching pattern of dilated bronchioles and peribronchiolar inflammation give the appearance of a budding tree (Fig. 5-8). Some variants have the same diagnostic value. They include clusters of centrilobular nodules linked together by fine linear opacities or branching tubular or Y-shaped opacities without nodules (Figs. 5-9 and 5-10). When the bronchiole is sectioned across its axis the filled dilated lumen may appear as a single well-defined

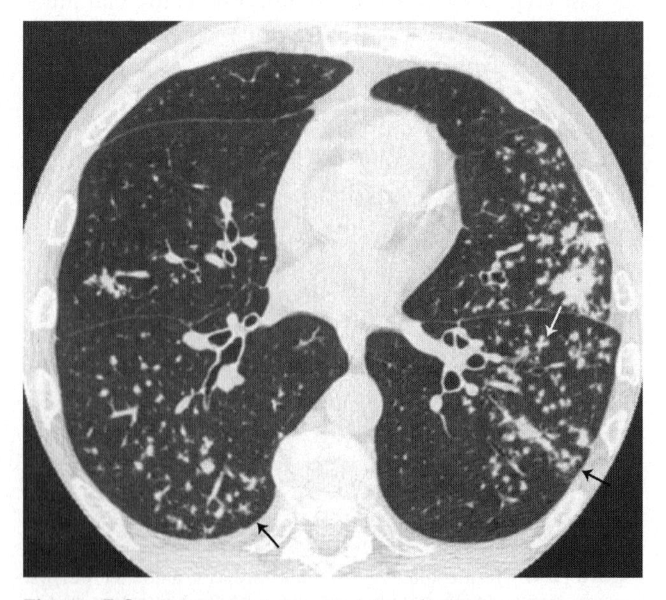

Figure 5-8 Tree-in-bud sign. Endobronchial spread of tuberculosis. Bilateral patchy areas of small centrilobular, nodular, and/or linear branching opacities. Note also the presence of larger nodules and an airspace consolidation in the left upper lobe.

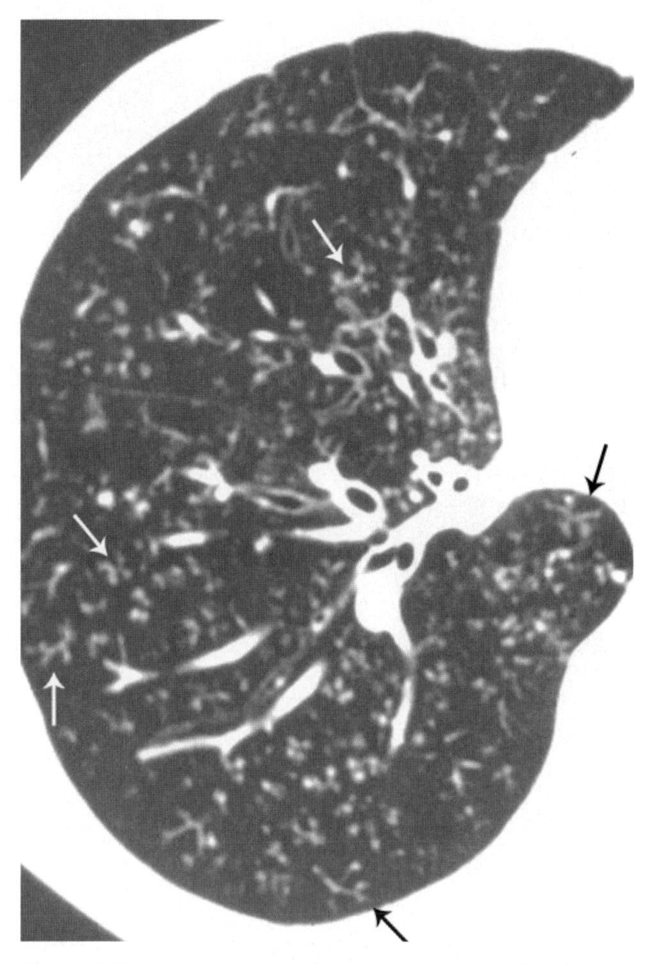

Figure 5-9 Tree-in-bud sign. Thin-section CT targeted on the right lung in a patient with diffuse aspiration bronchiolitis secondary to esophagobronchial fistula seen as a complication of cancer of esophagus. There are multiple small centrilobular nodular and/or branching linear opacities. Some arrows show typical tree-in-bud sign.

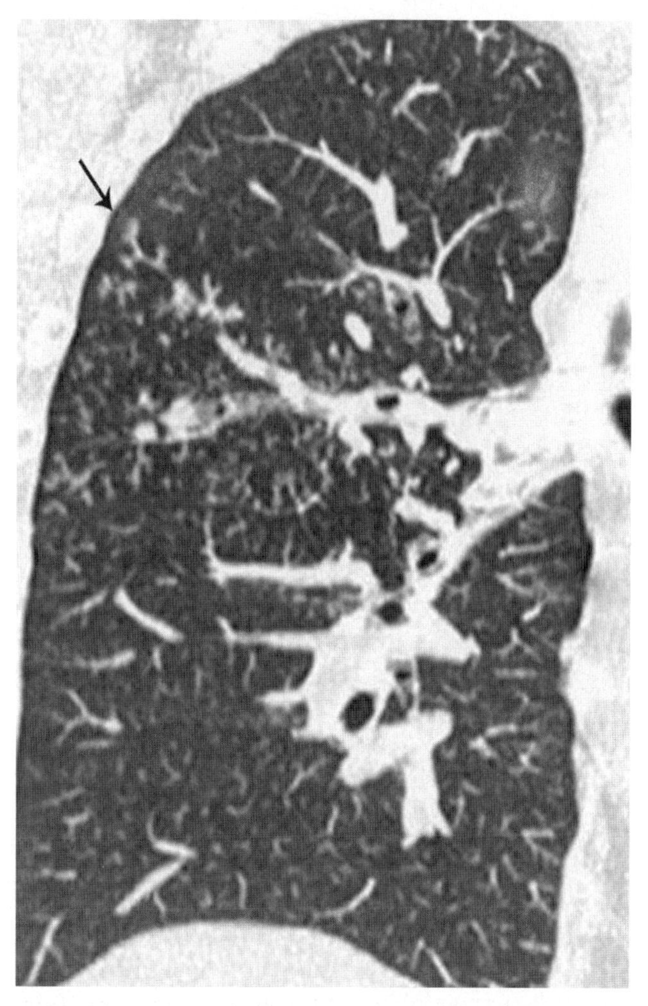

Figure 5-10 Tree-in-bud sign. A 5-mm-thick coronal slab using the multiplanar volume reformation combined with maximum intensity projection technique after thin-collimation multidetector CT acquisition. Multiple areas of small centrilobular, nodular, and/or linear branching opacity become apparent in the posterior segment of the right upper lobe *(arrow)*. This helped the endoscopist perform a selective bronchial aspiration, which permitted the diagnosis of tuberculosis.

centrilobular nodule a few millimeters in diameter. In every case, the key feature is the centrilobular location of these opacities, at least 3 mm from the pleura.

The tree-in-bud sign is characteristic of acute or chronic infectious bronchiolitis (34). It can also be seen in diffuse panbronchiolitis, diffuse aspiration bronchiolitis, and bronchiolitis obliterans with intraluminal polyps featuring bronchiolar filling with granulation tissue (35).

The tree-in-bud sign is distinguished from abnormal centrilobular perivascular interstitial thickening by its more irregular appearance, a lack of tapering, and the bulbous or knobby appearance of the tips of small branches. Some difficulties in interpretation may occur. Bronchiolar filling with tumor cells, observed in bronchioloalveolar cell carcinoma or tumor emboli within small centrilobular arteries, can produce centrilobular nodules and branching lines (36–39). In the same way, peribronchiolar nodules resulting from sarcoidosis that occur in relation to the centrilobular arteries occasionally may mimic the appearance of the tree-in-bud sign (7,35). Hopefully, other typical features of sarcoidosis usually also are present.

The frequent association of tree-in-bud sign with other findings of airway disease facilitates the diagnosis of small airway disease. They include areas of air-filled bronchiolar dilatation; ill-defined centrilobular nodules, reflecting areas of inflammation; bronchiolar wall thickening; and bronchiectasis.

Poorly Defined Centrilobular Nodules

The presence of ill-defined centrilobular nodules in patients who have bronchiolar disease usually reflects the presence of peribronchiolar inflammation in the absence of airway filling with secretion (40) (Fig. 5-11). Unfortunately this pattern is not specific to small airway disease and may also suggest a vascular or interstitial disease (41). When the finding is patchy in distribution, the list of entities potentially responsible is wide, including inflammatory/infectious bronchiolitis, asbestosis, silicosis, Langerhans cell histiocytosis,

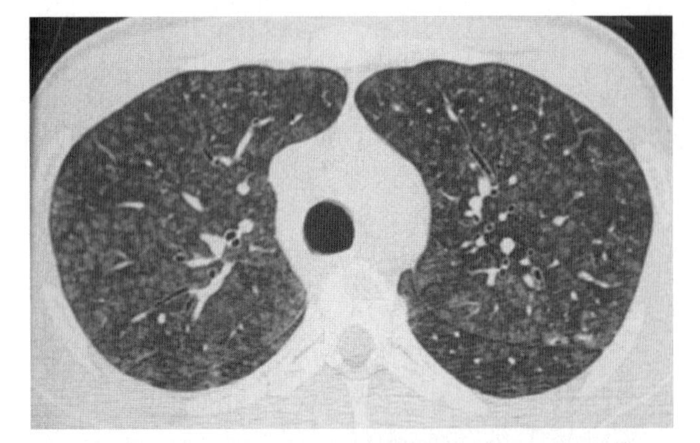

Figure 5-11 Poorly defined centrilobular nodules. Subacute hypersensitivity pneumonitis (bird fancier's lung). Thin-section CT scan shows diffuse and homogeneous distribution throughout the lungs of the small centrilobular opacities expressing the inflammation in the bronchial and peribronchial areas.

vasculitis, pulmonary hypertension, sarcoidosis, or, rarely, BOOP. When the distribution of nodules is diffuse and homogeneous, the pattern is suggestive of bronchiolar disease or vascular entities, including pulmonary edema, pulmonary hemorrhage, and capillary hemangiomatosis. Differential diagnosis with bronchiolar disease is based on associated findings, such as pleural effusion in edema and enlargement of proximal pulmonary arteries. Bronchiolar possibilities include respiratory bronchiolitis, bronchiolitis associated with hypersensitivity pneumonitis, and follicular bronchiolitis (7,40). Despite the large number of diseases potentially responsible for this pattern, in most cases the differential diagnosis is simplified by detailed clinical information, including occupational and environmental histories.

Focal Ground-Glass Opacities, Airspace Consolidation, or Both

Unilateral or bilateral patchy areas of airspace consolidation containing air bronchogram are a nonspecific radiologic pattern. In the clinical context of small airway disease, they are suggestive of BOOP, reflecting the filling of the distal airspaces with granulation tissue. Consolidation affects mainly the peribronchial or subpleural lung regions (Fig. 5-12) (42, 43). Small centrilobular nodular opacities may be associated, reflecting the presence of intrabronchiolar granulation tissue or peribronchiolar consolidation. In case of infectious bronchiolitis, focal areas of consolidation, reflecting areas of bronchopneumonia, can be seen in association with small centrilobular and linear opacities (Fig. 5-8) (15,44).

Ground-glass opacity can be seen in association with respiratory bronchiolitis (15,45,46), respiratory bronchiolitis associated with interstitial lung disease (Fig. 5-13) (15,47,48), and BOOP (42,43). In respiratory bronchiolitis, the abnormality is bilateral, may be diffuse or patchy, and tends to involve predominantly or exclusively the upper lung zones. Ground-glass opacity is also often seen in association

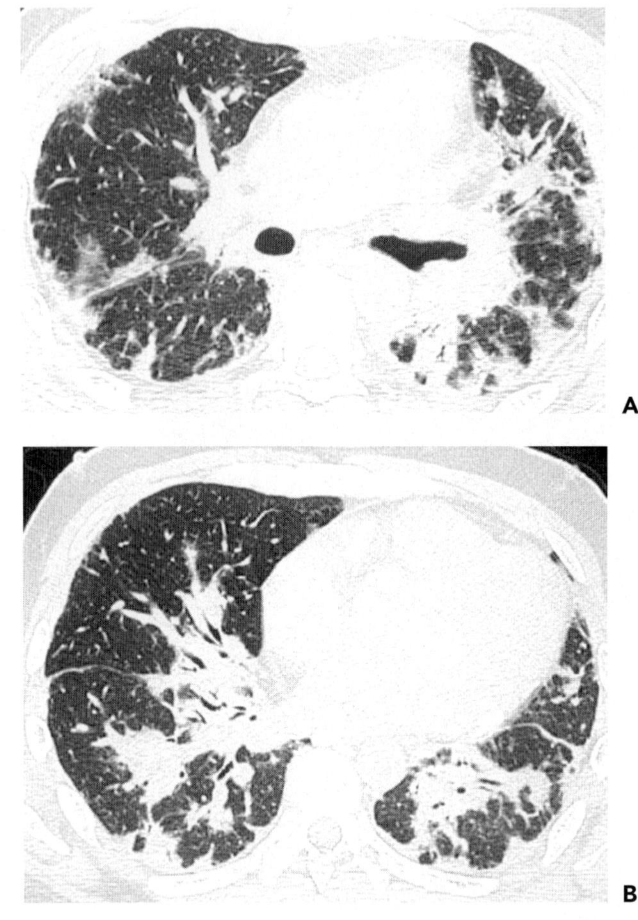

Figure 5-12 Airspace consolidation. Cryptogenic organizing pneumonia. Bilateral areas of airspace consolidation having both peripheral and peribronchovascular predominant distribution. **A:** Thin-section CT at the level of upper lobes and superior segments of lower lobes. **B:** Thin-section CT scan at the level of lower lobes.

with airspace consolidation in BOOP. In immunocompromised patients who have BOOP, ground-glass opacity is occasionally the only abnormality on thin-section CT scans (42). Extensive bilateral areas of ground-glass

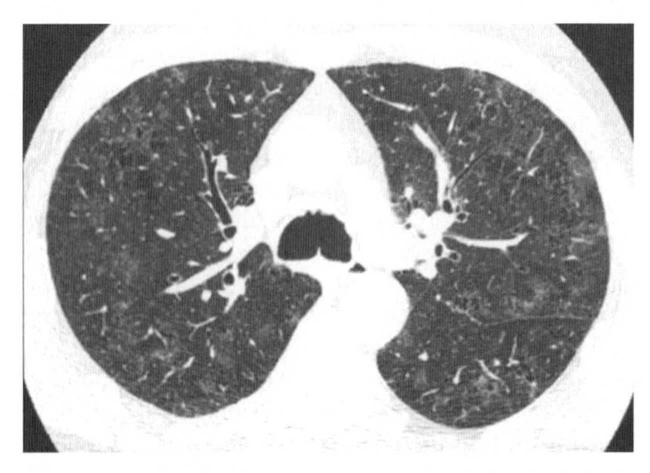

Figure 5-13 Ground-glass opacity. RB-ILD. Thin-section CT at the level of the main bronchi in a heavy smoker suffering from chronic dyspnea and cough. Patchy areas of ground-glass attenuation are present within the peripheral part of the lungs. Multiple spaces of centrilobular emphysema and bronchial wall thickening are also present. The abnormalities are related to RB-ILD.

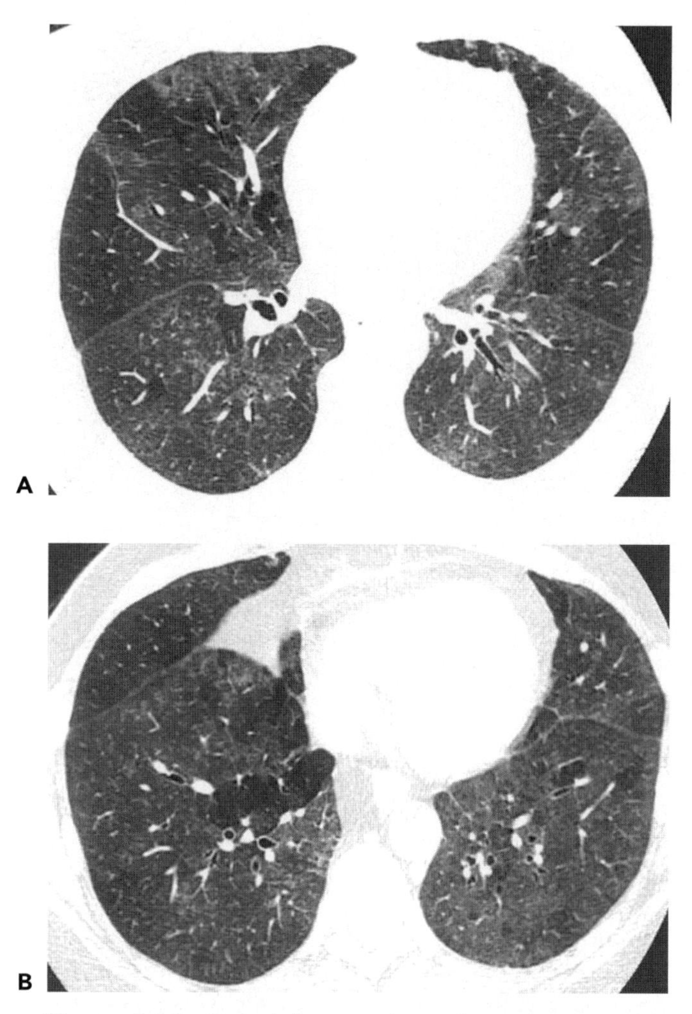

Figure 5-14 Ground-glass opacity and mosaic attenuation pattern. Subacute hypersensitivity pneumonitis (bird fancier's lung). **A** and **B:** Two thin-section CT scans through the mid **(A)** and lower **(B)** parts of the lung. Multiple patchy areas of ground-glass attenuation are associated with small, poorly defined centrilobular nodules. Notice also the presence of some secondary pulmonary nodules appearing hypoattenuated and free of nodules, reflecting the presence of air trapping.

attenuation, more or less associated with poorly defined centrilobular nodular opacities, is a CT pattern frequently observed in acute or subacute hypersensitivity pneumonitis (Fig. 5-14) (49).

Decreased Lung Attenuation and Mosaic Perfusion

Areas of decreased lung attenuation associated with vessels of decreased caliber observed in bronchiolar disease reflect bronchiolar obstruction resulting in a decrease of perfusion (50). In acute bronchiolar obstruction, this decrease of perfusion represents a physiologic reflex of hypoxic vasoconstriction (51), but in the chronic state vascular remodeling takes place and the reduced caliber becomes irreversible. Although the vessels within areas of decreased attenuation on thin-section CT may be of markedly reduced caliber, they are not distorted as in emphysema. The lung areas of decreased attenuation related to decreased perfusion can be patchy or widespread. They are poorly defined or sharply demarcated, giving a geographical outline, representing a collection of affected secondary pulmonary lobules. Redistribution of blood flow to the normally ventilated areas causes increased attenuation of lung parenchyma in these areas. The patchwork of abnormal areas of low attenuation and normal lung or less diseased areas, appearing normal in attenuation or hyperattenuated, gives the appearance of mosaic attenuation (Fig. 5-15). The vessels in the abnormal hypoattenuated areas are reduced in caliber, whereas the vessels in normal areas are increased in size, and the resulting pattern is called "mosaic perfusion." The difference in vessel size between low- and high-attenuation areas allows one to distinguish the mosaic perfusion pattern from mosaic attenuation due to an infiltrative lung disease with patchy distribution, in which the vessels have the same caliber in both high-attenuation and normal-attenuation areas (52,53). However, the decreased vessel size may be subtle and difficult to observe in some patients with mosaic perfusion (Fig. 5-16) (54).

Mosaic perfusion pattern is not always the result of bronchiolar disease and can also be caused by direct vascular obstruction (52). The obstructed pulmonary arteries are responsible for the low-attenuation areas, whereas redistribution of blood to surrounding normal lung areas results in increased attenuation. Vascular diseases leading to mosaic perfusion pattern seen on CT images include mainly chronic thromboembolic disease

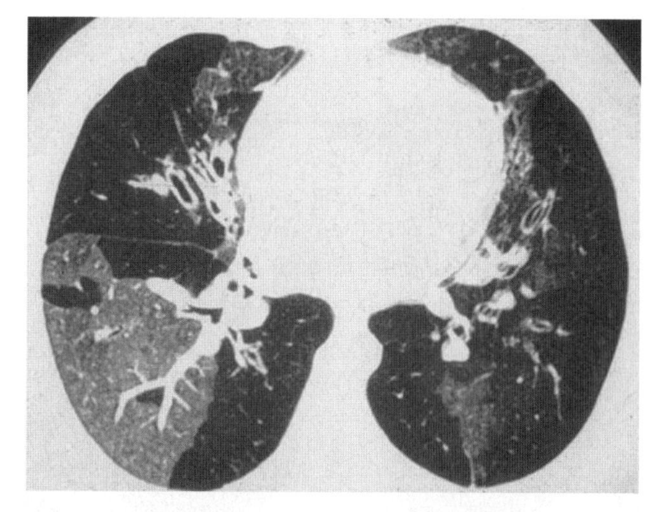

Figure 5-15 Mosaic perfusion pattern. Postinfectious obliterative bronchiolitis. Thin-section CT scan in a 14-year-old boy suffering from shortness of breath at exercise. The hyperattenuated area contains enlarged vessels, reflecting the pulmonary blood flow distribution toward the normal ventilated areas. Hypoattenuated areas are extended in both lungs and contain few and small pulmonary vessels. Bronchiectasis is also present in the right middle lobe and the left lower lobe. The demarcation between normal and abnormal areas is well defined, reflecting the limits between segments and lobules. (Courtesy of Christopher Flower.)

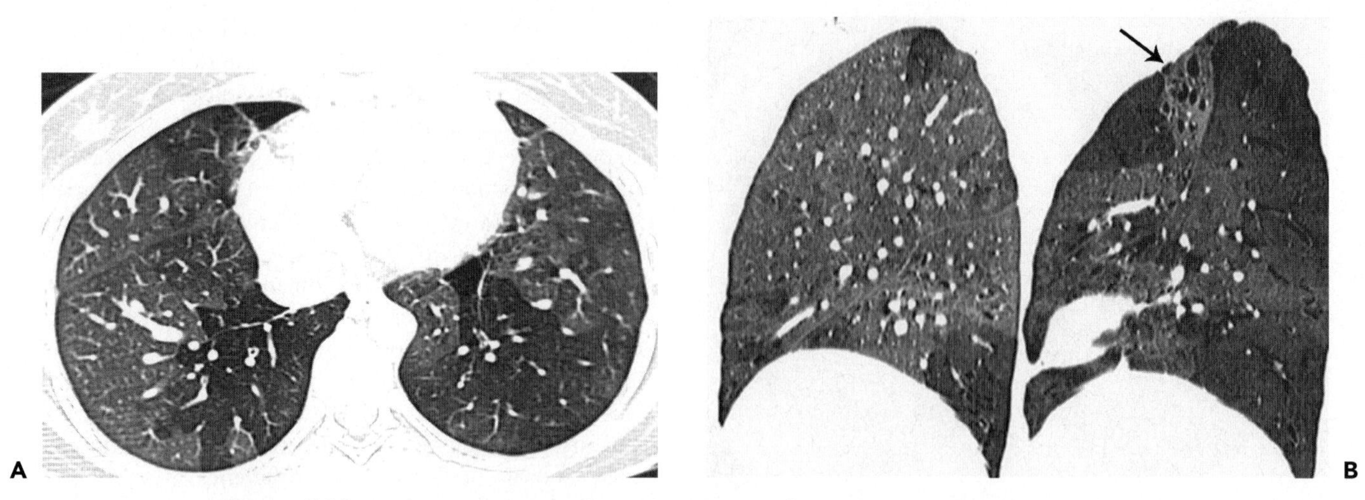

Figure 5-16 Mosaic perfusion pattern at MDCT. Postinfectious bronchiolitis. Thin-collimation MDCT acquisition. **A:** Thin-section CT at the level of the lower part of the lungs showing patchy areas of hypoattenuation in the lower lobes and the right middle lobe. **B:** Lateral reformation after thin-collimation multidetector row CT acquisition using the multiplanar volume reformation and minimum-intensity projection techniques in combination. Left (sagittal reformation of the right lung) and right (sagittal reformation of the left lung) images show well-demarcated areas of hypoattenuation and decreased perfusion, reflecting the territories where the lesions of obliterative bronchiolitis are situated. Notice the presence of bronchiectasis in the apicoposterior segment of the left upper lobe *(arrow)*.

(55,56) and, less often, primary pulmonary hypertension (57), pulmonary capillary hemangiomatosis (58), pulmonary venoocclusive disease (59), polyarteritis nodosa (52), scleroderma (57), and intimal sarcoma of the pulmonary arteries (60). The differential diagnosis between a bronchiolar and a vascular cause can be based on the presence or absence of air trapping on expiratory CT, respectively (54,61). When caused by bronchiolar obstruction, mosaic perfusion is accentuated on expiratory CT because the low-attenuation areas show air trapping (Fig. 5-17). In chronic vascular occlusive disease, air trapping theoretically does not occur. However, in a study by Worthy et al. (52) applying the previously mentioned criteria to distinguish diseases that may cause mosaic pattern of lung attenuation on CT scans, two observers made a correct diagnosis in 90% of infiltrative lung disease cases, 91% of airway disease, and only 32% of vascular disease. The difficulty in the diagnosis of vascular disease was the result of the presence of expiratory air trapping in a certain number of cases (52). This phenomenon was

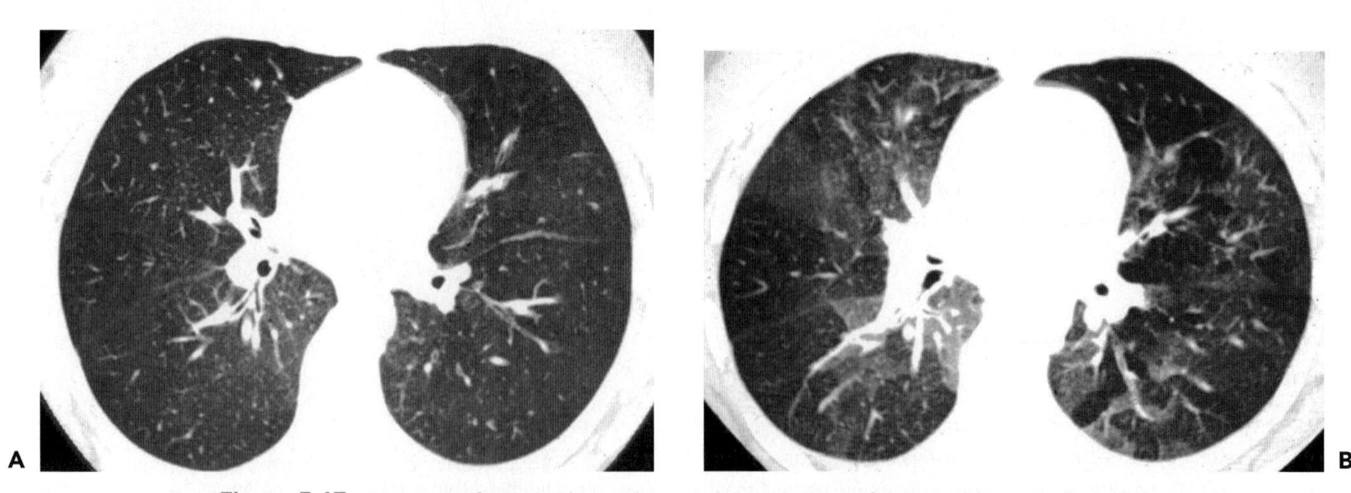

Figure 5-17 Mosaic perfusion and expiratory air trapping. Postinfectious obliterative bronchiolitis. Thin-section CT scan performed at full inspiration **(A)** and full expiration **(B)** of the middle parts of the lungs. On inspiratory scan, mosaic perfusion pattern is difficult to perceive. There is only mild hypoattenuation in the periphery of the left lung and the peripheral part of the right upper and lower lobes. At expiration, the contrast in attenuation between normal and abnormal areas is accentuated. The normally ventilated areas increase in attenuation at expiration as normally expected, whereas the abnormal areas do not, because of air trapping.

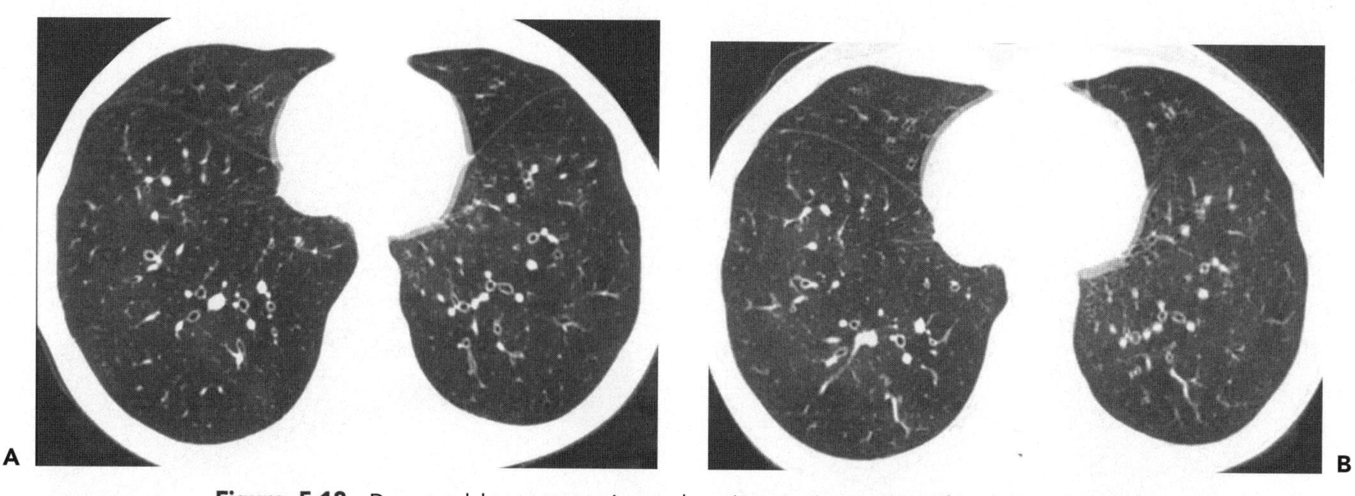

Figure 5-18 Decreased lung attenuation and expiratory air trapping. Thin-section CT scans obtained at full inspiration **(A)** and full expiration **(B)** in a patient presenting with post–bone marrow transplantation obliterative bronchiolitis. **A:** On inspiratory scan, there is a diffuse decrease in attenuation throughout the lungs with a paucity of pulmonary vessels in the periphery, expressing a severe and diffuse distribution of the bronchiolar obstructive lesions. Notice also the presence of bronchial wall thickening and slight dilatation of the bronchial lumen within the lower lobes. **B:** On expiratory scans, there is no significant increase in attenuation of the lung parenchyma. The cross-sectional areas of the lungs are not very different from those at inspiration, expressing the presence of bilateral and diffuse expiratory air trapping.

confirmed recently by Arakawa et al. (62), who found expiratory air trapping in six of nine patients with chronic embolism. Air trapping was associated with the presence of proximal arterial stenosis ($p < .01$), and the area showed less contrast enhancement than did the adjacent lung ($p < .05$).

Air trapping at expiratory CT is defined as "retention of excess gas (air) in all or part of the lung, especially during expiration, either as a result of complete or partial airway obstruction or as a result of local abnormalities in pulmonary compliance," according to the Nomenclature Committee of the Fleischner Society (63). The air is trapped and the cross-sectional area of the affected parts of the lung does not decrease in size on expiratory CT. Usually the regional inhomogeneity of the lung density seen at end-inspiration on thin-section CT scans is accentuated on sections obtained at end, or during, expiration because the high-attenuation areas increase in density and the low-attenuation areas remain unchanged (Fig. 5-17). In the case of more global involvement of the small airways, the lack of regional homogeneity of the lung attenuation is difficult to perceive on inspiratory scans, and as a result, mosaic perfusion becomes visible only on expiratory scans. In patients with particularly severe and widespread involvement of the small airways, the patchy distribution of hypoattenuation and mosaic pattern is lost. Inspiratory scans appear with an apparent uniformity of decreased attenuation in the lungs, and scans taken at end-expiration may appear unremarkable. In these patients, the most striking features are paucity of pulmonary vessels and lack of change of the cross-sectional areas of the lung at comparable levels on inspiratory and expiratory scans (Fig. 5-18).

Mosaic perfusion pattern associated with expiratory air trapping is seen on thin-section CT scans in patients who have obliterative bronchiolitis, regardless of etiology (15,64,65); bronchiolitis associated with hypersensitivity pneumonitis (49,66); and asthma (67,68).

Lobular Areas of Expiratory Air Trapping

Focal areas of low attenuation may appear on expiratory CT scans, whereas no lung attenuation abnormality is depicted on inspiratory CT scans (Fig. 5-19). This

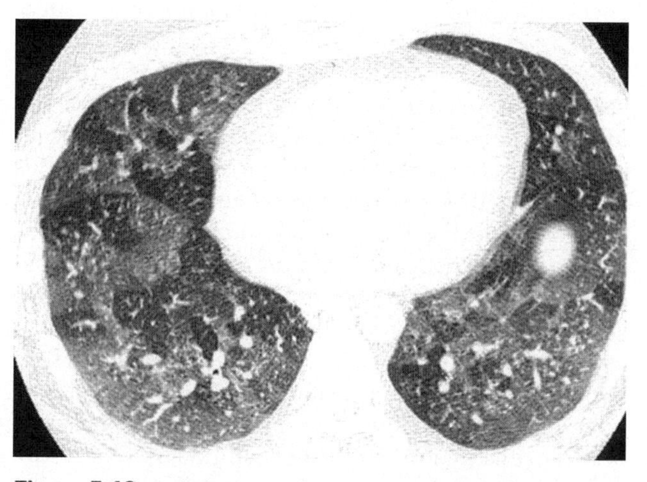

Figure 5-19 Lobular areas of expiratory air trapping. Early stage of sarcoidosis. Thin-section CT obtained at full expiration. Several lobular areas in both lungs did not increase in attenuation as normally expected. There was no abnormality depictable on inspiratory scans performed at the same anatomic level.

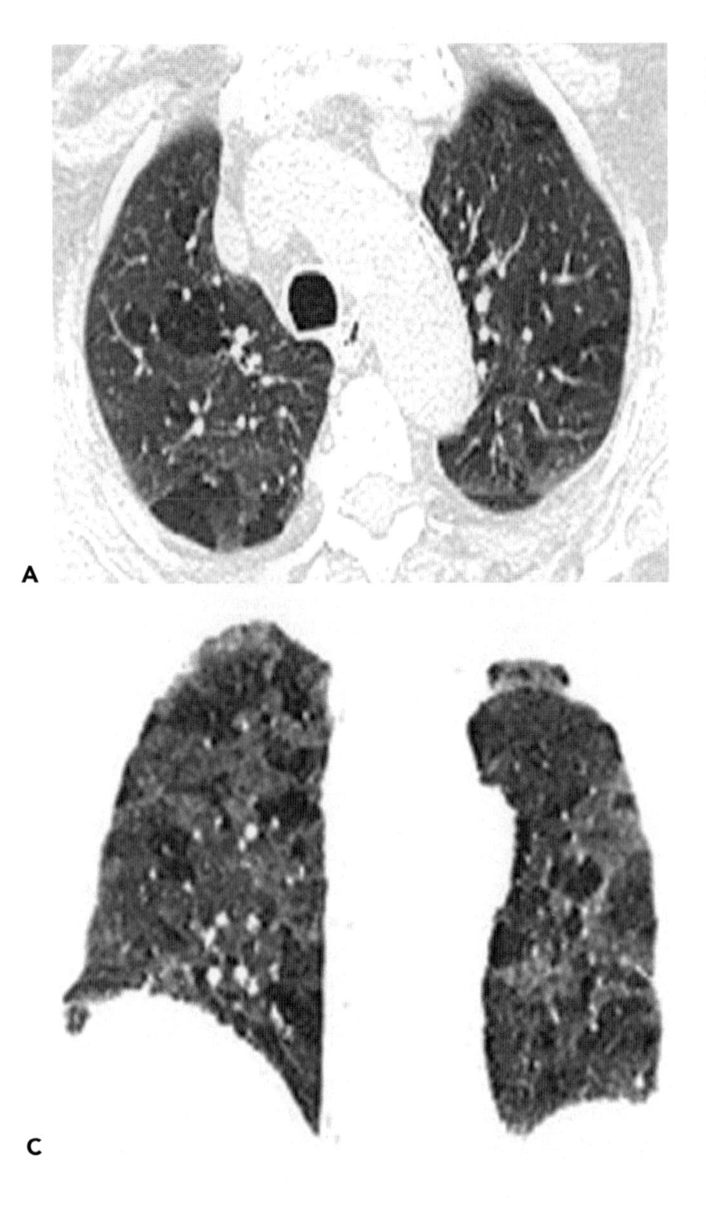

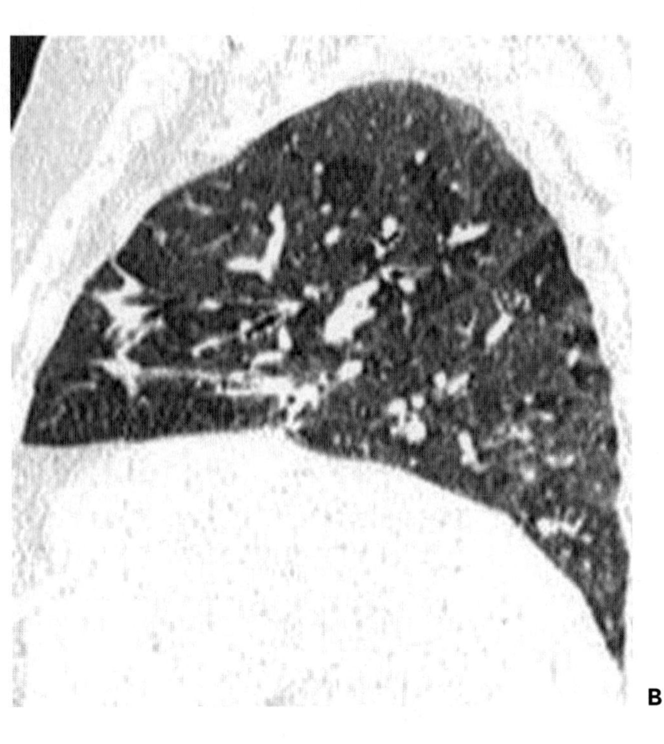

Figure 5-20 Lobular areas of air trapping at MDCT. Mild persistent asthma. Low-dose thin-collimation MDCT acquisition performed at maximum expiration. **A:** Axial thin-section CT shows lobular areas of air trapping in the upper lobe. **B:** Sagittal reformation of the right lung displays the upper and posterior distribution of lobular areas of air trapping. **C:** Coronal reformation with minimal intensity projection technique displays the extent of air trapping in both lungs.

phenomenon reflects the presence of air trapping in areas where partial airway obstruction is present (69–72). These areas are commonly well demarcated, reflecting the geometry of individual or joined lobules. This pattern is frequently observed in smokers and in patients with asthma (Fig. 5-20), obliterative bronchiolitis, bronchiolitis associated with hypersensitivity pneumonitis (Fig. 5-21), or sarcoidosis (Fig. 5-19). In addition, this pattern may also be seen in patients with acute pulmonary embolism (73). Arakawa et al. (73) found in a series of 41 patients with acute pulmonary embolism one or more areas of air trapping in 72% of the patients. This air trapping was seen not only in areas with pulmonary embolism but also in areas without embolism. The proposed mechanism of bronchoconstriction in acute pulmonary embolism includes bronchoactive amines released from platelet aggregations in the thrombus or a change in parasympathetic nervous system tension, which centralizes the bronchial smooth muscle tension.

The diagnostic value of the pattern of lobular areas of air trapping on expiratory CT scans depends on the extent and location of air-trapping areas. In approximately 50% of asymptomatic subjects, lobular areas of air trapping may be depicted on expiratory CT scans in dependent portions of the lungs irrespective of the patient's position (70,72,74–76). Lee et al. (74) showed that the frequency of air trapping observed on expiratory CT scans of asymptomatic subjects increases with age ($p < .05$), and the degree of air trapping has a significant correlation with age ($r = 0.523$, $p < .001$).

The physiologic presence of focal areas of low attenuation on expiratory CT must be taken into account in the interpretation of air trapping (64,75). Usually, dependent lung regions show a greater increase in lung density during expiration than do nondependent lung regions. As a result, the anteroposterior attenuation gradients normally seen on inspiratory scans are significantly greater on expiratory scans. The anteroposterior lung attenuation

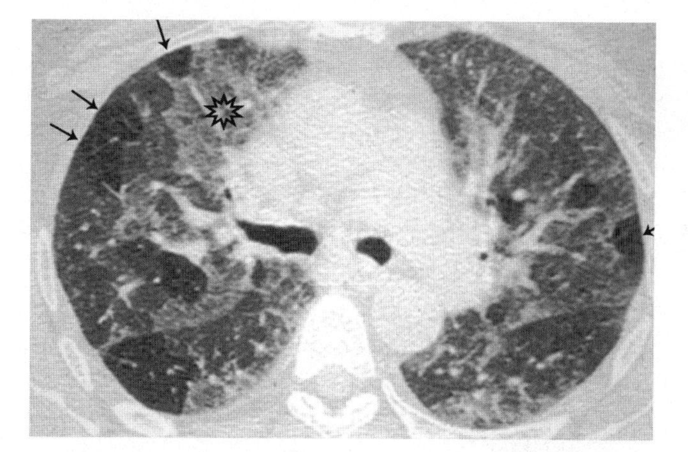

Figure 5-21 Ground-glass, mosaic perfusion, and lobular areas of air trapping ("head cheese" pattern). Subacute hypersensitivity pneumonitis. Expiratory thin-section CT at the level of the upper part of the lungs, showing patchy areas of ground-glass attenuation *(star)*, combined with normal areas and some lobules appearing hypoattenuated because of air trapping *(arrows)*.

gradient can have a lobar component on expiratory scan; the posterior aspect of the upper lobe, anterior to the major fissure, often appears denser than the anterior aspect of the lower lobe, behind the major fissure. Some focal areas of low attenuation may also be seen near the tip of the lingula. All these physiologic low-attenuation areas involve less than 25% of the cross-sectional area of one lung at one scan level. As a result, air trapping can be considered abnormal when it affects nondependent areas or dependent lung areas greater than 25% of the lung cross-sectional area or a lung volume equal to or greater than a pulmonary segment and is not limited to the superior segment of the lower lobe.

The combination of ground-glass attenuation areas, mosaic perfusion pattern, and lobular areas of expiratory air trapping in a given patient expresses the association of interstitial and airway disease and has been called "head cheese pattern" (40). This pattern is suggestive of hypersensitivity pneumonitis, respiratory bronchiolitis–associated intersitial lung disease (RB-ILD), and sarcoidosis.

CT TECHNIQUE

So far we have based the recommended CT technique for assessing the small airways on high-resolution CT scans performed at full-suspended inspiration and full-suspended expiration. The inspiratory and expiratory thin-section CT scans are sampled at 10-mm and 30-mm intervals, respectively, from the apex of the lung to the diaphragm. A current alternative, multidetector computed tomography (MDCT) volumetric acquisitions during a single breath hold using thin collimation (1.25 mm), is performed over the entire lungs with the following parameters: 100 to 120 kVp and 100 to 150 mAs at full inspiration, and 100 to 120 kVp and 40 to 80 mAs at full expiration. Reconstruction of axial images is performed with 0.6-mm overlap if multiplanar reformations are requested (64,77).

Multiplanar Volume Reconstruction and Maximum- and Minimum-Intensity Projection Techniques

Multiplanar reformations are the easiest reconstruction to generate and can be interactively performed in real time at the console or workstation. Whereas the thickness of the displayed planar image is 0.6 to 0.8 mm, depending on the dimension of the field of view, multiplanar volume reconstruction (MPVR) consists of a slab with a thickness of several pixels and is a less noisy reformation. MPVRs may also form the basis of intensity projection techniques. With minimum-intensity projection (MinIP) technique, pixels encode the minimum voxel value encountered by each ray (Fig. 5-16B). Airways are visualized because air contained within the bronchial tree is lower in attenuation than surrounding pulmonary parenchyma. MPVR-MinIP technique may be used in the detection of air bronchograms in focal areas of airspace consolidation or of ground-glass opacification (77). Increasing the contrast between areas of normal lung attenuation and areas of lung hypoattenuation may facilitate the depiction of mosaic perfusion pattern (Fig. 5-22) (77). Its application on expiratory CT scans can facilitate assessment of the presence and extent of expiratory air trapping (Fig. 5-22). Several studies have shown that MinIP images improve the detection of air trapping and are associated with increased observer confidence and agreement as compared with thin sections alone (78,79).

In maximum intensity projection (MIP) technique, pixels encode the maximum voxel value encountered by each ray. The thickness of the slab is selected interactively at the console or workstation. This is beneficial in the display of small centrilobular nodular and/or linear opacities (tree-in-bud sign) or poorly defined centrilobular nodules. The technique consists of increasing the profusion of nodules in the volume of interest by increasing the thickness of the slab and simultaneously keeping the same spatial resolution as that of a thin-section CT scan (Figs. 5-10 and 5-23). The use of MPVR–MIP has been proved to increase the number of bronchiolar centrilobular opacities compared with single thin-section CT scans in patients with infectious or inflammatory bronchiolitis (80).

Texture Analysis

Although thin-section CT is an accurate imaging technique for the detection of constrictive bronchiolitis, features on thin-section CT images can be subtle, particularly in the early stages of disease, and diagnosis is subject to interobserver variability. To refine the differential diagnosis of obstructive lung disease, it is necessary to take into account the textural appearance of lung parenchyma with abnormally low attenuation. Chabat et al. (81) developed an automated method for the differentiation of centrilob-

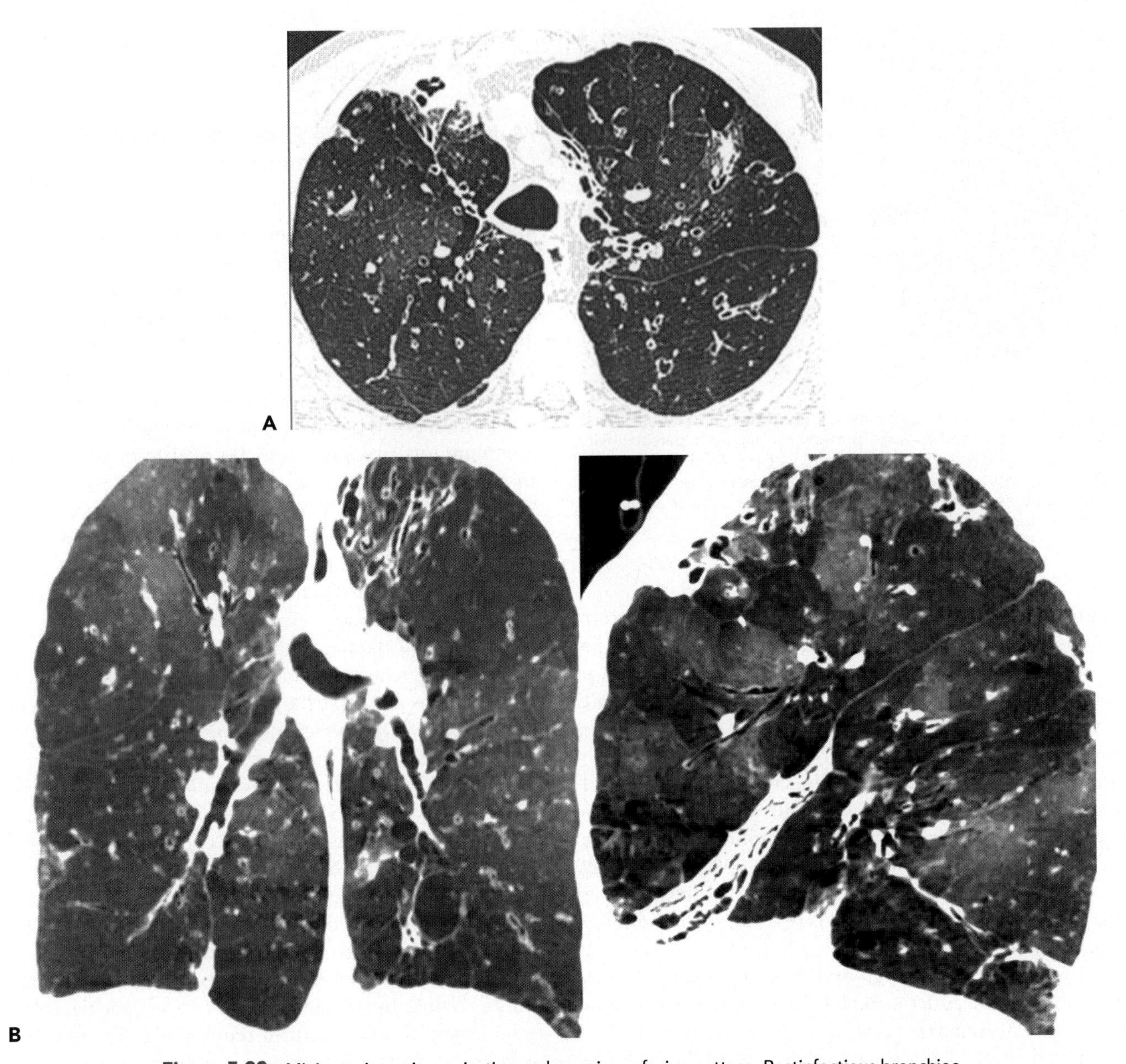

Figure 5-22 Minimum-intensity projection and mosaic perfusion pattern. Postinfectious bronchiectasis and obliterative bronchiolitis. **A:** Thin-section axial CT scan at the level of the upper part of the lungs. Distortion and enlargement of the lumen of the trachea with bilateral cylindrical bronchiectasis in the upper lobes and the superior segment of the left lower lobe. Slight heterogeneity in lung attenuation. **B:** Multiplanar volume reformation combined with minimum intensity projection technique after thin–collimation MDCT acquisition. The coronal *(left)* and sagittal *(right)* reformations reinforce the detection of mosaic perfusion pattern and help assess the extent of decreased attenuation areas in both lungs. Notice the presence of a nonaerated collapse of the right middle lobe associated with bronchiectasis *(right)*.

ular emphysema, panlobular emphysema, constrictive bronchiolitis, and normal lung on the basis of texture features. The proposed technique discriminates well among patterns of obstructive lung disease on the basis of parenchymal texture alone, with good sensitivity and good specificity (Fig. 5-24).

Expiratory CT

The most commonly used technique for the assessment of air trapping at CT is based on postexpiratory thin-section CT scans obtained during suspended respiration following a forced exhalation. Each of the postexpiratory scans is compared with the inspiratory scan that most closely duplicates its level to detect air trapping. Dynamic CT acquisition during continuous expiration, which can be used to collect data at a fixed level during expiration, is a second technique. Electron beam CT initially was performed with a scanning time of 100 msecond per image, to assess the dynamic changes in lung attenuation and in architecture during expiration with minimal motion artifacts (82). More recently a dynamic expiratory maneuver performed during helical CT acquisition was described in a small number of

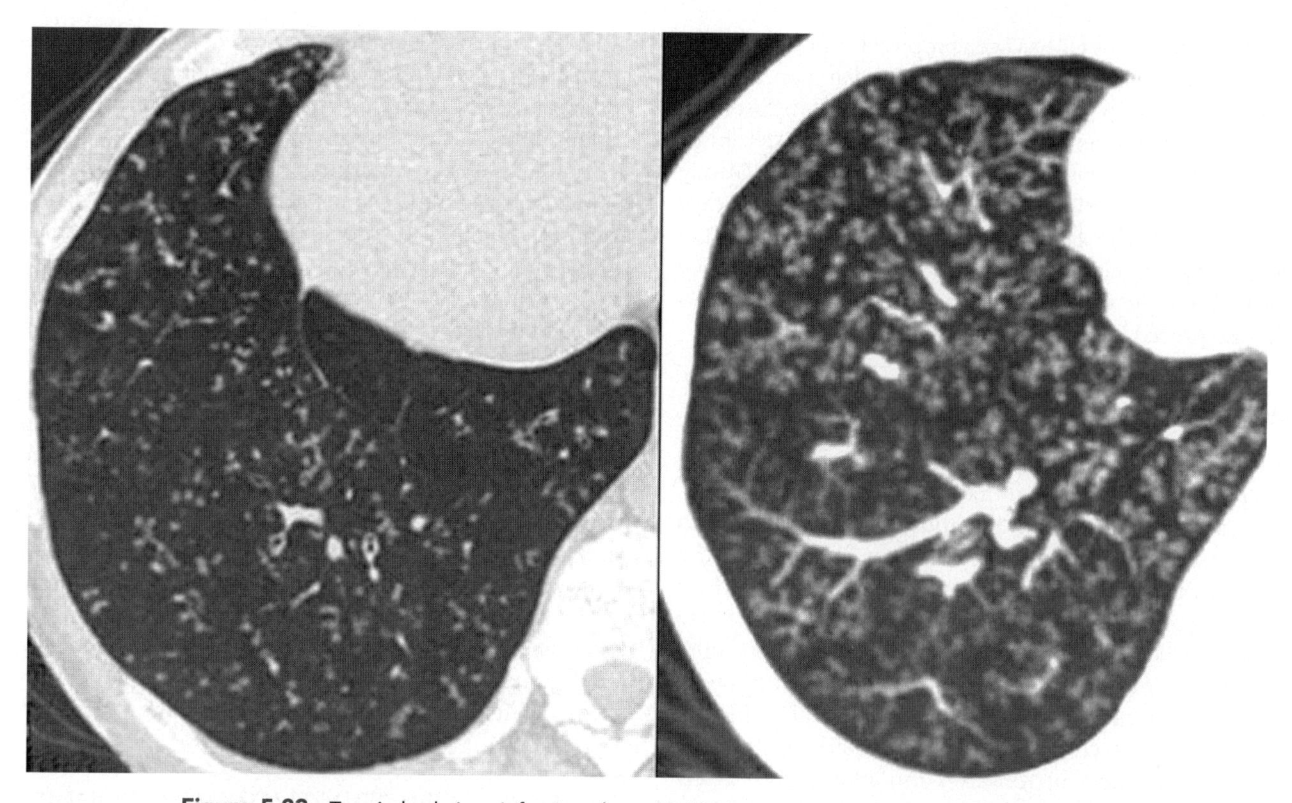

Figure 5-23 Tree-in-bud sign. Infectious bronchiolitis in a patient with ciliary dyskinesia. *Left:* Thin-section CT targeted on the right lower lobe showing multiple small centrilobular, nodular and linear branching opacities in many lobules of the right lower lobe. *Right:* A 7-mm-thick axial slab using the multiplanar volume reformation and maximum-intensity projection technique, increasing the profusion of the small centrilobular opacities and keeping the same spatial resolution of thin-section CT scan in infectious bronchiolitis.

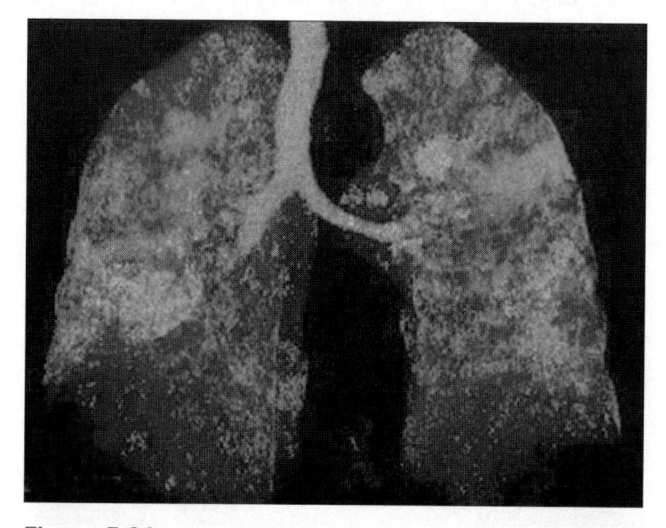

Figure 5-24 Three-dimensional (3D) display of expiratory air trapping. Same patient as in Figure 5-20. The areas of hypoattenuation resulting from expiratory air trapping are automatically segmented and highlighted and taken into account in the 3D reconstruction.

patients with good results despite a longer scanning time per image (83,84). Motion artifacts, which increase as temporal resolution decreases, represent the major limitations of continuous expiratory CT. The use of 180-degree linear interpolation algorithms with a 0.5-second rotation time provides images representing scanning periods of about 250 msecond. Motion artifacts are at maximum during the early phase of expiration and at a minimum during its late phase, which allows good visualization of lobular air trapping with helical CT.

Patients can have greater difficulty maintaining the residual volume after an exhalation than during an active exhalation when they have to continue the expiratory effort until the end of the acquisition. With Lucidarme et al. (84), we compared continuous expiratory CT performed with helical scanner and suspended end-expiration CT for the assessment of air trapping in a series of 49 patients who had a chronic airway disease. For the 39 of those 49 patients (80%) with areas of air trapping on at least one expiratory CT scan, the air trapping extent and the relative contrast scores obtained with continuous expiratory CT were significantly higher than those obtained with suspended end-expiratory CT. The improvement provided by continuous expiratory CT can be explained by a small increase in the degree of expiration, which leads to a better detection of air trapping. On the basis of this information, when suspended end-expiration CT images are ambiguous or when patients have difficulty performing the suspended end-expiration maneuver adequately, continuous expiratory CT can be performed using MDCT over the lungs to improve the conspicuity and the apparent extent of air trapping (Fig. 5-20). Using low-dose CT, this technique has become routine in some institutions to depict air trapping (85).

Lateral decubitus CT has been proposed as a helpful alternative in the detection and visualization of air trapping in a small number of patients with suboptimal, inconclusive, or uninterpretable supine expiratory CT scans. Lateral decubitus positioning causes the dependent hemithorax to be relatively splinted, thereby restricting movement of the thoracic cage on that side. The lateral decubitus position allows the observer to take advantage of gravitational gradients, thereby accentuating the differences in lung attenuation (86). This has also proved to be helpful in children (87).

Quantitative Assessment of Air Trapping

The extent of air trapping present on expiratory scans can be measured using a semiquantitative scoring system that estimates the percent of lung that appears abnormal on each scan. In the scoring system proposed by Stern et al. (82), estimates of air trapping were made at each level and for each lung on a four-point scale: 0: no air trapping; 1: 1% to 25%; 2: 26% to 50%; 3: 51% to 75%; and 4: 76% to 100% of cross-sectional areas of lung affected. The air-trapping score is the summation of these numbers for the different levels studied. According to Ng et al. (88), this scoring system allows good interobserver and intraobserver agreement. Interestingly, observer variation increased when a finer scoring system than the one described by Ng et al. was used (nearest 5% instead of a coarser five-point scale). Using a grid superimposed on the CT images can also reduce interobserver variation. The extent of expiratory air trapping at CT has proved to be correlated with the degree of airflow obstruction at pulmonary function tests (PFTs) in patients with small airway disease (89).

Objective density measurement of the lung can be expressed in several ways. An automatic technique may be used to obtain an accurate and reproducible assessment of the extent of air trapping. This extent assessment can be expressed as a mean density of the voxels included in a chosen region of interest (ROI) (90), as a histogram that shows the distribution of attenuation values within the ROI (91), as a density mask that highlights, or as a calculation that summarizes the pixels with a density below a certain critical value. In the density mask technique, all the pixels included in areas of air trapping are segmented by thresholding at −910 HU and are highlighted and automatically counted (Fig. 5-22). This permits calculation of the pixel index, which is defined as the percentage of pixels in both lungs on a single scan that show an attenuation lower than a predetermined threshold value. To increase the precision of the anatomic segmentation of areas of decreased lung attenuation, Chabat et al. (93) developed a model-based iterative deconvolution filter and adaptive clustering algorithms to compensate for the nondependent–dependent lung attenuation gradient. They validated their technique in a series of 15 patients with obliterative bronchiolitis and 8 normal subjects. The automated quantification of the areas of decreased attenuation on expiratory CT scans was within 8.2% from the average scoring of two experienced observers.

Using multislice CT with a 1-mm slice thickness over the lungs performed at full expiration, an exhaustive assessment of the volume of air trapping may be provided as well as a 3D visualization of distribution of air trapping. Acquisition performed at maximum expiration can be insured by spirometrically triggering CT scans at 10% of the vital capacity. Using this method, quantitative assessment of CT images with respect to lung attenuation, lung cross-sectional surface, or lung volume can be performed with excellent precision (94). Kohz et al. (95) obtained highly reproducible lung density measurements using spirometrically controlled CT.

Expressing lung density on a histogram has the advantage that changes in the distribution of attenuation values are detectable when mean attenuation is unchanged. Mean lung density, however, is easier to obtain and compare. Using this method, density changes between full inspiration and full expiration can be compared, and expiratory/inspiratory ratios can be calculated (96). The density mask has the advantage that it combines density measurement with the visual assessment of pathology so that it is possible to allow for regional abnormalities, such as hyperinflation and fibrosis, that influence mean lung attenuation.

SPECIFIC CLINICOPATHOLOGIC FORMS OF SMALL AIRWAY DISEASE

Acute Infectious Bronchiolitis

Acute infectious bronchiolitis is most often caused by viruses (Fig. 5-25), *Mycoplasma pneumoniae,* and *Chlamydia* species (6). It occurs most frequently in infants and children. It can occur in adults, however, and particularly in those who are immunocompromised or suffering from chronic airway disease (Fig. 5-24). Infectious bronchiolitis may also be caused by endobronchial spread of tuberculosis

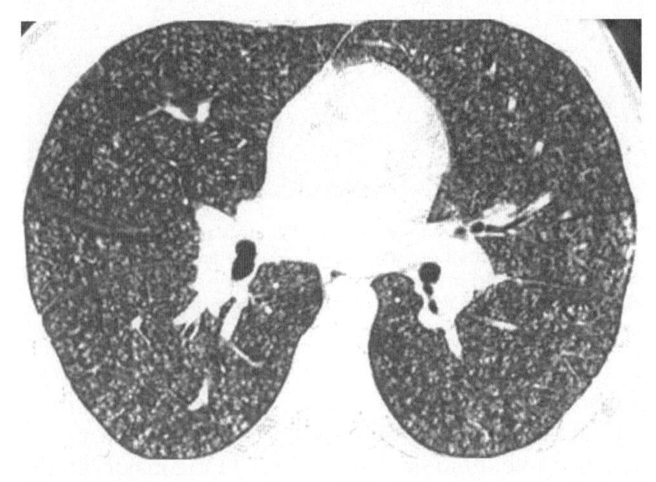

Figure 5-25 Acute viral bronchiolitis. Thin-section CT at the level of the midpart of the lungs shows the presence of small centrilobular nodular opacities diffusely and homogeneously distributed throughout the lungs. (Courtesy of Christian Herold.)

or infection by *Mycobacterium avium-intracellulare* (97) (Figs. 5-8 and 5-10).

In immunocompromised patients, infection of the airways may also result from *Aspergillus*. Acute *Aspergillus* bronchopneumonia, also called airway invasive aspergillosis, is characterized histologically by necrosis and neutrophilic infiltrate that is centered on the small bronchi and bronchioles (44).

The radiographic findings of acute infectious bronchiolitis usually consist of a nodular, reticular, or reticulonodular pattern followed by patchy areas of consolidation (98). The hallmark of the disease on thin-section CT scans is tree-in-bud pattern, which correlates pathologically with the presence of an intraluminal exudate and inflammatory cell infiltrate within the walls of terminal and respiratory bronchioles (Figs. 5-10 and 5-26) (34). Distribution of centrilobular opacities may be either diffuse and homogeneous throughout the lungs or, more often, patchy and heterogeneous.

In some cases, focal areas of ground-glass attenuation or consolidation are present and associated with or superimposed on the tree-in-bud appearance (Fig. 5-8) (44). They frequently have a lobular distribution and express extension of infection from the airways into the adjacent lung parenchyma and resulting in bronchopneumonia. CT findings in conjunction with clinical findings are usually sufficient to allow presumptive therapy with antibiotics, pending the results of sputum culture.

With postprimary tuberculosis, bronchogenic spread of infection can be identified on thin-section CT scans in 95% of cases (99–101). According to Im et al. (102), the most common thin-section CT findings are 2- to 4-mm centrilobular nodules and sharply marginated linear branching opacities which, with thin-section CT-pathologic correlation, have been shown to represent caseous necrosis within and around terminal and respiratory bronchioles (102). Other CT findings include 5- to 8-mm poorly defined nodules, lobular consolidation, and interlobular septal thickening.

In patients with pulmonary infection to *Mycobacterium avium-intracellulare*, the pattern is quite similar to that of endobronchial spread of tuberculosis (97,103,104). Bronchiectasis is more common and more extensive in patients with *Mycobacterium avium-intracellulare*. Tree-in-bud pattern may also be seen in mycobacterial infection owing to other species such as *M. kansasii* and *M. xenopi* (105).

Diffuse Panbronchiolitis

Diffuse panbronchiolitis is a disease of unknown etiology and pathogenesis characterized by a chronic inflammation of the paranasal sinuses and respiratory bronchioles. Panbronchiolitis is defined histologically by an accumulation of mononuclear inflammatory cells in the walls of respiratory bronchioles, alveolar ducts, and, to a lesser extent, adjacent alveoli. Mucus and aggregates of neutrophils are seen in the airway lumen (Fig. 5-27) (106). This chronic inflammatory cell infiltration results in a bronchiolectasis and striking hyperplasia of lymphoid follicles in the walls of respiratory bronchioles.

Although the disease has been recognized almost exclusively in Japan and South Korea, a few cases have been described in North America and Europe (106,107).

Clinical manifestations include dyspnea on exertion and cough, often with sputum production. Sinusitis and progressive disease are common. Colonization with *Pseudomonas aeruginosa* frequently complicates the late stages of the disease. PFTs show marked obstruction and mild restrictive disease.

On chest radiographs, the abnormalities consist of diffuse nodules smaller than 5 mm in diameter and mild to moderate hyperinflation (106). The characteristic thin-section CT findings reflect the pathologic distribution of the disease. They include small centrilobular nodules and branching linear opacities (tree-in-bud pattern), bronchiolectasis, cylindrical bronchiectasis, and mosaic areas of decreased lung attenuation (108,109). The presence of these findings is related to the stage of the disease: the earliest finding is

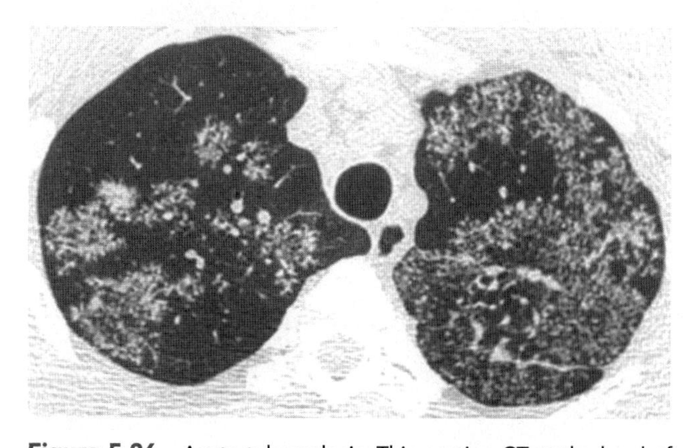

Figure 5-26 Acute tuberculosis. Thin-section CT at the level of the upper part of the lungs showing bilateral patchy areas of small centrilobular and linear branching opacities (tree-in-bud sign).

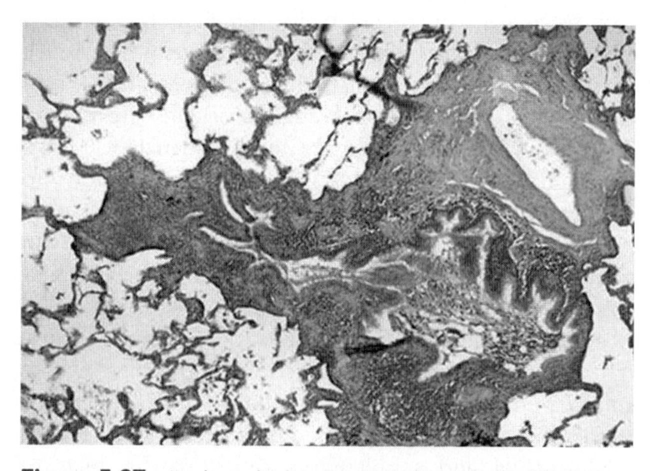

Figure 5-27 Panbronchiolitis; sagittal biopsy (×20, HE.) Dilatation and inflammatory cell infiltration of the respiratory bronchiole. Hyperplasia of lymphoid follicles. (Courtesy of Jung-Gi Im.)

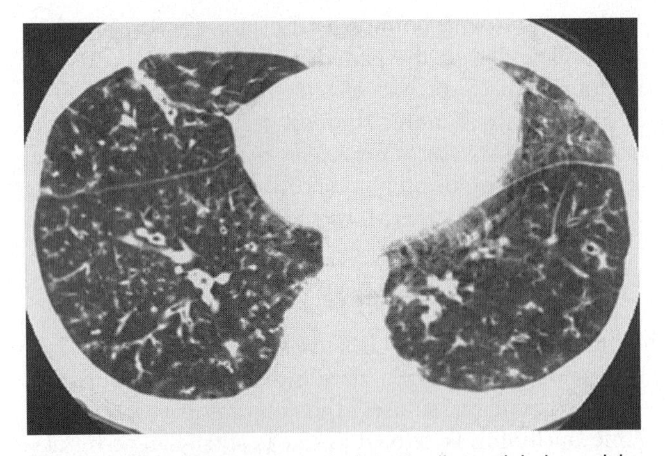

Figure 5-28 Diffuse panbronchiolitis. Small centrilobular nodules and branching linear opacities in the periphery of the lungs. Notice the presence of bronchial wall thickening, bronchial dilatation, decreased lung attenuation in the periphery of the lungs, and linear scars in the right middle lobe (Courtesy of Jung-Gi Im.)

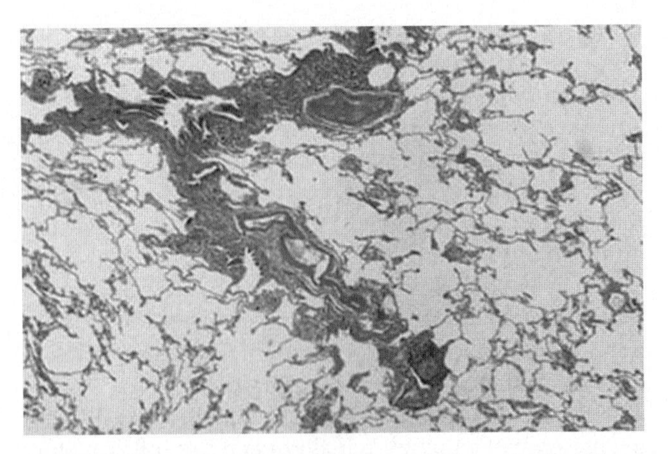

Figure 5-29 Follicular bronchiolitis—pathology. Surgical biopsy (×20, HE) in a case of Sjögren disease. The wall of this terminal bronchiole contains several lymphoid follicles and some degree of inflammation.

tree-in-bud sign followed by thick-walled, centrilobular lucencies. These findings have been demonstrated to correspond to bronchiolar wall and peribronchiolar inflammation and fibrosis, bronchiolar dilatation, the presence of intraluminal secretions, and dilated air-filled bronchioles (Fig. 5-28). Late abnormalities include large, cystic spaces, bullae and evidence of air trapping, large lung volume and decreased attenuation of the peripheral parts of lung parenchyma.

In addition, CT has been useful in following the evolution of disease. In a study by Akira et al. (110) of 17 patients, tree-in-bud pattern progressed to dilatation of proximal airways in 5 untreated patients, whereas the lesions decreased in number and size after erythromycin therapy in 12 patients.

Follicular Bronchiolitis

Follicular bronchiolitis is characterized histologically by a lymphocytic infiltrate of the bronchioles that is often associated with the presence of hyperplastic lymphoid follicles with reactive germinal centers distributed along the bronchioles and, to a lesser extent, along the bronchi (Fig. 5-29). Most often follicular bronchiolitis occurs in the clinical context of connective tissue disease, particularly rheumatoid disease and Sjögren's syndrome, immunodeficiency disorders, and hypersensitivity reactions. The exact relationship among follicular bronchiolitis, lymphocytic interstitial pneumonitis, and obliterative bronchiolitis, particularly in patients with rheumatoid arthritis in whom these pathologies may coexist, remains controversial.

The chest radiograph characteristically shows a diffuse reticulonodular pattern. Thin-section CT findings include small, poorly defined centrilobular nodules having a diffuse and homogeneous distribution (Fig. 5-30). Peribronchial and subpleural nodules, patchy areas of ground-glass attenuation, bronchial wall thickening, and patchy areas of low attenuation are variably associated (111).

Respiratory Bronchiolitis

Respiratory bronchiolitis is characterized histologically by the association of accumulation of pigment-laden macrophages in the respiratory bronchioles and adjacent alveoli (Fig. 5-31) and thickening of the respiratory bronchiolar walls by inflammatory cells and fibrous tissue. The lesion is one of the earliest pathologic reactions to cigarette smoking.

Respiratory bronchiolitis is frequently identified as an incidental finding in asymptomatic smokers (112,113). Smokers occasionally present with cough, dyspnea, crackles, and a combined restrictive and obstructive pattern on lung function testing. In such cases, the clinicopathologic syndrome has been called respiratory bronchiolitis–associated interstitial lung disease (RB-ILD) (114). Patients with this syndrome constitute a subset of individuals who have a more severe form of cigarette smoke–induced respiratory bronchiolitis in which inflammation and fibrosis extend into the peribronchiolar parenchyma. This entity has also

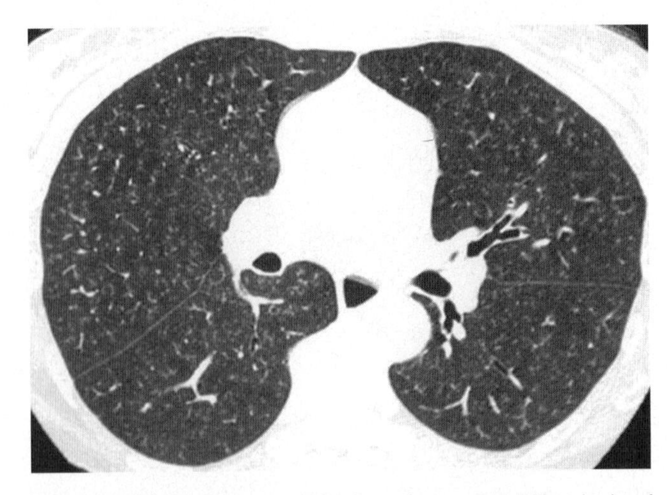

Figure 5-30 Follicular bronchiolitis. Thin-section CT at the level of the midpart of the lungs in a patient with Sjögren's syndrome showing multiple tiny centrilobular nodules in both lungs.

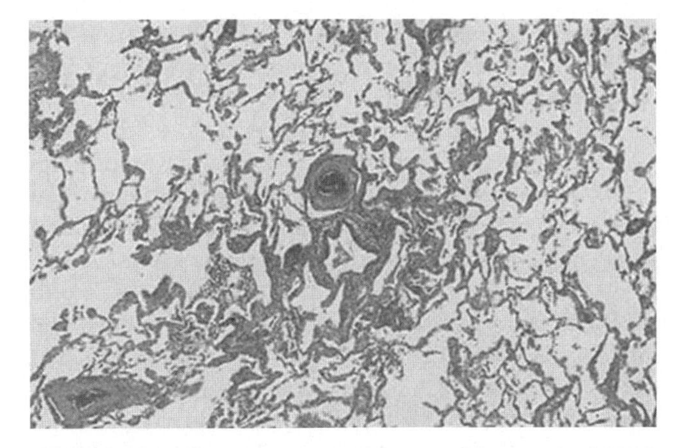

Figure 5-31 Respiratory bronchiolitis. Surgical biopsy (×20, HE). Fibrosis of the bronchial and adjacent alveolar walls. Numerous pigmented macrophages are present in the bronchioles and alveoli lumens.

been considered to be a part of a histologic spectrum of disease that includes a desquamative interstitial pneumonia (DIP). Patients with DIP have more diffuse involvement with a greater likelihood of developing parenchymal fibrosis and progressive lung disease.

Most patients with respiratory bronchiolitis have normal chest radiograph and CT scans. In a small number of patients, thin-section CT scans may show poorly defined centrilobular nodules (Fig. 5-32) or ground-glass opacity having a diffuse distribution or, more often, a predominant or exclusive distribution within the upper lobes (30,88,89).

Most patients with RB-ILD have abnormalities evident on both chest radiographs and thin-section CT scans (48,115). The radiographic features include ground-glass opacity with or without associated fine reticular or reticulonodular opacities. On thin-section CT scan, the abnormality consists of diffuse or patchy areas of ground-glass attenuation, or poorly defined centrilobular nodular opacities, or both (48,115,116) (Figs. 5-13 and 5-33). These opacities are often superimposed on a background of centrilobular emphysema, and bronchial wall thickening is also often present. Occasionally a fine reticular pattern is superimposed on areas of ground-glass attenuation, expressing the presence of fibrosis. The clinical symptoms and radiologic abnormalities observed in patients with RB-ILD may regress after smoking cessation and corticosteroid therapy.

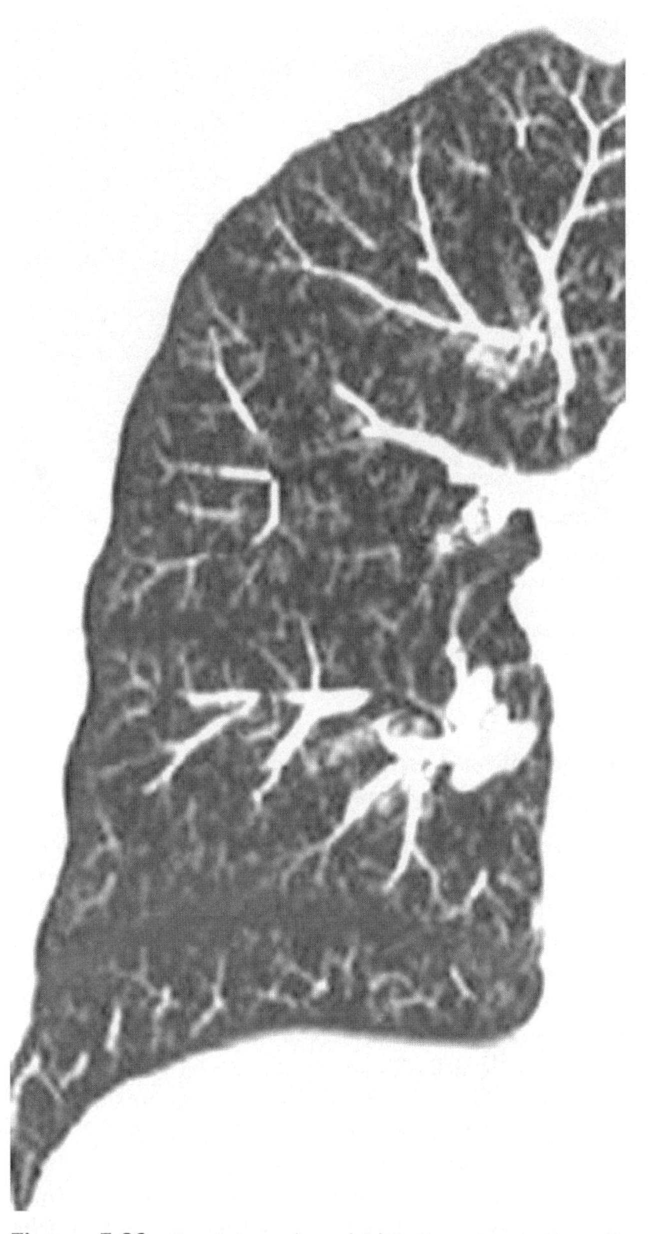

Figure 5-32 Respiratory bronchiolitis in an asymptomatic heavy smoker. Multiplanar volume reformation (7-mm-thick coronal slab) combined with maximum-intensity projection technique and targeted on the right lung shows multiple small, poorly defined centrilobular nodules in the upper and mid parts of the lungs. These abnormalities were not depicted on single thin-section CT scan.

Diffuse Aspiration Bronchiolitis

Diffuse aspiration bronchiolitis is a new clinical entity characterized by a chronic inflammation of bronchioles induced by recurrent aspiration of foreign particles (117). In elderly patients, neurologic disorders and dementia are commonly associated diseases. Oropharyngeal dysphagia is present in half of patients. This entity, however, may occur in any patient with dysphagia, irrespective of age (118). Clinical presentations are signs of bronchorrhea, bronchospasm, wheezing, and dyspnea, closely associated with oral food intake. Histologic findings are characterized by localization of chronic mural inflammation with foreign body reaction in bronchioles. HRCT findings include disseminated small centrilobular linear branching opacities with the tree-in-bud appearance (Fig. 5-34). Some patchy lobular areas of airspace consolidation may also be present, reflecting focal areas of BOOP or bronchopneumonia.

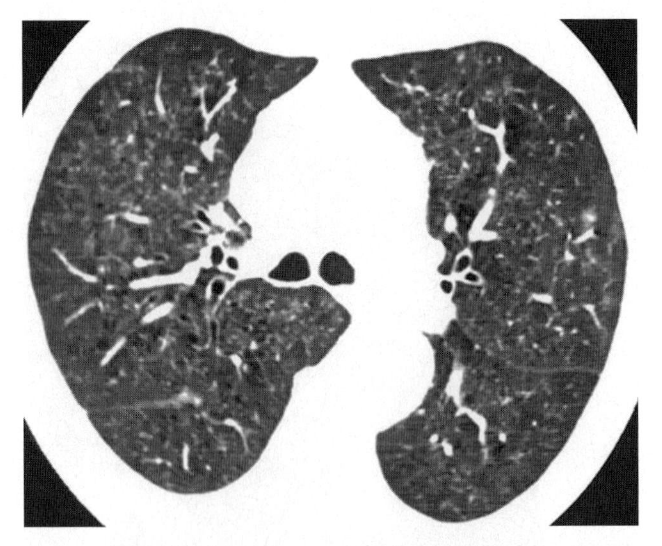

Figure 5-33 RB-ILD. Heavy smoker suffering from chronic cough and shortness of breath at exercise. Some restriction is present at pulmonary function tests. Thin-section CT shows patchy areas of small ill-defined centrilobular nodules associated with some ground-glass opacities predominant in the upper parts of the lungs.

Bronchiolitis Associated with Hypersensitivity Pneumonitis

Hypersensitivity pneumonitis, also called extrinsic allergic alveolitis (EAA), is an allergic lung disease caused by the inhalation of organic dusts of plants or animal origin or of some chemicals. The organism or protein complex that causes hypersensitivity pneumonitis is small, probably no more than 1 to 2 μm in most cases. In susceptible individuals, the position of these organic dusts in the terminal and respiratory bronchioles and in the alveoli results in both alveolitis and bronchiolitis and causes inflammatory granulomatous bronchiolitis of variable degrees.

Although more than 50 different substances have been associated with hypersensitivity pneumonitis, most individuals in whom the disease develops are farmers (the causative agent being thermophilic *Actinomycetes*) and bird fanciers or workers (the antigen being bird protein derived from feces and feathers) (119).

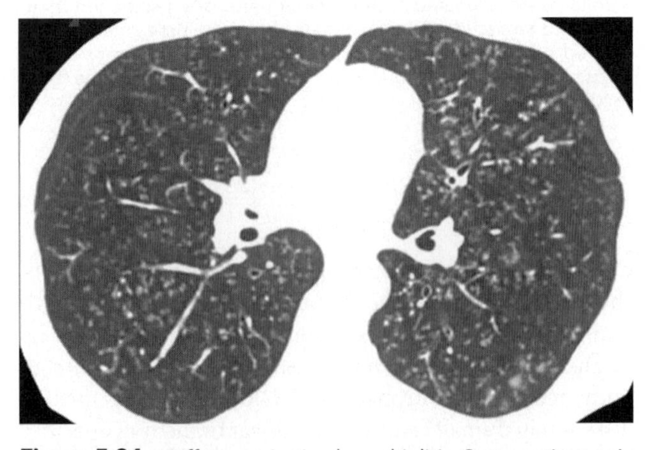

Figure 5-34 Diffuse aspiration bronchiolitis. Same patient as in Fig. 5-9. Thin-section CT scan showing bilateral widespread areas of small centrilobular, nodular, and branching linear opacities (tree-in-bud sign).

Histologic abnormalities tend to be more severe in the vicinity of terminal and proximal respiratory bronchioles (120). Mononuclear (predominantly lymphocytic) infiltration is present in both alveolar interstitium and the walls of small membranous and respiratory bronchioles. Poorly formed granulomas and isolated or small clusters of multinucleated giant cells are common in the peribronchiolar interstitium. A proteinaceous exudate and fibroblastic tissue occasionally are present within the alveolar spaces. In severe cases, bronchiolar epithelium ulceration and obliterative bronchiolitis may be seen. Repeated and chronic exposure may induce interstitial lung fibrosis (121).

The clinical features are divided into three phases: acute, subacute, and chronic, with an important overlap between them. The radiologic features vary according to the phase of the disease (122–124). In the acute phase, heavy exposure to the antigen may result in pulmonary edema with diffuse airspace consolidation. In the subacute phase, the radiologic pattern is made of bilateral ground-glass opacities and poorly defined nodules, reflecting the presence of alveolitis and bronchiolitis, respectively. On thin-section CT scans, the nodules are small, poorly defined, and centrilobular. The distribution of abnormalities is homogeneous and diffuse or tends to involve mainly the middle and lower lung zones (Fig. 5-11). Another common finding is the presence of lobular areas of decreased attenuation and perfusion (mosaic perfusion pattern), showing air trapping on expiratory CT scans (Figs. 5-14 and 5-21) (66). These abnormalities are probably the result of bronchiolar obstruction by plugs of fibroblastic tissue.

In the chronic phase of the disease, the radiologic features include not only those expressing evidence of active disease but also intralobular interstitial thickening, irregular interlobular septal thickening, traction bronchiectasis, and honeycombing (125,126). It has been shown that the extent of low-attenuation areas correlates significantly with the severity of pulmonary obstruction measured by the increase of the residual volume, whereas ground-glass opacity and reticular pattern correlate with restrictive lung function changes (49).

Bronchiolitis Obliterans with Organizing Pneumonia (BOOP)

BOOP can be seen in association with a number of etiologies, including connective tissue diseases, drugs, infection, and aspiration. However, BOOP is most commonly idiopathic; thus, the disease is currently classified among the idiopathic interstitial pneumonias rather than bronchiolitis and is called cryptogenic organizing pneumonia (COP) (114). Patients with COP usually present with a 1- to 3-month history of nonproductive cough, low-grade fever, and increasing shortness of breath.

The main radiologic pattern visible on both chest radiographs and thin-section CT scans in patients with secondary BOOP or COP is patchy areas of airspace consolidation (42,43,127). On chest radiographs, the opacities are most often peripheral and pleural based. They may decrease in size in one area and appear in previously unaffected areas. The size of the individual opacities varies from 2 to 3 cm to an entire lobe. Their margins are ill defined and may contain air bronchograms. Lung volume is normal or decreased. Small pleural effusions may also be present. Airspace consolidation may be associated with a reticulonodular pattern or appear as multiple nodular opacities (128,129).

Occasionally the pattern is composed of a focal area of consolidation or reticular or reticulonodular opacities. The thin-section CT scans of most patients show areas of airspace consolidation containing air bronchograms or small nodules, or both. Areas of ground-glass attenuation may also be present. More than half of patients have a predominant subpleural and peribronchovascular distribution of areas of airspace consolidation (Fig. 5-12).

In some patients airspace consolidation appears as large nodular opacities with irregular margins related to the pleura with parenchymal lines (Fig. 5-35) or broad and large parenchymal bands containing air bronchograms (Figs. 5-36 and 5-37) (130–132). The parenchymal bands may extend either radially along the line of the bronchi toward the pleura, being intimately related to the bronchi, or running parallel to the peripheral pleura, having no relationship to the bronchi (132). These parenchymal bands may be curvilinear, or appear as a crescent or ring shape (133,134) (atoll sign) (Fig. 5-37). The association of central ground-glass opacity and surrounding airspace consolidation of crescent or ring shape (reverse halo sign) has proved to be relatively specific to make a diagnosis of COP on CT (135).

Bronchiolar involvement often is not apparent on thin-section CT because it is hidden by airspace consolidation. It

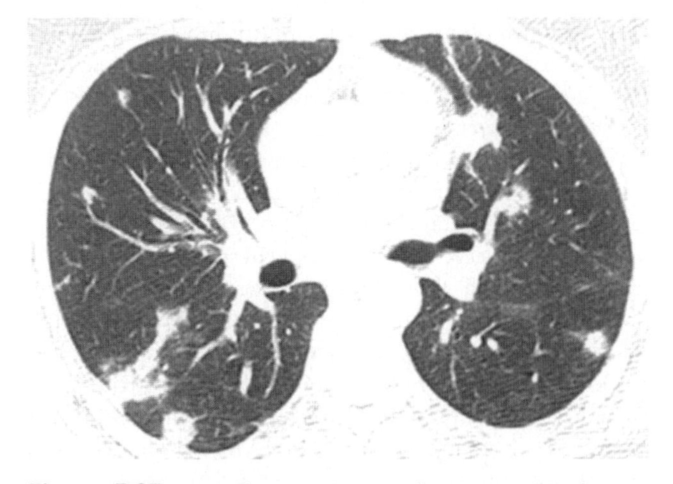

Figure 5-35 Postinfectious BOOP. Thin-section CT showing multiple bilateral rounded areas of airspace consolidation having either a subpleural or a peribronchovascular distribution.

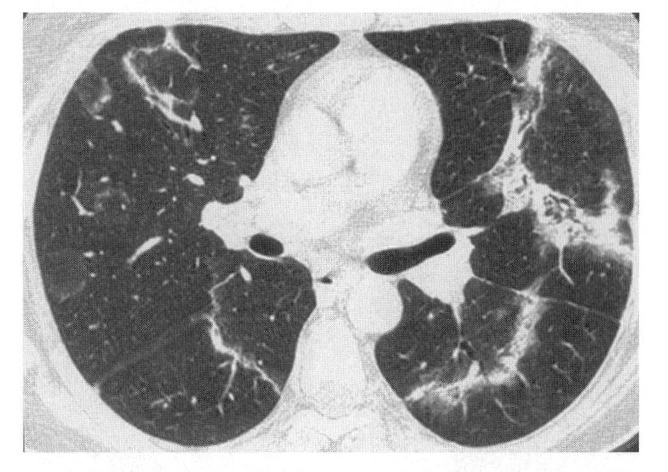

Figure 5-36 Cryptogenic organizing pneumonia. Thin-section CT showing linear bands containing air bronchograms running throughout the left upper lobe and the superior segment of the left lower lobe. Notice also the presence of linear opacities in the right lung.

may appear, in the absence of organizing pneumonia, as small centrilobular and branching linear opacities. Ground-glass attenuation and nodules are more common in immunocompromised patients (42,136).

Occasionally, BOOP may appear on CT as a pattern of multiple cavitary lung nodules (137,138) or as a solitary pulmonary nodule with irregular or spiculated margins, simulating bronchial carcinoma (139). A halo of ground-glass opacity and cavitation may be present (139,140). In a study including thin-section CT scans of 129 patients with a pathologically proved idiopathic interstitial pneumonia (usual interstitial pneumonia, $n = 30$; COP, $n = 24$; desquamative interstitial pneumonia, $n = 23$; acute interstitial pneumonia, $n = 20$; and nonspecific interstitial pneumonia, $n = 27$), two blinded observers made a correct diagnosis in 19 of 24 patients (79%) with COP. This diagnosis was made with a high level of confidence in 15 patients (62%) (141).

Whatever the clinical and radiologic presentations, BOOP responds well to steroids, and the radiologic abnormalities are reversible in almost all cases (142).

Obliterative (Constrictive) Bronchiolitis

Obliterative bronchiolitis is the result of a variety of causes and, rarely, is idiopathic (Table 5-2). Affected patients usually present with progressive shortness of breath and functional evidence of airflow obstruction. The chest radiograph is often normal. In a small number of patients, mild hyperinflation, subtle peripheral attenuation of the vascular markings, widespread and conspicuous abnormalities in lung attenuation, and central bronchiectasis may be seen (143,144). Thin-section CT is superior to radiographs in demonstrating the presence and extent of abnormalities (145,146). The main thin-section CT findings usually consist of areas of decreased lung attenuation associated

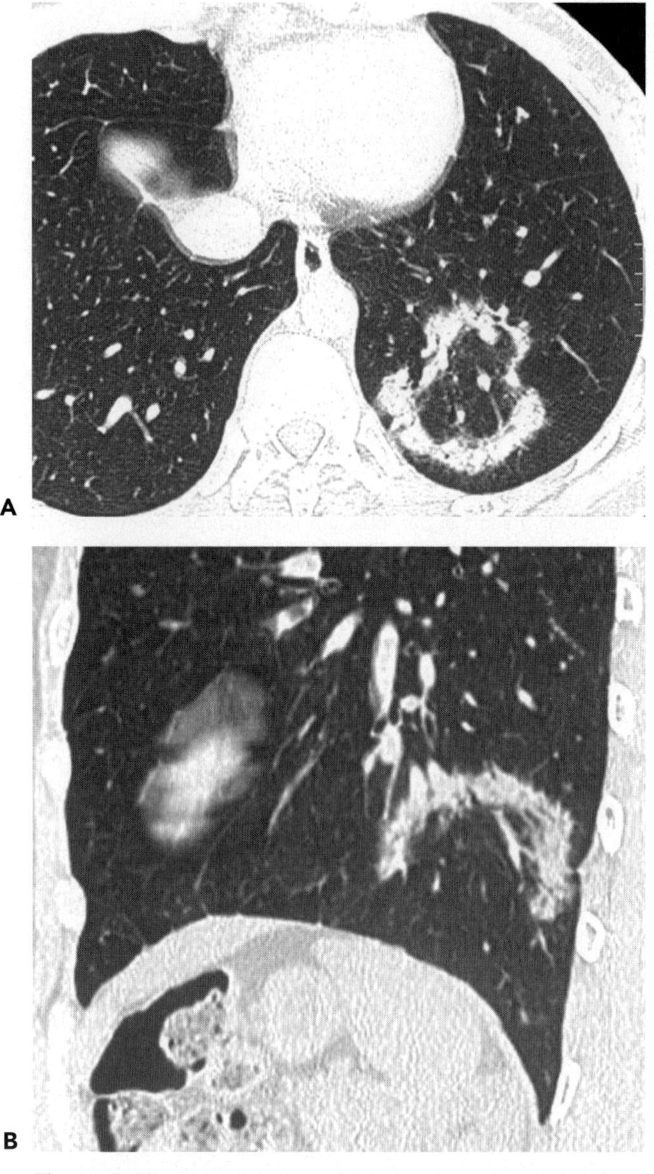

Figure 5-37 Postinfectious BOOP. Curvilinear band of airspace consolidation in the left lower lobe giving a ring shape. The sagittal reformation **(B)** confirms the curvilinear shape of airspace consolidation and explains the ring appearance on axial CT image **(A).**

with vessels of decreased caliber on inspiratory scans and air trapping on expiratory scans (Fig. 5-17) (147,148). Because the lesions of bronchiolar narrowing or obstruction are heterogeneously distributed throughout the lungs, redistribution of blood flow to areas of normal lung or less diseased areas results in a pattern of mosaic perfusion (Figs. 5-15 and 5-16). Bronchial wall thickening and bronchiectasis, both central and peripheral, are also commonly present (Figs. 5-15 and 5-23) (148,149). Sometimes inspiratory CT scans are unremarkable and focal and multifocal areas of air trapping on expiratory CT scans are the only depictable CT abnormality (71,147). Conversely when the airway lesions are severe and diffuse, the patchy difference in attenuation is absent in both inspiratory and respiratory CT scans (Fig. 5-18). In such cases, the differential diagnosis with other pulmonary parenchymal or airway abnormalities that result in chronic airflow obstruction may become difficult. Copley et al. (150), in a study of thin-section CT scans of 105 patients with obstructive pulmonary disease (asthma, $n = 35$; centrilobular emphysema, $n = 30$; panlobular emphysema, $n = 21$; and obliterative bronchiolitis, $n = 19$) and in 33 healthy subjects assessed by two independent observers, demonstrated high sensitivity (92%), specificity (94%), and accuracy (93%) of CT in the identification of obliterative bronchiolitis. There were only few misdiagnoses between patients with obliterative bronchiolitis and those with panlobular emphysema. Both conditions are characterized by bronchial wall thickening and generalized decreased attenuation of the lung parenchyma and bronchial dilatation. However, the observers were able to assess the entire lung and identify areas of mosaic attenuation in patients with less severe obliterative bronchiolitis. There were also significantly higher frequency and greater extent of parenchymal destruction in patients with panlobular emphysema. Long lines reflecting limited thickened interlobular septa were significantly more frequent in patients with panlobular emphysema.

Postinfectious Obliterative Bronchiolitis

Most often, postinfectious obliterative bronchiolitis represents the sequelae of a previous infection, occurring in infancy or childhood (viral infection resulting from adenovirus or syncytial respiratory virus or *M. pneumoniae*) (Table 5-3). Sometimes the disease is recognized or at least suspected in childhood in the investigation of repeated respiratory infections (151,152). In many cases, though, the condition does not become apparent until adulthood. According to the extent of the lesions, dyspnea at exercise may be present or absent. Often, the diagnosis is made during a CT evaluation performed on an asymptomatic patient. The majority of cases of postinfectious obliterative bronchiolitis are self-limiting with no long-term consequences.

Swyer-James or MacLeod syndrome is a variant form of postinfectious obliterative bronchiolitis in which the obliterative bronchiolar lesions affect predominantly one lung (6). The patients are asymptomatic or present with a history of repeated lower respiratory tract infections. The characteristic radiographic findings include decreased vascularity and hyperlucency in the affected lung. On suspended full inspiratory radiographs the volume of affected lung is normal or reduced, and expiratory chest radiographs show air trapping. On thin-section CT scans, decreased lung attenuation and perfusion are extended throughout the affected lung, involving one or more lobes and more or less associated with central thin-walled bronchiectasis (153,154). On expiratory CT scans air trapping is present (Fig. 5-38). In many cases, CT shows that similar changes are present in the contralateral lung but to a lesser extent, indicating that the process was much more heterogeneous than suspected (154).

TABLE 5-3
AGENTS CAUSING POSTINFECTIOUS CONSTRICTIVE BRONCHIOLITIS

Common	Uncommon
Adenovirus	Corona virus
Respiratory syncytial virus (RSV)	Rubeola virus
Mycoplasma	Mumps
Varicella	Rhinovirus
Influenza A and B	Parvovirus B19
Parainfluenza	Enteroviruses
Cytomegalovirus (CMV)	

Bronchiolitis Related to Toxic Gases, Fumes, and Dusts

A variety of inorganic agents may cause inhalation lung injury of which bronchiolitis may be the major manifestation or a minor component (Table 5-4). Acute exposure to smoke, sulfur dioxide (SO_2), the oxides of nitrogen, and a variety of other gases and fumes can cause bronchiolitis associated with severe airflow obstruction. Cough and dyspnea appear minutes or hours after exposure and may be accompanied by the development of pulmonary edema. At this stage, pathologic changes include necrosis of bronchiolar epithelium and acute inflammatory exudate. If patients survive, this acute phase of the disease is followed by the pathologic changes of predominant obliterative bronchiolitis (155). This occurs in 2 to 5 weeks with increased airflow obstruction, fever, chills, cough, and dyspnea. When the concentration of gas or fumes is not too high, acute symptoms may be minimal, and there can be a symptom-free period before the development of obliterative bronchiolitis. Thin-section CT scans show patchy or, more often, diffuse areas of decreased lung attenuation with expiratory air trapping. Bronchial wall thickening and bronchiolectasis are also present.

Bronchiectasis

Thin-section CT has shown that areas of decreased attenuation visible as mosaic perfusion pattern and air trapping on expiratory CT and reflecting obliterative bronchiolitis are very common in patients with severe bronchiectasis and can even precede the development of bronchiectasis (Figs. 5-15 and 5-23) (156). Im et al. (53) examined 48 consecutive patients with lobular low-attenuation areas of the lung on thin-section CT and found that the majority (85%) had bronchiectasis. Small airway narrowing, which causes these areas of low attenuation, is very likely responsible for the obstructive pulmonary function changes. This was suggested in a study performed by Roberts et al. (157). These authors examined the inspiratory and expiratory features on the CT scans of 100 patients with bronchiectasis

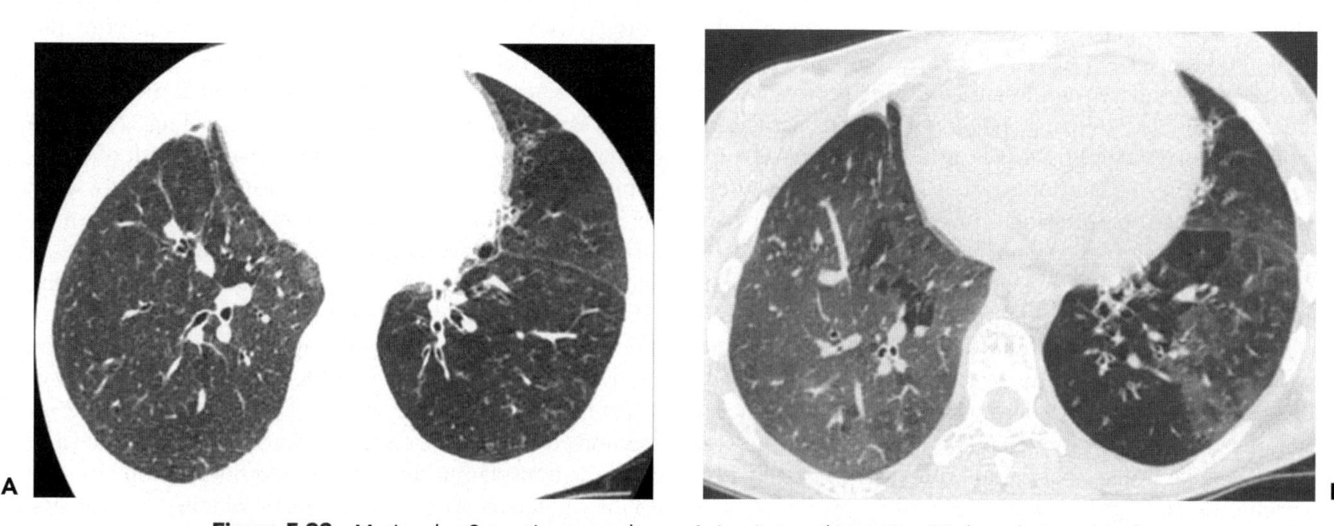

Figure 5-38 MacLeod or Swyer-James syndrome. **A:** Inspiratory thin-section CT shows large areas of decreased lung attenuation associated with oligemia in the left lower lobe and the lingula. **B:** Expiratory thin-section CT at the same anatomic level shows air trapping and bronchiectasis in the left lower lobe and the lingula. Some lobules in the right lower lobe also show air trapping.

TABLE 5-4
INHALED AND INGESTED AGENTS THAT CAN CAUSE OBLITERATIVE BRONCHIOLITIS

Inhaled	Ingested
Ammonia	Sauropus androgynus*
Chlorine	
Fire smoke	
Hydrogen bromide	
Hydrogen selenide	
Oxides of nitrogen	
Sulfur dioxide	
Thionyl chloride	

*Yang CF, Wu MT, Chiang AA, et al. Correlation of high-resolution CT and pulmonary function in bronchiolitis obliterans: a study based on 24 patients associated with consumption of sauropus androgynus. *AJR J Roentegenol* 1997;168:1045–1050.

undergoing concurrent lung function tests. They demonstrate that the extent of CT evidence of small airway disease (decreased lung attenuation and expiratory air trapping) was the strongest independent determinant of airflow obstruction. In contrast, the obstructive defect found at pulmonary function tests was not related to the degree of collapse of large airways on expiratory CT or the extent of mucous plugging of the airways (157).

Obliterative Bronchiolitis Associated with Organ Transplantation

Obliterative bronchiolitis is an important complication of bone marrow, lung, and heart-lung transplantation. Most patients present with a history of cough and progressive breathlessness. Lung function testing reveals progressive airflow obstruction.

Most patients who have obliterative bronchiolitis in the setting of bone marrow transplantation have evidence of chronic graft-versus-host disease (GVHD) elsewhere in the body, and it has been suggested that the bronchiolitis may represent a primary manifestation of this process in the lungs (Fig. 5-18). After lung and lung-heart transplantation, obliterative bronchiolitis is a feature of chronic rejection (158). The diagnosis of obliterative bronchiolitis in these patients is based on histologic findings, but because of the patchy distribution of the small airway involvement, in a substantial number of patients bronchial biopsy cannot provide material for histologic proof. As a result, the International Society for Heart and Lung Transplantation has proposed a clinical diagnosis of "bronchiolitis obliterans syndrome," defined as a decline in the forced expiration volume in 1 sec (FEV_1) to a level of 80% or less of the best postoperative value that is unexplained except by the chronic allograft dysfunction (159).

Thin-section CT scan has been used to predict bronchiolitis obliterans syndrome in both adults and children (160–170). Leung et al. (147) obtained inspiratory and expiratory thin-section CT images and spirometry in 21 lung transplant recipients. On inspiratory scans, bronchiectasis and mosaic pattern of lung attenuation were present in 4 and 7 of the 11 patients with pathologic and functional evidence of obliterative bronchiolitis, respectively, and 2 and 1 of 10 patients without obliterative bronchiolitis ($p < .05$), respectively. On expiratory scans, air trapping was found in 10 of 11 patients with obliterative bronchiolitis compared with 2 of 10 patients without obliterative bronchiolitis ($p < .002$). Bankier et al. (166) demonstrated reproducible anatomic distribution and extent of air trapping at sequential expiratory thin-section CT examination in heart-lung transplant recipients. They examined a larger group of patients and performed a visual quantification of the air trapping (167). They found that the extent of air trapping increased with bronchiolitis obliterans syndrome severity. In addition, a threshold of 32% of air trapping turned out to be optimal for distinguishing between patients with and those without bronchiolitis obliterans syndrome and provided sensitivity, specificity, and accuracy of 83%, 89%, and 88%, respectively. Patients without bronchiolitis obliterans syndrome who had air trapping exceeding 32% of the parenchyma were at a significantly increased risk of developing bronchiolitis obliterans syndrome. Conversely, Choi et al. (168) found no correlation between the extent of air trapping and bronchiolitis obliterans syndrome stage in either single- or bilateral-lung transplant recipients. Along the same lines, Konen et al. (165) reported that the value of air trapping before the clinical appearance and during the early stages of bronchiolitis obliterans syndrome is lower than has been previously reported. They reviewed the thin-section CT scans of 26 lung transplant recipients who did and 26 lung transplant recipients who did not develop bronchiolitis obliterans syndrome. CT scans obtained in patients with bronchiolitis obliterans syndrome were divided into three groups: group A consisted of the last scans obtained before the clinical appearance of bronchiolitis obliterans syndrome; groups B and C consisted of, respectively, the first and last scans obtained after the clinical appearance of bronchiolitis obliterans syndrome. The sensitivities of air trapping for the diagnosis of bronchiolitis obliterans syndrome in groups A, B, and C were 50%, 44%, and 64%, respectively; specificities were 80%, 100%, and 80%, respectively. Sensitivities of mosaic perfusion were 4%, 20%, and 36%, respectively; specificities were 100%, 96%, and 96%, respectively. Sensitivities of bronchiectasis were 25%, 24%, and 32%, respectively; specificities were 80%, 80%, and 96%, respectively. Sensitivities of bronchial wall thickening were 4%, 24%, and 40%, respectively; specificities were 96%, 84%, and 80%, respectively. Interestingly, Knollman et al. (169) in a series of 49 lung transplant recipients examined at least 8 months after surgery did not find the contribution of visual analysis of CT scans significant to the prognosis but demonstrated the potential role of spirometrically gated lung CT. Mean lung attenuation was significantly lower in patients who developed bronchiolitis obliterans syndrome within 1 year after the CT study than in patients with persistent normal lung function.

The usefulness of expiratory thin-section CT in detecting airway obstruction and air trapping was also assessed in pediatric lung transplant recipients (170). In a population of 21 pediatric lung transplant recipients, the sensitivity of expiratory CT for enabling the diagnosis of bronchiolitis obliterans syndrome was 100%, the specificity 71%, the positive predictive value 64%, and the negative predictive value 100% (170). Expiratory CT scores correlated strongly with scores based on PFTs. Dilatation of the lower lobe bronchi is another sign of obliterative bronchiolitis in lung transplantation patients. The percentage of dilated bronchi has been shown to increase with increasing pulmonary dysfunction (149).

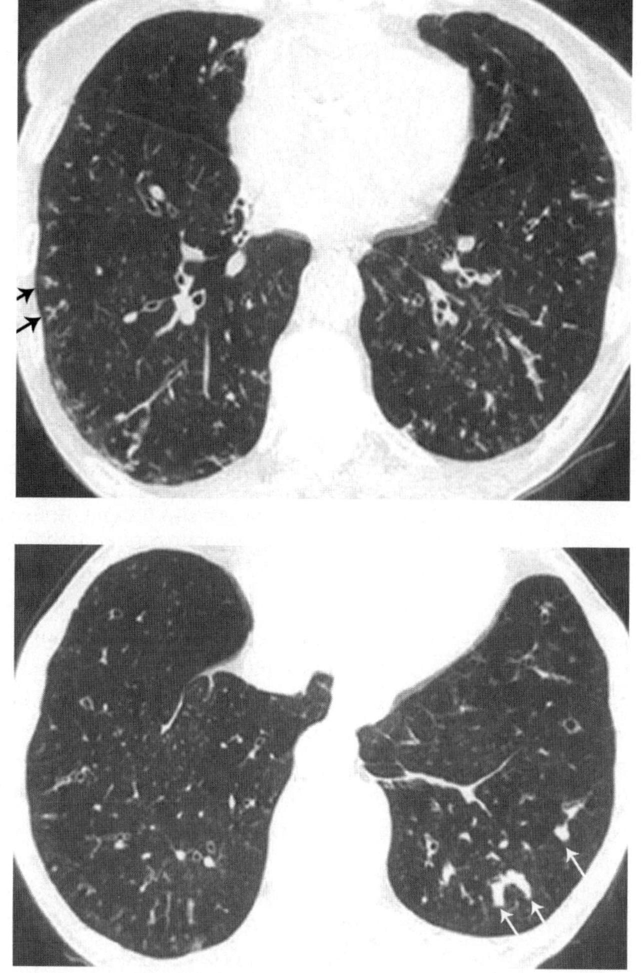

Figure 5-39 Rheumatoid arthritis and obstructive pulmonary disease. Thin-section CT scans (**A** and **B**) at the level of lower parts of the lungs show bilateral cylindrical bronchiectasis and diffuse decreased lung attenuation reflecting obliterative bronchiolitis. Notice the presence of some small centrilobular opacities (**A,** *black arrows*); linear band and mucoid impaction in dilated bronchi within the left lower lobe (**B,** *white arrows*).

Obliterative Bronchiolitis Associated with Rheumatoid Arthritis and Sjögren's Syndrome

Rheumatoid arthritis (RA) is strongly associated with airway disease (171,172). Bronchiectasis can be recognized in up to 35% of patients with RA; obliterative bronchiolitis is present in many patients and can even be the dominant presenting feature, often with a rapidly progressive disease (Fig. 5-39) (173,174). Penicillamine has been incriminated as a contributive causative agent. In a CT study of 84 patients, 30% showed features of bronchiectasis and bronchiolectasis presumed to reflect small airway involvement (174). Perez et al. (175) prospectively evaluated, with thin-section CT and pulmonary function tests, 50 patients with RA without radiographic evidence of RA-related lung changes. Thin-section CT demonstrated bronchial and/or lung abnormalities in 70% of patients, consisting of air trapping (32%), cylindrical bronchiectasis (30%), mild heterogeneity in lung attenuation (20%), and/or centrilobular areas of high attenuation (6%). Pulmonary function tests demonstrated airway flow obstruction in 18% and small airway disease in 8% of patients, both correlated with the presence of bronchiectasis and bronchial wall thickening and were not related to rheumatologic data.

In Sjögren's syndrome, obliterative bronchiolitis is rarely the dominant presenting feature. However, Taouli et al. (176) found signs of large and/or small airway disease in 54% of a group of 35 patients with primary Sjögren's syndrome. The authors found a significant correlation between the extent of air trapping and FEV_1. In another study, air trapping on expiratory CT was found in 32% of patients with Sjögren's syndrome (177).

Obliterative Bronchiolitis Associated with Neuroendocrine Cell Hyperplasia

Neuroendocrine cell hyperplasia is defined by a purely intraepithelial proliferation of the neuroendocrine cells, often associated with multiple pulmonary tumorlets consisting of nodular proliferation of airway neuroendocrine cells that extends beyond the epithelium into the adjacent wall or lung parenchyma. The vast majority of

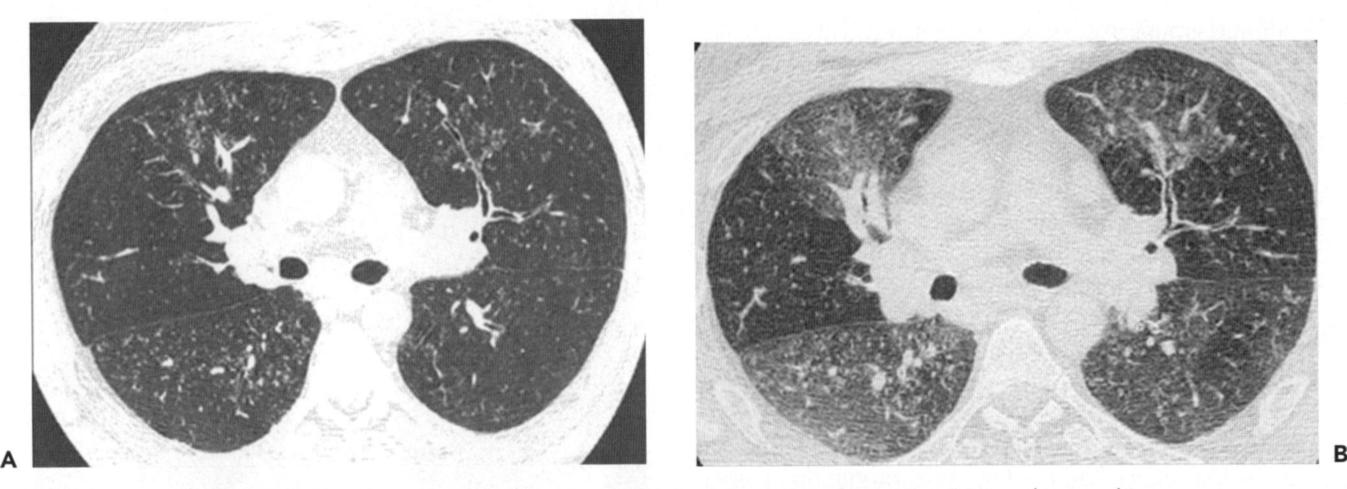

Figure 5-40 Expiratory air trapping in sarcoidosis. **A:** Inspiratory thin-section CT scan shows multifocal areas of centrilobular nodules in both lungs. Bronchial wall thickening and subcarinal and right hilar lymphadenopathy are also present. **B:** Expiratory thin-section CT scan performed at the same anatomic level as **A** shows areas of air trapping in the right and left upper lobes and the superior segment of the left lower lobe.

pulmonary tumorlets behave in a benign fashion. Although this abnormality may be identified in otherwise normal lung, evidence of concomitant pulmonary disease is frequent, the most common associated conditions being bronchiectasis and carcinoid tumor. The characteristic growth within and around small airways, focally associated with significant luminal obliteration by fibrous tissue, may lead to a pattern of obliterative bronchiolitis. Cough and progressive dyspnea associated with obstructive pulmonary function changes have been reported in some patients with neuroendocrine cell hyperplasia (178,179). Rarely the airway narrowing is extensive enough to cause respiratory failure (180). Decreased lung attenuation and expiratory air trapping are depicted on thin-section CT scans, and some tiny nodules occasionally may be present, reflecting the visibility of pulmonary tumorlets (179,180).

Small Airway Involvement in Sarcoidosis

In sarcoidosis, the granulomas present in the lungs typically show a perilymphatic distribution. As a result, sarcoid granulomas are concentrated not only along the subpleural interlobular and peribronchovascular interstitium but also around the small airways. Peribronchiolar granulomata may cause small airway obstruction, particularly at an early stage of the disease. This may result in a pattern of mosaic perfusion and patchy areas of air trapping, even in patients in whom inspiratory CT scans show none of the typical features of pulmonary involvement (Fig. 5-40). Air trapping may occur in any lung zone and involve either individual lobules or segments (181). It may even be the only CT finding of pulmonary sarcoidosis (Fig. 5-19) (182). In one study, air trapping on expiratory CT was noted in 95% of patients with sarcoidosis but was not specific for a given stage of the disease (183). In this study, the extent of air trapping correlated significantly with airflow obstruction at pulmonary function tests (183), whereas the other CT findings (nodules, septal thickening, traction bronchiectasis, lung distortion, and ground-glass opacity) did not correlate with pulmonary function. By contrast, in another study, including a larger proportion of patients having a more advanced fibrotic stage of the disease, Hansell et al. (184) showed that the presence and extent of a reticular pattern was the main determinant of functional impairment, particularly airflow obstruction.

Small Airway Disease in Smokers and Chronic Obstructive Pulmonary Disease

When the lungs of smokers are compared with those of nonsmokers at autopsy, smokers' lungs show narrowing and inflammatory changes in membranous and respiratory bronchioles (185). The airway narrowing is correlated with decreased maximal expiratory flow and increased total airway resistance (186,187). Disease of the small airways is one of the abnormalities that leads to airway obstruction in patients with chronic obstructive pulmonary disease (COPD) (188). The peripheral location of increased airway resistance in patients who have COPD has been demonstrated pathologically and *in vivo* using micromanometer-tipped catheters introduced into the peripheral airways. Although the mechanism for the increased airway resistance in these patients is incompletely understood, it appears to be related to one or more of several abnormalities, such as a loss of the alveolar attachment to the outer wall of the small airways resulting from pulmonary emphysema, chronic inflammation and fibrosis of the airway wall resulting in a thickening of all the components of the wall, a diffuse narrowing of the lumen, localized areas of bronchiolar stenosis, and accumulation of mucus in the airway lumen secondary to goblet cell hyperplasia and impaired mucociliary clearance (6).

Thin-section CT has proved its ability in demonstrating the presence of small airway abnormalities in asymptomatic smokers before the development of an obstructive lung disease. In a prospective study of 175 healthy adult volunteers (current smokers, ex-smokers, and nonsmokers) with overall normal function tests, Rémy-Jardin et al. (189) detected lung parenchymal changes in current smokers and ex-smokers that were not present, or present to a lesser degree, in nonsmokers. About 20% to 25% of the smokers showed multiple areas of ground-glass attenuation and small nodules, which were significantly more extensive than in ex-smokers (4%) and nonsmokers (0%). Emphysema was also seen significantly more often in smokers than in the other two groups. Differences among the three groups for other findings, such as the presence of bronchial wall thickening, dependent areas of attenuation, septal lines, and subpleural small nodules, were not significant. In a CT pathologic correlation study in heavy smokers having a thoracotomy for lung resection, Rémy-Jardin et al. (45) showed that the areas of ground-glass attenuation corresponded to histologic findings of respiratory bronchiolitis. The parenchymal small nodules corresponded to bronchiolectasis with peribronchiolar fibrosis. These abnormalities were predominantly seen in the upper lung zones, and the presence of emphysema and abnormal bronchial wall thickening were the only CT features associated with significantly lower values of functional parameters.

Since the introduction of expiratory thin-section CT, several studies have attempted to demonstrate that air trapping observed at CT in healthy volunteers is related to smoking and intensity of smoking and can be observed before pulmonary function deteriorates (72,74,190,191). Verschakelen et al. (72) examined 30 healthy subjects with a smoking history and normal pulmonary function tests. Areas of focal air trapping were found in 7 nonsmokers, 7 ex-smokers, and 10 current smokers. The scores of focal air trapping were not significantly different between smokers and ex-smokers but were significantly lower in nonsmokers and showed a significant correlation with pack-years. Lee et al. (74) performed prospectively thin-section CT of the lung at end-inspiration and end-expiration in 82 asymptomatic subjects (27 smokers, 55 nonsmokers) without any history of pulmonary disease. The overall frequency of air trapping was 52%. Comparing smokers and nonsmokers, the frequency of air trapping was significantly higher ($p < .05$) in smokers with smoking history of more than 10 pack-years. In another study, Tanaka et al. (190) performed inspiratory and expiratory thin-section CT scans of the lung in 50 subjects with normal pulmonary function, including 26 nonsmokers and 24 smokers (14 current and 10 ex-smokers; 11 mild and 13 heavy smokers). The overall frequency of air trapping was 64%. Lobular air trapping involving one or two adjacent secondary pulmonary lobules in one or two regions per lung level was seen in 10 subjects (20%); mosaic air trapping defined by three or more areas of lobular air trapping that alternate with normal areas was seen in 14 subjects (28%). Extensive air trapping, defined by contiguous areas of air trapping larger than three adjacent pulmonary lobules and being subsegmental, segmental, or lobar in distribution, was seen in eight subjects (16%). There was no significant difference in the visual grade and semiquantitative grade ratio of air trapping among the nonsmokers, current smokers, and ex-smokers or among the nonsmokers, mild smokers, and heavy smokers. For these authors, air trapping depicted at CT in subjects with normal pulmonary function tests had no correlation with the subject's current smoking status or cigarette consumption (190). Mastora et al. (191) evaluated prospectively the frequency and morphologic characteristics of air trapping in 250 volunteers including 144 smokers, 47 ex-smokers, and 59 nonsmokers. The overall frequency of air trapping was 62%. Lobular air trapping was depicted in 117 subjects (47%), without significant differences among smokers ($n = 91$), ex-smokers ($n = 33$), and nonsmokers ($n = 31$). Segmental and lobar air trapping depicted in 38 subjects (15%) was significantly ($p < .001$) more frequent among smokers (26%) and ex-smokers (27%) than nonsmokers (0.8%). No relationship was found between air trapping and functional indexes of small airway disease when the CT pattern of air trapping was considered. The strongest relationship between CT abnormalities and functional alterations at the small airway level was between inspiratory CT features of bronchiolitis, ground-glass opacities, ill-defined small nodules, bronchiolectasis, and airflow at low lung volumes.

Pelinkovic et al. (192) evaluated overall lung attenuation changes during inspiration and expiration in smokers and nonsmokers and correlated them with pulmonary function tests and measurement on CT scans of cross-sectional area changes. They found that healthy, asymptomatic male smokers had a significantly higher lung attenuation at inspiration and a smaller cross-sectional area increase of the lung during inspiration than the healthy, asymptomatic nonsmokers. These changes could be related to the decreased compliance of the smokers' lungs resulting from small airway disease.

Two studies followed healthy volunteers over several years and examined sequential changes in structural and functional abnormalities of the lung on CT scans. Rémy-Jardin et al. (193) found significant differences in CT findings between the initial CT examination and the subsequent CT examination performed after a minimum follow-up period of 4 years, but only in the group of persistent current smokers. Those patients showed a significantly higher frequency of emphysema and ground-glass attenuation. In current smokers in whom small nodules were present at the initial CT, no change was seen in one third of patients, small nodules appeared with a higher profusion in one third of patients, and in the remaining one third of patients small nodules were replaced by emphysema. Subjects with emphysema and/or areas of ground-glass attenuation at the initial CT had a significantly more rapid decline in lung function than did those with an initial normal CT scan. Soejima et al.

(194) performed an annual inspiratory and expiratory thin-section CT for 5 years in a group of current smokers, ex-smokers, and nonsmokers and calculated the mean lung attenuation, the highest frequency CT value, and the relative area of low attenuation with CT values less than −912 HU. In distinction, in nonsmokers, only the percentage of the relative area of low attenuation in the middle or lower lung zones exhibited an annual increase. In current smokers, the percentage of the relative area of low attenuation in the upper lung zone increased, while inspiratory mean lung attenuation and the highest frequency CT value in the middle and lower lung zones became more positive. In ex-smokers, the percentage of low attenuation in any lung zone increased. Although this annual increase in the extent of low attenuation area in the upper lung zones was larger for ex-smokers than for nonsmokers, and there was little difference between past and current smokers. Annual changes on expiratory CT scans were few in all groups.

In patients with COPD, the extent of lung hypoattenuation at expiration probably reflects air trapping more than reduction of the alveolar wall surface. However, expiratory air trapping in these patients may be the result of either airway obstruction caused by a loss of alveolar attachment to the airways directly owing to emphysema or of intrinsic bronchial and bronchiolar abnormalities associated with cigarette smoking.

Asthma

Asthma is a chronic inflammatory condition involving the airways. This inflammation causes a generalized increase in existing bronchial hyperresponsiveness to a variety of stimuli. This is commonly used in practice to confirm the clinical diagnosis of asthma. In susceptible individuals, this inflammation induces recurrent episodes of wheezing, chest tightness, breathlessness, and coughing usually associated with widespread but variable airflow obstruction that is often reversible either spontaneously or with treatment. The chronic inflammation process leads to structure changes, such as new vessel formation, airway smooth muscle thickening, and fibrosis, which may result in irreversible airway narrowing.

The clinical indications for CT in patients with asthma include: to detect bronchiectasis in patients with suspicion of allergic bronchopulmonary aspergillosis (ABPA); to document the presence and extent of emphysema in smokers with asthma; and to identify conditions that may be confused with asthma, such as hypersensitivity pneumonitis (195). CT abnormalities on airway and lung parenchyma, including airway wall thickening, bronchiectasis, centrilobular opacities, mucoid impaction, decreased lung attenuation, mosaic perfusion, and air trapping, have been reported in several studies (68,76,92,196), but only a few of them compared the frequency of the findings observed in asthmatics with a control group (68,76,196,197). Park et al. (76) demonstrated that only three findings were significantly more frequent in asthmatic patients than in normal individuals: bronchial wall thickening, bronchial dilatation, and expiratory air trapping. The prevalence of these thin-section CT abnormalities increases with increasing severity of symptoms (197). Considerable variation exists, however, in the reported frequency of abnormalities. This variation is related to differences in diagnostic criteria and patient selection.

Abnormal expiratory air trapping has been observed in 50% of asthmatic patients (76) (Fig. 5-20). This reflects the luminal obstruction of the airways and is potentially, but not always, reversible. CT may depict air trapping before lung function deteriorates. Goldin et al. (198) showed significant leftward shifts in the frequency distribution of lung parenchymal attenuation values measured by 3-mm-thick CT scans of lungs before and after methacholine challenge in mildly asthmatic patients. These effects returned to normal after the administration of albuterol. Beigelman-Aubry et al. (199) demonstrated, in a small group of mild intermittent asthmatics, the presence of baseline bronchial constriction on CT scans performed at spirometrically controlled lung volume (65% total lung capacity). In the same patients, air trapping on expiratory CT scans appears after methacholine inhalation. In these patients, both bronchial constriction and expiratory air trapping appear partly or fully reversible after inhalation of a short-acting bronchodilator (salbutamol). By contrast, Laurent et al. (200) showed, in moderate persistent asthmatics, an absence of change in air trapping scores after inhalation of salbutamol, suggesting that the air trapping may reflect permanent changes resulting from small airway remodeling.

Focal and diffuse areas of decreased lung attenuation seen in 20% to 30% of asthmatic patients are likely the result of a combination of air trapping and pulmonary oligemia owing to alveolar hypoventilation (68,196) (Fig. 5-41). Laurent et al. (200) compared the inspiratory and expiratory thin-section CT findings of 22 patients classified with moderate asthma with 22 healthy volunteers (10 smokers and 12 nonsmokers). Mosaic perfusion was found in 23% of the asthmatics, 5% of the smokers, and 0% of the nonsmokers. Air trapping scores were significantly higher in the asthmatics than in nonsmoking control subjects but not in smokers. In severe persistent asthma, diffuse decreased lung attenuation and expiratory air trapping make the pattern difficult to distinguish from that of obliterative bronchiolitis (150,201). The presence and extent of bronchial dilatation, vascular attenuation, and decreased lung attenuation seem to favor the diagnosis of obliterative bronchiolitis (150).

The ability to follow up bronchial reactivity and lung attenuation at expiration by CT over time in cohorts of patients receiving different treatments can provide an independent tool to assess and monitor current and new therapy in asthmatic patients. In addition, the current challenge for CT in asthma is also to assess the degree of inflammation in small airways and to evaluate airway wall remodeling. Beigelman-Aubry et al. (199) assessed lung attenuation in a series of patients with mild intermittent asthma and in normal volunteers at select lung volume (65% of total lung capacity), monitored by pneumota-

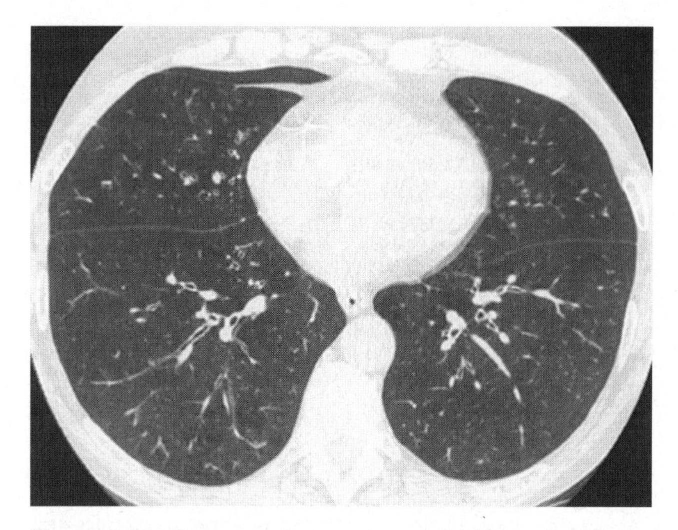

Figure 5-41 Severe persistent asthma. Axial thin-section CT scan at full inspiration. Diffuse decreased lung attenuation and bronchial wall thickening in both lungs.

chography. They showed in asthmatics abnormally higher lung attenuation compared with normal subjects. They hypothesized that the peribronchial and small airway inflammation occurring in asthma explains the attenuation and gradient increases. The observation that these increased attenuation values were not affected by methacholine and salbutamol challenges supports the hypothesis that bronchoconstriction played only a small or no role in attenuation changes and that distal inflammation was a more likely contributor. Smooth muscle hypertrophy and hyperplasia defining airway wall remodeling are responsible for the faster and higher decrease related to age of FEV_1 in asthmatics than in controls (202). Bronchial wall thickness measured at CT has proved to be prominent in patients with more severe asthma. This fact correlated with the duration and severity of the disease and the degree of airflow obstruction (200). This observation supports the concept that quantitative assessment of bronchial wall area at CT could be used to assess airway wall remodeling in asthmatic patients for longitudinal studies to evaluate the effects of new therapies. Such longitudinal prospective studies need to be carried out to monitor changes in the degree of small airway inflammation and airway wall remodeling.

CONCLUSION

The clinical diagnosis of small airway disease is quite difficult. The chest radiograph is normal or may show nonspecific findings. Thin-section CT has become the imaging modality of choice to perform after chest radiograph in patients with clinical suspicion of small airway disease. Thin-section CT may show direct signs of involvement of the small airways (tree-in-bud sign, ill-defined centrilobular nodules), expressing bronchiolar exudation and/or bronchiolar wall and peribronchiolar inflammation, or indirect signs (decreased lung attenuation, mosaic perfusion pattern, and expiratory air trapping), expressing the consequence of the obstruction of the lumen of the small airway on lung ventilation and perfusion. Comparison of images at full inspiration and full expiration is the most sensitive method to detect obstruction of the small airways. In patients presenting with chronic airflow obstruction, thin-collimation CT is highly accurate for the diagnosis of obliterative bronchiolitis. Good correlation exists between the extent of decreased lung attenuation and air trapping at CT and the degree of airflow obstruction at pulmonary function tests. Low-dose thin-collimation multidetector row CT acquisition over the entire lungs at full inspiration and full expiration may contribute to quantifying the extent of small airway disease.

ACKNOWLEDGMENTS

We thank warmly Catherine Beigelman-Aubry, Frédérique Capron, and Michel Brauner for their contributions in preparing the figures for this chapter.

REFERENCES

1. Wright JL, Cagle P, Churg A, et al. Diseases of the small airways. *Am Rev Respir Dis* 1992;146:240–262.
2. Miller WS. *The lung,* 2nd ed. Thomas, Springfield, IL 1947.
3. Plopper CG, Ten Have-Opbroek AAW. Anatomical and histological classification of the bronchioles. In: Epier GR, ed. *Diseases of the bronchioles.* New York: Raven Press, 1994:15–25.
4. Hansen JE, Ampaya EP Bryant GH, Navin JJ. Branching pattern of airways and air spaces of a single human terminal bronchiole. *J Appl Physiol* 1975;38:983–989.
5. Weibel ER, Taylor CR. Design and structure of the human lung. In: Fishman AP, ed. *Pulmonary diseases and disorders,* 2nd ed. New York: McGraw-Hill, 1988:11–60.
6. Fraser RS, Muller NL, Colman N, Paré PD, eds. *Diagnosis of diseases of the chest,* 4th ed. Philadelphia: WB Saunders, 1999.
7. Gruden JF, Webb WR, Warnock M. Centrilobular opacities in the lung on high-resolution CT: diagnostic considerations and pathologic correlation. *AJR Am J Roentgenol* 1994;162:569–574.
8. Itoh H, Murata K, Konishi J, et al. Diffuse lung disease: pathologic basis for the high-resolution computed tomography findings. *J Thorac Imaging* 1993;8:176–188.
9. Murata K. Itoh H, Todo G, et al. Centrilobular lesions of the lung: demonstration by high-resolution CT and pathologic correlation. *Radiology* 1986;161:641–645.
10. Colby TV. Bronchiolitis: pathologic considerations. *Am J Clin Pathol* 1998;109:102–109.
11. Myers JL, Colby TV. Pathologic manifestations of bronchiolitis, constrictive bronchiolitis, cryptogenic organizing pneumonia, and diffuse panbronchiolitis. *Clin Chest Med* 1993;14:611–622.
12. Hwang JH, Kirn TS, Lee KS, et al. Bronchiolitis in adults: pathology and imaging. *J Comput Assist Tomogr* 1997;21:913–919.
13. Poletti V, Zompatori M, Cancellieri A. Clinical spectrum of adult chronic bronchiolitis. *Sarcoidosis Vasc Diffuse Lung Dis* 1999;16:183–196.
14. Worthy SA, Muller NL. Small airway diseases. *Radiol Clin North Am* 1998;36:163–173.
15. Muller NL, Miller RR. Diseases of the bronchioles: CT and histopathologic findings. *Radiology* 1995;196:3–12.
16. Epler GR, Colby TV. The spectrum of bronchiolitis obliterans. *Chest* 1983;83:161–162.
17. Epler GR, Colby TV, McLoud TC, et al. Bronchiolitis obliterans organizing pneumonia. *N Engl J Med* 1985;312:152–158.
18. Kohli-Seth R, Killu C, Amolat MJ, et al. Bronchiolitis obliterans organizing pneumonia after orthotopic liver transplantation. *Liver Transpl* 2004;10:456–459.
19. Radzikowska E, Szczepulska E, Chabowski M, Bestry I. Organising pneumonia caused by transtuzumab (Herceptin) therapy for breast cancer. *Eur Respir J* 2003;21:552–555.
20. Evans A, Steward CG, Lyburn ID, Grier DJ. Imaging in haematopoietic stem cell transplantation. *Clin Radiol* 2003;58:201–214.

21. DeAngelo AJ, Ouellette D. Bronchiolitis obliterans organizing pneumonia in an orthotopic liver transplant patient. *Transplantation* 2002;73:544–546.
22. Herraez I, Gutierrez M, Alonso N, Allende J. Hypersensitivity pneumonitis producing a BOOP-like reaction: HRCT/pathologic correlation. *J Thorac Imaging* 2002;17:81–83.
23. Erasmus JJ, McAdams HP, Rossi SE. High-resolution CT of drug-induced lung disease. *Radiol Clin North Am* 2002;40:61–72.
24. Ferriby D, Stojkovic T. Clinical picture: bronchiolitis obliterans with organising pneumonia during interferon beta-1a treatment. *Lancet* 2001;357:751.
25. Cameron RJ, Kolbe J, Wilsher ML, Lambie N. Bronchiolitis obliterans organising pneumonia associated with the use of nitrofurantoin. *Thorax* 2000;55:249–251.
26. Crestani B, Valeyre D, Roden S, et al. Bronchiolitis obliterans organizing pneumonia syndrome primed by radiation therapy to the breast. The Groupe d'Etudes et de Recherche sur les Maladies Orphelines Pulmonaires (GERM"O"P) *Am J Respir Crit Care Med* 1998;158:1929–1935.
27. Worthy SA, Flint JD, Muller NL. Pulmonary complications after bone marrow transplantation: high-resolution CT and pathologic findings. *Radiographics* 1997;17:1359–1371.
28. Kanda Y, Takahashi T, Imai Y, et al. Bronchiolitis obliterans organizing pneumonia after syngeneic bone marrow transplantation for acute lymphoblastic leukemia. *Bone Marrow Transplant* 1997;19:1251–1253.
29. Verberckmoes R, Verbeken E, Verschakelen J, Vanrenterghem Y. BOOP (bronchiolitis obliterans organizing pneumonia) after renal transplantation. *Nephrol Dial Transplant* 1996;11:1862–1863.
30. Diehl JL, Gisselbrecht M, Meyer G, et al. Bronchiolitis obliterans organizing pneumonia associated with chlamydial infection. *Eur Respir J* 1996; 9:1320–1322.
31. Imasaki T, Yoshii A, Tanaka S, et al. Polymyositis and Sjögren's syndrome associated with bronchiolitis obliterans organizing pneumonia. *Intern Med* 1996;35:231–235.
32. Piperno D, Donne C, Loire R, Cordier JF. Bronchiolitis obliterans organizing pneumonia associated with minocycline therapy: a possible cause. *Eur Respir J* 1995;8:1018–1020.
33. Du Bois RM, Geddes DM. Obliterative bronchiolitis, cryptogenic organizing pneumonia and bronchiolitis obliterans organizing pneumonia: three names for two different conditions. *Eur Respir J* 1991;4:774–777.
34. Aquino SL, Gamsu G. Webb WR, Kee ST. Tree-in-bud pattern: frequency and significance on thin section CT. *J Comput Assist Tomogr* 1996; 20:594–599.
35. Collins J, Blankenbaker D, Stern EJ. CT patterns of bronchiolar disease: what is tree in bud? *AJR Am J Roentgenol* 1998;171:365–370.
36. Akira M, Atagi S, Kawahara M, et al. High-resolution CT findings of diffuse bronchioloalveolar carcinoma in 38 patients. *AJR Am J Roentgenol* 1999;173:1623–1629.
37. Kushihashi T, Munechika H, Ri K, et al. Bronchioalveolar adenoma of the lung: CT-pathologic correlation. *Radiology* 1994;193:789–793.
38. Franquet T, Gimenez A, Prats R, et al. Thrombotic microangiopathy of pulmonary tumors: a vascular cause of tree-in-bud pattern on CT. *AJR Am J Roentgenol* 2002;179:897–899.
39. Hwang JH, Kim TS, Han J, et al. Primary lymphoma of the lung simulating bronchiolitis: radiologic finding. *AJR Am J Roentgenol* 1998;170:220–221.
40. Webb WR, Muller NL, Naidich DP, eds. *High resolution CT of the lung,* 3rd ed. Philadelphia: Lippincott Williams & Wilkins, 2001.
41. Collins J. CT signs and patterns of lung disease. *Radiol Clin North Am* 2001;39:1115–1135.
42. Lee KS, Kullnig P, Hartman TE, Muller NL. Cryptogenic organizing pneumonia: CT findings in 43 patients. *AJR Am J Roentgenol* 1994;162:543–546.
43. Muller NL, Staples CA, Miller RR. Bronchiolitis obliterans organizing pneumonia: CT features in 14 patients. *AJR Am J Roentgenol* 1990;154:983–987.
44. Logan PM, Primack SL, Miller RR, Muller NL. Invasive aspergillosis of the airways: radiographic, CT, and pathologic findings. *Radiology* 1994; 193:383–388.
45. Rémy-Jardin M, Rémy J, Gosselin B, et al. Lung parenchymal changes secondary to cigarette smoking: pathologic-CT correlations. *Radiology* 1993;186:643–651.
46. Gruden JF, Webb WR, Warnok M. CT findings in a proved case of respiratory bronchiolitis. *AJR Am J Roentgenol* 1993;161:44–46.
47. Holt RM, Schmidt RA, Godwin JD, Raghu G. High-resolution CT in respiratory bronchiolitis-associated interstitial lung disease. *J Comput Assist Tomogr* 1993;17:46–50.
48. Park JS, Brown KK, Tuder RM, et al. Respiratory bronchiolitis-associated interstitial lung disease: radiologic features with clinical and pathologic correlations. *J Comput Assist Tomogr* 2002;26:13–20.
49. Hansell DM, Wells AU, Padley SP, et al. Hypersensitivity pneumonitis: correlation of individual CT patterns with functional abnormalities. *Radiology* 1996;199:123–128.
50. Webb WR. High-resolution computed tomography of obstructive lung disease. *Radiol Clin North Am* 1994;32:745–747.
51. Guckel C, Wells AU, Taylor DA, et al. Mechanism of mosaic attenuation of the lungs on computed tomography in induced bronchospasm. *J Appl Physiol* 1999;86:701–708.
52. Worthy SA, Muller NL, Hartman TE, et al. Mosaic attenuation pattern on thin-section CT scans of the lung: differentiation among infiltrative lung, airway, and vascular diseases as a cause. *Radiology* 1997;205:465–470.
53. Im JG, Kirn SH, Chung MJ, et al. Lobular low attenuation of the lung parenchyma on CT: evaluation of forty-eight patients. *J Comput Assist Tomogr* 1996;20:756–762.
54. Arakawa H, Webb WR, McCowin M, et al. Inhomogeneous lung attenuation at thin-section CT: diagnostic value of expiratory scans. *Radiology* 1998;206:89–94.
55. King MA, Bergin CJ, Yeung DW, et al. Chronic pulmonary thromboembolism: detection of regional hypoperfusion with CT. *Radiology* 1994;191:359–363.
56. Schwickert HC, Schweden F, Schild HH, et al. Pulmonary arteries and lung parenchyma in chronic pulmonary embolism: preoperative and postoperative CT findings. *Radiology* 1994;191:351–357.
57. Sherrick AD, Swensen SJ, Hartman TE. Mosaic pattern of lung attenuation on CT scans: frequency among patients with pulmonary artery hypertension of different causes. *AJR Am J Roentgenol* 1997;169:79–82.
58. Primack SL, Muller NL, Mayo JR, et al. Pulmonary parenchymal abnormalities of vascular origin: high-resolution CT findings. *Radiographics* 1994;14:739–746.
59. Mandel J, Mark EJ, Hales CA. Pulmonary veno-occlusive disease. *Am J Respir Crit Care Med* 2000;162:1964–1973.
60. Dennie CJ, Veinot JP, McCormack DG, Rubens FD. Intimal sarcoma of the pulmonary arteries seen as a mosaic pattern of lung attenuation on high-resolution CT. *AJR Am J Roentgenol* 2002;178:1208–1210.
61. Stern EJ, Swensen SJ, Hartman TE, Frank MS. Mosaic pattern of lung attenuation: distinguishing different causes. *AJR Am J Roentgenol* 1995; 165:813–816.
62. Arakawa H, Stern EJ, Nakamoto T, et al. Chronic pulmonary thromboembolism. Air trapping on computed tomography and correlation with pulmonary function tests. *J Comput Assist Tomogr* 2003;27: 735–742.
63. Austin JH, Muller NL, Friedman PJ, et al. Glossary of terms for CT of the lungs: recommendations of the Nomenclature Committee of the Fleischner Society. *Radiology* 1996;200:327–331.
64. Grenier PA, Beigelman-Aubry C, Fetita C, et al. New frontiers in CT imaging of airway disease. *Eur Radiol* 2002;12:1022–1044.
65. Waitches GM, Stern EJ. High-resolution CT of peripheral airways diseases. *Radiol Clin North Am* 2002;40:21–29.
66. Small JH, Flower CD, Traill ZC, Gleeson FV. Air-trapping in extrinsic allergic alveolitis. *Clin Radiol* 1996;51:684–688.
67. King GG, Muller NL, Pare PD. Evaluation of airways in obstructive pulmonary disease using high-resolution computed tomography. *Am J Respir Crit Care Med* 1999;159:992–1004.
68. Lynch DA, Newell JD, Tschomper BA, et al. Uncomplicated asthma in adults: comparison of CT appearance of the lungs in asthmatic and healthy subjects. *Radiology* 1993;188:829–833.
69. Stern EJ, Frank MS. Small-airways disease of the lungs: findings at expiratory CT. *AJR Am J Roentgenol* 1994;163:37–41.
70. Desai SR, Hansell DM. Small airways disease: expiratory computed tomography comes of age. *Clin Radiol* 1997;52:332–337.
71. Arakawa H, Webb WR. Air trapping on expiratory high-resolution CT scans in the absence of inspiratory scan abnormalities: correlation with pulmonary function tests and differential diagnosis. *AJR Am J Roentgenol* 1998;170:1349–1353.
72. Verschakelen JA, Scheinbaum K, Bogaert J, et al. Expiratory CT in cigarette smokers: correlation between areas of decreased lung attenuation, pulmonary function tests and smoking history. *Eur Radiol* 1998; 8:1391–1399.
73. Arakawa H, Kurihara Y, Sasaka K, et al. Air trapping on CT of patients with pulmonary embolism. *AJR Am J Roentgenol* 2002;178:1201–1207.
74. Lee KW, Chung SY, Yang I, et al. Correlation of aging and smoking with air trapping at thin-section CT of the lung in asymptomatic subjects. *Radiology* 2000;214:831–836.
75. Webb WR, Stern EJ, Kanth N, Gamsu G. Dynamic pulmonary CT: findings in healthy adult men. *Radiology* 1993;186:117–124.
76. Park CS, Muller NL, Worthy SA, et al. Airway obstruction in asthmatic and healthy individuals: inspiratory and expiratory thin-section CT findings. *Radiology* 1997;203:361–367.
77. Grenier PA, Beigelman-Aubry C, Fetita C, Martin-Bouyer Y. Multidetector-row CT of the airways. In: Schoepf UJ, ed. *Multidetector-row CT of the thorax.* Berlin: Springer-Verlag, 2004:63–80.
78. Fotheringham T, Chabat F, Hansell DM, et al. A comparison of methods for enhancing the detection of areas of decreased attenuation on CT caused by airways disease. *J Comput Assist Tomogr* 1999;23:385–389.
79. Wittram C, Batt J, Rappaport DC, Hutcheon MA. Inspiratory and expiratory helical CT of normal adults: comparison of thin section scans and minimum intensity projection images. *J Thorac Imaging* 2002; 17:47–52.
80. Rémy-Jardin M, Rémy J. Spiral CT of parenchymal lung disease. In: Rémy-Jardin M, Rémy J, eds. *Spiral CT of the chest.* Berlin: Springer-Verlag, 1996:151–159.
81. Chabat F, Yang Gi, Hansell DM. Obstructive lung diseases: texture classification for differentiation at CT. *Radiology* 2003;228:871–877.
82. Stern EJ, Webb WR, Gamsu G. Dynamic quantitative computed tomography. A predictor of pulmonary function in obstructive lung diseases. *Invest Radiol* 1994;29:564–569.

83. Johnson JL, Kramer SS, Mahboubi S. Air trapping in children: evaluation with dynamic lung densitometry with spiral CT. *Radiology* 1998; 206:95–101.
84. Lucidarme O, Grenier PA, Cadi M, et al. Evaluation of air trapping at CT: comparison of continuous—versus suspended—expiration CT techniques. *Radiology* 2000;216:768–772.
85 Gotway MB, Lee ES, Reddy GP, et al. Low-dose, dynamic, expiratory thin-section CT of the lungs using a spiral CT scanner. *J Thorac Imaging* 2000;15:168–172.
86. Franquet T, Stern EJ, Gimenez A, et al. Lateral decubitus CT: a useful adjunct to standard inspiratory-expiratory CT for the detection of air-trapping. *AJR Am J Roentgenol* 2000;174:528–530.
87. Choi SJ, Choi BK, Kim HJ, et al. Lateral decubitus HRCT: a simple technique to replace expiratory CT in children with air trapping. *Pediatr Radiol* 2002;32:179–182.
88. Ng CS, Desai SR, Rubens MB, et al. Visual quantitation and observer variation of signs of small airways disease at inspiratory and expiratory CT. *J Thorac Imaging* 199914:279–285.
89. Lucidarme O, Coche E, Cluzel P, et al. Expiratory CT scans for chronic airway disease: correlation with pulmonary function test results. *AJR Am J Roentgenol* 1998;170:301–307.
90. Goddard PR, Nicholson EM, Laszlo G, Watt I. Computed tomography in pulmonary emphysema. *Clin Radiol* 1982;33:379–387.
91. Wegener OH, Koeppe P, Oeser H. Measurement of lung density by computed tomography. *J Comput Assist Tomogr* 1978;2:263–273.
92. Newman KB, Lynch DA, Newman LS, et al. Quantitative computed tomography detects air trapping due to asthma. *Chest* 1994;106:105–109.
93. Chabat F, Desai SR, Hansell DM, Yang GZ. Gradient correction and classification of CT lung images for the automated quantification of mosaic attenuation pattern. *J Comput Assist Tomogr* 2000;24:437–447.
94. Kalender WA, Rienmuller R, Seissler W, et al. Measurement of pulmonary parenchymal attenuation: use of spirometric gating with quantitative CT. *Radiology* 1990;175:265–268.
95. Kohz P, Stabler A, Beinert T, et al. Reproducibility of quantitative, spirometrically controlled CT. *Radiology* 1995;197:539–542.
96. Kubo K, Eda S, Yamamoto H, et al. Expiratory and inspiratory chest computed tomography and pulmonary function tests in cigarette smokers. *Eur Respir J* 1999;13:252–256.
97. Primack SL, Logan PM, Hartman TE, et al. Pulmonary tuberculosis and Mycobacterium avium-intracellulare: a comparison of CT findings. *Radiology* 1995;194:413–417.
98. Rosmus HH, Parc JA, Masson AM, Fraser RG. Roentgenographic patterns of acute mycoplasma and viral pneumonitis. *J Can Assoc Radiol* 1968;19:74–77.
99. Im JG, Itoh H, Han MC. CT of pulmonary tuberculosis. *Semin Ultrasound CT MR* 1995;16:420–434.
100. Leung AN. Pulmonary tuberculosis: the essentials. *Radiology* 1999; 210:307–322.
101. Im JG, Itoh H, Shim Y, et al. Pulmonary tuberculosis: CT findings—early active disease and sequential change with anti-tuberculous therapy. *Radiology* 1993;186:653–660.
102. Hatipoglu ON, Osma E, Manisali M, et al. High-resolution computed tomographic findings in pulmonary tuberculosis. *Thorax* 1996;51:397–402.
103. Patz EF, Swensen SJ, Erasmus J. Pulmonary manifestations of nontuberculous mycobacterium. *Radiol Clin North Am* 1995;33:719–729.
104. Lynch DA, Simone PM, Fox MA, et al. CT features of pulmonary mycobacterium avium complex infection. *J Comput Assist Tomogr* 1995;19:353–360.
105. Hollings NP, Wells AU, Wilson R, Hansell DM. Comparative appearances of non-tuberculous mycobacteria species: a CT study. *Eur Radiol* 2002;12:2211–2217.
106. Homma H, Yamanaka A, Tanimoto S, et al. Diffuse panbronchiolitis: a disease of the transitional zone of the lung. *Chest* 1983;83:63–69.
107. Fitzgerald JE, King TE Jr, Lynch DA, et al. Diffuse panbronchiolitis in the United States. *Am J Respir Crit Care Med* 1996;154:497–503.
108. Nishimura K, Kitaichi M, Izumi T, Itoh H. Diffuse panbronchiolitis: correlation of high-resolution CT and pathologic findings. *Radiology* 1992; 184:779–785.
109. Akira M, Kitatani F, Lee YS, et al. Diffuse panbronchiolitis: evaluation with high-resolution CT1. *Radiology* 1988;168:433–438.
110. Akira M, Higashihara T, Sakatani M, Hara H. Diffuse panbronchiolitis: follow-up CT examination. *Radiology* 1993;189:559–562.
111. Howling SJ, Hansell DM, Wells AU, et al. Follicular bronchiolitis: thin-section CT and histologic findings. *Radiology* 1999;212:637–642.
112. Hartman TE, Tazelaar HD, Swensen SJ, Muller NL. Cigarette smoking: CT and pathologic findings of associated pulmonary diseases. *Radiographics* 1997;17:377–390.
113. Moon J, du Bois RM, Colby TV, et al. Clinical significance of respiratory bronchiolitis on open lung biopsy and its relationship to smoking related interstitial lung disease. *Thorax* 1999;54:1009–1014.
114. ATS/ERS International Multidisciplinary Consensus Classification of Idiopathic Interstitial Pneumonias. *Am J Respir Crit Care Med* 2002;165:277–304.
115. Heyneman LE, Ward S, Lynch DA, et al. Respiratory bronchiolitis, respiratory bronchiolitis-associated interstitial lung disease, and desquamative interstitial pneumonia: different entities or part of the spectrum of the same disease process? *AJR Am J Roentgenol* 1999;173: 1617–1622.
116. Essadki O, Chartrand-Lefebvre C, Briere J, Grenier P. Respiratory bronchiolitis: CT findings in a pathologically proven case. *Eur Radiol* 1998; 8:1674–1678.
117. Matsuse T, Oka T, Kida K, Fukuchi Y. Importance of diffuse aspiration bronchiolitis caused by chronic occult aspiration in the elderly. *Chest* 1996;110:1289–1293.
118. Matsuse T, Teramoto S, Matsui H, et al. Widespread occurrence of diffuse aspiration bronchiolitis in patients with dysphagia, irrespective of age. *Chest* 1998;114:350–351.
119. Selman-Lama M, Perez-Padilla R. Airflow obstruction and airway lesions in hypersensitivity pneumonitis. *Clin Chest Med* 1993;14:699–714.
120. Coleman A, Colby TV. Histologic diagnosis of extrinsic allergic alveolitis. *Am J Surg Pathol* 1988;12:514–518.
121. Matar LD, McAdams HP, Sporn TA. Hypersensitivity pneumonitis. *AJR Am J Roentgenol* 2000;174:1061–1066.
122. Silver SF, Muller NL, Miller RR, Lefcoe MS. Hypersensitivity pneumonitis. Evaluation with CT. *Radiology* 1989;173:441–445.
123. Hansell DM, Moskovic E. High-resolution computed tomography in extrinsic allergic alveolitis. *Clin Radiol* 1991;43:8–12.
124. Rémy-Jardin M, Rémy J, Wallaert B, Muller NL. Subacute and chronic bird breeder hypersensitivity pneumonitis: sequential evaluation with CT and correlation with lung function tests and bronchoalveolar lavage. *Radiology* 1993;189:111–118.
125. Adler BD, Paddle SP, Muller NL, et al. Chronic hypersensitivity pneumonitis: high-resolution CT and radiographic features in 16 patients. *Radiology* 1992;185:91–95.
126. Lynch DA, Newell JD, Logan PM, et al. Can CT distinguish hypersensitivity pneumonitis from idiopathic pulmonary fibrosis? *AJR Am J Roentgenol* 1995;165:807–811.
127. Alasaly K, Muller N, Ostrow DN, et al. Cryptogenic organizing pneumonia. A report of 25 cases and a review of the literature. *Medicine (Baltimore)* 1995;74:201–211.
128. Muller N, Guerry-Force ML, Staples C, et al. Differential diagnosis of bronchiolitis obliterans with organizing pneumonia and usual interstitial pneumonia: clinical, functional, and radiologic findings. *Radiology* 1987;162; 151–156.
129. Chandler PW, Shin MS, Friedman SE, et al. Radiographic manifestations of bronchiolitis obliterans with organizing pneumonia vs usual interstitial pneumonia. *AJR Am J Roentgenol* 1986;147:899–906.
130. Akira M, Yamamoto S, Sakatani M. Bronchiolitis obliterans organizing pneumonia manifesting as multiple large nodules or masses. *AJR Am J Roentgenol* 1998;170:291–295.
131. Oikonomou A, Hansell DM. Organizing pneumonia: the many morphological faces. *Eur Radiol* 2002;12:1486–1496.
132. Murphy JM, Schnyder P, Verschakelen J, et al. Linear opacities on HRCT in bronchiolitis obliterans organising pneumonia. *Eur Radiol* 1999; 9:1813–1817.
133. Zompatori M, Poletti V, Battista G, Diegoli M. Bronchiolitis obliterans with organizing pneumonia (BOOP), presenting as a ring-shaped opacity at HRCT (the atoll sign). A case report. *Radiol Med* 1999;97:308–310.
134. Voloudaki AE, Bouros DE, Froudarakis ME, et al. Crescentic and ring-shaped opacities. CT features in two cases of bronchiolitis obliterans organizing pneumonia (BOOP). *Acta Radiol* 1996;37:889–892.
135. Kim SJ, Lee KS, Ryu YH, et al. Reversed halo sign on high-resolution CT of cryptogenic organizing pneumonia: diagnostic implications. *AJR Am J Roentgenol* 2003;180:1251–1254.
136. Logan PM, Miller RR, Muller NL. Cryptogenic organizing pneumonia in the immunocompromised patient: radiologic findings and follow-up in 12 patients. *Can Assoc Radiol J* 1995;46:272–279.
137. Haro M, Vizcaya M, Texido A, et al. Idiopathic bronchiolitis obliterans organizing pneumonia with multiple cavitary lung nodules. *Eur Respir J* 1995;8:1975–1977.
138. Froudarakis M, Bouros D, Loire R, et al. BOOP presenting with haemoptysis and multiple cavitary nodules. *Eur Respir J* 1995;8:1972–1974.
139. Murphy J, Schnyder P, Herold C, Flower C. Bronchiolitis obliterans organising pneumonia simulating bronchial carcinoma. *Eur Radiol* 1998; 8:1165–1169.
140. Heller I, Biner S, Isakov A, et al. TB or not TB: cavitary bronchiolitis obliterans organizing pneumonia mimicking pulmonary tuberculosis. *Chest* 2001;120:674–678.
141. Johkoh T, Muller NL, Cartier Y, et al. Idiopathic interstitial pneumonias: diagnostic accuracy of thin-section CT in 129 patients. *Radiology* 1999; 211:555–560.
142. Lohr RH, Boland BJ, Douglas WW, et al. Organizing pneumonia. Features and prognosis of cryptogenic, secondary, and focal variants. *Arch Intern Med* 1997;157:1323–1329.
143. Breatnach E, Kerr I. The radiology of cryptogenic obliterative bronchiolitis. *Clin Radiol* 1982;33:657–661.
144. Skeens JL, Fuhrman CR, Yousem SA. Bronchiolitis obliterans in heart-lung transplantation patients: radiologic findings in 11 patients. *AJR Am J Roentgenol* 1989;153:253–256.
145. Sweatman MC, Millar AB, Strickland B, Turner-Warwick M. Computed tomography in adult obliterative bronchiolitis. *Clin Radiol* 1990;41:116–119.
146. Morrish WF, Herman SJ, Weisbrod GL, Chamberlain DW. Bronchiolitis obliterans after lung transplantation: findings at chest radiography and high-resolution CT. *Radiology* 1991;179:487–490.

147. Leung AN, Fisher K, Valentine V, et al. Bronchiolitis obliterans after lung transplantation: detection using expiratory HRCT. *Chest* 1998; 113:365–370.
148. Worthy SA, Flint JD, Muller NL. Pulmonary complications after bone marrow transplantation: high-resolution CT and pathologic findings. *Radiographics* 17:1359–1371.
149. Lentz D, Bergin CJ, Berry GJ, et al. Diagnosis of bronchiolitis obliterans in heart-lung transplantation patients: importance of bronchial dilatation on CT. *AJR Am J Roentgenol* 1992;159:463–467.
150. Copley SJ, Wells AU, Müller NL, et al. Thin-section CT in obstructive pulmonary disease: discriminatory value. *Radiology* 2002;223:812–819.
151. Zhang L, Irion K, da Silva Porto N, Abreu e Silva F. High-resolution computed tomography in pediatric patients with postinfectious bronchiolitis obliterans. *J Thorac Imaging* 1999;14:85–89.
152. Chang AB, Masel JP, Masters B. Post-infectious bronchiolitis obliterans: clinical, radiological and pulmonary function sequelae. *Pediatr Radiol* 1998;28:23–29.
153. Marti-Bonmati L, Ruiz Perales F, Catala F, et al. CT findings in Swyer-James syndrome. *Radiology* 1989;172:477–480.
154. Moore AD, Godwin JD, Dietrich PA, et al. Swyer-James syndrome: CT findings in eight patients. *AJR Am J Roentgenol* 1992;158:1211–1215.
155. Tasaka S, Kanazawa M, Mori M, et al. Long-term course of bronchiectasis and bronchiolitis obliterans as late complication of smoke inhalation. *Respiration* 1995;62:40–42.
156. Hansell DM, Wells AU, Rubens MB, Cole PJ. Bronchiectasis: functional significance of areas of decreased attenuation at expiratory CT. *Radiology* 1994;193:369–74.
157. Roberts HR, Wells AU, Milne DG, et al. Airflow obstruction in bronchiectasis: correlation between computed tomography features and pulmonary function tests. *Thorax* 2000;55:198–204.
158. Estenne M, Hertz MI. Bronchiolitis obliterans after human lung transplantation. *Am J Respir Crit Care Med* 2002;15;166:440–444.
159. Cooper JD, Billingham M, Egan T, et al. A working formulation for the standardization of nomenclature and for clinical staging of chronic dysfunction in lung allografts. International Society for Heart and Lung Transplantation. *J Heart Lung Transplant* 1993;12:713–716.
160. Miller WT Jr, Kotloff RM, Blumenthal NP, et al. Utility of high resolution computed tomography in predicting bronchiolitis obliterans syndrome following lung transplantation: preliminary findings. *J Thorac Imaging* 2001;16:76–80.
161. Lee ES, Gotway MB, Reddy GP, et al. Early bronchiolitis obliterans following lung transplantation: accuracy of expiratory thin-section CT for diagnosis. *Radiology* 2000;216:472–477.
162. Lau DM, Siegel MJ, Hildebolt CF, Cohen AH. Bronchiolitis obliterans syndrome: thin-section CT diagnosis of obstructive changes in infants and young children after lung transplantation. *Radiology* 1998; 208:783–788.
163. Ooi GC, Peh WC, Ip M. High-resolution computed tomography of bronchiolitis obliterans syndrome after bone marrow transplantation. *Respiration* 1998;65:187–191.
164. Worthy SA, Park CS, Kim JS, Muller NL. Bronchiolitis obliterans after lung transplantation: high-resolution CT findings in 15 patients. *AJR Am J Roentgenol* 1997;169:673–677.
165. Konen E, Gutierrez C, Chaparro C, et al. Bronchiolitis obliterans syndrome in lung transplant recipients: can thin section CT findings predict disease before its clinical appearance? *Radiology* 2004;231:467–473.
166. Bankier AA, van Muylem A, Scillia P, et al. Air trapping in heart-lung transplant recipients: variability of anatomic distribution and extent at sequential expiratory thin-section CT. *Radiology* 2003;229:737–742.
167. Bankier AA, van Muylem A, Knoop C, et al. Bronchiolitis obliterans syndrome in heart-lung transplant recipients: diagnosis with expiratory CT. *Radiology* 2001;218:533–539.
168. Choi YW, Rossi SE, Palmer SM, et al. Bronchiolitis obliterans syndrome in lung transplant recipients: correlation of computed tomography findings with bronchiolitis obliterans syndrome stage. *J Thorac Imaging* 2003;18:72–79.
169. Knollman FD, Ewert R, Wündrich T, et al. Bronchiolitis obliterans syndrome in lung transplant recipients: use of spirometrically gated CT. *Radiology* 2002;225:655–662.
170. Siegel MJ, Bhalla S, Gutierrez FR, Hildebolt C, Sweet S. Post-lung transplantation bronchiolitis obliterans syndrome: usefulness of expiratory thin-section CT for diagnosis. *Radiology* 2001;220:455–462.
171. Hayakawa H, Sato A, Imokawa S, et al. Bronchiolar disease in rheumatoid arthritis. *Am J Respir Crit Care Med* 1996;154:1531–1536.
172. Akira M, Sakatani M, Hara H. Thin-section CT findings in rheumatoid arthritis-associated lung disease: CT patterns and their courses. *J Comput Assist Tomogr* 1999;23:941–948.
173. McDonagh J, Greaves M, Wright AR, et al. High resolution computed tomography of the lungs in patients with rheumatoid arthritis and interstitial lung disease. *Br J Rheumatol* 1994;33:118–122.
174. Rémy-Jardin M, Rémy J, Cortet B, et al. Lung changes in rheumatoid arthritis: CT findings. *Radiology* 1994;193:375–382.
175. Perez T, Rémy-Jardin M, Cortet B. Airways involvement in rheumatoid arthritis: clinical, functional, and HRCT findings. *Am J Respir Crit Care Med* 1998;157:1658–1665.
176. Taouli B, Brauner MW, Mourey I, et al. Thin-section chest CT findings of primary Sjögren's syndrome: correlation with pulmonary function. *Eur Radiol* 2002;12:1504–1511.
177. Franquet T, Diaz C, Domingo P, et al. Air trapping in primary Sjögren syndrome: correlation of expiratory CT with pulmonary function tests. *J Comput Assist Tomogr* 1999;23:169–173.
178. Aguayo SM, Miller YE, Waldron JA Jr, et al. Brief report: idiopathic diffuse hyperplasia of pulmonary neuroendocrine cells and airways disease. *N Engl J Med* 1992;327:1285–1288.
179. Miller MA, Mark GJ, Kanarek D. Multiple peripheral pulmonary carcinoids and tumorlets of carcinoid type, with restrictive and obstructive lung disease. *Am J Med* 1978;65:373–378.
180. Brown MJ, English J, Müller NL. Bronchiolitis obliterans due to neuroendocrine hyperplasia: high-resolution CT—pathologic correlations. *AJR Am J Roentgenol* 1997;168:1561–1562.
181. Gleeson FV, Traill ZC, Hansell DM. Expiratory CT evidence of small airways obstruction in sarcoidosis. *AJR Am J Roentgenol* 1996; 166:1052–1054.
182. Bartz RR, Stern EJ. Airways obstruction in patients with sarcoidosis: expiratory CT scan findings. *J Thorac Imaging* 2000;15:285–289.
183. Davies CW, Tasker AD, Padley SP, et al. Air trapping in sarcoidosis on computed tomography: correlation with lung function. *Clin Radiol* 2000;55:217–221.
184. Hansell DM, Milne DG, Wilsher ML, Wells AU. Pulmonary sarcoidosis: morphologic associations of airflow obstruction at thin-section CT. *Radiology* 1998;209:697–704.
185. Cosio MG, Hale KA, Niewoehner DE. Morphologic and morphometric effects of prolonged cigarette on the small airways. *Am Rev Respir Dis* 1980;122:265–321.
186. Niewoehner DE, Knoke JD, Kleinerman J. Peripheral airways as a determinant of ventilatory function in the human lung. *J Clin Invest* 1977; 60:139–151.
187. Niewoehner DE, Kleinerman J. Morphologic basis of pulmonary resistance in the human lung and effects of aging. *J Appl Physiol* 1974; 36:412–418.
188. Hogg JC, Macklem PT, Thurlbeck WM. Site and nature of airway obstruction in chronic obstructive lung disease. *N Engl J Med* 1968; 278:1355–1360.
189. Rémy-Jardin M, Rémy J, Boulenguez C, et al. Morphologic effects of cigarette smoking on airways and pulmonary parenchyma in healthy adult volunteers: CT evaluation and correlation with pulmonary function tests. *Radiology* 1993;186:107–115.
190. Tanaka N, Matsumoto T, Miura G, et al. Air trapping at CT: high prevalence in asymptomatic subjects with normal pulmonary function. *Radiology* 2003;227:776–785.
191. Mastora I, Rémy-Jardin M, Sobaszek A, et al. Thin-section CT finding in 250 volunteers: assessment of the relationship of CT findings with smoking history and pulmonary function test results. *Radiology* 2001; 218:695–702.
192. Pelinkovic D, Lorcher U, Chow KU, et al. Spirometric gated quantitative computed tomography of the lung in healthy smokers and nonsmokers. *Invest Radiol* 1997;32:335–343.
193. Rémy-Jardin M, Edme JL, Boulenguez C, et al. Longitudinal follow-up study of smoker's lung with thin-section CT in correlation with pulmonary function tests. *Radiology* 2002;222:261–270.
194. Soejima K, Yamaguchi K, Kohda E, et al. Longitudinal follow-up study of smoking-induced lung density changes by high-resolution computed tomography. *Am J Respir Crit Care Med* 2000;161:1264–1273.
195. Lynch DA. Imaging of asthma and allergic bronchopulmonary mycosis. *Radiol Clin North Am* 1998;36:129–142.
196. Grenier P, Mourey-Gerosa I, Benali K, et al. Abnormalities of the airways and lung parenchyma in asthmatics: CT observations in 50 patients and inter- and intra-observer variability. *Eur Radiol* 1996;6:199–206.
197. Paganin F, Seneterre E, Chanez P, et al. Computed tomography of the lungs in asthma: influence of disease severity and etiology. *Am J Respir Crit Care Med* 1996;153:110–114.
198. Goldin JG, McNitt-Gray MF, Sorensen SM, et al. Airway hyperreactivity: assessment with helical thin-section CT. *Radiology* 1998;208:321–329.
199. Beigelman-Aubry C, Capderou A, Grenier PA, et al. Mild intermittent asthma: CT assessment of bronchial cross-sectional area and lung attenuation at controlled lung volume. *Radiology* 2002;223:181–187.
200. Laurent F, Latrabe V, Raherison C, et al. Functional significance of air trapping detected in moderate asthma. *Eur Radiol* 2000;10:1404–1410.
201. Jensen SP, Lynch DA, Brown KK, et al. High-resolution CT features of severe asthma and bronchiolitis obliterans. *Clin Radiol* 2002;57: 1078–1085.
202. Lange P, Parner J, Vestbo J, et al. A 15-year follow-up study of ventilatory function in adults with asthma. *N Engl J Med* 1998;339:1194–1200.

Functional Imaging of the Airways

6

Advances in thoracic imaging, until recently, have been focused primarily on improved depiction of structural changes. The introduction of high-resolution computed tomography (HRCT) scanning of the lungs and, more recently, multidetector helical scanners, together with newer volumetric image analysis tools, has greatly advanced anatomic imaging of the airways and the lung parenchyma.

Static structural images, however, do not begin to reflect the highly physiologic nature of the lungs: the cyclic flow of inspired gas from the upper airway into the distal airspaces, the changing caliber and wall thickness of airways during the respiratory cycle, the ongoing exchange of oxygen and carbon dioxide across the alveolar-capillary wall, the auto-regulation and matching of regional ventilation and perfusion, the flow of expired gas from the alveoli back to the upper airway, and the rhythmic motions of the heart, diaphragms, and chest wall. Although we marvel at what we have been able to image, these important functions have been largely invisible to the eyes of the radiologist, as dark matter and dark energy are to the astronomer and cosmologist.

Functional imaging of the lungs has largely been indirect, relegated to correlating the structural changes depicted on these scans with conventional pulmonary function tests (PFTs). For example, CT-based grading of emphysema has been correlated with spirometric measures of airflow obstruction and decreased diffusion capacity, and likewise grading of interstitial lung disease with PFT measures of restrictive physiology.

Direct functional imaging of the lungs until recently has been largely limited to nuclear medicine techniques, including standard ventilation and perfusion scintigraphy and, to a lesser extent, single-photon emission tomography (SPECT) and positron emission tomography (PET). The introduction of both static inspiratory-expiratory CT scanning and dynamic imaging with electron beam CT (EBCT), as well as with multirow detectors for helical CT, enabled evaluation of abnormal tracheobronchial collapse and/or gas trapping. HRCT has been used to measure the caliber and wall thickness of bronchi in response to pharmacologic agents such as methacholine and bronchodilators in studies of airway reactivity in asthma. These techniques represent important initial steps in using CT to evaluate airway function.

We are witnessing the emergence of a number of exciting, new approaches to direct imaging of pulmonary ventilation, principally using magnetic resonance (MR) and CT techniques (Tables 6-1 and 6-2). The introduction of new MR contrast agents, including the hyperpolarized noble gases ^{3}helium and ^{129}xenon among others, along with more rapid pulse sequences, have enabled direct imaging of gas wash-in, distribution in the lungs, and washout with unprecedented spatial and temporal resolution. Likewise, dynamic, high-resolution, contrast-enhanced CT ventilation scanning using stable nonradioactive xenon gas recently has been shown to be feasible.

These new techniques offer a number of substantial advantages over traditional methods of assessing pulmonary function. Although conventional PFTs have become an indispensable tool in pulmonary medicine, and have revealed a wealth of information about lung physiology in normal and diseased states, they are limited to global measurements of total lung function. The image-based methods, on the other hand, can provide quantitative displays of regional lung function, not only of individual lungs but also of lobes, segments, and even smaller regions. This represents a major step forward, since the physiology of both the normal lung and virtually all lung

TABLE 6-1
MR VENTILATION AGENTS

MR Ventilation Agents
Hyperpolarized ^{3}helium
Hyperpolarized ^{129}xenon
^{19}Fluorine
Oxygen
Aerosolized gadolinium agents
Air (regional mechanics)

disorders is heterogeneous to some degree (Fig. 6-1). Common examples include centrilobular emphysema, which is commonly upper zone predominant; usual interstitial pneumonia, a typically basilar disease with temporal and spatial heterogeneity in its pathologic evolution (Fig. 6-2); asthma and small airway disease, in which the airway abnormalities are heterogeneously distributed both spatially and temporally; pulmonary embolism, which involves select pulmonary vascular distributions; and adult respiratory distress syndrome (ARDS), in which the lung involvement and resulting mechanical impairment are typically heterogeneously distributed.

Moreover, these new methods are able to image other physiologic parameters that were previously unavailable on a region-by-region basis, such as alveolar oxygen partial pressures, airway gas diffusion rates, alveolar–capillary gas diffusion, direct ventilation–perfusion matching, and regional lung biomechanics. In addition, these multiparametric functional maps can be coregistered and overlaid on the high-resolution anatomic displays, providing exciting new ways to visualize structure–function relationships in the lung. Furthermore, this new functional information can be used to determine morphometric features of alveolar microstructure, such as alveolar size, shape, and wall thickness, which are beyond the anatomic resolution capability of current clinical scanners. Thus, with these new imaging developments we have moved from extrapolating function from structure to revealing lung microstructure from function.

Although many of these new methods are investigational and/or in an early stage of clinical application, they offer the potential not only to localize sites of disease for therapy but also possibly to detect the onset of disease before the onset of visible structural changes or detection by less sensitive global PFT measurements. These evolving functional imaging techniques also hold promise as a means to monitor new therapies, such as surgical and mechanical approaches to advanced emphysema, new medical treatments for asthma and chronic interstitial disease, or tailoring of mechanical ventilatory parameters in ARDS.

In this chapter, we describe and illustrate these new functional imaging techniques and their applications to the evaluation of normal and diseased airways. Although clearly molecular imaging technologies, including PET and optical methods, which are currently in their infancy, represent another major future direction in the functional

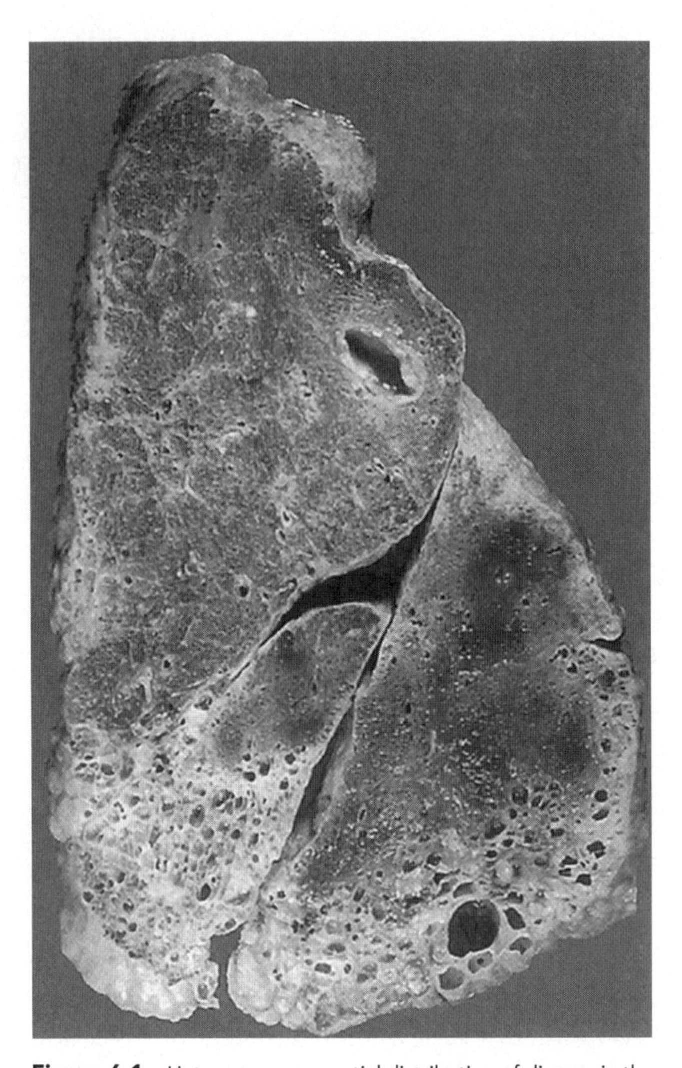

Figure 6-1 Heterogeneous spatial distribution of disease in the lung. Sagittal slice of the right lung with usual interstitial pneumonia shows severe fibrosis and honeycomb change in the basal aspects of the lower and middle lobes. Less marked disease can be seen in the subpleural region of the anterior portion of the upper lobe and posterior portion of the lower. (From Muller NL, Fraser RS, Lee KS, Johkoh T. *Diseases of the lung. Radiologic and pathologic correlations*. Philadelphia: Lippincott Williams & Wilkins, 2003, with permission.)

TABLE 6-2
CT VENTILATION AGENTS

CT Ventilation Agents
Air (inspiratory–expiratory HRCT, dynamic CT)
Xenon (stable, nonradioactive gas)
Aerosolized iodinated agents
SF6

CT, computed tomography; HRCT, high-resolution computed tomography; SF6, sulfur hexafluoride.

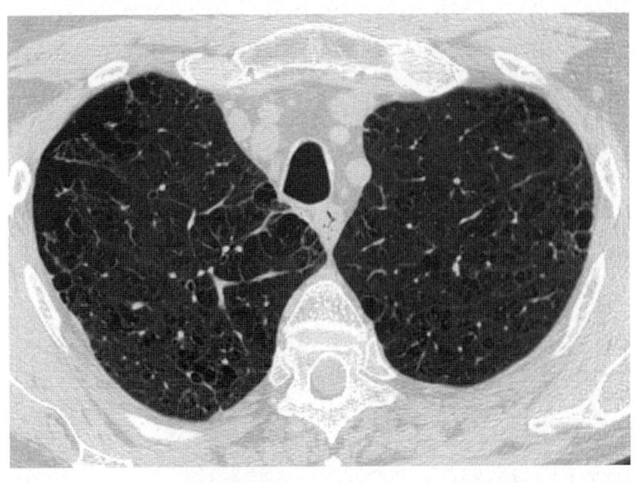

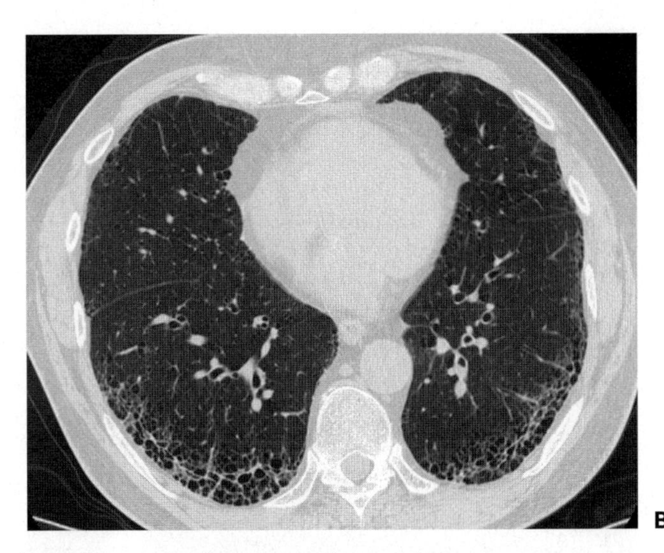

Figure 6-2 **A** and **B:** Regional distribution of pathology is illustrated in this patient with centrilobular emphysema in the upper lung zones **(A),** and pulmonary fibrosis with honeycombing resulting from idiopathic pulmonary fibrosis (IPF) in the lower lung zones **(B).** Conventional PFTs may indicate mixed obstructive and restrictive physiologies but, unlike CT, cannot spatially separate these processes.

imaging of lung disease, we focus here on physiologic imaging primarily using CT and MR.

THE UPPER AIRWAY

The upper airway is an important, albeit underemphasized component of the respiratory tract. Not only is the upper airway the portal of entry for ventilation, but also the entire tidal volume during each breath must traverse a rather small aperture along the small-diameter segments of the retropharyngeal and retroglossal airway (Fig. 6-3). Interestingly, the upper airway must be rigid enough to withstand collapse by the negative intraluminal pressure generated during inspiration, and yet it must be sufficiently compliant to allow for the marked shape changes that are needed for swallowing and phonation. Thus, the upper airway is a finely controlled apparatus in which the caliber of the airway lumen is maintained by active dilator muscle activity counterbalancing the inspiratory negative intraluminal pressure.

Upper airway imaging studies using both ultrafast MR and EBCT, in conjunction with physiologic monitoring of respiration, are providing new insights into the biomechanical functioning of the normal upper airway, as well as clues to the pathophysiology of obstructive sleep apnea (OSA), a common respiratory disorder (1). Furthermore, these upper airway imaging techniques are helping to elucidate the mechanisms underlying the efficacy of various therapeutic interventions for this disorder. Dynamic imaging during both wakefulness and sleep has provided the opportunity to analyze the behavior of upper airway structures during respiration as well as airway closure associated with apneic events. Although upper airway imaging currently serves primarily as a powerful research tool, clinical indications for upper airway imaging in OSA are emerging. For example, MR imaging may be considered for preoperative evaluation of patients undergoing surgical treatment (uvulopalatopharyngoplasty) or CT scanning with volumetric reconstructions in patients undergoing maxillomandibular advancement (1).

Respiratory-related dynamic upper airway imaging has been performed with CT, MR, and nasopharyngoscopy. EBCT studies in normal persons and in patients with OSA during wakefulness have revealed that (Fig. 6-4): (a) at the onset of inspiration, there is a small increase in upper airway area, presumably reflecting increased activity of the upper airway dilator muscles; (b) during most of inspiration, the airway area remains relatively constant, suggesting a balance between upper airway dilator muscle action and the negative intraluminal pressure; (c) in early expiration, upper airway caliber increases owing to positive airway pressure expanding the passive airway; this expansion is relatively larger in patients with OSA, reflecting a more distensible airway; and (d) at end-expiration, airway caliber rapidly decreases because neither the expiratory positive intraluminal pressure nor the phasic inspiratory active dilator muscle activity is available to distend the airway. This end-expiratory collapse is particularly evident in OSA patients, suggesting greater collapsibility of the apneic airway. These transluminal cross-sectional changes are greater in the lateral dimension, reflecting the behavior of the lateral pharyngeal muscular walls, compared with the anteroposterior dimension which relates to the position of the soft palate and the tongue (2,3).

These data, obtained via imaging, suggest that the upper airway may be particularly susceptible to collapse at the end of expiration. Shephard et al. (4) using EBCT also found that airway caliber was smallest at the end of expiration in apneics. Of note, these data suggest that airway closure is occurring at end-expiration, before the generation of negative

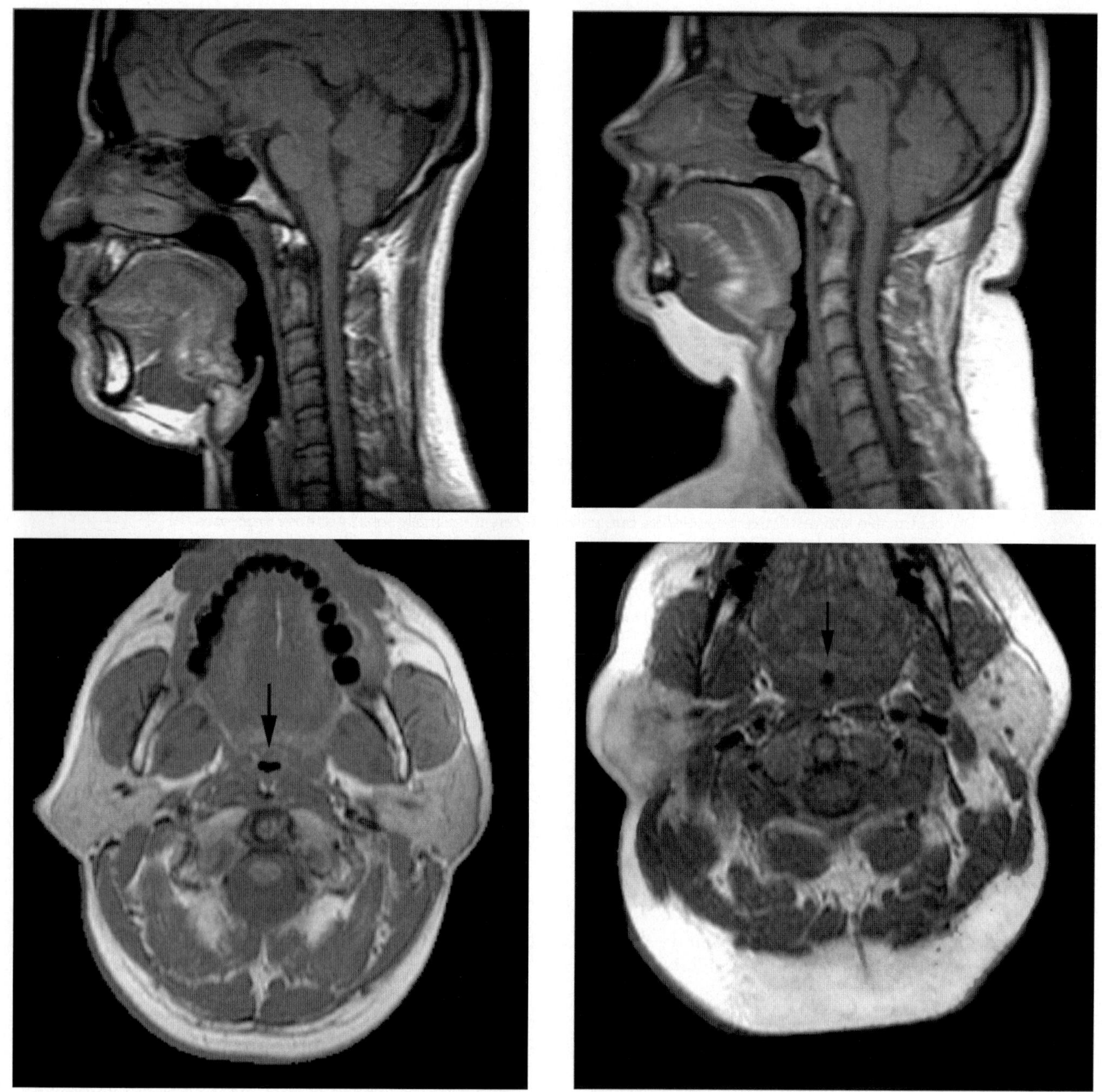

Figure 6-3 **A:** Midsagittal MR image of the upper airway in a normal subject. **B:** Midsagittal MR image of the upper airway in a patient with obstructive sleep apnea (OSA), demonstrating airway narrowing. Note increased submental and posterior subcutaneous fat. Comparison of an axial MR image in the retropalatal region of a normal subject **(C)** and a patient with sleep apnea **(D).** The patient with sleep apnea has a smaller airway area and width and a larger lateral pharyngeal wall.

pressure during inspiration. Imaging studies obtained during sleep have also supported these findings. Studies of airway closure during sleep with nasopharyngoscopy (5) revealed that airway narrowing occurred during expiration, again indicating the importance of end-expiration in the genesis of obstructive apneas. Application of positive airway pressure near the end of expiration to prevent this narrowing of the airway may thus be beneficial in OSA.

CT studies have revealed that the respiratory-related changes in upper airway caliber are predominantly in the lateral rather than the anteroposterior dimension, implying that the lateral walls play an important role in modulating airway caliber (2,3). Cine MRI has also confirmed these CT findings, demonstrating an inverse relationship between airway caliber and the size of the lateral pharyngeal walls (6). The latter were relatively constant in inspiration,

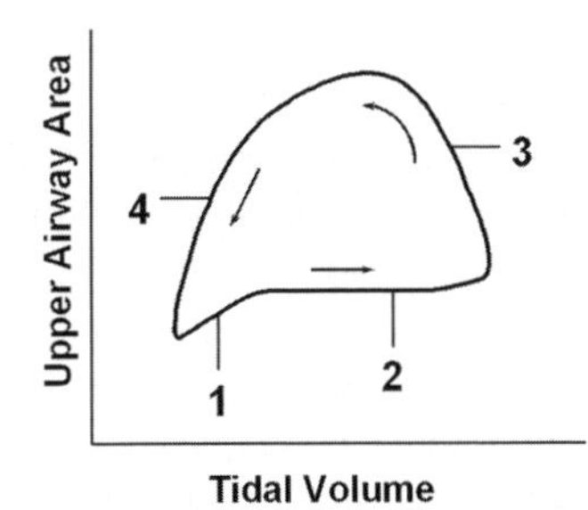

Figure 6-4 Diagram of the changes in upper airway area as a function of tidal volume during the respiratory cycle in an apneic patient. Airway narrowing is maximal at end-expiration. (See text for description of each phase.)

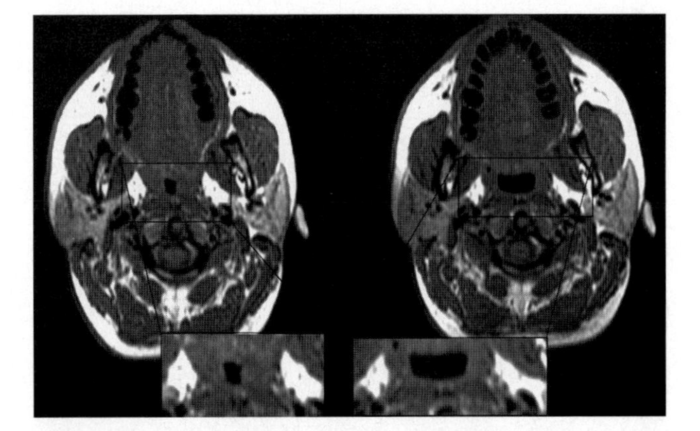

Figure 6-5 Effect of CPAP on the upper airway. Axial MR image at the retropalatal region in a normal subject with 0 cm H_2O of CPAP *(left)* and CPAP of 15 cm H_2O *(right)*. Airway enlargement is demonstrated predominantly in the lateral dimension with the application of 15 cm H_2O of CPAP. The anterior–posterior dimension is not significantly changed.

thinned in early expiration, and thickened toward the end of expiration. Contrary to expectations, these data indicated that the lateral pharyngeal airway muscles are more important than the tongue and soft palate in mediating respiratory cycle–related dynamic changes in upper airway cross-sectional areas.

MR studies using magnetic tagging stripes can be performed to track the motion of the soft tissues surrounding the airway, providing a more detailed visualization of the biomechanical effects of upper airway muscles in modulating airway caliber and shape. Furthermore, MR imaging can now be performed during electrode stimulation of specific muscles to further elucidate the role of various upper airway muscles in controlling the configuration of the airway (7).

The majority of CT and MR imaging studies, although not all, have shown a smaller upper airway in apneics compared with normals (Fig 6-3) (1). Airway narrowing is greatest in the retropalatal region in normals and OSA patients. CT and MR studies have shown that the upper airway in normals has a horizontal orientation (elliptical with the major axis in the coronal plane) in contrast to the apneic airway, which has an anteroposterior orientation (elliptical with lateral narrowing) (Fig. 6-3) (2,8). This lateral narrowing of the apneic airway is associated with increased thickness of the lateral pharyngeal walls. The basis for this increased thickness is unclear. Possible factors include fatty infiltration of the tissues, edema, muscle hypertrophy, or contracted muscles associated with radial and longitudinal airway collapse.

Furthermore, the total volume of parapharyngeal fat is greater in obese patients with apnea, contributing to the lateral narrowing (9–12). The mechanism whereby obesity predisposes to sleep apnea remains controversial, however. Craniofacial bony abnormalities as well as increased soft palate and tongue volume have also been observed in OSA, further compromising upper airway size.

Continuous positive airway pressure (CPAP) is a highly effective noninvasive therapy for OSA, presumably by acting as a pneumatic splint. CT (13) and MR (14) imaging studies in normals and in patients with OSA during the application of varying levels of nasal CPAP, together with compliance modeling, have demonstrated maximum effective compliance along the lateral walls of the retropalatal segment of the airway (Fig. 6-5). Such studies again indicate that the lateral wall muscles play an important role in modulating upper airway caliber and appear most susceptible to collapse.

The abnormal configuration of the upper airway in OSA patients may adversely affect the upper airway muscle activity and predispose the apneic to airway closure during sleep. In addition to dynamic upper airway imaging, studies performed during both wakefulness and sleep have led to further advancements in our understanding of the pathogenesis of sleep apnea. Imaging studies during sleep are particularly relevant because sites of upper airway narrowing during wakefulness do not exactly correlate with the site of obstruction during sleep. Several studies using conventional CT and/or EBCT have evaluated airway caliber in apneic patients during sleep. Horner et al. (15) demonstrated that airway obstruction during sleep was the result of posterior displacement of the soft palate and tongue as well as lateral displacement of the pharyngeal walls. Investigations using EBCT have demonstrated multiple sites of airway occlusion in the retropalatal and retroglossal regions during apneic events (16) Suto et al. (17) also demonstrated retropalatal airway closure in both normals and apneics during sleep using sagittal ultrafast MRI. State-dependent changes in airway caliber and surrounding soft tissue structures in normal subjects have been studied using MRI. The volume of the retropalatal airway was found to be reduced by 19% in normals during sleep (Fig. 6-6) (18). The narrowest portion of the airway was in the retropalatal region.

THE TRACHEA

From the upper airway, inspired gas is conducted via the trachea into the bronchial tree. The tracheal cartilages protect the anterior and lateral walls of the intrathoracic

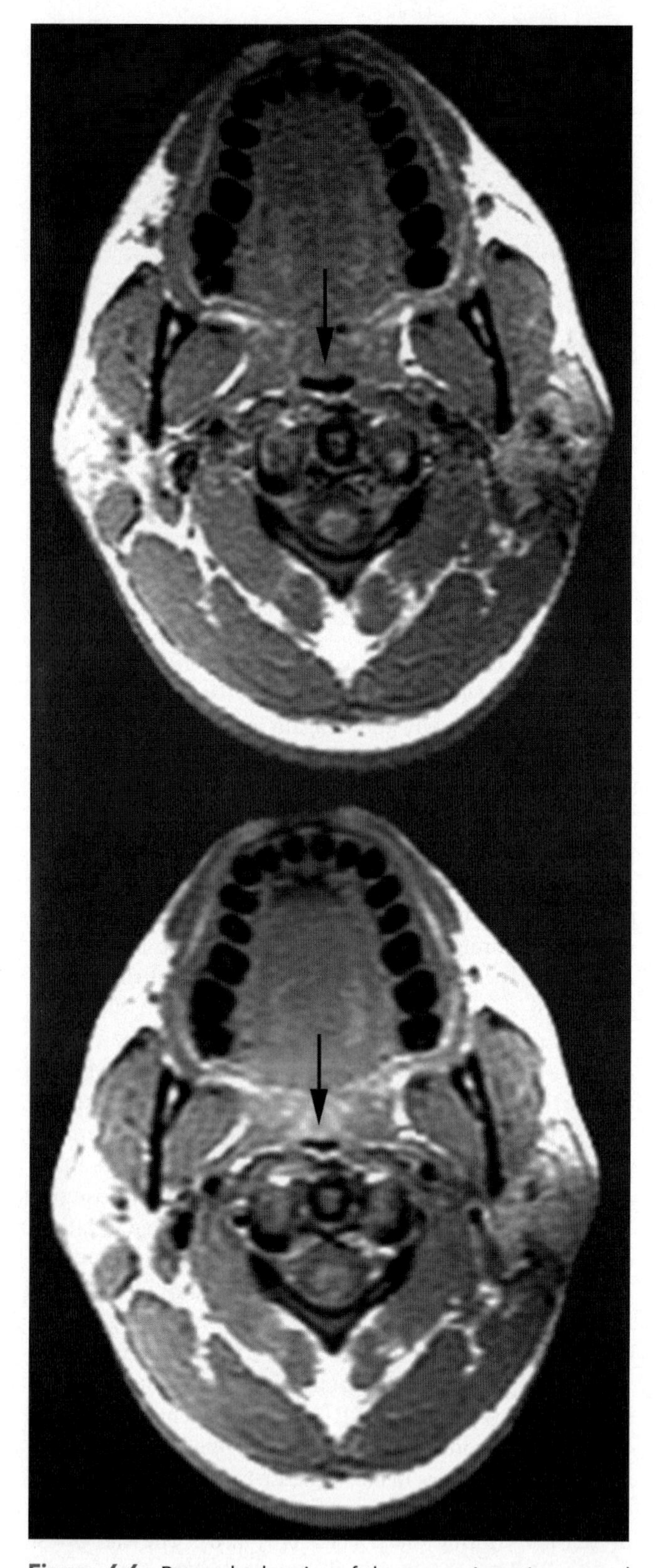

Figure 6-6 Retropalatal region of the upper airway in a normal subject during wakefulness *(top)* and sleep *(bottom)*. Anterior–posterior and lateral airway narrowing is demonstrated during sleep. Thickening of the lateral pharyngeal walls occurs during sleep, reducing airway cross-sectional area.

trachea from collapse during expiration, although the posterior membranous portion is susceptible to the intraluminal tracheal pressure changes occurring with respiration. Using EBCT in normal subjects, Stern et al. (19) found that the tracheal airway surface decreased 35% from full inspiration to expiration (280 mm^2 to 178 mm^2). Normal bowing of the posterior membranous trachea is thus observed in expiration.

In tracheobronchomalacia, damage to the tracheal cartilage with resultant loss of the normal structural integrity of the airway wall leads to an increase in tracheal compliance and increased flaccidity. The latter is most evident during coughing or forced expiration. The coronal diameter of the trachea substantially exceeds the sagittal diameter, resulting in a so-called lunate configuration (Fig. 6-7).

Dynamic expiratory multislice CT scanning has now become a feasible alternative to bronchoscopy for the diagnosis of suspected tracheobronchomalacia (20). Such dynamic expiratory CT may demonstrate collapse of greater than 75% of the airway lumen. Some patients may even show complete collapse of the trachea. The marked bowing of the posterior tracheal wall, which may be focal or diffuse, gives rise to an oval or crescent shape (21).

In patients with chronic obstructive pulmonary disease (COPD), the high downstream resistance can result in excessive dynamic tracheal transmural pressure gradients. These may cause tracheal caliber changes of greater than 50% with expiration, despite normal intrinsic tracheal compliance. Thus, a decrease of greater than 70% in the cross-sectional area of the tracheal lumen in expiration should be used in diagnosing tracheomalacia (19).

Patients with COPD may also show a decrease in the amount of bronchial cartilage (22–24). This has been found to be most severe in segmental and subsegmental bronchi and more prevalent in the lower than the upper lobes. CT may thus demonstrate an exaggerated expiratory bronchial collapse in patients with COPD.

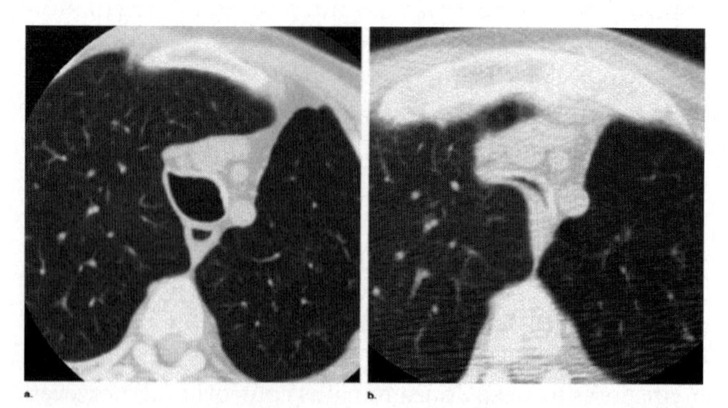

Figure 6-7 Tracheobronchomalacia. A 62-year-old man with chronic cough and progressive dyspnea. **Left:** CT scan of upper thoracic trachea shows an accentuated coronal diameter, also referred to as a "lunate" configuration. **Right:** Low-dose (40 mA) dynamic expiratory CT scan at a similar level shows excessive narrowing of the tracheal lumen, consistent with tracheobronchomalacia. (From Zheng J, Hasegawa I, Feller-Kopman D, Boiselle PM. Dynamic expiratory volumetric CT imaging of the central airways: comparison of standard dose and low-dose techniques. 2003 AUR Memorial Award. *Acad Radiol* 2003;10:719–724, with permission.)

THE PROXIMAL BRONCHI

CT has clearly revolutionized our ability to image structural changes in the central airways. Using careful CT acquisition, display, and quantitative analysis methods, HRCT and multislice CT can now be used to image structural changes in the airways in response to variations in lung volumes as well as their responses to pharmacologic stimuli such as methacholine and β agonists (Fig. 6-8). Unlike conventional PFT measurements, which are limited to a global assessment of all the airways in aggregate, new imaging methods using CT can localize the relative contributions of various generations of the airways to the overall pulmonary physiology. Conventional spirometric lung function tests (e.g., forced expiratory volume in 1 second [FEV_1] and forced vital capacity [FVC]) reflect only a gross average function of the airways and cannot evaluate regional or individual airway changes (25). The latter are likely important in understanding and treating disorders with impairment of airflow.

The ability to directly visualize airway responses to various stimuli and treatments as well as to changes in lung volume would be a great contribution to our understanding of airway pathophysiology. HRCT has become a most important diagnostic and investigational radiologic tool for the evaluation of airway function (Fig. 6-8). It has been used to measure dynamic changes in airway caliber *in vivo* that are not detectable by conventional global lung measurements such as airway and lung resistance (26,27). HRCT is uniquely capable of addressing questions regarding airway responsiveness *in vivo* that cannot be answered by other techniques (28–33). However, the ability to study bronchial function with imaging is challenging. These imaging methods rely on accurate and reproducible measurements of airway luminal areas and wall thickness to be able to compare the airways before and after acute interventions (e.g., bronchoprovocation, bronchodilatation, response to changes in lung volumes) and to carry out longitudinal studies, such as in chronic airway remodeling in asthma.

Such measurements include airway luminal cross-sectional area and bronchial wall thickness. Obtaining such measurements accurately has been problematic for four principal reasons: (1) the measurements vary with the obliquity of the CT slice through airways; thus, images that are truly perpendicular to the local long axis of the airway throughout the entire branching central airways are required (Fig. 6-9); (2) normal physiologic changes in airway caliber occur during the respiratory cycle, so that imaging of the airways at select, reproducible lung volumes is necessary; (3) an accurate and reproducible means to define the inner

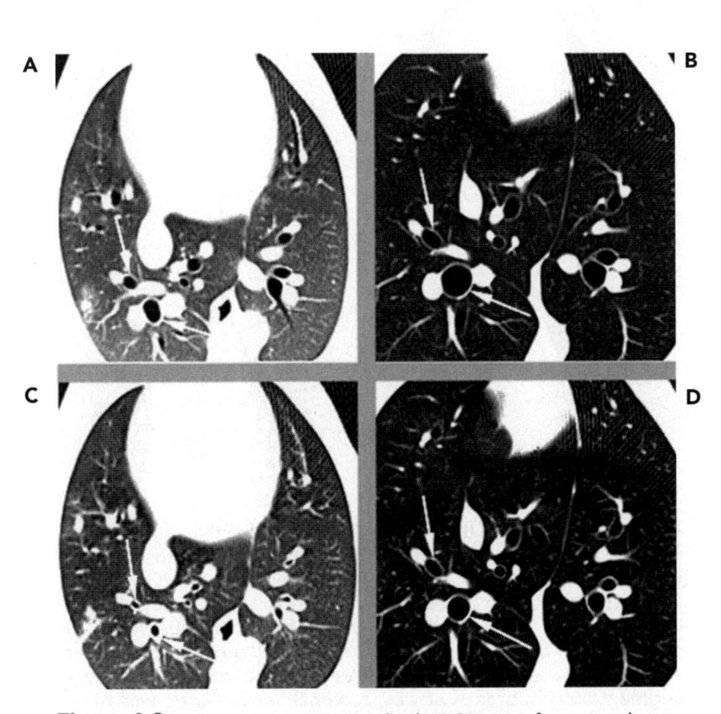

Figure 6-8 Airway reactivity. Matched HRCT scans from one dog at baseline (**A** and **B**) and after challenge with aerosolized methacholine (**C** and **D**). Images were acquired at low lung volume (FRC). (**A** and **C**) and at high lung volume (TLC) (**B** and **D**). The arrows show the same airways matched under all conditions. (From Brown RH, Mitzner W, Wagner E, et al. Airway distention with lung inflation measured by HRCT. *Acad Radiol* 2003;10:1097–1103, with permission.)

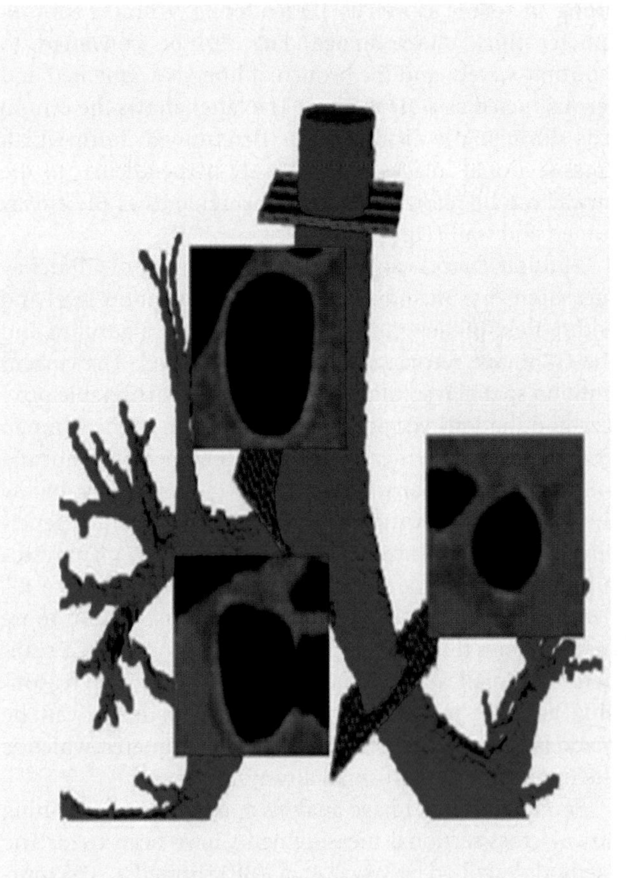

Figure 6-9 Regional airway geometric parameters are calculated from 3D images along planes selected to be perpendicular to the regional airway long axis. (From Hoffman EA, Reinhardt JM, Sonka M, et al. Characterization of the interstitial lung diseases via density-based and texture-based analysis of computed tomography images of lung structure and function. *Acad Radiol* 2003;10:1104–1118, with permission.)

and outer edges of the airway walls is required; this can be challenging for the smaller, more peripheral airways at the limits of spatial resolution and even in the more central airways because of inherent blurring in the image reconstruction; and (4) the precise location (segment, generation) along the airway tree at which measurements are made must be specified, so that serial measurements of precisely the same airway are obtained repeatedly. Recent advances in CT scanner technology as well as dedicated image analysis tools have begun to address these issues.

Initial airway reactivity studies with HRCT used 2D slices, analyzing those airways that by chance were felt to be imaged in true cross section (34). However, the in-plane resolution with a 2D-based analysis is insufficient to visualize airways with diameters smaller than 1 mm and to quantify changes in airway dimensions in airways smaller than 1.5 mm. Nonetheless, valuable results have been obtained (34–36) despite methodologic limitations that likely introduced errors in the measurements.

Current multislice helical scanners with increasing numbers of detector rows can now rapidly acquire image volumes through the entire lungs in less than 10 seconds. These datasets allow for subcentimeter image reformations along any plane as well as 3D rendering. With the submillimeter thick slices, image data can be converted to isotropic voxels, and the bronchial lumens segmented and reconstructed as a 3D volume. The latter allows the central axis through the airways to be determined, from which cross-sectional images that are truly perpendicular to the airway can be reformatted for measurements of the airway lumen and wall (Fig. 6-9) (20).

Multiple factors can influence the accuracy of CT airway measurements, including slice thickness, window level and width, field-of-view, and the reconstruction algorithm and the CT image reconstruction algorithm used. The current limit on spatial resolution is dependent on achievable pixel size and the intrinsic point spread function of the scanner. The wall thickness, measured morphometrically, of normal 1.5-mm diameter airways is 0.15 to 0.20 mm, just below the lower limit of current clinical CT scanners, which generally achieve a pixel size of 0.25×0.25 mm (37). This resolution will continue to improve with new multislice CT detector technology, and certainly spatial resolution more than 10 times this can be achieved with new micro-CT scanners. The smallest visible normal airways on which reasonably accurate measurements of lumen diameter can be made is in the range of 1.5 to 2.0 mm diameter, which is the upper size limit of small airways.

Several different image analysis approaches to obtaining airway cross-sectional measurements have been used. The method described by Wood et al. (38) showed a 20% overestimation of diameters for airways larger than 2 mm in diameter. The method of Amirav et al. (35), using the "full width at half maximum" principle, is relatively operator independent and achieved a coefficient of variation (SD/mean) of 4.4% for airways of 6.3-mm diameter and 16.6% for 1.3-mm diameter airways. Small airways have very thin walls, typically on the order of 10% to 15% of inner diameter (39). The full width at half maximum method can yield inaccurate measurements for these very small, thin-walled airways.

More recently, sophisticated model-based methods for accurate and automated edge detection and measurements of the airway walls have been developed (40–43). Reinhardt et al. developed an improved, more accurate edge detection program that takes into account the point spread function of the particular scanner as well as the slice selection and reconstruction algorithm used and applies a model-based deconvolution to account for blur in the scanning process (41,42). The method is accurate for a wide range of relevant airway sizes down to 1 to 15 mm inner diameter. Inner and outer airway wall borders can be detected to subvoxel resolution (41).

An airway analysis algorithm capable of fully automated segmentation of the first five to six airway generations has been described (39). After segmentation, the program executes skeletonization and branch point localization to automatically identify the 3D center line of individual branches (Fig. 6-10). The program can match two airway

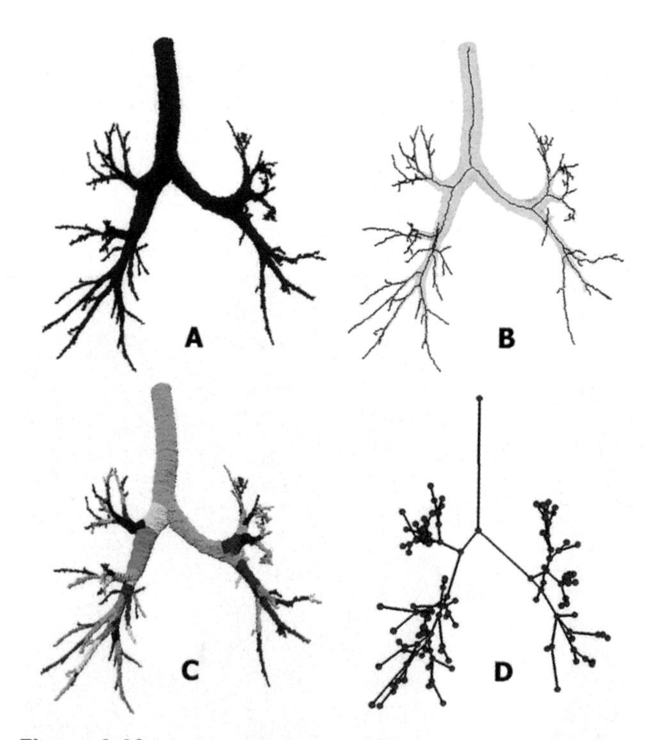

Figure 6-10 **A** to **D:** 3D airway analysis algorithm. **A:** Adaptive region growing-based airway segmentation. **B:** Extraction of center lines, topologically and geometrically correct thinning. **C:** Partitioning segmented tree via isotropic label propagation. **D:** Mathematical graph representation of the individual tree. The tree shown in **D** is stored in an XML file, which provides associated measures for each part of the tree. These measures include segment length, branch angles, regional luminal area, wall thickness, segment luminal volume, segment surface area, regional minimum diameter, and the diameter of the orthogonal as well as regional maximum diameter. (From Hoffman EA, Reinhardt JM, Sonka M, et al. Characterization of the interstitial lung diseases via density-based and texture-based analysis of computed tomography images of lung structure and function. *Acad Radiol* 2003;10:1104–1118, with permission.)

trees with 150 to 200 branch points in less than 2 seconds. It has been validated with phantom and *in vivo* scans with a high degree of agreement between the automated computer method and human experts.

Furthermore, a method to automatically label the various portions of the airway tree has been established (Fig. 6-10). The algorithm can be applied to multiple scans of the same subject to track changes in airway dimensions along an airway path, in addition to changes in airway dimensions with varying lung volumes.

Scanning at controlled, specified lung volumes is critical to match and compare exactly the same airways on serial studies of an individual and to eliminate lung-volume dependent changes in airway lumen and wall caliber. Such spirometric control of the scans has not been widely used. Intrascan inconsistencies may contribute to the apparent "heterogeneity" in airway lumen and wall measurements made throughout an individual bronchial tree.

Recently, a pneumotachometer-based CT lung volume controller has been developed (Fig. 6-11) (44). The device monitors the volume of expired gas and can trigger a high-frequency balloon valve to occlude the airway and hold the subject's lung volume at a fixed percent of the vital capacity, or the subject can relax against various levels of positive end-expiratory pressure (PEEP) and scanning can be performed during prolonged expiratory pauses (42). The pneumotachometer signal then also initiates the CT scan acquisition (45,46). Other approaches to monitoring lung volumes in connection with CT gating have included mouth-based air flow methods using an ultrasound probe, turbine, and a chest wall–based inductance plethysmograph (39).

Moreover, respiration is a dynamic process, and many pathophysiologic disorders in lungs manifest themselves only during active breathing. Examples are dynamic compression of the airways and frequency dependence

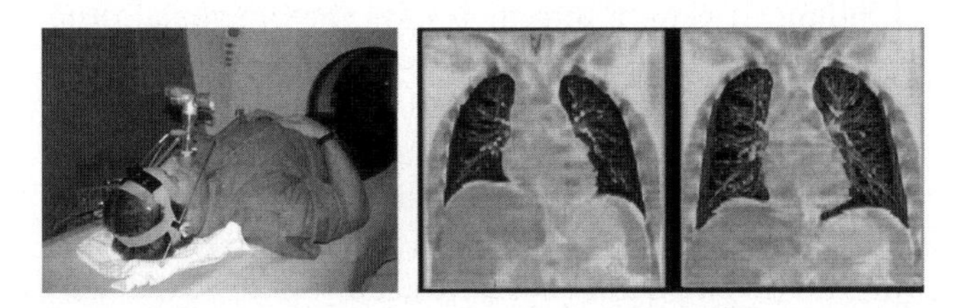

Figure 6-11 By use of a pneumotachometer or other lung volume–tracking device *(left image)* to follow respiration, axial scans can be gated to specific points within the respiratory cycle. Using multislice CT, a set of axial sections are obtained at multiple points within a respiratory cycle and then the table is advanced to acquire the adjacent set of slices at the same lung volumes of the next respiratory cycle. Two images at right show a volume rendering of the 3D lung and a coronal section sampled from the center of the stacked image data set. Note that every four slices used to produce these 3D images were from a different respiratory cycle than the adjacent four slices, and yet anatomy is depicted as being continuous from apex to base of lungs. (From Hoffman EA, Reinhardt JM, Sonka M, et al. Characterization of the interstitial lung diseases via density-based and texture-based analysis of computed tomography images of lung structure and function. *Acad Radiol* 2003;10:1104–1118, with permission.)

of compliance. Furthermore, many dyspneic patients have difficulty breath holding. Ideally for physiologic studies of the airways, full 3D helical imaging through the lungs at multiple phases of the respiratory cycle is desirable, analogous to CT cardiac imaging with retrospective gating. The latter uses the speed and reproducibility of the cardiac cycle to build up images at multiple phases from portions of successive heart beats. This is not yet possible for respiration, however, given the much greater length of the respiratory cycle, the greater cycle-to-cycle variations in respiration compared with cardiac motion, and radiation dose considerations. Nonetheless, new strategies for multiphasic helical scanning to capture several phases of the respiratory cycle have recently been demonstrated (Fig. 6-11). Specifically, Hoffman et al. (39) have described a scheme using a four-slice multidetector CT scanner in which the lungs are scanned at two points in the respiratory cycle while moving the table location by a combined thickness of two of the four slices between each gated scan acquisition. The process is then repeated for the two volume locations with sequential respiratory cycles until the entire lungs are imaged.

Despite these technical advancements, most CT studies of airway reactivity to date have relied on more traditional 2D HRCT methods (33,35,37,47–49). These CT studies of airway reactivity are providing new information regarding the pathophysiology of asthma, including the sites of bronchoconstriction during acute episodes as well as the structural and functional changes associated with airway remodeling resulting from the inflammatory changes of chronic asthma.

Asthma is characterized by reversible obstruction of airways owing to bronchial hyperresponsiveness associated with airway inflammation involving both proximal and distal airways (50). It is a chronic inflammatory condition associated with widespread but variable airflow obstruction that is often reversible (20). Airway reactivity, the hallmark of asthma, refers to the ability of the airways to reversibly change their diameter in response to stimuli (20).

HRCT findings involving the airways in asthmatics are variable and frequently subtle but include airway wall thickening, bronchial narrowing, bronchiectasis, centrilobular opacities, and mucoid impaction (50). In addition, mosaic perfusion and air trapping are commonly present (51–59). The majority of patients with chronic asthma have bronchial wall thickening (51,52,57,60,61). Airway wall remodeling, which occurs in chronic asthma and likely is the result of chronic inflammation, is associated with structural changes in the airway walls. These include subepithelial fibrosis, mucous gland hyperplasia, and smooth muscle hypertrophy and hyperplasia (20,61,62).

Okazawa et al. (63) measured bronchial wall thickness and the site of methacholine-induced bronchoconstriction in asthmatics versus controls using HRCT. The asthmatics showed wall thickening. Following methacholine, there was significant heterogeneous bronchoconstriction found in all size airways, with the greatest change observed in airways

2 to 4 mm in diameter. The bronchial wall area normally decreases on bronchoconstriction; however, this decrease in wall thickness is not seen in the airways of asthmatics. Similar findings were also observed by Kee et al. (64).

CT studies of dynamic changes of airway narrowing and hyperresponsiveness have demonstrated spatial heterogeneity in response, with maximum narrowing in intermediate-sized airways in animal models (2- to 6-mm diameter in dogs) and human subjects (2- to 4-mm diameter) following carbachol challenge and lung deflation. In addition, airway wall area decreased with narrowing in response to pharmacologically induced airway smooth muscle contraction (37).

Airway reactivity studies in pigs have demonstrated that HRCT can detect changes in peripheral (<2 mm) airways challenged with methacholine before such changes are reflected in more conventional PFTs (35). HRCT airway reactivity studies in human asthmatic subjects have shown that the central airways have a greater response to methacholine than do the peripheral airways (Fig. 6-12); conversely, the peripheral airways of asthmatics show greater response to β agonists (34,36,64a). These results are consistent with a higher density of cholinergic receptors in the central airways than in the peripheral airways and a greater prevalence of β receptors peripherally. The data, when compared with previous studies showing heterogeneity in response throughout various locations in the bronchial tree of asthmatics, emphasize the need for careful, objective computer-based quantification of airways together with carefully developed imaging protocols controlling for lung volumes during scan acquisition to ensure that the same airways are compared preintervention and postintervention (34,41,65).

A study by Beigelman-Aubry et al. (49) using spirometrically controlled CT at 65% total lung capacity (TLC) showed that patients with mild intermittent asthma have baseline bronchoconstriction compared with normal subjects. Furthermore, inhalation of salbutamol following a methacholine challenge resulted in bronchial cross-sectional areas comparable to those of controls as well as above their own baseline values. This baseline bronchoconstriction may be the result of increased muscle tone or impaired stretching.

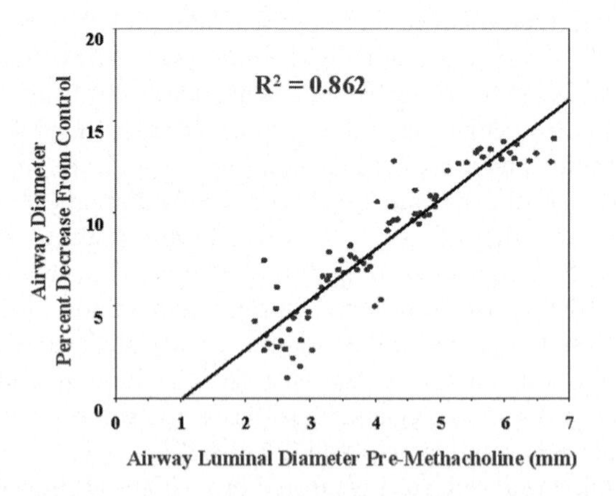

Figure 6-12 Airway reactivity using quantitative HRCT. Graph of airway narrowing in response to methacholine challenge as a function of baseline airway cross-sectional diameter in asthmatic subjects. Note linear relationship between the percent decrease in airway diameter with methacholine and the baseline airway diameter, indicating greater bronchoconstriction in the larger (central) airways. (Courtesy of Eric A. Hoffman, PhD, University of Iowa.)

Asthma may be related to the inability to sufficiently distend airways with lung inflation. This inability may be secondary to increased stiffness of smooth muscle preventing distension, airway remodeling with collagen deposition (66), or decreased distensibility resulting from air trapping and leading to increased lung volume at functional residual capacity (FRC). Airways normally dilate with inspiration and constrict in response to inhaled stimuli such as methacholine and histamine. In healthy subjects, deep inspirations to TLC have been shown to have both a bronchoprotective effect (prevention of subsequent spasmogen-induced bronchoconstriction) and a bronchodilator effect (25,67–69). These effects of deep inspiration, however, are impaired in asthmatic patients compared with healthy subjects.

HRCT studies have shown that after constriction induced by methacholine, a deep inspiration resulted in bronchodilation in normals but further bronchoconstriction in asthmatics (27). In asthmatics with severe airflow obstruction, the ability to distend the airways on HRCT with deep inspiration is significantly decreased.

These studies suggest that HRCT measurements of airway distensibility in human subjects may provide insights into the pathophysiology, progression of disease, and response to therapy in asthmatic patients (25).

THE PERIPHERAL AIRWAYS

Despite dramatic developments in HRCT and helical CT for anatomic imaging of the lungs, radiologic techniques including CT cannot directly resolve the individual distal airways and airspaces at the gas exchange level in the lung parenchyma. However, functional imaging techniques are available to visualize ventilation and gas exchange in the lung parenchyma. This has traditionally been performed with nuclear medicine techniques. More recently, however, MR- and CT-based methods have been developed that have greatly expanded our ability to image a variety of functional parameters related to ventilation. These exciting methods, many of which are still under development, provide quantitative imaging of regional lung function with high temporal and spatial resolution.

NUCLEAR MEDICINE

Scintigraphy has been the traditional functional imaging study to evaluate perfusion and ventilation and V/Q. It is sensitive, although nonspecific, with low spatial and temporal resolution. Inhaled radionuclide gases, including ^{133}Xe, ^{127}Xe, and ^{81}Kr, are distributed through the smaller airways. Aerosols such as technetium ^{99}m diethylenetriamine pentacetic acid (DTPA) have particle sizes of 0.1 to 3 μ (70) but suffer from deposition in the larger central airways (71). An ultrafine dispersion of Tc-^{99}m–labeled carbon particles (Technegas), with particle sizes of approximately 0.005 μ (72), has deeper penetration but low anatomic resolution for the distal airways.

The resolution of the nuclear medicine studies has been improved with SPECT, which can provide cross-sectional images as well as quantification of ventilation, perfusion, and V/Q (73,74). Using a three-headed SPECT camera with a continuous repetitive rotating mode, tomographic images at equilibrium and during wash-out at 30-second intervals for 5 minutes can be acquired using ^{133}Xe gas. The regional wash-out is quantified by calculating the half-time (T1/2) and mean transit time (MTT) (75). The SPECT data are reconstructed into a 3D image with a color surface-rendering technique. A 3D fusion image of the 3-minute wash-out image is embedded within the equilibrium image, the latter delineating the lung contours, to display the size, extent, and distribution of areas of abnormal gas trapping. These can be further quantified using the T1/2 and MTT kinetic parameters. This technique has been applied to evaluate the lungs of patients with emphysema before and after lung volume reduction surgery (LVRS) (76,77), as well as in asthmatic patients pretherapy and posttherapy for asthma and correlated with FEV_1 (77).

Three-dimensional surface displays of dynamic ^{133}Xe ventilation and Tc-^{99}m MAA SPECT perfusion have also been performed in patients pre-LVRS and post-LVRS (78). Furthermore, respiratory-gated Tc-^{99}m Technegas SPECT ventilation and SPECT perfusion functional scans have been reliably coregistered with CT images. These coregistered SPECT–CT images have allowed accurate identification of the location and extent of V/Q deficits related to the underlying CT anatomy, thus coupling the functional and structural abnormalities (79).

Further refinements in V/Q imaging have been made possible with PET, with a resolution of 5 to 10 mm, although temporally slow (approximately 30 seconds) relative to the respiratory cycle (80,81). After intravenous bolus injection during a breath hold and subsequent wash-out from the lungs on resumption of breathing, $^{13}N_2$ PET has been able to show the topographic distribution of regional perfusion as well as regional-specific alveolar ventilation (ventilation per unit alveolar gas volume) and alveolar V/Q ratios (82,83). When these V/Q measurements are combined into a whole-lung distribution, they have been validated against global arterial blood gases (ABGs). Three-dimensional PET data in sheep before and after methacholine bronchoconstriction and pulmonary embolism have shown excellent correlation with ABGs and demonstrate V/Q heterogeneity in the lungs at length scales smaller than the spatial resolution of the imaging method (83). The PET V/Q work has been largely limited to investigational studies.

With regard to other airway applications of nuclear medicine techniques, [18F]-fluorodeoxyglucose-PET (^{18}FDG-PET) has been used in imaging of disease activity in patients with pneumoconiosis, sarcoid, asthma, and infection (84). Pharmaceutical compounds can be labeled with radioisotopes to study their distribution of deposition and pharmacokinetics. New compounds can also be mixed with Tc-^{99}m-DTPA aerosols, assuming they have similar particle deposition (85,86). PET (^{11}C) labeling of inhalational pharmaceuticals, such as for the treatment of asthma, also has been used to show the distribution of the inhaled agents in connection with the design and use of these drugs (87,88). The agents have also been labeled with ^{18}FDG PET (89).

PET has also been used to label the β-adrenoceptors in the lung to quantify the receptors and correlate their density with the bronchodilator response to β-agonist therapy (90,91).

Beyond the classical ventilation and perfusion agents, a wide range of radiopharmaceutical agents can be traced in the lungs. These have the potential to label the basic components involved in inflammation as well as in the development of pulmonary fibrosis (92). ^{18}FDG PET has also been used on a limited basis to image allergen-invoked airway inflammation in atopic asthma (93). PET imaging using a fluorinated analog of proline amino acid (cis-4-[(18)F] fluoro-L-proline) has been used as a label of active pulmonary fibrosis in a rabbit model of experimental silicosis (94).

Molecular Imaging

The most exciting new imaging applications for the study of the airways are those of so-called molecular imaging. A new generation of imaging devices now makes it possible to obtain structural and functional images of the lungs in small animals, including mouse and rat models. These include micro-PET; micro x-ray CT; high-field, small-bore MR scanners; highly sensitive cooled charge-coupled device (CCD) cameras for bioluminescence and fluorescence optical imaging, as well as advances in ultrasound (95). These can be used to study not only ventilation and perfusion but also lung inflammation and even gene transfer. Fusion of images such as PET and CT allow for structure–function and function–function relationships to be studied on a regional basis. These emerging techniques have tremendous potential for studying lung biologic structure and function from the macroscopic down to the molecular level.

Recently developed micro-PET instruments enable PET imaging in mouse models and small animals with spatial resolution to 2 mm. The technique provides a uniquely powerful means to monitor activity of the inflammatory process in the lung. A promising new approach to imaging airway diseases such as asthma is the integration of the functional–metabolic data obtained from PET with the anatomic airway data acquired from CT. Micro-CT units can now scan the lungs at resolutions down to the 10 μ range. Such combined PET–CT imaging studies could be used to spatially map the distribution of active inflammation along the airway.

An example of this emerging molecular imaging of the airways is the imaging of reporter gene expression in the lungs with PET. Pulmonary gene transfer has been carried out in rats via the intratracheal instillation of an adenoviral vector containing a fusion gene that encodes for mutant Herpes simplex virus type-1 thymidine kinase and an enhanced green fluorescent protein. A PET-labeled substrate for the mutant kinase is used (96). PET is able to image the magnitude and spatial distribution of the transgene expression and can thus provide useful information about the efficacy of various gene transfer delivery strategies within the lung (97,98).

CT IMAGING: AIR AS A CONTRAST AGENT

CT has a unique characteristic whereby changes in air content in the lung due to ventilation result in a corresponding change in regional CT density as well as lung volume. Thus air itself can be used in CT as a contrast agent for indirect measurements of ventilation.

Regional air content can be quantified using CT attenuation values (34,99). The lung can be regarded as comprising structures equal in density to only air or water (the density of lung tissue and blood, at 1.055, being very close to that of water). Simplistically, if a voxel with 100% air measures −1,000 HU, then a voxel measuring −600 HU would be considered to contain 60% air (40% tissue). More precisely, the following equation can be used to calibrate lung density values to quantify the regional content of air in the lung:

$$\text{Voxel \% air content} = ([1 - CT_x - CT_{air}]/[CT_{water} - CT_{air}]) \times 100$$

where CTx = original grayscale of lung voxel to be converted; CTair = grayscale value to voxels with a region of known 100% air content (lumen of trachea or proximal bronchi); CTwater = region of known 100% "water" (chamber of heart or lumen of great vessels).

With the additional use of a bolus injection of a radiopaque contrast agent together with rapid scanning, it is also possible to determine the percentage of blood and tissue within the "water" compartment in the region of interest.

Using the previous equation without contrast injection, a voxel in the lung periphery can be assigned a percent air content value, with the remainder of the voxel comprising lung tissue and blood.

The majority of CT studies have used the changes in regional lung density at various phases of inspiration to infer regional ventilation and density changes in expiration to evaluate gas trapping.

CT Volumetry

Perhaps the most direct application of using air as a contrast agent for CT is CT-based measurement of lung volumes, or so-called CT volumetry. Lung volumes have traditionally been measured by spirometry with body plethysmography and helium dilution. None of these conventional global methods, however, can provide volume information for specific sub-lung regions. CT volumetry is based on the current ability to scan the entire lungs at a specified state of lung inflation monitored by spirometry (92). Dedicated lung extraction software using automated segmentation can now be used to accurately and reproducibly derive lung volumes, and these measurements compare well with plethysmographic measurements (100,101). However, in one study inspiratory helical CT consistently underestimated TLC by 15% (100), and expiratory helical CT overestimated residual volume (RV) by almost 1 L. This may be related to supine positioning for CT versus sitting erect for PFTs. Further refinements using 3D reconstructions have been able to reduce errors to approximately 3% (102). Unlike conventional PFTs, CT can provide volume measurements of individual lungs and even lung regions (103).

Determination of changes in small areas of the lung with varying degrees of inflation is more challenging, however, and relies on the ability to track accurately the motion of individual points in the lung. This is now becoming possible using new nonrigid image registration analysis software programs, which are discussed further in the section on pulmonary mechanics. Volumetry of ventilated airspaces can also be obtained via MR hyperpolarized gas imaging, also discussed later.

Inspiratory–Expiratory HRCT

The use of lung density changes in different phases of respiration has had its primary application in inspiratory–expiratory HRCT scans, which have become the most commonly used CT functional imaging study in clinical practice. Expiratory HRCT is discussed elsewhere in this text, particularly as it relates to small airway disease.

Expiratory HRCT is a highly useful and relatively simple method to detect air trapping, a hallmark of small airway obstruction (104). (Gas trapping can also be caused by regional abnormality in pulmonary compliance.) On expiration the attenuation of normal lung increases as a consequence of decreased gas volume, whereas regions of air trapping remain essentially unchanged in density (Figs. 6-13 and 6-14). Likewise, the area (or volume) of normal lung decreases on expiration, while those regions with air trapping remain unchanged in size (56,105–108). Normally, the dependent lung regions show the greatest expiratory increase in density (109).

Constriction of pulmonary vessels can also be seen within the areas of decreased lung density. Bronchiolar obstruction causes hypoxic vasoconstriction, which results in areas of decreased lung attenuation. These low-attenuation regions

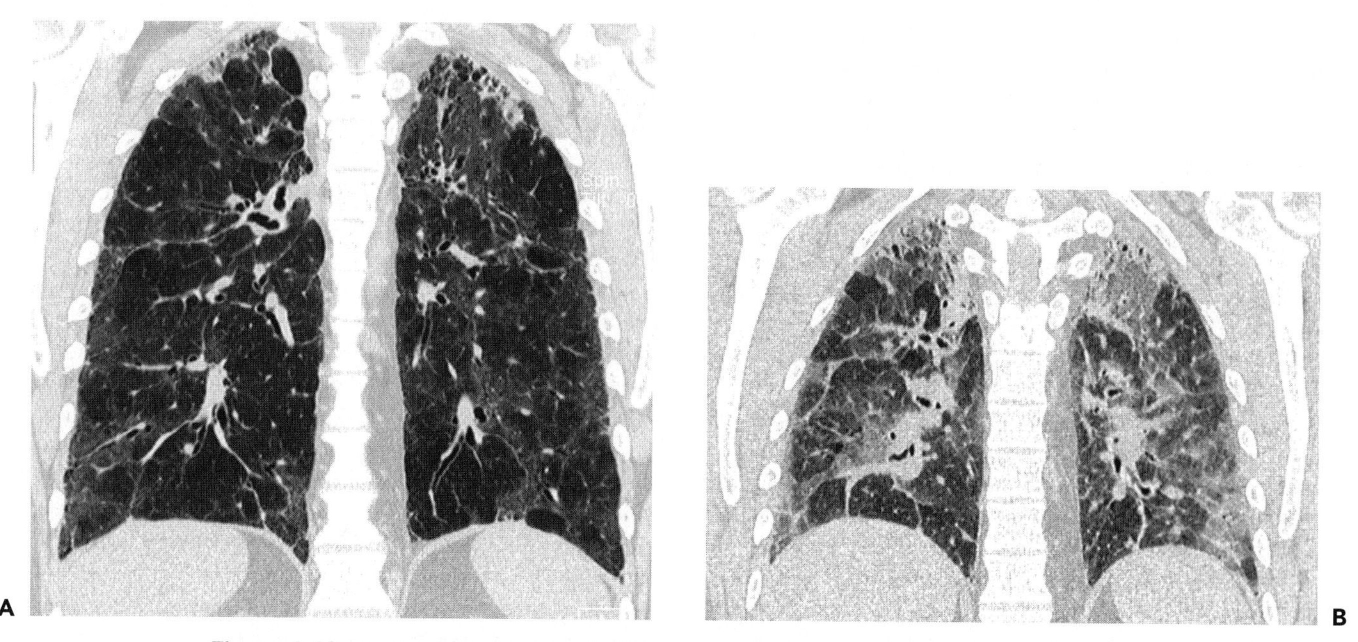

Figure 6-13 **A:** Coronal inspiratory HRCT image acquired during a breath hold using a 16-row detector multislice CT scanner. Mosaic attenuation pattern is present, in addition to upper lobe scarring in this patient with sarcoidosis. **B:** Coronal expiratory HRCT scan demonstrates multiple regions of gas trapping. The full volume and distribution of gas trapping can be determined.

can be patchy or diffuse and are generally poorly marginated but can have well-demarcated geographic outlines (50). Redistribution of blood flow leads to increased attenuation in the normal adjacent areas of lung. The appearance of this patchwork variation in CT density is referred to as a "mosaic attenuation" pattern (110); corresponding regional differences in vessel size constitute a "regional perfusion" pattern. Expiratory CT often can differentiate bronchiolar from infiltrative or vascular causes of a mosaic attenuation pattern (e.g., chronic thromboembolic disease) (111), because the mosaic attenuation is accentuated on expiration in cases of bronchiolar (small airway) disease. The findings of air trapping may be confused with emphysema in patients with severe obstructive airway disease, because the hypoxic vasoconstriction leads to decreased lung attenuation on both inspiratory and expiratory HRCT scans (53,57).

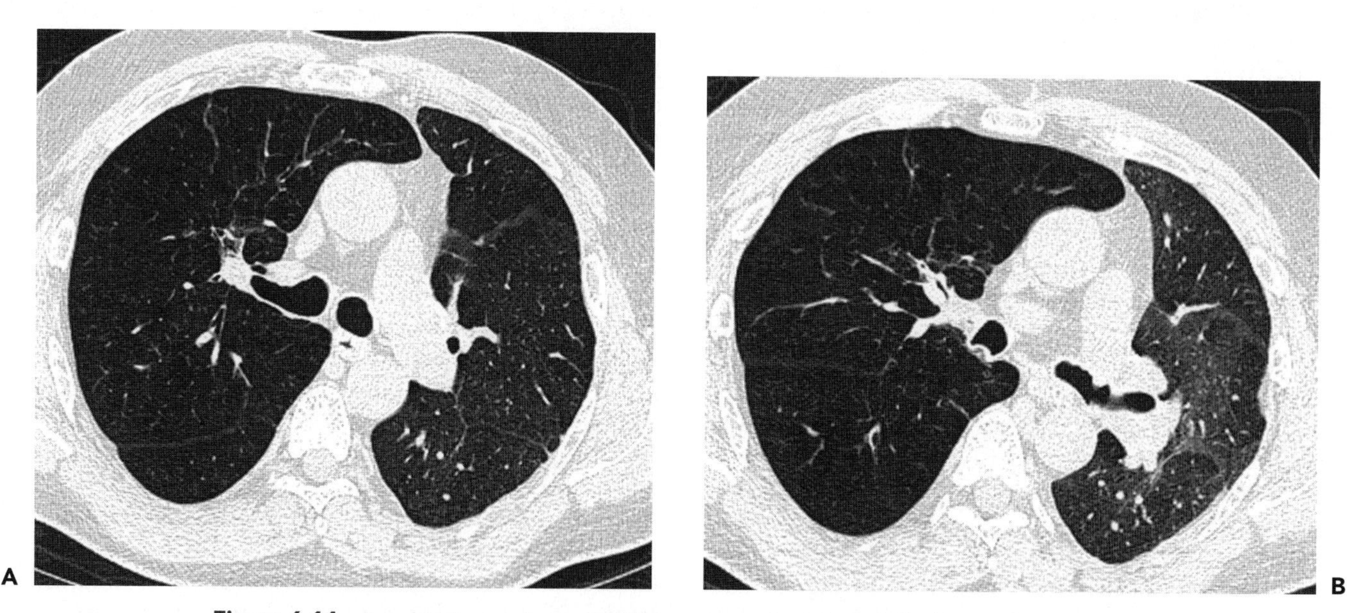

Figure 6-14 **A** and **B:** Two expiratory HRCT images acquired dynamically during a forced exhalation. The patient is post–left lung transplant for emphysema. Serial images were acquired at the same location in the midlungs, **(A)** at the start and **(B)** at the end of expiration. Gas trapping is evident in the transplanted left lung, a manifestation of bronchiolitis obliterans resulting from chronic rejection. Marked diffuse air trapping is also present in the emphysematous native right lung. There is resulting expiratory shift of the mediastinum to the left.

However, unlike in emphysema, the decreased vessels in hypoxic vasoconstriction are not distorted (50).

In 50% to 80% of normal subjects with normal PFTs, expiratory HRCT may show one or more areas of air trapping, often limited to one or a few adjacent secondary pulmonary lobules (107,112). These occur predominantly in the dependent parts of the lower lobes (113) and are seen more frequently with increasing age and smoking (107,113). Air trapping is generally considered abnormal when it affects a volume of lung equal to or greater than a pulmonary segment (114) and particularly when it involves nondependent areas of the lung.

Air trapping detected on expiratory HRCT has been observed in a number of pulmonary disorders, including constrictive (obliterative) bronchiolitis, asthma, sarcoid, hypersensitivity pneumonitis, bronchitis, bronchiectasis, and emphysema (104,108,115–120).

Expiratory HRCT can be performed using either *static* or *dynamic* imaging protocols. Static images are acquired during breath holding at the end of a forced expiration, with a limited number of gapped slices through the lungs. With the advent of multislice helical CT scanners, it is now possible to acquire thin slices through the entire volume of the lung during inspiratory and expiratory breath holds (Fig. 6-13). Although the clinical value of such scans is currently being investigated, these volumetric HRCT scans offer the potential to determine the full volume of air trapping and to visualize its 3D distribution (45,121,122). Furthermore, minimum-intensity projection (minIP) reconstructions can improve the detection of air trapping on these multislice acquisitions (117,121–124).

Dynamic expiratory HRCT, originally performed using EBCT (50 to 100 msecond/image) (112,125,126), can now be acquired with helical scanners during a forced expiration (127–129) (Fig. 6-14). In a study comparing dynamic expiratory HRCT with suspended expiratory HRCT in 49 patients with various airway disorders, air trapping was found to be significantly more extensive on the dynamic (continuous) expiratory HRCT (130). These scans should use a low-dose technique (40 ma) to decrease radiation exposure (131). The dynamic acquisition, particularly during the last phase of the expiratory maneuver, may be relatively free of motion artifacts and offers a useful alternative method to detect air trapping in patients who cannot suspend respiration at end-expiration or when the static images are equivocal (129).

The extent of air trapping on expiratory HRCT may be quantified using either objective automated methods or subjective semiquantitative scoring systems. The objective methods include the mean density of voxels (132), mean density expiratory–inspiratory ratios (133), histograms of the distribution of attenuation values (134), a density mask highlighting regions of predetermined density values (135,136), or a calculation summarizing pixels with densities above or below specified critical values (137). The density mask has the advantage of superimposing the quantitative air-trapping maps on the underlying HRCT images showing the lung pathology. These quantitative methods, however, may be limited by a lack of distinct differences between normal and abnormal lung, particularly when the small airway disease is heterogeneously distributed (50).

Several semiquantitative scoring systems that estimate the percentage of air trapping on each scan have been described (138). Although subjective, a visual scoring system may be reliable (120).

The findings of air trapping on expiratory HRCT have been shown to correspond well with PFTs (19,56,108, 115,130,137,139–143). The use of global PFT measurements as a reference standard is problematic, however, because expiratory HRCT may show limited focal or multifocal regions of air trapping that may not be sufficiently extensive to alter spirometric measurements. Thus, although many studies of obliterative bronchiolitis report a strong correlation between the extent of air trapping on end-expiratory CT (144–146) and PFTs indicating obstructive physiology, not all studies have shown this association (56,140). Likewise, the relationship between the extent of air trapping on expiratory HRCT and the PFTs of asthmatic patients has varied among studies (49,56,137,147).

Expiratory HRCT has also been used in studies of airway reactivity (49,56,147). Methacholine-induced air trapping on expiratory CT and its partial reversibility following salbutamol inhalation in asthmatic patients, together with the observation of a baseline bronchoconstriction, have indicated that the methacholine-induced bronchoconstriction in asthmatics involves primarily the small airways (49). Histograms of the frequency distribution of lung parenchymal attenuation values on HRCT before and after bronchial provocation with methacholine have been studied in patients with mild asthma versus control subjects (148). The histograms were repeated after reversal of the methacholine challenge with albuterol. The histograms of the controls and asthmatics were similar at baseline. After methacholine, the controls showed no significant changes in lung attenuation curves and less than 10% decrease in FEV_1. In contrast, the asthmatics showed a significant leftward shift in the histograms, with decreases in the median and lowest tenth percentile regions of the attenuation curves, together with a 20% to 30% decrease in FEV_1. Following albuterol administration, the control subjects showed no change in their spirometric measurements, lung attenuation values, or bronchial size, whereas in the asthmatics all of these parameters returned to their baseline levels.

Dynamic Cine CT

Rapid continuous scanning through the same volume of the lung over time can provide a dynamic display of regional lung aeration. Initially performed using the higher temporal resolution of EBCT, it is now possible to achieve temporal increments in sequential images of 100 mseconds using spiral CT (149). However, this has been limited to one or two contiguous slices, although it should be possible to scan larger volumes of the lungs dynamically with continued technical developments using cone beam geometry in multislice helical CT. These studies are limited by the high radiation dose and to some extent by the large amount of raw data accumulated for reconstruction.

Dynamic CT has been used to study the dynamic behavior of the lungs in ARDS in a porcine model (Fig. 6-15). Using 270 degrees of raw data for image reconstruction together with a sliding window reconstruction technique, rapid CT images were acquired at 250 mseconds/image over several respiratory cycles. CT density-derived indices of aeration were used to assess the regional response of the lungs to ventilatory interventions (150).

In ARDS, there is an inhomogeneous distribution of ventilation (and perfusion), with cyclical collapse and recruitment of atelectasis primarily in the basilar and dependent portions of the lung (151). Undesirable consequences of

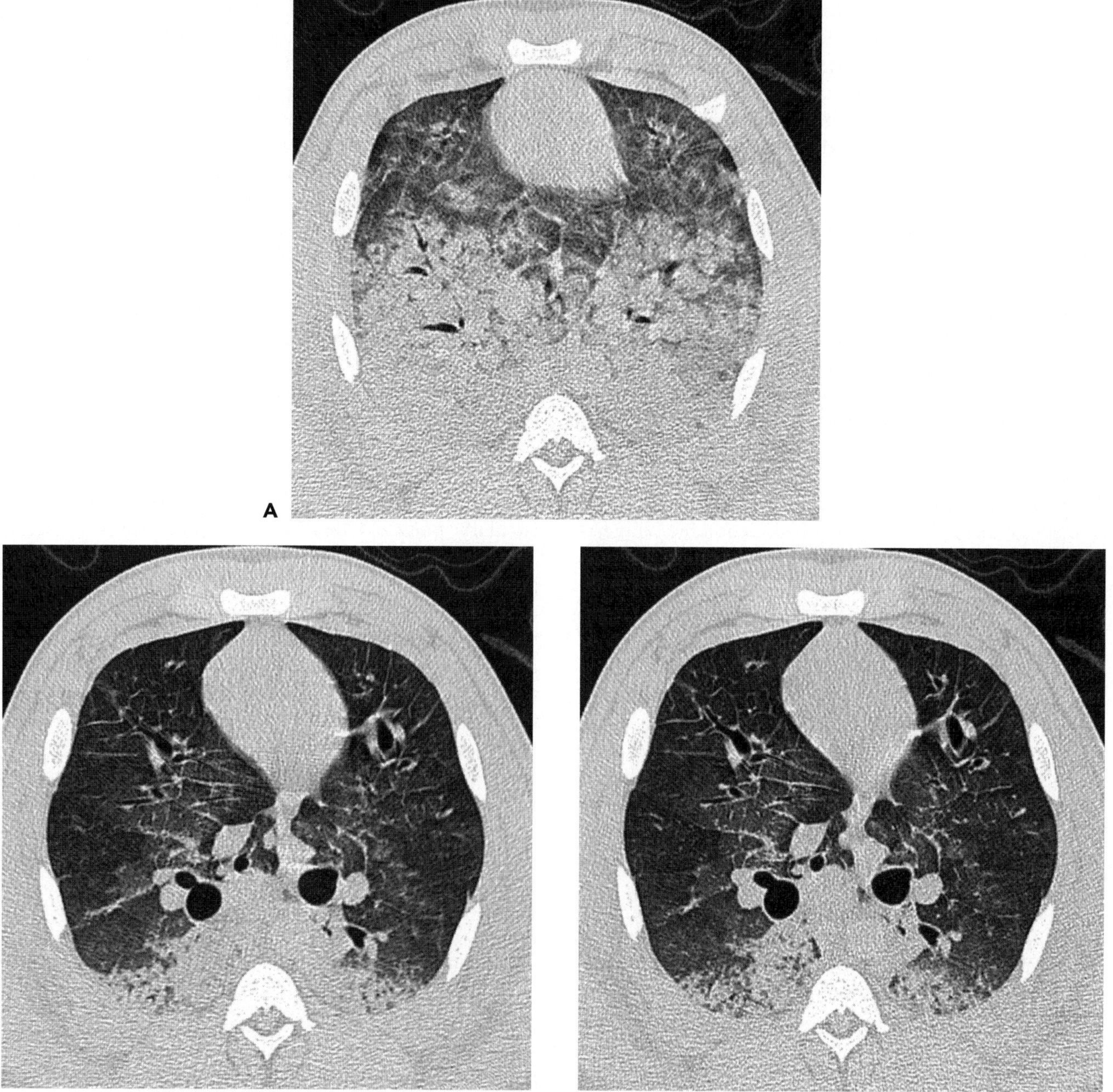

Figure 6-15 **A** to **C:** Dynamic cine CT demonstrating regional alveolar recruitment in a porcine model of ARDS. Images acquired during progressive increase in inspiratory pressure from 0 mbar to 50 mbar. Images depict recruitment of atelectatic regions of lung, particularly in the posterior dependent regions. The imaging sequence provides direct visualization of the anatomic distribution of atelectatic, normal, and hyperinflated lung components. In addition, quantitative time constants reflecting the rate of regional aeration of the lungs can be derived, with the potential to optimize mechanical ventilatory parameters in ARDS. (Courtesy of Klaus Markstaller, MD, University of Mainz.)

this ventilatory pattern include (a) high sheer forces between the collapsed and aerated alveoli, (b) varying shunt fraction with each respiratory cycle (152,153), and (c) overdistention of aerated lung.

Treatment of ARDS has included mechanical ventilation with low tidal volumes as well as avoidance of high peak airway pressures. The clinical goal is to optimize the ventilatory parameters and thereby to minimize ventilator-associated lung injury.

CT has confirmed that the findings of ARDS are inhomogeneously distributed in the lung, including regions of atelectasis, hypoventilated lung, and well-aerated lung, and these depend on the etiology of the ARDS, the ventilatory settings, and patient positioning (154–157). Although static CT can visualize and quantify the amount of atelectasis at a predefined air pressure, the lung aeration changes dynamically during the respiratory cycle and varies regionally and with different respiratory parameters. The dynamic CT technique, conversely, can depict and quantify the kinetics of regional alveolar recruitment during the respiratory cycle in ARDS with high spatial and temporal resolution. It has the potential to visualize the differential effects of mechanical ventilation on the atelectatic, normally ventilated, and overinflated lung (150,158,159). These various functional lung compartments are quantified based on their different density ranges on histograms, expressed as a fraction of the total lung area (149,151,160–162). Time constants of regional aeration (defined as time to reach 63.2% of total inspiration or expiration) have also been derived based on the dynamic CT density changes. These techniques have been performed in animal models (150,158), in anesthetized healthy volunteers (163), and in ARDS patients (164). The dynamic CT results could potentially be used to determine the optimal ventilatory parameters, including PEEP, plateau pressure, and respiratory rate. Although it is difficult and often impractical to transport ARDS patients to the CT scanner, further clinical trials to evaluate the potential benefit of CT-tailored ventilatory therapy seems warranted.

CONTRAST AGENTS AND TRACERS FOR MR AND CT IMAGING OF REGIONAL VENTILATION, GAS EXCHANGE, AND V/Q RATIO

Despite the tremendous amount of information that can be obtained with inspiratory–expiratory HRCT, dynamic cine CT, and multislice spiral CT, there is a significant limitation in using air as a CT contrast agent for ventilation. Unenhanced CT cannot differentiate residual air remaining in the alveoli at end-expiration from newly replenished air introduced in inspiration. Although CT can assess the density and volume changes occurring during the respiratory cycle, it cannot directly visualize the ventilatory exchange of gas (165). True ventilation CT aims to quantify the regional distribution of inspired air in a time-resolved fashion (103). There is thus a need for imaging techniques and contrast agents that can directly track gas flow into and out of lungs. Fortunately, new MR- and CT-based methods to do this are now available.

HYPERPOLARIZED ^{3}HELIUM MR

Proton MR imaging using conventional pulse sequences yields very little signal from the lung parenchyma because air has a low proton density (approximately 20% to 30%). In addition, alveolar microstructure consisting of the numerous sponge-like alveolar spaces and walls results in highly heterogeneous magnetic susceptibility, given the differences in potential to magnetize tissue versus air. This results in magnetic field gradients that diphase the MR signal (leading to a very short T2* of lung), causing its rapid decay. This limitation can be overcome to some extent with the faster pulse sequences now available, such as ultrafast gradient echo with very short TE (time to echo) times and single-shot fast spin echo (166). Furthermore, respiratory and cardiovascular motion adds to the challenge of imaging the lungs with proton MR.

MR imaging of the lungs has changed dramatically with the advent of hyperpolarized noble gases. ^{3}He and ^{129}Xe, nonradioactive noble gases, have low spin density and thus generate little signal in thermal equilibrium in a strong magnetic field. However, the population of nuclear spin states of these gases can be enhanced and the resulting signal increased by a factor of 100,000 by "hyperpolarization" via optical pumping with high-energy lasers using circularly polarized light of the appropriate wavelength. There are two major techniques for this hyperpolarization process: (a) spin exchange, which uses an optically pumped rubidium vapor as an intermediary to transfer polarization to the ^{3}He and (b) metastability exchange, which does not require the rubidium and is performed at low pressure; in this case, the gas must then be stored in a compressed state to maintain the polarization. The metastability method can achieve a higher percentage of polarization.

Following the hyperpolarization, the gas is maintained in glass cells to protect it from contact with any paramagnetic or ferromagnetic substances. It is also shielded with a magnetic field for storage and transfer. The hyperpolarization is destroyed irreversibly by contact with oxygen, being weakly paramagnetic, as well as by the radiofrequency (RF) pulses used in MR imaging.

The hyperpolarized ^{3}He can be inhaled either from collapsible bags or as a measured bolus delivered via PC-controlled application device (165). The gas may be administered as a ^{3}He-nitrogen mixture or as pure ^{3}He. ^{3}He imaging requires MR scanners with broadband RF systems, using dedicated RF coils tuned to the resonant frequency of ^{3}He.

The signal from the ^{3}He emanates from the gas itself, as opposed to paramagnetic effects on tissue, as is the case for other commonly used MR contrast agents such as gadolinium. Hyperpolarized ^{3}He not only produces high-signal images of ventilated airspaces of the lung with

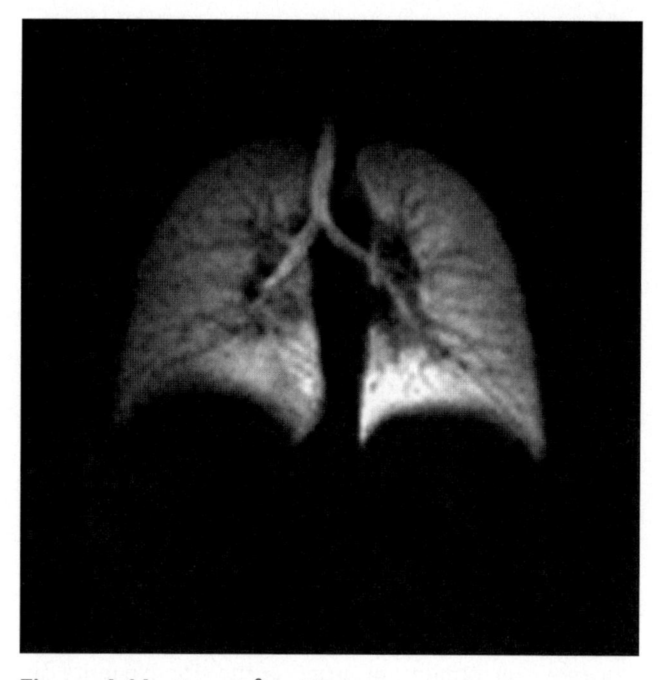

Figure 6-16 Normal ^{3}He MR image, showing homogeneous signal of the gas throughout the lungs.

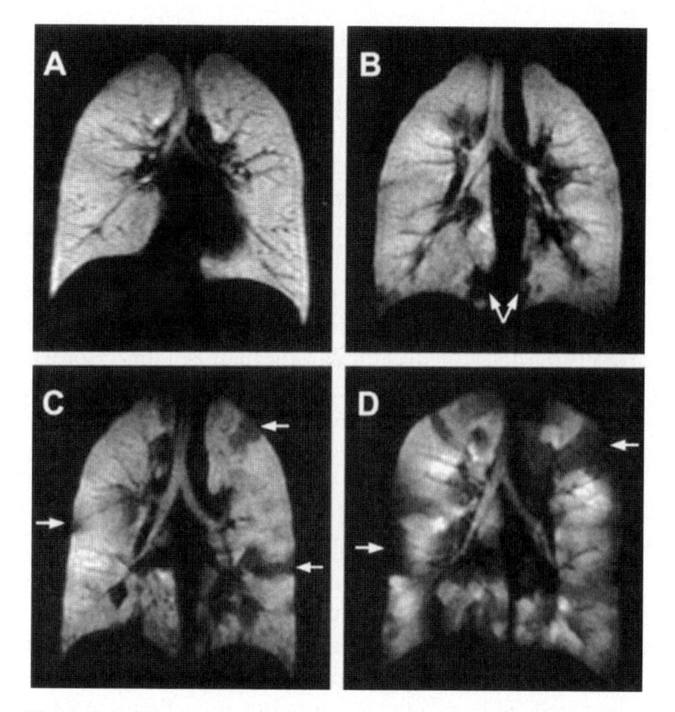

Figure 6-17 Coronal MR images obtained immediately after inhalation of hyperpolarized ^{3}He gas in a healthy volunteer **(A)**, and in patient with mild (FEV_1 of 132% of predicted value) asthma **(B)**, moderate (FEV_1 of 83% of predicted value) asthma **(C)**, and severe (FEV_1 of 34% of predicted value) **(D)** asthma. The distribution of the gas is homogeneous in the normal volunteer, and ventilation defects are seen with increasing numbers in the asthmatic patients with increasing severity (*arrows* point to several defects). (From Samee S, Altes T, Powers P, et al. Imaging the lungs in asthmatic patients by using hyperpolarized helium-3 magnetic resonance: assessment of response to methacholine and exercise challenge. *J Allergy Clin Immunol* 2003;111:1205–1211, with permission.)

spatial and temporal resolution greater than that of nuclear medicine, it also can provide novel functional parameters of ventilation including alveolar PO_2, diffusion, and alveolar V/Q ratios. The lack of ionizing radiation allows multiple-scan strategies. Moreover, the gas is inert with negligible solubility and thus has no adverse biologic effects (except for the hypoxic content of pure ^{3}He or a ^{3}He-nitrogen mixture).

^{3}He is currently regarded as an investigational agent for imaging. Because it is a byproduct of tritium decay, the gas is of limited availability and thus expensive, appreciable drawbacks to its widespread clinical use.

Static Helium Images

Static images reflecting the distribution of ^{3}He gas are obtained following a single breath inhalation of approximately 300 mL ^{3}He.

Normal lungs demonstrate near homogeneous signal (Fig. 6-16) (167–169). Normally, there may be a few small areas of signal void limited to the dependent portions of the lungs (165,168,170,171), reflecting collapse or air trapping in a few secondary pulmonary lobules. This is analogous to normal areas of dependent atelectasis and air trapping seen on CT scans of normal subjects. Larger regions of helium signal void referred to as "ventilation defects" are the result of functional or structural abnormalities (Fig. 6-17).

Among smokers, such defects are present even in subjects with apparently normal PFTs and normal chest radiographic findings (80,172). They are more numerous than in nonsmokers (165,172). The clinical and prognostic significance of these defects is currently uncertain. They may prove useful in the early detection of smoking-related lung disease, particularly with the advent of emerging new therapies for emphysema, such as retinoic acid, protease inhibitors, and antiinflammatory agents.

Patients with asthma demonstrate peripheral defects (Fig. 6-17), which may be transient. They may undergo partial or complete resolution following bronchodilator therapy (Fig. 6-18). Larger defects are seen associated with more symptomatic asthma with abnormal lung function (Fig. 6-18) (80,168). A study of patients with moderate or

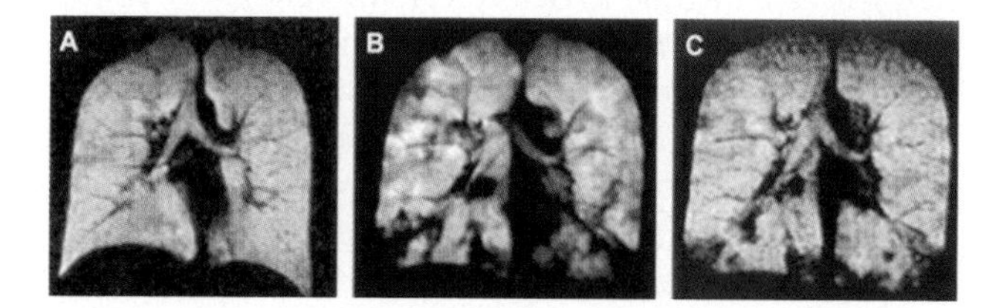

Figure 6-18 Methacholine challenge. **A:** Baseline coronal hyperpolarized ^{3}He MR image of the lungs in a patient with mild asthma (FEV_1 of 118% of predicted value) shows relative homogenous distribution of the gas in the lungs. **B:** Image obtained after methacholine challenge testing (FEV_1 of 73% of predicted value) demonstrates a large number of ventilation defects. **C:** Image obtained after inhalation of albuterol shows improvement of the ventilation defects. (From Samee S, Altes T, Powers P, et al. Imaging the lungs in asthmatic patients by using hyperpolarized helium-3 magnetic resonance: assessment of response to methacholine and exercise challenge. *J Allergy Clin Immunol* 2003;111:1205–1211, with permission.)

severe asthma has shown that the number of defects is inversely related to the percent predicted FEV$_1$ (173). In this study the number of defects increased following methacholine challenge and also after exercise. Such ventilation defects on ^{3}He MR may be seen even in well-controlled asthmatic subjects who are asymptomatic and with normal spirometry, reflecting the chronic airway inflammation in asthma (168). ^{3}He MR may thus provide an opportunity to monitor and quantify the extent of irreversible abnormalities in regional ventilation between bouts of acute asthma. These irreversible defects reflect the chronic nature of this disorder, which can be progressive and associated with airway remodeling and deterioration in lung function.

In patients with cystic fibrosis, the ^{3}He scans have been found to be more sensitive than the Brasfield chest radiographic score and correlated with PFTs (170). Defects have been seen in patients with mild disease and normal spirometry (174). Thus ^{3}He MR could play a role in monitoring response to therapy in these patients.

Bronchiolitis obliterans secondary to chronic rejection following lung transplantation is a common complication associated with significant mortality in patients at least 5 years posttransplant. Therapy is important in delaying further decline in lung function. The clinical diagnosis of this disorder is difficult. Such patients may be asymptomatic with slowly evolving obstructive physiology on PFTs (175). Transbronchial biopsy is not sensitive and CT may be normal. ^{3}He MR can demonstrate ventilation defects in patients with mild bronchiolitis obliterans that are more extensive than the abnormalities seen on scintigraphy. Only 65% of the ^{3}He defects had corresponding abnormalities identified on CT (165,176).

Defects are observed among patients with COPD, with or without emphysema (170,171,177,178). These patients also demonstrate long-time constants for wash-in on dynamic ^{3}He studies and abnormal helium diffusion with emphysema (see later). In the presence of emphysema, both multiple, frequently large ^{3}He defects and a heterogeneous ventilation pattern are seen, which correlate with the CT findings of emphysema.

Such static helium studies to date indicate that this is a very sensitive method to detect regional ventilatory abnormalities. However, the helium defects themselves appear to be nonspecific. Another drawback of the static ^{3}He technique is its inability to demonstrate air trapping (175). However, as indicated later, such gas trapping can be readily identified using a dynamic ^{3}He imaging sequence.

Other airway applications of static ^{3}He MR have included imaging of the upper airway and trachea (169). Three-dimensional reconstructions of the helium lung images can be used to obtain ^{3}He MR volumetry, which can quantify the volumes of ventilated lung. These have been well-correlated with global spirometry in normal subjects, patients with fibrosis, and patients with unilateral lung transplants. However, unlike the global PFTs, the MR volumetry can be used to quantify the volume of individual ventilated lungs, such as the native and grafted lungs in a single-lung transplant (165,179,180). Finally, such static hyperpolarized ^{3}He scans have been able to localize air leaks from the lung parenchyma into the pleura in an animal model with pneumothorax (181).

Dynamic Helium Imaging

Using newer rapid-pulse sequences, dynamic ^{3}He images can now be obtained with temporal resolutions in the range of 5.4 to 120 mseconds per frame (Fig. 6-19) (182–186). These pulse sequences include interleaved echo-planar imaging (EPI) and radial and spiral techniques. Such dynamic helium imaging may be considered to provide "regional spirometry" (80,179,187). These rapid scans show the dispersion of ^{3}He through the lungs during a complete respiratory cycle. In normal subjects, the hyperpolarized helium shows rapid inflow through the central airways, followed by synchronous and homogeneous distribution into the distal airspaces (165,185).

With motion correction of these rapid imaging sequences, quantitative measures of the ^{3}He dynamics can be calculated. These parameters include (a) tracheal transit time, (a) tracheo-alveolar time interval, (c) alveolar rise time, and (d) alveolar signal amplitude (187). The time to peak enhancement of the trachea and the lung parenchyma can also be measured (185). In emphysema, the dynamic helium sequence demonstrates an irregular and asynchronous distribution pattern, with areas of slow or absent uptake (Fig. 6-19), slow wash-out, and areas of gas trapping (80,182). The distribution may become more uniform during rebreathing. The slow decay of the signal in some areas may relate to regions with low alveolar Po$_2$ (see later) in addition to gas trapping. Dynamic helium imaging, in combination with the diffusion measurements described later, could provide regional functional information that would be useful in the preoperative evaluation of patients with emphysema who are being considered for LVRS. In single-lung transplants, dynamic helium imaging has shown preferential (earlier and more prolonged) flow of gas into the normal transplanted lung compared with the diseased transplanted lung (187).

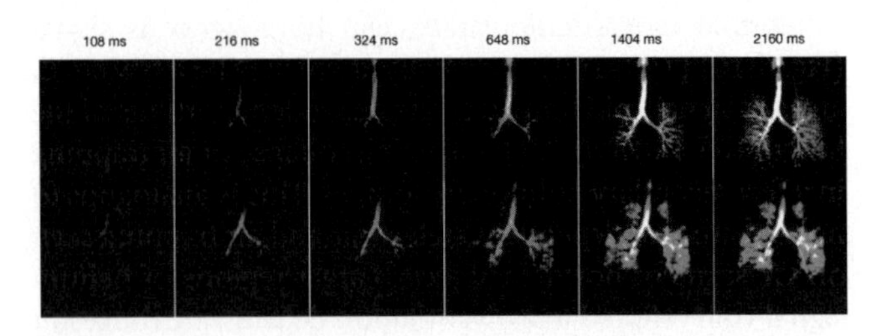

Figure 6-19 Dynamic ^{3}He MR imaging. The upper series shows radial projection images (128 views per frame) selected at intervals from the first part of an inhalation in a healthy normal subject. The time course of passage of gas down the trachea into the bronchi is clearly resolved. The lower series shows a dynamic time sequence in a patient with COPD with areas of slow ventilation in both lungs, particularly in the upper lobes. (From Mills GH, Wild JM, Eberle B, Van Beek EJR. Functional magnetic resonance imaging of the lung. *Br J Anaesth* 2003;91:16–300, with permission.)

Quantification of Regional Ventilation Using ^{3}He MR

Helium imaging can also be used to quantify and map relative ventilation on a regional basis. This is done by repetition of the imaging after sequentially incrementing the number of helium breaths. The rate of rise of signal intensity versus the number of helium-containing breaths is calculated as the fresh new helium gradually replaces the alveolar volume of air. From these wash-in curves, a rate constant (r) can be derived, which is a measure of the local fractional ventilation. This method has been used to obtain fractional ventilation maps and histograms of their frequency distribution in a rat model of elastase-induced emphysema (Fig. 6-20) (188) as well as in a murine model of asthma (189).

Diffusion-Weighted ^{3}He Imaging

Helium atoms, being of relatively low atomic weight, have high rates of diffusion. Diffusion referred to here is that of Brownian motion at the atomic level, rather than the more common notion of bulk gas diffusion across the alveolar-capillary membrane. With the use of bipolar gradients to diphase the spins of moving atoms, diffusion-weighted ^{3}He MR images can be produced (190). Diffusion-weighted MR sequences can thus provide a measure of the apparent diffusion coefficient (ADC) of the helium gas, which is a measure of the distance the atoms can travel within a unit time.

With unrestricted motion, the ^{3}He atoms will move approximately 0.4 mm in 1 msecond (or 0.88 cm^2/second) (191). This translates to a displacement of up to several millimeters during the echo time of a typical gradient-echo pulse sequence (175). Thus in open spaces such as the trachea, the diffusion of the gas atoms is rapid, reflected in a high value of the ADC. On the other hand, the restricted spatial architecture of normal alveoli, acini, and bronchioles results in low values for the ADC ($\leq$0.2 cm^2/second) (192–195).

In pulmonary disorders associated with abnormal enlargement of the distal airways and alveoli, including

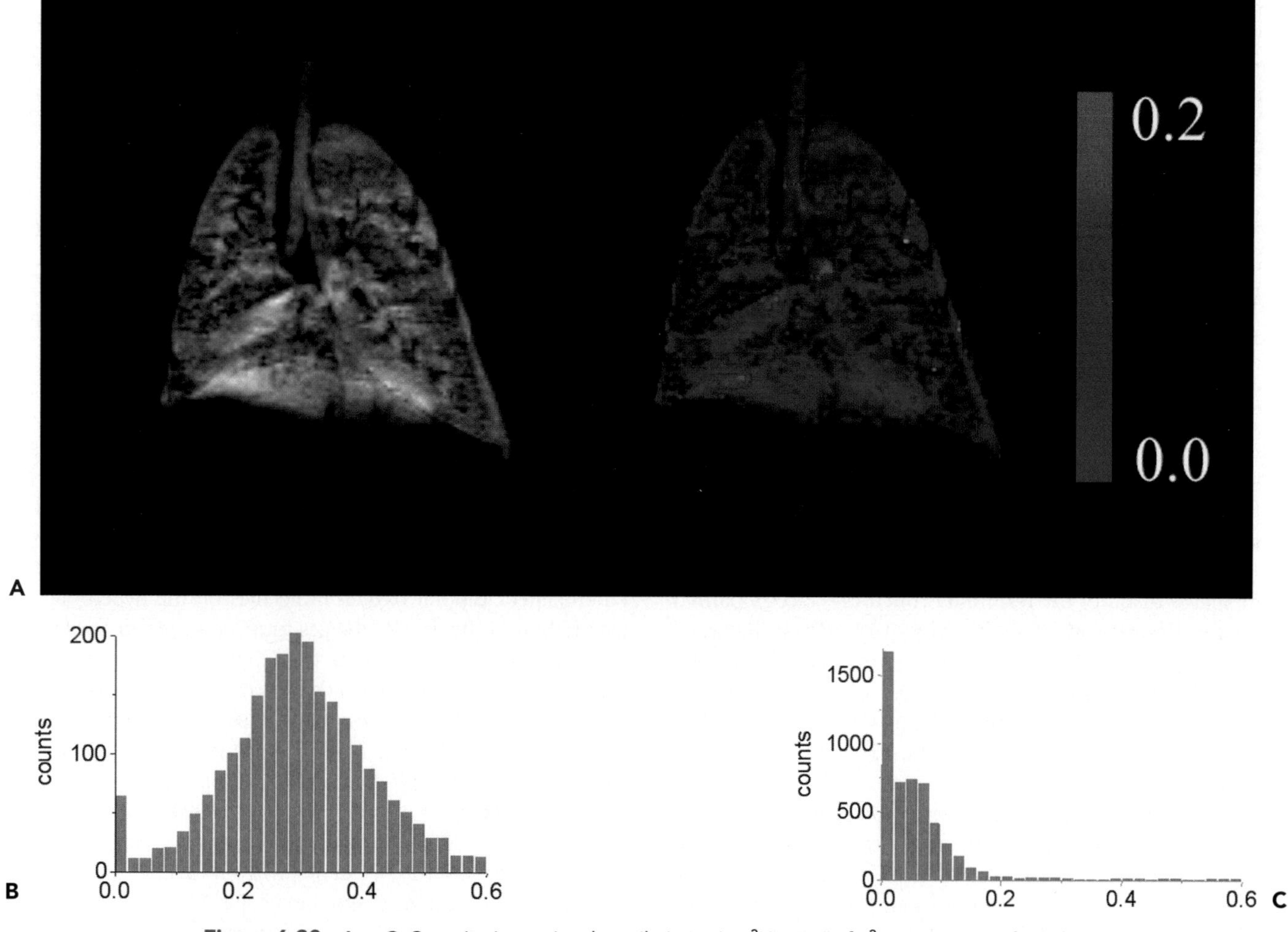

Figure 6-20 **A** to **C:** Quantitative regional ventilation using ^{3}He. **A:** *(Left)* ^{3}He MR image of emphysematous rat lung. *(Right)* Corresponding fractional ventilation color map. (Values exceeding the indicated range are depicted in orange.) **B:** Histogram of the distribution of regional ventilation in a normal rat. **C:** Histogram of the distribution of regional ventilation in an emphysematous rat. Note the shift toward increased lung units with lower regional fractional ventilation in the emphysematous rat compared with the normal rat.

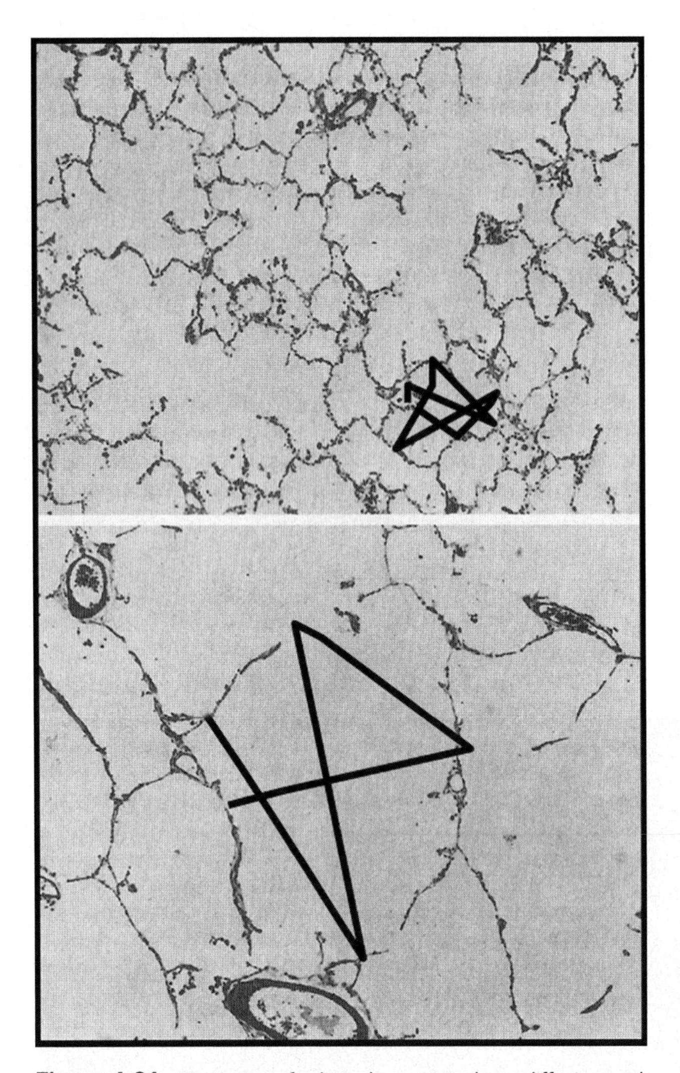

Figure 6-21 Depiction of relatively restricted gas diffusion path *(black line)* in normal alveoli *(top)* compared with longer diffusion path in the enlarged alveoli of emphysema *(bottom)*. The latter results in an increased measured ADC using diffusion-weighted ^{3}He.

emphysema as well as the traction bronchiectasis and honeycombing associated with advanced pulmonary fibrosis, the ADC values are abnormally elevated (196). Emphysema is defined by permanent enlargement of the airspaces distal to the terminal bronchioles, accompanied by the destruction of their walls (197). These enlarged airspaces enable longer diffusion paths (Fig. 6-21), and thus the ADC values increase to 0.4 to 0.9 cm^2/second, based on animal and human studies (196,198,199). The ADC values in emphysema may be up to 2.5 times larger than normal (198).

Moreover, the ADC values, which are spatially homogeneous in normal lung, are heterogeneously distributed in emphysema (200). The degree of heterogeneity can be assessed by maps as well as frequency histograms of the ADC values (Fig. 6-22) (200,201). The values correlate with FEV_1 (200). In a comparison of diffusion-weighted ^{3}He MR with CT using a visual grading system for emphysema in heavy smokers, smokers with FEV_1 greater than 70% of predicted, and normal controls, the MR studies showed more extensive emphysematous changes than did CT. The findings thus suggest a greater sensitivity for diffusion-weighted MR, although the specificity remains unknown (202). Diffusion-weighted ^{3}He may prove useful in very early detection of emphysema in smokers or those with α_1-antitrypsin deficiency. Early detection is of increasing importance with the advent of potential new therapies being developed for emphysema such as retinoic acid, antiprotease therapy, and others.

Normal diffusion is anisotropic, because alveoli and distal air passages are nonspherical, with diffusion being greater along the longitudinal axis of these airways. Measuring the ADC values of ^{3}He in all three orthogonal axes can therefore provide information not only about the size but also about the shape of the airspaces at the acinar level in health and disease. The mean longitudinal ADC is three times greater than the mean transverse ADC in normals. This is in contrast to emphysema, in which both the longitudinal and transverse ADCs are increased, reducing the anisotropy and indicative of abnormal sphericity of the alveolar spaces (191). Thus, rather remarkably, diffusion-weighted helium MR can be used to assess alveolar microstructure even beyond the anatomic resolution of HRCT performed on current clinical multislice CT scanners.

Alveolar Po_2 Measurements from ^{3}He

Using measurements of Po_2 in inspired and expired gas, together with oximetry of arterial and mixed venous blood, the global oxygen uptake of the lungs can be determined and the venous admixture ("shunt") fraction can be estimated (80). However, these methods do not provide any spatial localization of these parameters, and analysis of regional alveolar gas is difficult. Indirect measures of alveolar and corresponding end-capillary Po_2 are derived using inspired Po_2, arterial Pco_2, and the gas exchange ratio (80). ^{3}He MR now offers a novel, noninvasive approach for determining regional alveolar Po_2.

The ^{3}He signal decays during the course of a sustained breath hold, resulting from depolarization by both the RF pulses used for MR imaging as well as the effect of the weakly paramagnetic dipolar oxygen molecules on the hyperpolarized helium. (This is why the gas must be stored in oxygen-free glass cells.) With respect to the latter, the rate of the oxygen-induced helium signal decay is dependent on the alveolar Po_2 (203). This effect of oxygen was initially considered a major impediment for ^{3}He imaging, until it was realized that it could be exploited to provide an instantaneous measurement of the intraalveolar Po_2 (187,204). As has often been the case in science, when a disadvantage is well characterized and understood, it can be turned into an advantage.

Fortunately, imaging sequences have been designed (using either two inhalations or, more recently, a single breath-hold technique) that can isolate and quantify the effect of Po_2 versus the RF pulses on ^{3}He signal decay. Regional Po_2 can be measured at the onset of a breath hold as well as at multiple times during the breath hold to

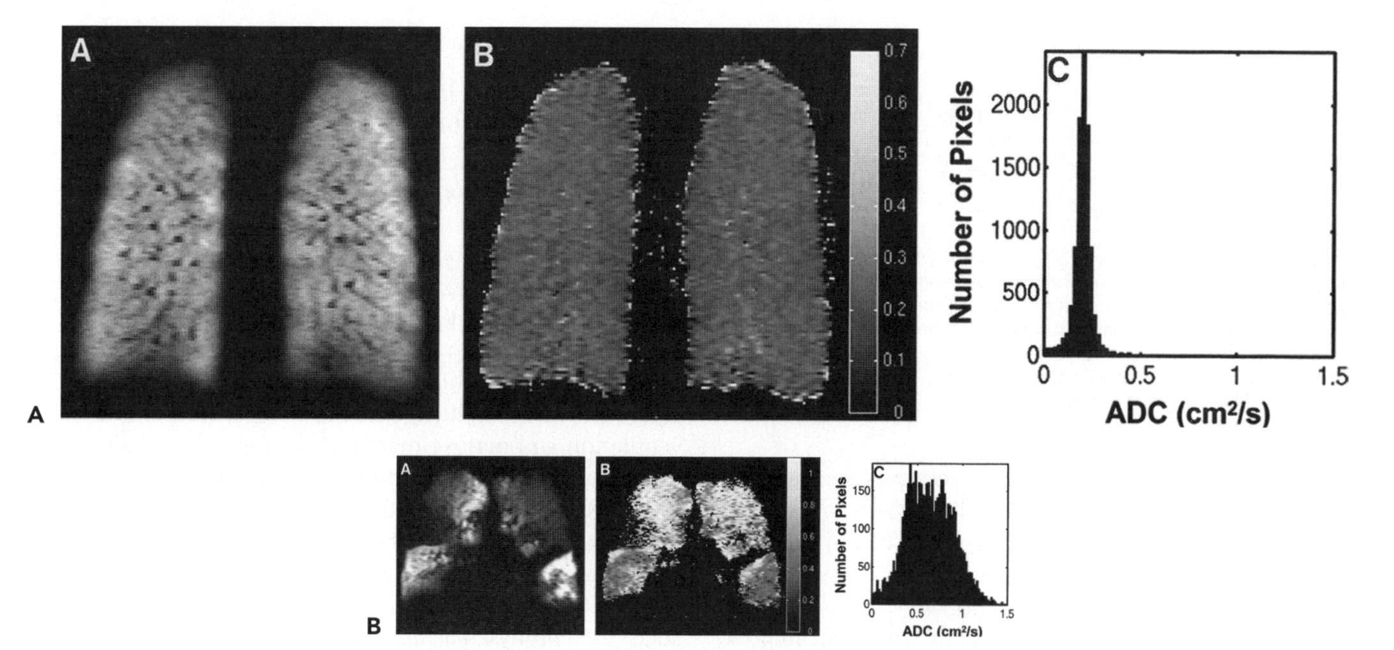

Figure 6-22 **A** and **B:** ^{3}He diffusion in a normal subject compared with a patient with emphysema. **A:** Coronal ventilation (A, *left*) and ADC (B, *middle*) ^{3}He MR images and the corresponding ADC histogram (C, *right*) in a representative volunteer. The signal intensities in **A** and **B** are homogeneous, and **C** depicts the low values for the mean ADC (0.21 cm^2/second) and SD (0.06 cm^2/second) in this image section. **B:** Coronal ventilation (A, *left*) and ADC (B, *middle*) ^{3}He MR images and the corresponding ADC histogram (C, *right*) in a patient with severe emphysema. Inhomogeneous signal intensities and several ventilation defects are seen in **A**. Compared with normal, **B** shows a general increase in the ADCs, particularly in the upper portions of the lung, which is reflected by an increase in the mean (0.64 cm^2/second), and a wider range of ADCs, which is reflected by an increase in the SD (0.27 cm^2/second) and in the width of the histogram in **C**. (From Salerno M, deLange E, Altes T, et al.: Emphysema: hyperpolarized helium3 diffusion MR imaging of the lungs compared with spirometric indexes—initial experience. *Radiology* 2002;222:252–260, with permission.)

determine its rate of decrease. The rate of PO_2 depletion resulting from alveolar-capillary oxygen transfer is a reflection of pulmonary perfusion (see later).

The ^{3}He-based MR measurements of regional alveolar PO_2 have been made in phantoms for validation, in animal models, and in humans (Fig. 6-23) (204–208). Studies have shown that the mean ^{3}He MR-derived PO_2 approximates the end-tidal PO_2 in healthy subjects (204) and is between that of end-tidal gas and arterial blood in patients (205).

Pulmonary Perfusion via ^{3}He MR

Alveolar oxygen consumption during a breath hold is governed by capillary perfusion rates together with end-capillary and precapillary oxygen concentration gradients (Fick's principle). Thus, alveolar perfusion rates can be calculated using ^{3}He MR to determine the alveolar PO_2 depletion rate, together with the results of venous blood gases (209). (This assumes the alveolar-capillary oxygen transfer rate is perfusion-limited, i.e., end-capillary oxygen concentration is determined by the P_AO_2.)

^{3}He MR may therefore be used not only for measuring regional alveolar PO_2 but also to measure the corresponding regional pulmonary perfusion. In areas of lung with absent or diminished perfusion (e.g., in pulmonary embolism and other parenchymal pathology), the rate of oxygen uptake by

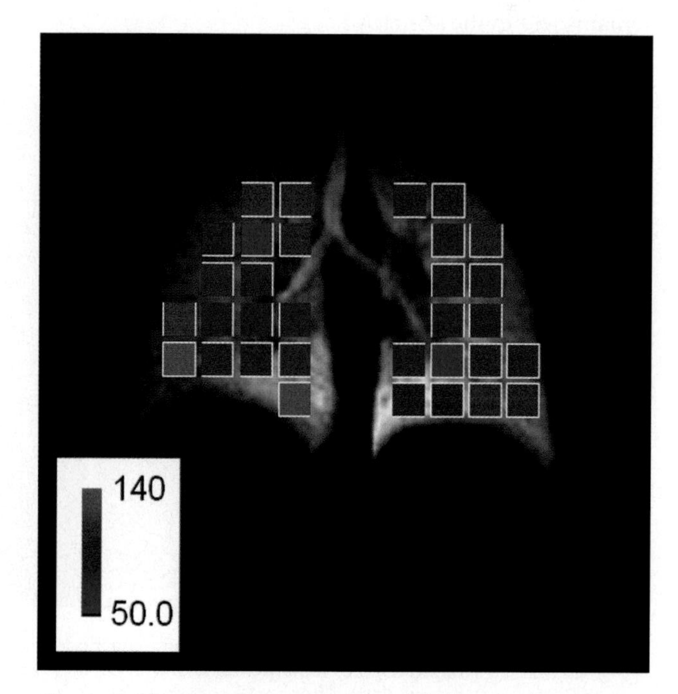

Figure 6-23 Map of regional P_AO_2 (in torr) derived from ^{3}He MR in a normal human subject.

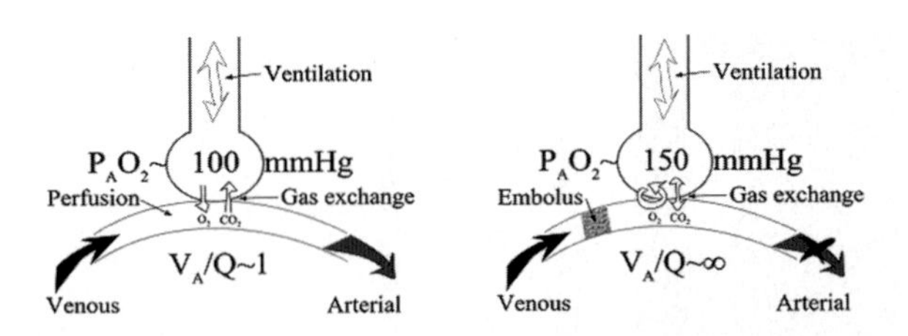

Figure 6-24 Diagrams of V_A/Q relationships in an alveolar-capillary unit. *Left* represents normal gas exchange, and *right* depicts altered gas exchange in pulmonary embolism. Note the resulting increased alveolar Po_2 owing to obstructed perfusion in pulmonary embolism. (From Ishii M, Fischer M, Emami K, et al. Hyperpolarized 3helium MR imaging of pulmonary function. *Radiol Clin N Am* 2005;43:235–246, with permission.)

regional blood flow will be reduced, resulting in an abnormally high regional alveolar Po_2 (Fig. 6-24) and consequently a lower ^{3}He MR signal (Fig. 6-25). In addition, the Po_2 will fall relatively slowly during the breath hold. Indeed, a correlation between the initial Po_2 and its rate of decline has been observed, consistent with matching of ventilation and perfusion (204). ^{3}He MR-based P_AO_2 measurements can thus be used to map perfusion throughout the lungs and have depicted areas of V/Q mismatch in pulmonary embolism (210,211). Preliminary results suggest that the ^{3}He-derived perfusion measurements agree with those obtained using microspheres, the gold standard for measuring pulmonary perfusion.

Thus, helium MR can be used to evaluate both pulmonary ventilation and perfusion. (Methods to further calculate V/Q ratios directly from the helium data are discussed further next.) It is rather extraordinary that pulmonary perfusion as well as oxygen exchange across the alveolar-capillary membrane can be assessed using hyperpolarized helium MR despite the fact that the helium gas remains within the airspaces!

Regional V/Q Calculation from ^{3}He MR

Matching of pulmonary ventilation and perfusion is a critical parameter in enabling optimal gas exchange, a primary function of the lung. Autoregulatory mechanisms such as hypoxic vasoconstriction and hypocapnic bronchoconstriction act to maintain a normal V/Q ratio. Hypoxemia in most pulmonary disorders is the result of disturbances in this matching. For example, in chronic interstitial lung disease, hypoxemia is primarily the consequence of such V/Q mismatching, rather than diffusion impairment resulting from the thickened, reorganized alveolar walls. Even in the normal lung, because of the effects of gravity, ventilation and perfusion are not homogeneously distributed spatially, and the multiple inert gas elimination technique (MIGET), which is the gold standard for assessing V/Q ratios in the lung, demonstrates the presence of units in the lung with a range of V/Q values, although with a mean value close to 1.0. In the presence of lung disorders such as emphysema and pulmonary embolism, the frequency of lung units with V/Q ratios substantially less than or greater than 1.0 can increase markedly.

Although the MIGET technique is a powerful physiologic tool, it provides no topographic location of the various lung V/Q "units" being measured. In fact, until recently no techniques have been available to map V/Q ratios throughout the lungs with a high degree of spatial resolution. Nuclear medicine ventilation and perfusion scintigraphic imaging has been the fundamental imaging-based method to assess regional V/Q ratios in the lungs. The technique, however, suffers from relatively poor spatial resolution. SPECT imaging improves on this resolution by providing tomographic capability. This is improved even further with PET using ^{13}N-N2, with subcentimeter resolution. The latter technique, however, is not generally available except on an investigational basis.

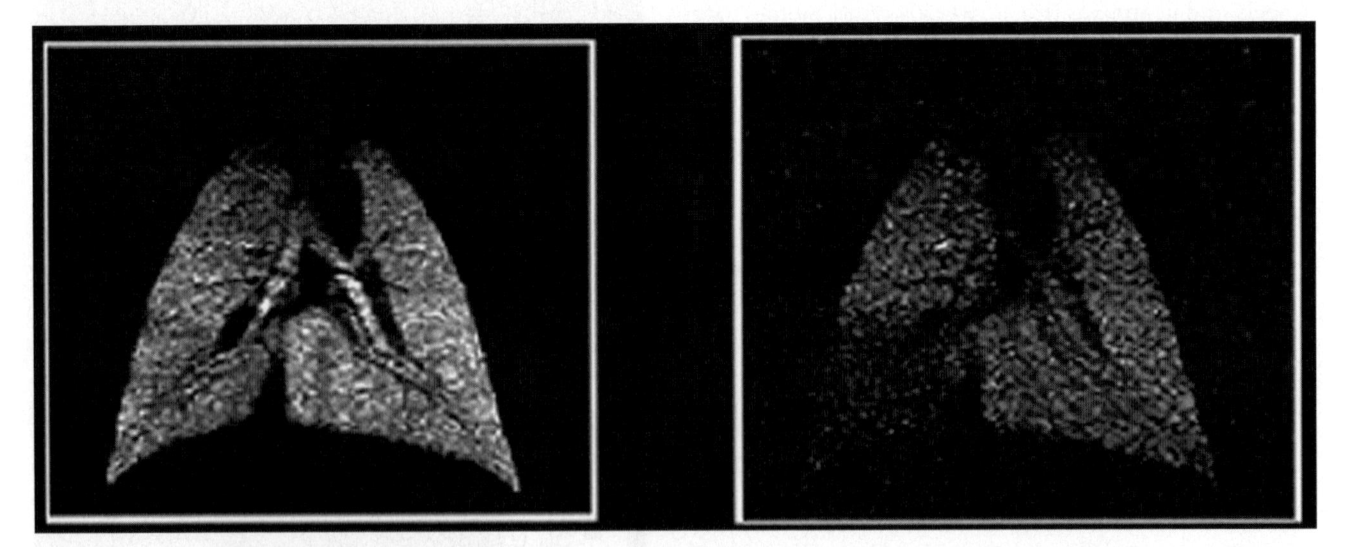

Figure 6-25 ^{3}He MR images in a pig model of pulmonary embolism. Balloon catheter occlusion of the right lower lobar pulmonary artery. Initial ventilation image shows homogeneous distribution of the gas *(left)*. After an 18-second delay, there is more rapid decay of the helium signal in the right lower lobe apparent as a wedge-shaped defect *(right)*. This defect results from the destructive effect of the higher regional alveolar Po_2 on the helium signal distal to the simulated pulmonary embolism (see diagrams in Fig. 6-24).

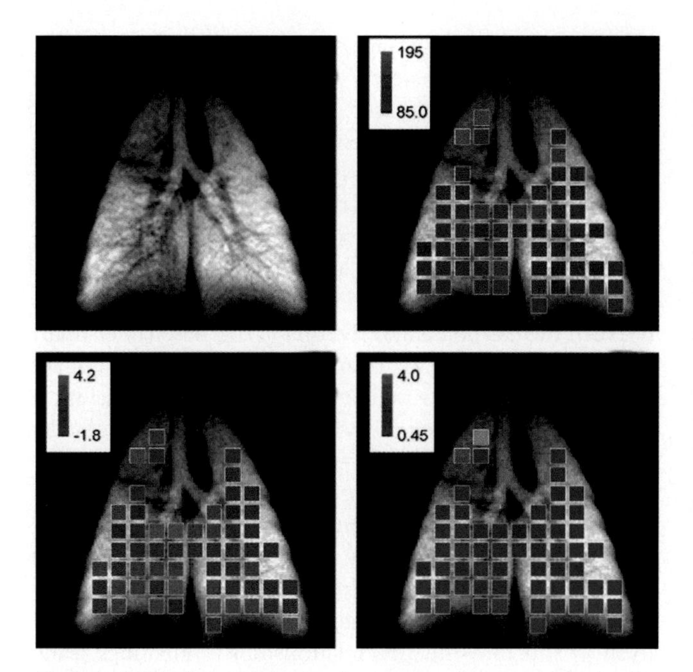

Figure 6-26 ^{3}He MR **(A)**, and corresponding regional alveolar P_{O_2} **(B)**, alveolar P_{O_2} depletion rate **(C)**, and calculated regional ventilation–perfusion ratio map **(D)** in a healthy pig. The parametric maps were all derived from the ^{3}He MR gas behavior. (From Ishii M, Fischer M, Emami K, et al. Hyperpolarized 3helium MR imaging of pulmonary function. *Radiol Clin N Am* 2005;43:235–246, with permission.)

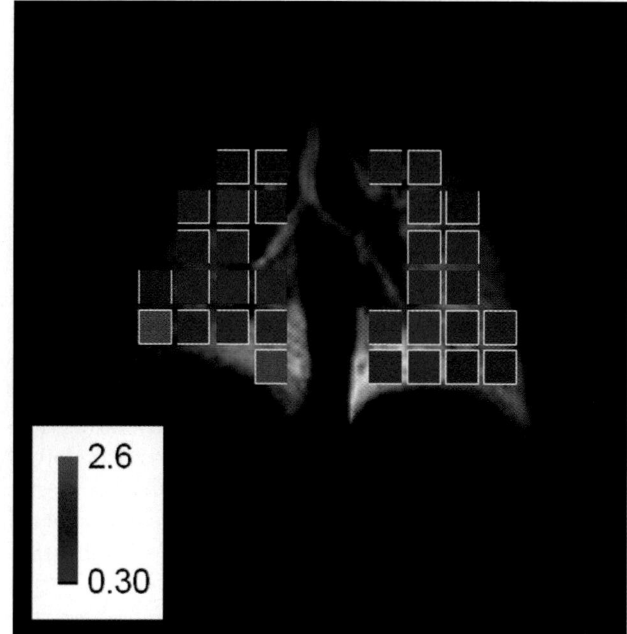

Figure 6-28 Map of regional V/Q ratios in a healthy human subject. This corresponds to the alveolar P_{O_2} map in Fig. 6-21. The average V_A/Q ratio for the entire lung was 0.93. V_A/Q ratios in the 32 regions depicted ranged from 0.32 to 2.6. Thus, despite normal regional heterogeneity in the V/Q values, there is close matching of ventilation and perfusion globally.

Now advances in MR and CT imaging are making it possible to assess V/Q ratios in the lungs to an even smaller scale. Until recently, this was carried out using MR by registering images of ventilation (obtained with ^{3}He or oxygen) with those of perfusion (using either gadolinium contrast agents or arterial spin tagging). Sophisticated coregistration algorithms have been applied to superimposing these scans to obtain V/Q maps (212). Such registration, however, can be challenging. With the advent of oxygen-sensitive hyperpolarized ^{3}He MR imaging, ^{129}Xe MR imaging, and xenon-enhanced CT imaging, exciting new approaches to direct measurements of regional V/Q relationships with very high topographic resolution are being demonstrated. The MR methods have been carried out on both animals and human subjects on an investigational basis, whereas the CT technique has been limited to animal models to date.

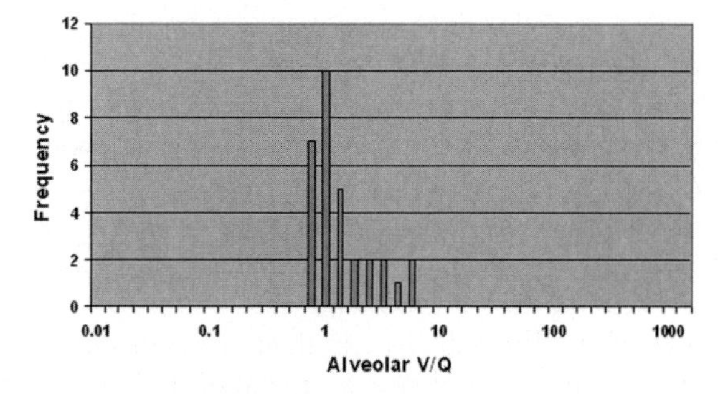

Figure 6-27 Frequency distribution of regional V_A/Q ratios in a porcine model of pulmonary embolism (balloon catheter–induced perfusion abnormality). Note regions with high alveolar V/Q values exceeding 1.0.

The principles by which helium and xenon gases are used to determine V/Q are distinctly different, however.

As described earlier, ^{3}He can be used to calculate regional alveolar P_{O_2}. We also indicated that the rate of P_{O_2} depletion during a breath hold can be used to derive the corresponding pulmonary perfusion. To obtain V_A/Q (alveolar V/Q) using hyperpolarized ^{3}He, the alveolar P_{O_2} is first measured (213) and used together with blood gas concentrations in conventional gas-exchange equations to derive the regional V_A/Q ratio (214–216). The method is essentially the reverse of a more traditional technique used to calculate regional P_AO_2 from an assumed V_A/Q ratio.

Spatial maps and histograms of the frequency distribution of both regional P_AO_2 and regional V/Q have been obtained recently in animal models (Fig. 6-26), including a porcine model of pulmonary embolism (Fig. 6-27), as well as in healthy human subjects (Fig. 6-28) (215). The frequency distributions of V_A/Q ratios derived from ^{3}He are comparable to those obtained using MIGET, the gold standard technique for global V_A/Q measurement (217).

Other approaches to direct measurements of regional V/Q using hyperpolarized ^{129}Xe MR and xenon-enhanced CT are described later.

HYPERPOLARIZED ^{129}XENON MR

^{129}Xe, like ^{3}He, is a noble gas that can be hyperpolarized for MR imaging via laser optical pumping. In fact xenon, rather than helium, was the first of these gases observed to yield images of the lung airspaces (218). Static gas-space imaging has been carried out in animals as well as in humans with spatial resolution of less than 1 cm^3 (219–221).

There are several important differences between ^{3}He and ^{129}Xe. ^{129}Xe is abundant and therefore inexpensive compared with ^{3}He, a considerable advantage. However, it has a lower gyromagnetic ratio and therefore generates less signal. ^{129}Xe is more difficult to polarize, and the polarization decays more rapidly than that of ^{3}He.

Another important difference between these noble gases is that ^{129}Xe, unlike ^{3}He, is highly soluble in blood and lipids. Although this is a problem in that higher concentrations of xenon are potentially anesthetic, it gives xenon unique properties that can be exploited for interesting MR-based physiologic imaging. The lipid solubility allows for a rapid exchange between gas in the alveoli and dissolved phases in the pulmonary interstitium. Moreover, the spectra from xenon within the gas, tissue, and blood compartments can be differentiated by their distinct chemical shift peaks on MR spectroscopy (Fig. 6-29) (222).

To facilitate gas exchange between air and blood, the human lung consists of approximately 300 million alveoli, forming a total surface area of approximately 100 m^2 (223–225). Although alveolar size varies throughout the respiratory cycle, at 75% TLC the alveoli reach a diameter of 200 to 300 μ and have an average wall thickness of 5 to 6 μ (225). Traveling from the alveolar space to a hemoglobin molecule inside an erythrocyte, a xenon atom must cross multiple barriers: the liquid alveolar lining, the alveolar epithelium, interstitium, the capillary endothelium, the capillary plasma, and finally the membrane and cytoplasm of a red blood cell (223). Despite these numerous membrane layers, the combined thickness of the air–blood barrier is only a fraction of 1 μ, reflecting the extreme thinness of each layer. Considering the average diffusion constant for xenon in tissue to be approximately 2×10^{-5} cm^2/second, a xenon atom requires about 10 mseconds to diffuse across the alveolar wall (223). Measurements of this diffusion constant can thereby be used to derive data on the thickness of the alveolar-capillary barrier (175,222,223,226). In addition, measurement of these kinetics can be used to quantify pulmonary perfusion as well as ventilation.

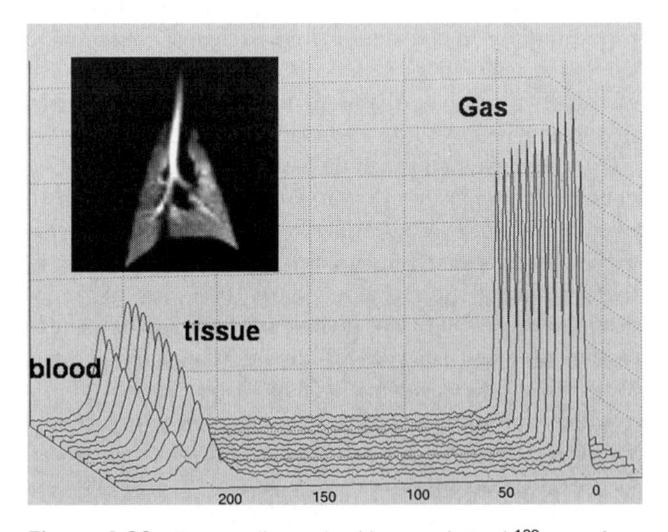

Figure 6-29 Temporally resolved hyperpolarized ^{129}xenon lung spectra. Note ability to separate peaks representing the ^{129}xenon in the gas phase (airspaces), tissue (interstitium), and blood (alveolar capillaries). By following the kinetics of gas transfer across the alveolar-capillary membrane, multiple parameters can be derived, including alveolar wall thickness and direct measurement of alveolar V/Q. (Courtesy of Bastiaan Driehuys, PhD., Duke University Medical Center)

Because of the large difference in the chemical shifts between the gas-phase and the dissolved-phase (interstitial) compartments, the ^{129}Xe polarization in the dissolved phase can be selectively destroyed by a series of frequency-selective RF pulses (223). During the delay between RF pulses, the depolarized xenon rapidly exchanges with the gas phase atoms, thereby reducing signal in the gas-phase compartment. This technique, referred to as xenon polarization transfer contrast (XTC) (223,227), can provide for measurements of regional lung tissue density, alveolar surface-to-volume ratio, and alveolar wall thickness. ^{129}Xe, therefore, can be a powerful tool to study structure–function relationships in the lungs at the level of the alveolar-capillary membrane.

As is the case for ^{3}He, measurements of ADC from diffusion imaging (and T2*) data using ^{129}Xe can be performed to yield information on alveolar size and shape (194,195). Furthermore, sensitivity to oxygen may allow for alveolar Po_2 measurements in a manner similar to ^{3}He.

Thus, as discussed for ^{3}He, ^{129}Xe MR can reveal features of microscopic alveolar fine structure below the spatial resolution of the scans. As noted earlier, dynamic structural images are often used to assess function, but as exemplified here, the converse can also take place, namely, the use of functional imaging to derive structure.

OXYGEN-ENHANCED MR

Molecular oxygen, being weakly paramagnetic as a result of its two unpaired outer electrons, can serve as another MR ventilation agent (Fig. 6-30). Unlike hyperpolarized helium, the signal obtained after inhalation of 100% oxygen does not come directly from the gas itself in the airspaces. Rather, the signal enhancement on T1-weighted proton images results from the T1-shortening effect of the oxygen on the pulmonary tissue. The oxygen diffuses across the alveolar-capillary membrane into the interstitium and dissolves in the capillary (pulmonary venous) blood. Thus, the oxygen can cause T1 shortening of both interstitial water and the blood. (The oxygen also has a T2 shortening effect on the hemoglobin in red blood cells, but this is a minor effect.) Inhalation of 100% oxygen results in a T1 shortening of the lung by 9% to 12% (228,229). Signal intensity in the lungs can increase by up to 18% compared with room air (229–231). The relaxivity (1/T1) of the lung shows excellent correlation with the arterial oxygen partial pressure (PaO_2) (232). Oxygen-enhanced MR imaging makes use of single-shot turbo spin-echo images with optimized inversion recovery to

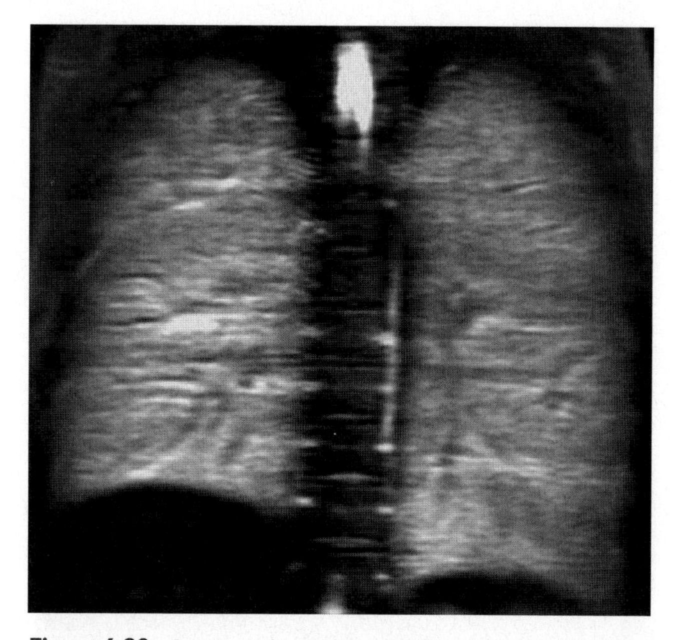

Figure 6-30 Oxygen-enhanced proton MR image showing homogeneous lung signal in a healthy volunteer. (From Kauczor H-U, Kanke A, van Beek EJR. Assessment of lung ventilation by MR imaging: current status and future perspectives. *Eur Radiol* 2002;12:1962–1970, with permission.)

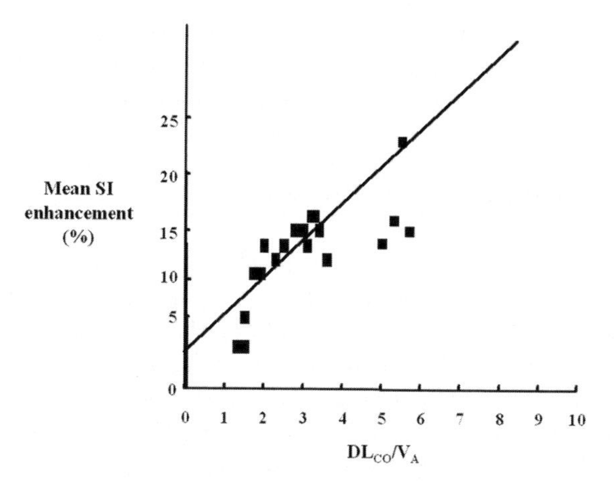

Figure 6-31 Linear correlation between mean lung signal intensity (SI) enhancement on oxygen-enhanced proton MR and pulmonary diffusing capacity for CO (D_LCO) ($r = 0.81$). This correlation is a consequence of the fact that the oxygen enhancement is dependent on diffusion of the weakly paramagnetic oxygen molecules into the interstitial water and capillary blood. (Courtesy of Y. Ohno, MD, Kobe University.)

obtain T1-weighting (166,233). Defects in the oxygen-enhanced MR lung images have been shown in animal models of airway obstruction (166,233). Using oxygen-enhanced MR in combination with MR perfusion imaging, V/Q mismatches have been demonstrated in both animal models and human subjects with pulmonary embolism (166,234). Dynamic imaging with a temporal resolution of 9 seconds showing the wash-in and wash-out of the oxygen enhancement and corresponding quantitative time constants has been reported (232).

Because the basis for the signal enhancement is related to the alveolar-capillary diffusion of oxygen, an excellent correlation between signal enhancement and D_LCO measurements of diffusing capacity in patients has been demonstrated (Fig. 6-31) (235–237). Thus, oxygen-enhanced MR may provide a relatively easily performed, noninvasive means to map regional diffusing capacity in the lungs. In addition, the mean slope of relative signal enhancement with oxygen has been strongly correlated with the FEV_1.

Significant advantages of oxygen-enhanced MR are that oxygen is widely abundant, inexpensive, and safe and that it can be used on routine proton MR scanners without the need for the additional sophisticated hardware and software that are required for hyperpolarized gas imaging. Oxygen is considerably easier to handle than the hyperpolarized gases. Furthermore, its physical characteristics closely approximate those of room air. There are several important drawbacks, however. Compared with hyperpolarized helium, the enhancement from oxygen has a very low signal-to-noise ratio. To compensate for this, the images are compiled by averaging over multiple respiratory cycles and by subtracting scans obtained while breathing 100% oxygen from those acquired while breathing room air. Another potential drawback of the oxygen-enhanced technique compared with hyperpolarized gas imaging is that ventilation is detected somewhat indirectly via the paramagnetic effects on the tissue, rather than the gas as the direct source of the signal.

OTHER MR VENTILATION CONTRAST AGENTS

Although hyperpolarized helium has been the principal MR contrast agent for ventilation studied to date, several other agents have also been considered. These include hyperpolarized ^{129}Xe, gadolinium aerosols, and fluorine MR.

Aerosolized Gadolinium

Gadolinium-based MR contrast agents in solution have been aerosolized for use in ventilation imaging. However, these agents have a tendency to deposit in the central airways and therefore have not been widely used.

Fluorine MR

Another approach to MR imaging of ventilation has been the use of fluorine MR.

After hydrogen protons, ^{19}F has the highest gyromagnetic ratio and is detectable with MR tuned to the Larmor frequency of fluorine rather than hydrogen. Highly fluorinated compounds have been used previously in the lung, including the perfluorocompounds, which have been used clinically for liquid ventilation and as oxygen-carrying blood substitutes, and sulfur hexafluoride (SF6). Here, ^{19}F atoms are bound within the fluorinated molecules.

Fluorine MR can be used to measure the T1 shortening of dissolved oxygen and thus the alveolar Po_2 (238). ^{19}F MR ventilation imaging has been performed in pigs (239).

XENON-ENHANCED CT

Stable xenon gas has a k edge close to that of iodine, allowing it to be detected by its density on CT images (Fig. 6-32) (240,241). As an offshoot of earlier work using xenon-enhanced CT scanning for evaluation of cerebral blood flow, xenon-enhanced CT imaging of the lungs has been shown to be feasible. Earlier studies were largely subjective and did not use the rapid respiratory and cardiac-gated CT scan capabilities now available on both EBCT and the newer multislice CT scanners. Recently, the ability to obtain accurate, quantitative CT images of regional-specific ventilation (ventilation per unit volume air in the lung) has been demonstrated on both EBCT and multislice CT scanners with a scan aperture of 500 msec-onds or less (Fig. 6-33). The current xenon-enhanced CT studies are limited to investigational studies in animal models. Phantom studies have shown a linear relationship between the CT density of the xenon gas and the concentration of the gas over a wide and clinically relevant range of concentrations. This relationship is 2.24 HU per percent increase in xenon concentration for multislice helical CT (240). Both static single-breath xenon-enhanced CT images and dynamic multibreath wash-out (Fig. 6-32) and wash-in imaging protocols have been demonstrated using spirometrically gated scanning. Because of the potential anesthetic effect of xenon, inhaled concentrations are kept below approximately 40%. Although the resulting CT signal is relatively lower than that of hyperpolarized helium, this is compensated for by subtracting the enhanced and the unenhanced images. These datasets are well registered because they are acquired at spirometrically controlled lung volumes.

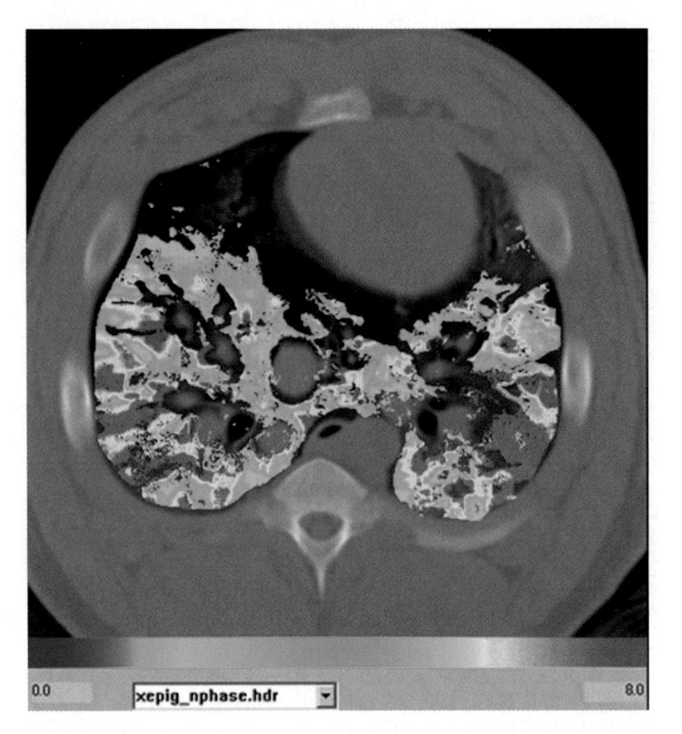

Figure 6-33 Functional map of specific ventilation derived from xenon-enhanced CT in a pig model. A powerful advantage of the CT-based method is its ability to display the quantitative map of regional ventilation directly within the high-resolution anatomic display provided by CT. (Courtesy of Eric A. Hoffman, PhD, University of Iowa.)

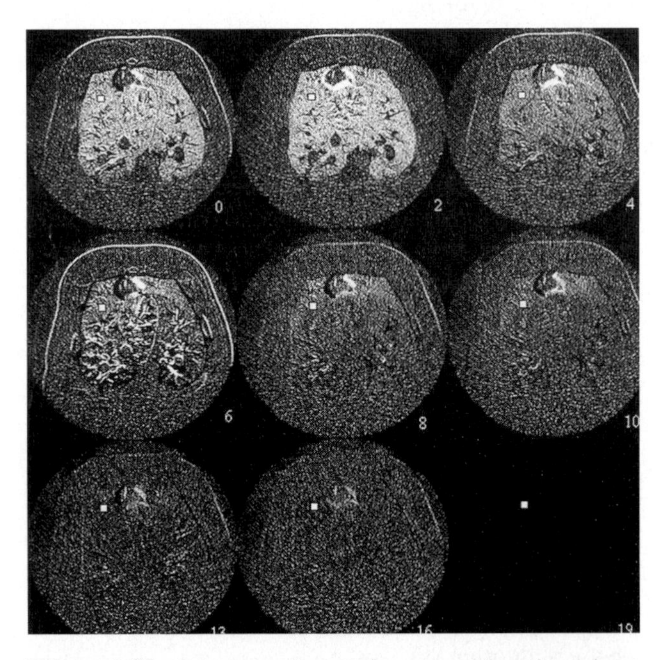

Figure 6-32 Subtraction images from a multibreath wash-out xenon-enhanced EBCT scan sequence. The lungs were equilibrated with a mixture of 66% xenon and 33% oxygen and then switched to breathing room air during image acquisition. The first image is the equilibrium image, followed by images taken over sequential breaths. The attenuation changes over time reflect tracer gas clearance. Note that the dependent lung regions clear the tracer gas more rapidly than do the nondependent lung regions. (From Tajik JK, Chon D, Won C, Tran BQ, Hoffman EA. Subsecond multisection CT of regional pulmonary ventilation. *Acad Radiol* 2002;9:130–146, with permission.)

Using the CT attenuation values before xenon gas inhalation, the distribution of air fraction in the lung can be mapped based on principles described earlier. Following xenon administration, specific ventilation can also be mapped. Initial results confirmed a greater calculated air fraction in the nondependent regions of the lung compared with the dependent areas, whereas the specific ventilation was greater in the dependent regions as expected (240). A very significant advantage of this technique is the ability to overlay the high-resolution functional ventilation maps onto the corresponding high-resolution anatomic displays available from CT (Fig. 6-33).

Moreover, with the use of bolus intravenous contrast enhancement, quantitative perfusion scans of the lungs can also now be obtained using CT (Fig. 6-34). Tight coregistration of spirometrically gated images of ventilation and perfusion is feasible and can be used to derive V/Q ratio maps (Fig. 6-34). Recently, however, a method to directly calculate

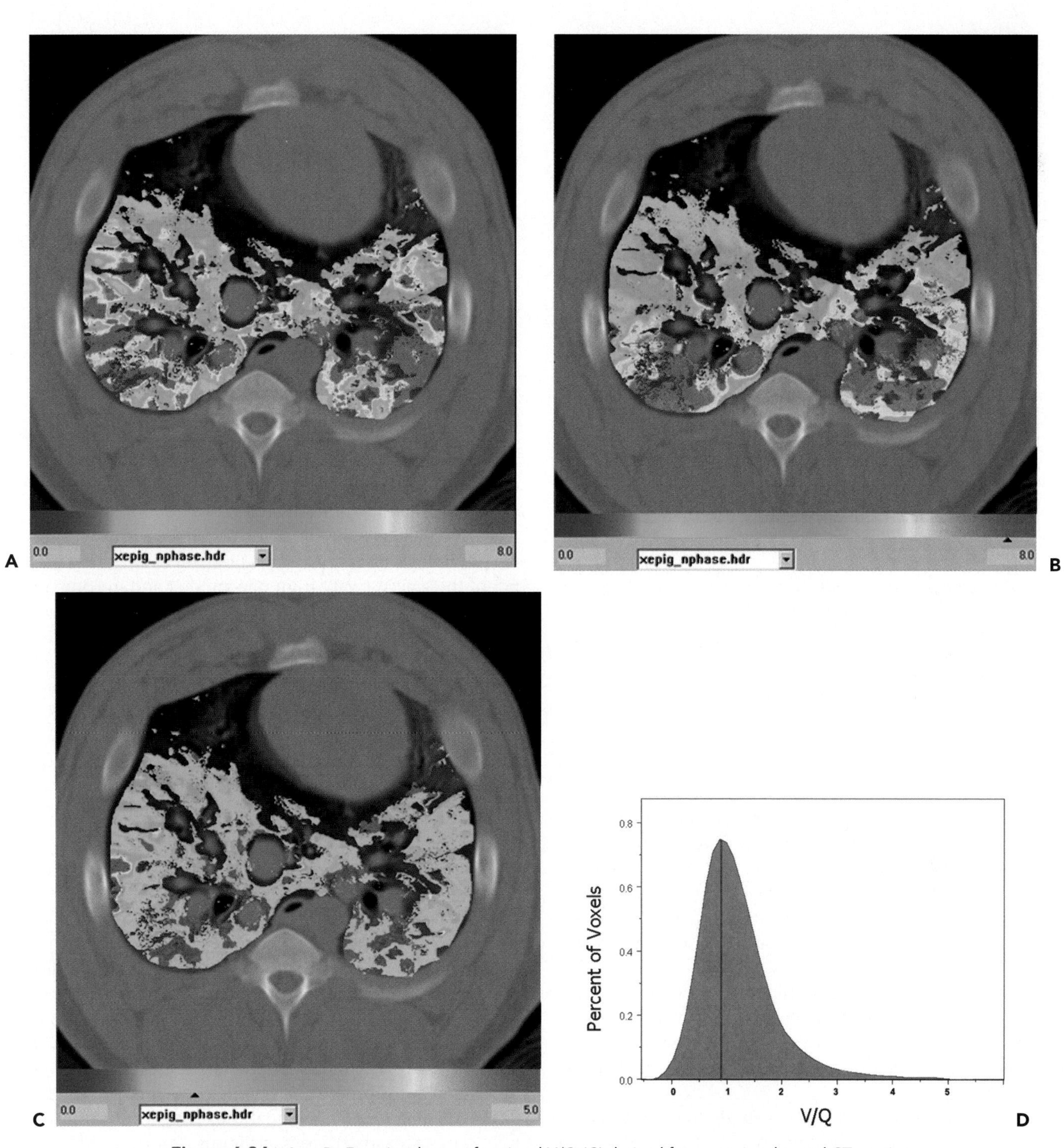

Figure 6-34 **A** to **D:** Functional map of regional V/Q **(C)** derived from xenon-enhanced CT ventilation **(A)** (this is same image as Fig. 6-33) and intravenous contrast-enhanced CT perfusion **(B)** maps in a pig model. Note that despite gravity-dependent spatial heterogeneity in both ventilation and perfusion, there is relatively greater homogeneity in the V/Q map, reflecting V/Q matching. This can also be seen in the histogram of the frequency distribution of the regional V/Q ratios **(D),** with a median V/Q close to 1.0 (0.85). The histogram is well correlated with similar measurements obtained with MIGET, although the latter, unlike CT, provides no spatial localization of the various V/Q values. (Courtesy of Eric A. Hoffman, PhD, University of Iowa.)

V/Q ratios from xenon-enhanced CT has been proposed (242). Based on the solubility of xenon in blood and the diffusion of the inhaled xenon gas into the pulmonary capillary blood, the xenon concentration in the lung is dependent on both regional perfusion and ventilation. Kreck et al. (242) have recently shown that sequential CT images obtained at end-inspiration during xenon wash-in can be used to measure both regional ventilation and perfusion simultaneously. Moreover, the very high spatial resolution of such functional CT V/Q scans is equivalent to that of the anatomic CT

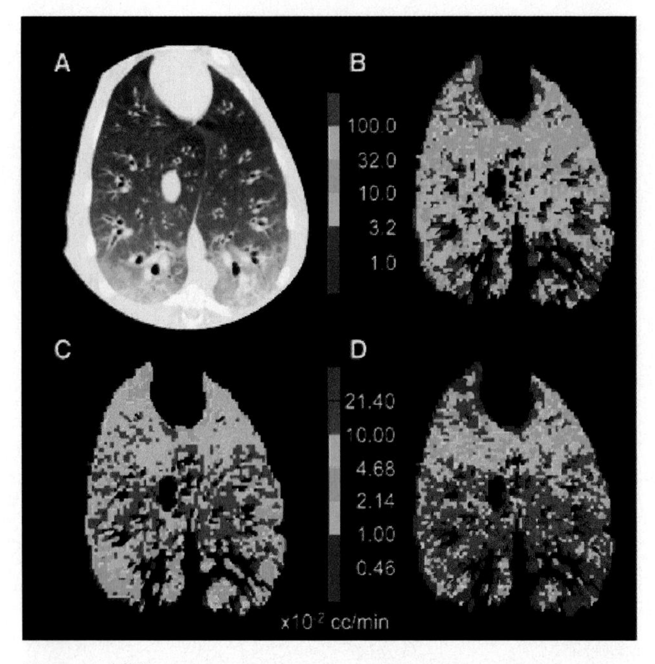

Figure 6-35 Xenon-enhanced CT direct mapping of V/Q in a sheep model. CT image **(A)** and corresponding V/Q **(B)**, V **(C)**, and Q **(D)** functional maps. Of note is the vertical gradient, isogravitational heterogeneity, and spatial clustering of V and Q. At this resolution scale, there is significantly greater spatial heterogeneity in perfusion than in ventilation. (From Kreck TC, Krueger MA, Altemeier WA, et al. Determination of regional ventilation and perfusion in the lung using xenon and computed tomography. *J Appl Physiol* 2001;91:1741–1749, with permission.)

images (Fig. 6-35). Xenon-enhanced CT can thus measure ventilation and perfusion in regions of lung 20- to 100-fold smaller than reported using either PET or microspheres (242). Using a sheep model, the radiodense xenon can be used to track tracer concentrations sequentially on CT through the alveolar space, end-capillary blood, and mixed venous blood.

Xenon-enhanced CT thus has the potential to provide *in vivo* measurements of regional ventilation and perfusion directly related to the underlying lung anatomy, providing a comprehensive assessment of pulmonary structure–function relationships.

Thus CT is joining MR in the rapidly advancing field of functional lung imaging. This is particularly significant because CT, rather than MR, is the standard clinical method for cross-sectional imaging of the lungs, with its superior spatial resolution for parenchymal detail.

OTHER CT VENTILATION CONTRAST AGENTS

Although nonradioactive xenon gas has been the primary CT contrast agent for ventilation investigated to date, several other agents have also been considered. These include aerosolized iodinated contrast and SF6.

Aerosolized Iodinated Contrast Agents

Limited studies investigating the use of aerosolized iodinated contrast agents for CT have been reported (243). As with MR, these are likely to suffer from the problem of central airways deposition.

FS6

The fluorine-containing compound FS6 has had limited use as another potential ventilation contrast agent for CT. CT scan density measurements during continuous breathing of an oxygen–SF6 mixture versus an oxygen–helium gas mixture have revealed regions of lung with slow time constants (density change/time) reflecting abnormal distribution of the denser gas in the small airways of patients with COPD (244).

It should be kept in mind that the physical characteristics, including density and viscosity, differ among the various ventilation agents discussed. For example, helium is less dense than air, whereas xenon and SF6 are heavier. Thus the physiologic behavior and resulting imaging characteristics of these agents vary from one another and in comparison to room air. For example, a potential limitation of using a xenon–oxygen mixture to investigate pulmonary physiology is that it has nearly four times the density of room air and a viscosity that is 20% greater. Low-density gases such as helium have decreased efficiency of oxygen exchange but increased efficiency of CO_2 exchange. Conversely, dense gases such as SF6 have the opposite effect. Precise quantitative comparisons of the relative behavior of these new contrast agents within the same individual are a subject for further research.

PULMONARY MECHANICS

Imaging has played a limited role as a physiologic tool for the direct measurement of pulmonary mechanics. Studies to date have focused principally on the diaphragm and chest wall. These studies have used static and dynamic MR and CT imaging to assess the action of inspiratory muscles via corresponding geometrical changes (245). Rapid MR imaging during tidal breathing has been used to show abnormal asynchronous motion of the diaphragm relative to the chest wall in patients with advanced emphysema, with subsequent improvement following LVRS (246,247). Such MR studies have also been correlated with SPECT xenon scintigraphic imaging of ventilation and measurements of air trapping in patients before and after LVRS, demonstrating improvements in chest wall and diaphragm motion together with surgical reduction in the volume of emphysematous lung (247).

As discussed earlier, dynamic cine CT imaging, in which a series of images are acquired rapidly over the same anatomic volume, has provided visualization of regional lung inflation and alveolar recruitment of atelectatic areas of the lung with the application of incremental PEEP pressures in ARDS (Fig. 6-15) (150). The temporal resolution of such scanning allows for derivation of regional inspiratory and expiratory time constants. As indicated previously, such information could potentially be used to customize mechanical ventilation to optimize alveolar recruitment while minimizing overinflation of more normal lung zones.

However, true quantitative imaging studies of regional lung mechanics has until recently been impractical because no methods were available to track the 3D motion of small regions of the lung with changes in lung inflation. This is no longer the case because both MR- and CT-based methods to measure regional lung inflation and lung tissue deformations on a small scale have become available.

The first of these methods uses magnetic tagging stripes to noninvasively label the lung tissue during the acquisition of MR images of the lung. The motion of these stripes can then be followed over time with changes in lung inflation. The technique was initially developed for myocardial wall motion studies and has recently been applied to the evaluation of local mechanical properties of the lung with very promising results (248,249). The technique is limited by the relatively low spatial resolution of the coarse grid intervals from which the estimated motion fields in the lung are derived (250). In addition, the tagging grid fades according to the T1 decay time of the tissue (which is shorter than the respiratory cycle duration) (248). Furthermore, the technique is difficult to apply in three dimensions (250).

Recently another MR-based method to derive a motion field (displacement vector at each point in the lung) over the entire respiratory cycle has been implemented (Fig. 6-36) (250). The motion is derived using the pulmonary vasculature and parenchymal structures as natural sources of spatial markers on a rapid MR imaging sequence. Regional parenchymal deformation and the associated finite strain tensor can be computed on a voxel-by-voxel basis. For example, in a study of normal subjects imaged during exhalation from TLC to RV, the posterior lung could be observed to displace superiorly and the anterior lung showed posterior and superior displacement. The calculated regional parenchymal strain appeared oriented toward the hilum with maximal strain at the midcycle of the expiratory phase (250).

Similar approaches have recently been applied to CT imaging. The higher spatial resolution of CT allows finer anatomic features in the lung to serve as intrinsic landmarks for motion analysis. However, relative to MR, the CT method is limited by ionizing radiation exposure.

An optical flow method (OFM) has recently been described to track the motion of intrinsic lung structures on serial CT images. OFM is a coarse-to-fine model–based motion estimation technique that can register sequential CT lung volumes. Using this image analysis tool, a CT dataset can be globally translated and rotated and then locally warped into alignment with a previously acquired volume (251). In the process of volume registration, which is carried out in all three dimensions, the OFM estimates the flow field, a map of the displacement between serial images. Moreover, displacement resulting from changes in lung inflation carries information on regional lung deformation. High-resolution displacement fields can then be generated from images acquired at different lung volumes (Fig. 6-37) and provide another means of studying regional lung mechanics. Again, knowledge of lung pressure together with the local volume changes computed from the 3D displacement fields allows for mapping of regional lung compliance (251). A similar voxel-based nonrigid registration algorithm to obtain a displacement vector field has also been recently reported (252).

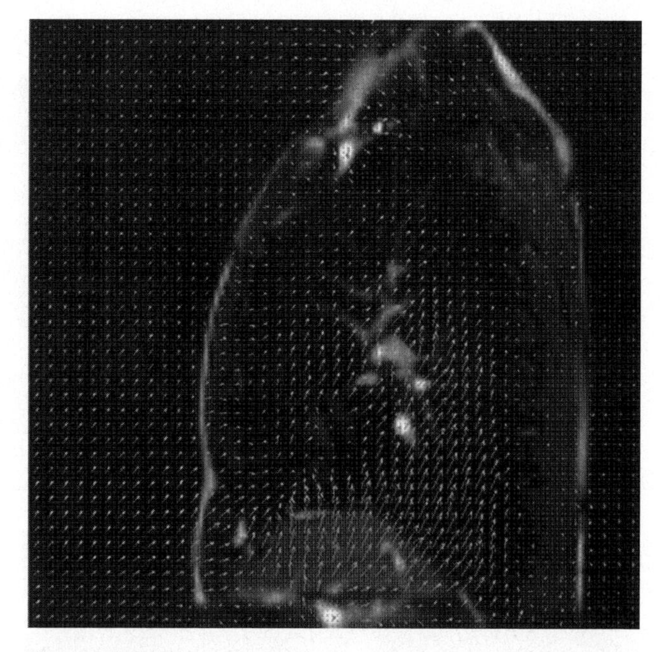

Figure 6-36 Lung biomechanics. Field of lung displacement vectors superimposed on sagittal MR image obtained using a rapid MR imaging sequence during respiration. The estimated lung motion between two consecutive frames was derived using nonrigid registration transformation between the images. The vector field provides a direct, quantitative measure of lung motion from which the induced strain can be derived and used to quantify regional tissue deformation. (From Gee J, Sundaram T, Hasegawa I, et al. Characterization of regional pulmonary mechanics from serial magnetic resonance imaging data. *Acad Radiol* 2003;10:1147–1152, with permission.)

Once again we are able to demonstrate the ability of new imaging techniques to provide unique physiologic information that was previously inaccessible on a regional basis. Determination of regional pulmonary compliance may have important clinical implications in evaluation of patients with emphysema, in which pulmonary compliance is abnormally increased, as well as in patients with chronic interstitial lung disease, which is associated with reduced lung compliance. The addition of this functional information provides a new dimension to the morphologic changes identified by HRCT and may have utility in directing and/or monitoring therapy in these patients. The true value of these

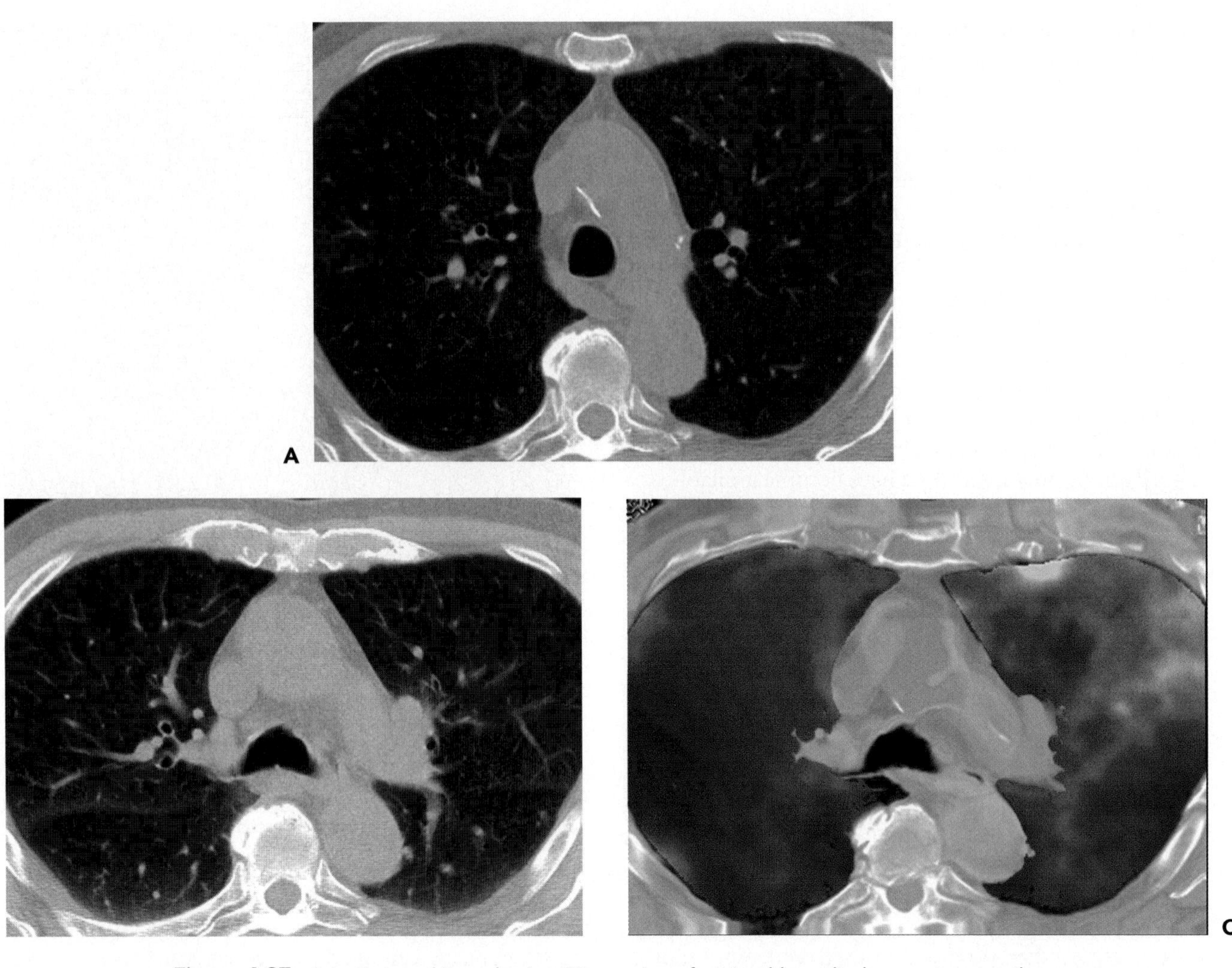

Figure 6-37 **A** to **C:** Lung biomechanics. CT mapping of regional lung displacements using the optical flow method (OFM). **A:** HRCT image at end-inspiration. **B:** HRCT image at end-expiration. **C:** This color map, superimposed on the end-expiration image, depicts the magnitude of regional 3D lung tissue displacement following a respiratory excursion. Black indicates stationary tissue; red, yellow, and white indicate increasing displacement. The OFM-derived displacement data can be used to map regional lung inflation, deformation (strain), and lung compliance. (From Dougherty L, Asmuth JC, Gefter WB. Alignment of CT lung volumes with an optical flow method. *Acad Radiol* 2003;10:249–254, with permission.)

new spatially resolved physiologic measurements, however, needs to be validated in clinical studies.

SUMMARY

Advances in functional imaging of the airways strengthen the prediction that the PFTs of this new millennium will be derived from imaging methods (253,254). Unlike global traditional PFTs, these new imaging techniques can quantify and localize regional lung physiology not only to individual lungs or lobes but also to even smaller regions. A principle function of the lung is gas exchange, which requires proper matching of ventilation and perfusion as well as normal biomechanical functioning of the lung tissue and chest wall. It is now possible to image and map the regional distribution of all three of these basic components of pulmonary function using state-of-the-art CT, MR, and nuclear medicine techniques, together with appropriate image acquisition protocols and newly emerging image analysis tools (254).

Furthermore, with PET and other molecular imaging approaches, we are advancing from imaging of macroscopic structure alone, to structure–function imaging down to the microscopic and even molecular levels. These emerging methods can image the distribution of inhaled pharmaceutical compounds, airway and tumor receptors, the components of the inflammatory process and fibrogenesis, and even gene expression. This molecular functional information can be coupled with the high-resolution structural information provided by multislice CT and micro-CT, providing a more comprehensive assessment of the airways.

New parameters of regional ventilation are now accessible, including measurements of alveolar P_{O_2}; alveolar size, shape, and wall thickness; alveolar-capillary gas diffusion; V/Q at a small spatial scale; regional spirometry; and pulmonary biomechanics. These new techniques may be used to identify those sites of the lungs that contribute maximally to hypoxemia.

The functional images may reveal lung pathology before structural abnormalities develop. In addition to early disease detection, physiologic imaging may provide improved monitoring of disease progression and the tailoring of therapies. Clinical applications include the evaluation of patients with asthma, emphysema, chronic interstitial lung disease, small airway disease, pulmonary embolism, and ARDS.

ACKNOWLEDGMENT

Gratitude is extended to the many colleagues and investigators who generously contributed their images, concepts, and data to this chapter.

REFERENCES

1. Schwab RJ, Gefter WB. Anatomic factors: insights from imaging studies. In: Packk AI, ed. *Sleep apnea: pathogenesis, diagnosis, and treatment.* New York: Marcel Dekker, 2002:1–30.
2. Schwab RJ, Gefter WB, Hoffman EA, et al. Dynamic upper airway imaging during respiration in normal subjects and patients with sleep disordered breathing. *Am Rev Respir Dis* 1993;148:1385–1400.
3. Schwab RJ, Gefter WB, Pack AI, Hoffman EA. Dynamic imaging of the upper airway imaging during respiration in normal subjects. *J Appl Physiol* 1993;74:1504–1514.
4. Shepard JW, Stanson AW, Sheedy PF, Westbrook PR. Fast-CT evaluation of the upper airway during wakefulness in patients with obstructive sleep apnea. In: Suratt PM, Remmers J, eds. *Proceedings of the First International Symposium on Sleep and Respiration.* New York: Alan R Liss, 1990:273–282.
5. Morrell MJ, Arabi Y, Zahn B, Badr MS. Progressive retropalatal narrowing preceding obstructive apnea. *Am J Respir Crit Care Med* 1998;158: 1974–1981.
6. Welch KC, Gefter WB, Ritter CT, et al. Dynamic respiratory related upper airway imaging during wakefulness in normal subjects and patients with sleep disordered breathing using MRI. *Am J Respir Crit Care Med* 1998; 157:A54.
7. Brennick MJ, Trouard TP, Gmitro AF, Fregosi RF. MRI study of pharyngeal airway changes during stimulation of the hypoglossal nerve branches in rats. *J Appl Physiol* 2001;90:1373–1384.
8. Rodenstein DO, Dooms G, Thomas Y, et al. Pharyngeal shape and dimensions in healthy subjects, snorers, and patients with obstructive sleep apnoea. *Thorax* 1990;45:722–727.
9. Schwab RJ, Gupta KB, Gefter WB, et al. Upper airway soft tissue anatomy in normals and patients with sleep disordered breathing. Significance of the lateral pharyngeal walls. *Am J Respir Crit Care Med* 1995; 152:1673–1689.
10. Shelton KE, Gay SB, Woodson H, Surratt PM. Pharyngeal fat in obstructive sleep apnea. *Am Rev Respir Dis* 1993;148:462–466.
11. Horner RL, Mohiaddin RH, Lowell DG, et al. Sites and sizes of fat deposits around the pharynx in obese patients with obstructive sleep apnoea and weight matched controls. *Eur Respir J* 1989;2:613–622.
12. Winter WC, Gampper T, Gay SB, Suratt PM. Enlargement of the lateral pharyngeal fat pad space in pigs increases upper airway resistance. *J Appl Physiol* 1995;79:726–731.
13. Kuna ST, Bedi DG, Ryckman C. Effect of nasal airway positive pressure on upper airway size and configuration. *Am Rev Respir Dis* 1988;138: 969–975.
14. Schwab RJ, Pack AI, Gupta KB, et al. Upper airway and soft tissue structural changes induced by CPAP in normal subjects. *Am J Respir Crit Care Med* 1996;154:1106–1116.
15. Horner RL, Shea SA, McIvor J, Guz A. Pharyngeal size and shape during wakefulness and sleep in patients with obstructive sleep apnoea. *Q J Med* 1989;72:719–735.
16. Stein MG, Gamsu G, DeGeer G, et al. Cine CT in obstructive sleep apnea. *AJR Am J Roentgenol* 1987;148:1069–1074.
17. Suto Y, Matsuo T, Kato T, et al. Evaluation of the pharyngeal airway in patients in sleep apnea: value of ultrafast MR imaging. *AJR Am J Roentgenol* 1993;160:311–314.
18. Trudo FJ, Gefter WB, Welch KC, et al. State related changes in upper airway caliber and surrounding soft tissue structures in normals. *Am J Respir Crit Care Med* 1998;158:1259–1270.
19. Stern EJ, Graham CM, Webb WR, Gamsu G. Normal trachea during forced expiration: dynamic CT measurements. *Radiology* 1993;187:27–31.
20. Grenier PA, Beigelman-Aubry C, Fetita C, Preteux F. Large airways at CT: bronchiectasis, asthma and COPD. In: Kauczor H-U, Ed. *Functional imaging of the chest.* Berlin: Springer, 2004:39–54.
21. Gilkeson RC, Ciancibello LM, Hejal RB, et al. Tracheo-bronchomalacia: dynamic airway evaluation with multidetector CT. *AJR Am J Roentgenol* 2001;176:205–210.
22. Maisel JC, Silvers GW, Mitchell RS, et al. Bronchial atrophy and dynamic expiratory collapse. *Am Rev Respir Dis* 1968;98:988–997.
23. Tandon MK, Campbell AH. Bronchial cartilage in chronic bronchitis. *Thorax* 1969;24:607–612.
24. Thurlbeck WM, Pun R, Toth J, et al. Bronchial cartilage in chronic obstructive lung disease. *Am Rev Respir Dis* 1974;109:73–80.
25. Brown RH, Mitzner W, Wagner E, et al. Airway distention with lung inflation measured by HRCT. *Acad Radiol* 2003;10:1097–1103.
26. Brown RH, Croisille P, Mudge B, et al. Airway narrowing in healthy humans inhaling methacholine without deep inspirations demonstrated by HRCT. *Am J Respir Crit Care Med* 2000;161:1256–1263.
27. Brown RH, Scichilone N, Mudge B, et al. High resolution computed tomographic evaluation of airways distensibility and the effects of lung inflation on airway caliber in healthy subjects and individuals with asthma. *Am J Respir Crit Care Med* 2001;163:994–1001.
28. Brown RH, Herold CJ, Hirshman CA, et al. Individual airway constrictor response heterogeneity assessed by high resolution computed tomography. *J Appl Physiol* 1993;74:2615–2620.
29. Brown RH, Herold C, Mitzner W, Zerhouni EA. Spontaneous airways constrict during breath holding studied by high-resolution computed tomography. *Chest* 1994;106:920–924.
30. Brown RH, Zerhouni EA, Mitzner W. Visualization of airway obstruction in vivo during lung vascular engorgement and edema. *J Appl Physiol* 1995;78: 1070–1078.
31. Brown RH, Mitzner W. Effect of lung inflation and airway muscle tone on airway diameter in vivo. *J Appl Physiol* 1996;80:1581–1588.
32. Brown RH, Zerhouni EA, Mitzner W. Variability in the size of individual airways over the course of one year. *Am J Respir Crit Care Med* 1995;151: 1159–1164.
33. Brown RH, Mitzner W, Bulut Y, et al. Effect of lung inflation in vivo on airways with smooth-muscle tone or edema. *J Appl Physiol* 1997;82:491–499.
34. Hoffman EA, McLennan G. Needs for assessment of pulmonary structure/ function relationships and clinical outcomes measures: quantitative volumetric CT of the lung. *Acad Radiol* 1997;4:758–776.
35. Amirav I, Kramer SS, Grunstein M, et al. Assessment of methacholine-induced airway constriction with ultrafast high-resolution computed tomography. *J Appl Physiol* 1993;75:2239–2250.
36. Casale TB, Chiplunkar R, Reed S, et al. Methacholine-induced airway constriction in vivo mimics in vitro cholinergic innervation. *J Respir Crit Care Med* 1996;153:A877.
37. King GG, Muller NL, Pare PD. Evaluation of airways in obstructive pulmonary disease using high-resolution computed tomography. *Am J Respir Crit Care Med* 1999;159:992–1004.
38. Wood SA, Zerhouni EA, Hoford JD, et al. Measurement of three-dimensional lung tree structures by using computed tomography. *J Appl Physiol* 1995; 79:1687–1697.
39. Hoffman EA, Reinhardt JM, Sonka M, et al. Characterization of the interstitial lung diseases via density-based and texture-based analysis of computed tomography images of lung structure and function. *Acad Radiol* 2003;10:1104–1118.
40. Reinhardt JM, Raab SA, D Souza, et al. Intra-thoracic airway measurement: ex vivo validation. *SPIE Medical Imaging* 1997;3033:69–80.
41. Reinhardt JM, D'Souza ND, Hoffman EA. Accurate measurement of intrathoracic airways. *IEEE Trans Med Imaging* 1997;16:820–827.
42. Saba O, Beck KC, Chon D, et al. Lung volume measurement reproducibility using gated-axial and spiral multi-row detector CT (MDCT). *Am J Respir Crit Care Med* 2003;167:A844.
43. Prêteux F, Fetita CI, Capderou A, et al. Modeling, segmentation, and caliber estimation of bronchi in high resolution computerized tomography. *J Electron Imaging* 1999;8:36–45.
44. Tran BQ, Tajik JK, Chiplunkar RA, et al. Lung volume control for quantitative x-ray CT. *J Biomed Engineering* 1996;24:S-66.
45. Kalender WA, Rienmuller R, Seissler W, et al. Measurement of pulmonary parenchymal attenuation: use of spirometric gating with quantitative CT. *Radiology* 1990;175:265–268.
46. Lamers RJ, Thelissen GR, Kessels AG, et al. Chronic obstructive pulmonary diseases: evaluation with spirometrically controlled CT lung densitometry. *Radiology* 1994;193:109–113.
47. McNamara AE, Muller NL, Okazawa M, et al. Airway narrowing in excised canine lungs measured by high-resolution computed tomography. *J Appl Physiol* 1992;73:307–316.
48. Brown RH, Georakopoulos I, Mitzner W. Individual canine airways responsiveness to aerosol histamine and methacholine in vivo. *Am J Respir Crit Care Med* 1998;157:491–497.
49. Beigelman-Aubry C, Capderou A, Grenier PA, et al. Mild intermittent asthma: CT assessment of bronchial cross-sectional area and lung attenuation at controlled lung volume. *Radiology* 2002;223:181–187.

50. Verschakelen J. Small airways, bronchiolitis, air trapping. In: Kauczor H-U, ed. *Functional imaging of the chest.* Berlin: Springer, 2004:55–82.
51. Lynch DA, Newell JD, Tschomper BA, et al. Uncomplicated asthma in adults: comparison of CT appearance of the lungs in asthmatic and healthy subjects. *Radiology* 1993;188:829–833.
52. Grenier P, Mourey-Gerosa I, Benali K, et al. Abnormalities of the airways and lung parenchyma in asthmatics: CT observations in 50 patients and inter- and intra-observer variability. *Eur Radiol* 1996;6:199–206.
53. Paganin F, Seneterre E, Chanez P, et al. Computed tomography of the lungs in asthma: influence of disease severity and etiology. *Am J Respir Crit Care Med* 1996;153:110–114.
54. Park CS, Müller NL, Worthy SA, et al. Airway obstruction in asthmatic and healthy individuals: inspiratory and expiratory thin-section CT findings. *Radiology* 1997;203:361–367.
55. Carr DH, Hibon S, Rubens M, et al. Peripheral airways obstruction on high-resolution computed tomography in chronic severe asthma. *Respir Med* 1998;92:448–453.
56 Lucidarme O, Coche E, Cluzel P, et al. Expiratory CT scans for chronic airway disease: correlation with pulmonary function test results. *AJR Am J Roentgenol* 1998;170:301–307.
57. Paganin F, Trussard V, Seneterre E, et al. Chest radiography and high resolution computed tomography of the lungs in asthma. *Am Rev Respir Dis* 1992;146:1084–1087.
58. Lynch DA. Imaging of asthma and allergic bronchopulmonary mycosis. *Radiol Clin North Am* 1998;36:129–142.
59. Gevenois PA, Scillia P, Maertelaer V de, et al. The effects of age, sex, lung size, and hyperinflation on CT lung densitometry. *AJR Am J Roentgenol* 1996;167:1169–1173.
60. Awadh N, Müller NL, Park CS, et al. Airway wall thickness in patients with near fatal asthma and control groups: assessment with high resolution computed tomography. *Thorax* 1998;53:248–253.
61. Niimi A, Matsumoto H, Amitani R, et al. Airway wall thickness in asthma assessed by computed tomography. *Am J Respir Crit Care Med* 2000;162: 1518–1523.
62. Lange P, Parner J, Vestbo J, et al. A 15-year follow-up study of ventilatory function in adults with asthma. *N Engl J Med* 1998;339:1194–1200.
63. Okazawa M, Muller N, McNamara AE, et al. Human airway narrowing measured using high resolution computed tomography. *Am J Respir Crit Care Med* 1996;154:1557–1562.
64. Kee ST, Fahy JV, Chen DR, et al. High-resolution computed tomography of airway changes after induced bronchoconstriction and bronchodilation in asthmatic volunteers. *Acad Radiol* 1996;3:389–394.
64a. Hoffman EA, Chiplunkar R, Casale TB. CT scanning confirms beta receptor distribution is greater for smaller vs. larger airways. *J Respir Crit Care Med* 1997;155:A855.
65. D'Souza ND, Reinhardt JM, Hoffman EA. ASAP: interactive quantification of 2D airway geometry. *SPIE Medical Imaging.* 1996;2709:197–208.
66. Roche WR, Beasley R, Williams JH, Holgate ST. Subepithelial fibrosis in the bronchi of asthmatics. *Lancet* 1989;1:520–524.
67. Kapsali T, Permutt S, Laube B, et al. Potent bronchoprotective effect of deep inspiration and its absence in asthma. *J Appl Physiol* 2000;89:711–720.
68. Scichilone N, Kapsali T, Permutt S, Togias A. Deep inspiration-induced bronchoprotection is stronger than bronchodilation. *Am J Respir Crit Care Med* 2000;162:910–916.
69. Scichilone N, Pygros G, Kapsali T, et al. Airways hyperresponsiveness and the effects of lung inflation. *Int Arch Allergy Immunol* 2001;124:262–266.
70. Dolovich MB, Cockcroft DW, Coates G. Aerosols in diagnosis: ventilation, airway penetrance, epithelial permeability, mucociliary transport and airway responsiveness. In: Moren F, Colovitch MB, Newhouse MT, Newman SP, eds. *Aerosols in medicine, principles, diagnosis and therapy.* Amsterdam: Elsevier Science, 1993:195–234.
71. White PG, Hayward MW, Cooper T. Ventilation agents—what agents are currently used? *Nucl Med Commun* 1991;12:349–352.
72. Burch WM, Sullivan PJ, McLaren CJ. Technegas—a new ventilation agent for lung scanning. *Nucl Med Commun* 1986;7:865–871.
73. Almquist H, Jonson B, Palmer J, et al. Regional V_A/Q ratios in man using 133Xe and single photon emission computed tomography (SPECT) corrected for attenuation. *Clin Physiol* 1999;19:475–481.
74. Sanchez-Crespo A, Petersson J, Nyren S, et al. A novel quantitative dual-isotope method for simultaneous ventilation and perfusion SPET. *Eur J Nucl Med Mol Imaging* 2002;29:863–875.
75. Suga K, Nishigauchi K, Kume N, et al. Dynamic pulmonary SPECT of xenon-133 gas washout. *J Nucl Med* 1996;37:807–814.
76. Suga K, Nishigauchi K, Shimizu K, et al. [Usefulness of 3-D dynamic pulmonary xenon-133 SPECT for thoracoscopic lung volume reduction surgery in patients with pulmonary emphysema]. *Nippon Acta Radiol* 1997; 57:215–216.
77. Suga K, Kume N, Nishigauchi K, et al. Three-dimensional surface display of dynamic pulmonary xenon-133 SPECT in patients with obstructive lung disease. *J Nucl Med* 1998;39:889–893.
78. Suga K, Nishigauchi K, Shimizu K, et al. Radionuclide imaging in emphysema after lung volume reduction surgery. *Clin Nucl Med* 1997;22:683–686.
79. Suga K, Yasuhiko K, Zaki, et al. Assessment of regional lung functional impairment with co-registered respiratory-gated ventilation/perfusion SPECT-CT images; initial experiences. *Eur J Nucl Med Mol Imaging* 2004;31: 240–249.
80. Mills GH, Wild JM, Eberle B, Van Beek EJR. Functional magnetic resonance imaging of the lung. *Br J Anaesth* 2003;91:16–30.
81. Schuster D. PET. *Semin Nucl Med* 1998;28:341–351.
82. Musch G, Layfield JD, Harris RS, et al. Topographical distribution of pulmonary perfusion and ventilation, assessed by PET in supine and prone humans. *J Appl Physiol* 2002;93:1841–1851.
83. Vidal Melo MF, Layfield D, Harris S, et al. Quantification of regional ventilation-perfusion ratios with PET. *J Nucl Med* 2003;44:1982–1991.
84. Alavi A, Gupta N, Alberini JL, et al. Positron emission tomography in nonmalignant thoracic disorders. *Semin Nucl Med* 2002;32:293–321.
85. Hirst PH, Bacon RE, Pitcairn GT, et al. A comparison of the lung deposition of budesonide from Easyhaler, Turbohaler and pMDI plus spacer in asthmatic patients. *Respir Med* 2001;95:720–727.
86. Hirst PH, Pitcairn GR, Richards JC, et al. Deposition and pharmacokinetics of an HFA formulation of triamcinolone acetonide delivered by pressurized metered dose inhaler. *J Aerosol Med* 2001;14:155–165.
87. Berridge MS, Lee Z, Heald DL. Pulmonary distribution and kinetics of inhaled [11C]triamcinolone acetonide. *J Nucl Med* 2000;41:1603–1611.
88. Lee Z, Berridge MS. PET imaging-based evaluation of aerosol drugs and their delivery devices: nasal and pulmonary studies. *IEEE Trans Med Imaging* 2002;21:1324–1331.
89. Yanai M, Hatazawa J, Ojima F, et al. Deposition and clearance of inhaled 18FDG powder in patients with chronic obstructive pulmonary disease. *Eur Respir J* 1998;11:1342–1348.
90. Hayes MJ, Qing F, Rhodes CG, et al. In vivo quantification of human pulmonary beta-adrenoceptors: effect of beta-agonist therapy. *Am J Respir Crit Care Med* 1996;154:1277–1283.
91. Qing F, Rhodes CG, Hayes MJ, et al. In vivo quantification of human pulmonary beta-adrenoceptor density using PET: comparison with in vitro radioligand binding. *J Nucl Med* 1996;37:1275–1281.
92. Hansell DM. General role of imaging in the evaluation of diffuse infiltrative and airways diseases. In: Kauczor H-U, ed. *Functional imaging of the chest.* Berlin: Springer, 2004:1–18.
93. Taylor IK, Hill AA, Hayes M, et al. Imaging allergen-invoked airway inflammation in atopic asthma with [18F]-fluorodeoxyglucose and positron emission tomography. *Lancet* 1996;347:937–940.
94. Wallace WE, Gupta NC, Hubbs AF, et al. Cis-4-[(18)F]fluoro-L-proline PET imaging of pulmonary fibrosis in a rabbit model. *J Nucl Med* 2002;43: 413–420.
95. Schuster DP, Kovacs A, Garbow J, et al. Recent advances in imaging the lungs of intact small animals. *Am J Respir Cell Mol Biol* 2004;30:129–138.
96. Richard JC, Factor P, Ferkol T, et al. Repetitive imaging of reporter gene expression in the lung. *Mol Imaging* 2003;2:342–349.
97. Richard JC, Factor P, Welch LC, Schuster DP. Imaging the spatial distribution of transgene expression in the lungs with positron emission tomography. *Gene Ther* 2003;10:2074–2080.
98. Richard JC, Zhou Z, Ponde DE, et al. Imaging pulmonary gene expression with positron emission tomography. *Am J Respir Crit Care Med* 2003;167: 1257–1263.
99. Hoffman EA, Gefter WB, Venegas J. Frontier pulmonary imaging. In: Fishman AP, ed. *Update: Pulmonary Diseases and Disorders.* New York: McGraw-Hill, 1992:323–340.
100. Kauczor HU, Heussel CP, Fischer B, et al. Assessment of lung volumes using helical CT at inspiration and expiration: comparison with pulmonary function tests. *AJR Am J Roentgenol* 1998;171:1091–1095.
101. Mergo PJ, Williams WF, Gonzalez-Rothi R, et al. Three-dimensional volumetric assessment of abnormally low attenuation of the lung from routine helical CT: inspiratory and expiratory quantification. *AJR Am J Roentgenol* 1998;170:1355–1360.
102. Hu S, Hoffman EA, Reinhardt JM. Automatic lung segmentation for accurate quantitation of volumetric x-ray CT images. *IEEE Trans Med Imaging* 2001;20:490–498.
103. van Beek EJR, Swift A, Wild JM. Analysis of distribution of ventilation. In: Kauczor H-U, ed. *Functional imaging of the chest.* Berlin: Springer, 2004: 119–154.
104. Arakawa H, Webb WR, McCowin M, et al. Inhomogenous lung attenuation at thin-section CT: diagnostic value of expiratory scans. *Radiology* 1998;206:89–94.
105. Stern EJ, Frank MS. Small-airways disease of the lungs: findings at expiratory CT. *AJR Am J Roentgenol* 1994;163:37–41.
106. Desai SR, Hansell DM. Small airways disease: expiratory computed tomography comes of age. *Clin Radiol* 1997;52:332–337.
107. Verschakelen JA, Scheinbaum K, Bogaert J, et al. Expiratory CT in cigarette smokers: correlation between areas of decreased lung attenuation, pulmonary function tests and smoking history. *Eur Radiol* 1998;8: 1391–1399.
108. Arakawa H, Webb WR. Air trapping on expiratory high-resolution CT scans in the absence of inspiratory scan abnormalities: correlation with pulmonary function tests and differential diagnosis. *AJR Am J Roentgenol* 1998;170:1349–1353.
109. Verschakelen J, Fraeyenhoven L van, Laureys G, et al. Differences in CT density between dependent and nondependent portions of the lung: influence of lung volume. *AJR Am J Roentgenol* 1993;161:713–717.
110. Austin JH, Muller NL, Friedman PJ, et al. Glossary of terms for CT of the lungs: recommendations of the Nomenclature Committee of the Fleischner Society. *Radiology* 1996;200:327–331.

111. Worthy SA, Müller NL, Hartman TE, et al. Mosaic attenuation pattern on thin-section CT scans of the lung: differentiation among infiltrative lung, airway and vascular diseases as a cause. *Radiology* 1997;205:465–470.
112. Webb WR, Stern EJ, Kanth N, et al. Dynamic pulmonary CT: findings in healthy adult men. *Radiology* 1993;186:117–124.
113. Lee KW, Chung SY, Yang I, et al. Correlation of aging and smoking with air trapping at thin-section CT of the lung in asymptomatic subjects. *Radiology* 2000;214:831–833.
114. Grenier P, Beigelman-Aubry C, Fétita C, et al. New frontiers in CT imaging of airway disease. *Eur Radiol* 2002;12:1022–1044.
115. Gleeson FV, Traill ZC, Hansell DM. Evidence on expiratory CT scans of small airway obstruction in sarcoidosis. *AJR Am J Roentgenol* 1996;166: 1052–1054.
116. Bartz RR, Stern EJ. Airways obstruction in patients with sarcoidosis: expiratory CT scan findings. *J Thorac Imaging* 2000;15:285–289.
117. Bhalla M, Naidich DP, McGuinness G, et al. Diffuse lung disease: assessment with helical CT—preliminary observations of the role of maximum and minimum intensity projection images. *Radiology* 1996;200: 341–347.
118. Rémy-Jardin M, Campistron P, Amara A, et al. Workflow issue with multislice CT (MSCT) of the thorax: usefulness of multiplanar reformations in the diagnostic approach of infiltrative lung disease. *Eur Radiol* 2002; 12(Suppl 1):134(abst).
119. Copley SJ, Wells AU, Müller NL, et al. Thin-section CT in obstructive pulmonary disease: discriminatory value. *Radiology* 2002;223:812–819.
120. Ng CS, Desai SR, Rubens MB, et al. Visual quantitation and observer variation of signs of small airways disease at inspiratory and expiratory CT. *J Thorac Imaging* 1999;14:279–285.
121. Fotheringham T, Chabat F, Hansell DM, et al. A comparison of methods for enhancing the detection of areas of decreased attenuation on CT caused by airways disease. *J Comput Assist Tomogr* 1999;23:385–389.
122. Wittram C, Batt J, Rappaport DC, et al. Inspiratory and expiratory helical CT of normal adults: comparison of thin section scans and minimum intensity projection images. *J Thorac Imaging* 2002;17:47–52.
123. Yang GZ, Hansell DM. CT image enhancement with wavelet analysis for the detection of small airways disease. *IEEE Trans Med Imaging* 1997;16: 953–961.
124. Rémy-Jardin M, Rémy J, Gosselin B, et al. Sliding thin slab, minimum intensity projection technique in the diagnosis of emphysema: histopathologic-CT correlation. *Radiology* 1996;200:665–671.
125. Stern EJ, Webb WR, Golden JA, et al. Cystic lung disease associated with eosinophilic granuloma and tuberous sclerosis: air trapping at dynamic ultrafast high-resolution CT. *Radiology* 1992;182:325–329.
126. Lynch DA, Brasch RC, Hardy KA, et al. Pediatric pulmonary disease: assessment with high-resolution ultrafast CT. *Radiology* 1990;176:243–248.
127. Im JG, Kim SH, Chung MJ, Koo JM, Han MC. Lobular low attenuation of the lung parenchyma on CT: evaluation of 48 patients. *J Comput Assist Tomogr* 1996;20:752–762.
128. Johnson JL, Kramer SS, Mahboubi S. Air trapping in children: evaluation with dynamic lung densitometry with spiral CT. *Radiology* 1998;206:95–101.
129. Lucidarme O, Grenier PA, Cadi M, et al. Evaluation of air trapping at CT: comparison of continuous versus suspended expiration CT techniques. *Radiology* 2000;216:768–772.
130. Chen D, Webb WR, Storto ML, et al. Assessment of air trapping using postexpiratory high-resolution computed tomography. *J Thorac Imaging* 1998; 13:135–143.
131. Gotway MB, Lee ES, Reddy GP, et al. Low-dose dynamic expiratory thin-section CT of the lungs using a spiral CT scanner. *J Thorac Imaging* 2000;15: 168–172.
132. Goddard PR, Nicholson EM, Laszlo G, et al. Computed tomography in pulmonary emphysema. *Clin Radiol* 1982;33:379–387.
133. Kubo K, Eda S, Yamamoto H, et al. Expiratory and inspiratory chest computed tomography and pulmonary function tests in cigarette smokers. *Eur Respir J* 1999;13:252–256.
134. Wegener OH, Koeppe P, Oeser H. Measurement of lung density by computed tomography. *J Comput Assist Tomogr* 1978;2:263–273.
135. Müller NL, Staples CA, Miller RR, et al. "Density mask": an objective method to quantitate emphysema using computed tomography. *Chest* 1988;94:782–787.
136. Adams H, Bernard MS, McConnochie K. An appraisal of CT pulmonary density mapping in normal subjects. *Clin Radiol* 1991;43:238–242.
137. Newman KB, Lynch DA, Newman LS, et al. Quantitative computed tomography detects air trapping due to asthma. *Chest* 1994;106:105–109.
138. Stern EJ, Webb WR, Gamsu G. Dynamic quantitative computed tomography: a predictor of pulmonary function in obstructive lung diseases. *Invest Radiol* 1994;29:564–569.
139. Knudson RJ, Standen JR, Kaltenborn WT, et al. Expiratory computed tomography for assessment of suspected pulmonary emphysema. *Chest* 1991;99:1357–1366.
140. Padley SPG, Adler BD, Hansell DM, et al. Bronchiolitis obliterans: high-resolution CT findings and correlation with pulmonary function tests. *Clin Radiol* 1993;47:236–240.
141. Hansell DM, Wells AU, Rubens MB, et al. Bronchiectasis: functional significance of areas of decreased attenuation at expiratory CT. *Radiology* 1994;193:369–374.
142. Heremans A, Verschakelen JA, Van Fraeyenhoven L, Demedts M. Measurement of lung density by means of quantitative CT scanning: a study of correlations with pulmonary function tests. *Chest* 1992;102:805–811.
143. Kauczor HU, Hast J, Heussel CP, et al. CT attenuation of paired HRCT scans obtained at full inspiratory/expiratory position: comparison with pulmonary function tests. *Eur Radiol* 2002;12:2757–2763.
144. Hansell DM, Rubens MB, Padley SPG, et al. Obliterative bronchiolitis: individual CT signs of small airways disease and functional correlation. *Radiology* 1997;203:721–726.
145. Gelb AF, Hogg JC, Muller NL, et al. Contribution of emphysema and small airways in COPD. *Chest* 1996;109:353–359.
146. Gelb AF, Zamel N, Hogg JC, et al. Pseudophysiologic emphysema resulting from severe small-airways disease. *Am J Respir Crit Care Med* 1998; 158:815–819.
147. Laurent F, Latrabe V, Raherison C, et al. Functional significance of air trapping detected in moderate asthma. *Eur Radiol* 2000;10:1404–1410.
148. Goldin JG, McNitt-Gray MF, Sorensen SM, et al. Airway hyperreactivity: assessment with helical thin-section CT. *Radiology* 1998;208:321–329.
149. Markstaller K, Arnold M, Döbrich M, et al. A software tool for automatic image-based ventilation analysis using dynamic chest CT-scanning in healthy and ARDS lungs. *Fortschr Rontgenstr* 2001;173:830–835.
150. Markstaller K, Eberle B, Kauczor HU, et al. Temporal dynamics of lung aeration determined by dynamic CT in a porcine model of ARDS. *Br J Anaesth* 2001;87:459–468.
151. Markstaller K. Respiration therapy. In: Kauczor H-U, ed. *Functional imaging of the chest.* Berlin: Springer, 2004:211–222.
152. Dreyfuss D, Saumon G. Ventilator-induced lung injury: lessons from experimental studies. *Am J Respir Crit Care Med* 1998;157:294–323.
153. Slutsky AS, Ranieri VM. Mechanical ventilation: lessons from the ARDSNet trial. *Respir Res* 2000;1:73–77.
154. Rommelsheim K, Lackner K, Westhofen P, et al. Respiratory distress syndrome of the adult in the computer tomograph. *Anasthesie, Intensivtherapie, Notfallmedizin* 1983;18:59–64.
155. Gattinoni L, Mascheroni D, Torresin A, et al. Morphological response to positive end expiratory pressure in acute respiratory failure: computerized tomography study. *Intensive Care Med* 1986;12:137–142.
156. Torresin A, et al. Adult respiratory distress syndrome profiles by computed tomography. *J Thorac Imaging* 1986;1:25–30.
157. Maunder RJ, Shuman WP, McHugh JW, et al. Preservation of normal lung regions in the adult respiratory distress syndrome: analysis by computed tomography. *JAMA* 1986;255:2463–2465.
158. Neumann P, Berglund JE, Mondejar EF, et al. Dynamics of lung collapse and recruitment during prolonged breathing in porcine lung injury. *J Appl Physiol* 1998; 85:1533–1543.
159. Neumann P, Berglund JE, Mondejar EF, et al. Effect of different pressure levels on the dynamics of lung collapse and recruitment in oleic acid-induced lung injury. *Am J Respir Crit Care Med* 1998;158:1636–1643.
160. Dambrosio M, Roupie E, Mollett JJ, et al. Effects of positive end-expiratory pressure and different tidal volumes on alveolar recruitment and hyperinflation. *Anesthesiology* 1997;87:495–503.
161. Vieira SR, Puybasset L, Richecoeur J, et al. A lung computed tomographic assessment of positive end-expiratory pressure-induced lung overdistension. *Am J Respir Crit Care Med* 1998;158:1571–1577.
162. Markstaller K, Kauczor HU, Eberle B, et al. Multi-rotation CT during continuous ventilation: comparison of different density areas in healthy lungs and in the ARDS lavage model. *Rofo Fortschr Geb Rontgenstr Neuen Bildgeb Verfahr* 1999;170:575–580.
163. Rothen HU, Neumann P, Berglund JE, et al. Dynamics of re-expansion of atelectasis during general anaesthesia. *Br J Anaesth* 1999;82: 551–556.
164. Markstaller K, Karmrodt J, Dobrich M, et al. Determination of different inspiratory time constants by dynamic CT in a patient with ARDS. *Eur J Anaesthesiol* 2002;19:62.
165. Kauczor H-U, Eberle B. Elucidation of structure-function relationships in the lung: contributions from hyperpolarized 3helium MRI. *Clin Physiol Funct Imaging* 2002;22:361–369.
166. Ohno Y, Chen Q, Hatabu H. Oxygen-enhanced magnetic resonance ventilation imaging of lung. *Eur J Radiol* 2001;37:164–171.
167. Kauczor HU, Hofmann D, Kreitner KF, et al. Normal and abnormal pulmonary ventilation: visualization at hyperpolarized He-3 MR imaging. *Radiology* 1996;201:564–568.
168. Altes TA, Powers PL, Knight-Scott J, et al. Hyperpolarized 3He MR lung ventilation imaging in asthmatics: preliminary findings. *J Magn Reson Imaging* 2001;13:378–384.
169. Bachert P, Schad LR, Bock M, et al. Nuclear magnetic resonance imaging of airways in humans with use of hyperpolarized 3He. *Magn Reson Med* 1996;36:192–196.
170. Kauczor HU, Ebert M, Kreitner KF, et al. Imaging of the lungs using 3He MRI: preliminary clinical experience in 18 patients with and without lung disease. *J Magn Reson Imaging* 1997;7:538–543.
171. Kauczor H, Surkau R, Roberts T. MRI using hyperpolarized noble gases. *Eur Radiol* 1998;8:820–827.
172. Guenther D, Eberle B, Hast J, et al. 3He MRI in healthy volunteers: preliminary correlation with smoking history and lung volumes. *NMR Biomed* 2000;13:182–189.

173. Samee S, Altes T, Powers P, et al. Imaging the lungs in asthmatic patients by using hyperpolarized helium-3 magnetic resonance: assessment of response to methacholine and exercise challenge. *J Allergy Clin Immunol* 2003;111:1205–1211.
174. Altes T, Froh DK, Salerno M, et al. Hyperpolarized helium-3 MR imaging of lung ventilation changes following airway mucus clearance treatment in cystic fibrosis. In: *Proceedings of the International Society of Magnetic Resonance Medicine,* 9th meeting, 2001.
175. Salerno M, Altes T, Mugler JP, et al. Hyperpolarized noble gas MR imaging of the lung: potential clinical applications. *Eur J Radiol* 2001;40:33–44.
176. Gast K, Viallon M, Eberle B, et al. MRI in lung transplant recipients using hyperpolarized 3He: comparison with CT. *J Magn Reson Imaging* 2002; 15:268–274.
177. DeLange EE, Mugler JP, Brookeman JR, et al. Lung air spaces: MR imaging evaluation with hyperpolarized 3He gas. *Radiology* 1999;210:851–857.
178. Kauczor HU, Kreitner KF. MRI of the pulmonary parenchyma. *Eur Radiol* 1999;9:1755–1764.
179. Markstaller K, Kauczor H, Puderbach M, et al. 3He-MRI-based vs. conventional determination of lung volumes in patients after unilateral lung transplantation: a new approach to regional spirometry. *Acta Anaesthesiol Scand* 2002;46:845–852.
180. Kauczor HU, Markstaller K, Puderbach M, et al. Volumetry of ventilated airspaces using 3He MRI: preliminary results. *Invest Radiol* 2001;36: 110–114.
181. Roberts DA, Rizi RR, Lipson DA, et al. Detection and localization of pulmonary air leaks using laser-polarized 3He MRI. *Magn Reson Med* 2000;44:379–382.
182. Gierada DS, Saam B, Yablonskiy D, et al. Dynamic echo planar MR imaging of lung ventilation with hyperpolarized 3He in normal subjects and patients with severe emphysema. *NMR Biomed* 2000;13:176–181.
183. Mugler JP, Brookeman JR, Knight-Scott J, et al. Interleaved echo-planar imaging of the lungs with hyperpolarized 3He. *Proc ISMRM* 1998;6:448.
184. Salerno M, Altes TA, Brookeman JR, et al. Dynamic spiral MRI of pulmonary gas flow using hyperpolarized 3He: preliminary studies in healthy and diseased lungs. *Magn Reson Med* 2001;46:667–677.
185. Schreiber WG, Weiler N, Kauczor HU, et al. Ultrafast MRI of lung ventilation using hyperpolarized helium-3. *Rofo Fortschr Geb Rontgenstr Neuen Bildgeb Verfahr* 2000;172:129–133.
186. Wild JM, Paley MNJ, Kasuboski L, et al. Dynamic radial projection MRI of inhaled hyperpolarized 3He gas. *Magn Reson Med* 2003;49:991–997.
187. Gast KK, Puderbach MU, Rodriguez I, et al. Dynamic ventilation 3He-magnetic resonance imaging with lung motion correction: gas flow distribution analysis. *Invest Radiol* 2002;37:126–134.
188. Spector ZZ, Fischer M, Emami K, et al. Quantitative and regional assessment of emphysema using polarized gas MRI. *Proceedings of the International Society of Magnetic Resonance in Medicine,* 2004.
189. Emami K, Haczu A, Fischer MC, et al. Measurement of regional ventilation in a model of airway hyper-responsiveness using polarized gas MRI. *Proceedings of the Society of Magnetic Resonance in Medicine,* 2004.
190. Moeller H, Chen X, Saam B, et al. MRI of the lungs using hyperpolarized noble gases. *Magn Reson Med* 2002;47:1029–1051.
191. Yablonsky DA, Sukstanskii AL, Leawoods JC, et al. Quantitative in vivo assessment of lung microstructure at the alveolar level with hyperpolarized 3He diffusion MRI. *Proc Natl Acad Sci U S A* 2002;99:3111–3116.
192. Chen XJ, Chawla MS, Cofer GP, et al. Hyperpolarized 3He NMR lineshape measurements in the live guinea pig lung. *Magn Reson Med* 1998;40:61–65.
193. Chen XJ, Chawla MS, Hedlund LW, et al. MR microscopy of lung airways with hyperpolarized 3He. *Magn Reson Med* 1998;39:79–84.
194. Chen XJ, Moller HE, Chawla MS, et al. Spatially resolved measurements of hyperpolarized gas properties in the lung in vivo. Part I: diffusion coefficient. *Magn Reson Med* 1999;42:721–728.
195. Chen XJ, Moller HE, Chawla MS, et al. Spatially resolved measurements of hyperpolarized gas properties in the lung in vivo. Part II: T*(2). *Magn Reson Med* 1999;42:729–37.
196. Hanisch G, Schreiber WG, Diergarten T, et al. Investigation of intrapulmonary diffusion by ^{3}He MRI. *Eur Radiol* 2000;10:S345.
197. Snider GL, Kleinerman J, Thurlbeck WM, Bengali ZH. The definition of emphysema. Report of a National Heart and Lung and Blood Institute, Division of Lung Diseases Workshop. *Am Rev Respir Dis* 1985;132:182–185.
198. Saam B, Yablonskiy D, Kodibagkar V, et al. MR imaging of diffusion of 3He gas in healthy and diseased lungs. *Magn Reson Med* 2000;44:174–179.
199. Chen X, Hedlund L, Moeller H, et al. Detection of emphysema in rat lungs using magnetic resonance measurements of 3He diffusion. *Proc Natl Acad Sci* 2000;97:11478–11481.
200. Salerno M, deLange E, Altes T, et al. Emphysema: hyperpolarized helium3 diffusion MR imaging of the lungs compared with spirometric indexes—initial experience. *Radiology* 2002;222:252–260.
201. Mugler J, Brookeman J, Knight-Scott J, et al. Regional measurement of the 3He diffusion coefficient in the human lung. *Proc Intl Soc Magn Reson Med* 1998;6:1906.
202. Salerno M, Mugler JP, DeLange EE, et al. Detection of early smoking related lung disease with diffusion-weighted hyperpolarized helium-3 lung imaging. RSNA 2003 Scientific Assembly and Annual Meeting Program, #881, p 526(abst).
203. Saam B, Happer W, Middleton H. Nuclear relaxation of 3He in the presence of O2. *Phys Rev A* 1995;52:862–865.
204. Eberle B, Weiler N, Markstaller K, et al. Analysis of intrapulmonary O(2) concentration by MR imaging of inhaled hyperpolarized helium-3. *J Appl Physiol* 1999;87:2043–2052.
205. Eberle B, Markstaller K, Lill J, et al. Oxygen-sensitive 3He magnetic resonance imaging of the lungs in patients after unilateral lung transplantation. *Am J Respir Crit Care Med* 2000;161:A718.
206. Moeller H, Hedlund L, Chen XJ, et al. Measurements of hyperpolarized gas properties in the lung. Part III: 3He T1. *Magn Reson Med* 2001;45:421–430.
207. Deninger AJ, Eberle B, Ebert M, et al. (3)he-MRI-based measurements of intrapulmonary p(O2) and its time course during apnea in healthy volunteers: first results, reproducibility, and technical limitations. *NMR Biomed* 2000;13:194–201.
208. Deninger A, Eberle B, Bermuth J, et al. Assessment of a single-acquisition imaging sequence for oxygen-sensitive 3He MRI. *Magn Reson Med* 2002;47:105–114.
209. Ishii M, Fischer MC, Yu J, et al. Regional lung perfusion mapping using hyperpolarized 3He MRI and validation to microsphere. *Proceedings of the International Society of Magnetic Resonance in Medicine,* 2004.
210. Eberle B, Markstaller K, Stepniak A, et al. 3Helium-MRI-based assessment of regional gas exchange impairment during experimental pulmonary artery occlusion. *Anesthesiology* 2002;96:A1309.
211. Fischer MC, Ishii M, Yu J, et al. Sensitivity of hyperpolarized 3He MRI in the detection of pulmonary embolism using glass beads occlusion in a porcine model. *Proceedings of the International Society of Magnetic Resonance in Medicine,* 2004.
212. Hasegawa I, Uematsu H, Gee J, Rogelj P, et al. Voxelwise mapping of magnetic resonance ventilation-perfusion ratio in a porcine model by multimodality registration: technical note. *Acad Radiol* 2003;10:1091–1096.
213. Deninger AJ, Eberle B, Ebert M, et al. Quantification of regional intrapulmonary oxygen partial pressure evolution during apnea by (3)He MRI. *J Magn Reson* 1999;141:207–216.
214. Olszowka AJ, Wagner PD. Numerical analysis of gas exchange. In: West JB, ed. *Pulmonary gas exchange.* Volume I: Ventilation, blood flow, and diffusion. New York: Academic Press, 1980:263–306.
215. Lipson DA, Fischer MC, Gefter W, et al. Human imaging of ventilation-perfusion ratios using hyperpolarized helium-3 MRI: preliminary results. *Proceedings of the International Society of Magnetic Resonance in Medicine,* 2004.
216. Rizi R, Baumgardner J, Edvinsson J, et al. RSNA 2003, Scientific Poster 504-P.
217. Rajaei S, Baumgardner JE, Ishii M, et al. Comparison of ventilation-perfusion obtained by polarized gas MRI with multiple inert gas elimination technique. *Proceedings of the International Society of Magnetic Resonance in Medicine,* 2004.
218. Albert MS, Cates GD, Driehuys B, et al. Biological magnetic resonance imaging using laser-polarized 129 Xe. *Nature* 1994;370:199–201.
219. Sakai K, Bilek AM, Oteiza E, et al. Temporal dynamics of hyperpolarized 129Xe resonances in living rats. *J Magn Reson B* 1996;111:300–304.
220. Albert MS, Tseng CH, Williamson D, et al. Hyperpolarized 129Xe MR imaging of the oral cavity. *J Magn Reson B* 1996;111:204–07.
221. Mugler JP III, Driehuys B, Brookeman JR, et al. MR imaging and spectroscopy using hyperpolarized 129Xe gas: preliminary human results. *Magn Reson Med* 1997;37:809–815.
222. Swanson SD, Rosen MS, Coulter KP, et al. Distribution and dynamics of laser-polarized 129Xe magnetization in vivo. *Magn Reson Med* 1999;42:1137–1145.
223. Ruppert K, Brookeman JR, Hagspiel KD, Mugler JP III. Probing lung physiology with xenon polarization transfer contrast (XTC). *Magn Reson Med* 2000;44:349–357.
224. Scheid P, Piper J. Diffusion. In: Crystal RG, ed. *The lung: scientific foundations.* Philadelphia: Lippincott-Raven, 1997:1681–1691.
225. Albertine KH. Structural organization and quantitative morphology of the lung. In: Cutillo AG, ed. *Application of magnetic resonance to the study of the lung.* New York: Futura, 1996:73–114.
226. Ruppert K, Brookeman JR, Hagspiel KD, et al. NMR of hyperpolarized 129Xe in the canine chest: spectral dynamics during a breath-hold. *NMR Biomed* 2000;13:220–228.
227. Ruppert K, Malta JF, Brookeman JR, et al. Exploring lung function with hyperpolarized (129)Xe nuclear magnetic resonance. *Magn Reson Med* 2004;51:676–687.
228. Edelman RR, Hatabu H, Tadamura E, et al. Noninvasive assessment of regional ventilation in the human lung using oxygen-enhanced magnetic resonance imaging. *Nat Med* 1996;2:1236–1239.
229. Loffler R, Muller CJ, Peller M, et al. Optimization and evaluation of the signal intensity change in multisection oxygen-enhanced MR lung imaging. *Magn Reson Med* 2000;43:860–866.
230. Mai VM, Liu B, Li W, et al. Influence of oxygen flow rate on signal and T(1) changes in oxygen-enhanced ventilation imaging. *J Magn Reson Imaging* 2002;16:37–41.
231. Muller CJ, Loffler R, Deimling M, et al. MR lung imaging at 0.2T with T1-weighted true FISP: native and oxygen-enhanced. *J Magn Reson Imaging* 2001;14:164–168.
232. Hatabu H, Tadamura E, Chen Q, et al. Pulmonary ventilation: dynamic MRI with inhalation of molecular oxygen. *Eur J Radiol* 2001;37:172–178.
233. Chen Q, Jakob PM, Griswold MA, et al. Oxygen-enhanced MR ventilation imaging of the lung. *MAGMA* 1998;7:153–161.

234. Chen Q, Levin DL, Kim D, et al. Pulmonary disorders: ventilation-perfusion MR imaging with animal models. *Radiology* 1999;213:871–879.
235. Ohno Y, Hatabu H, Takenaka D, et al. Oxygen-enhanced MR ventilation imaging of the lungs: preliminary experience in 25 subjects. *AJR Am J Roentgenol* 2001;177:185–194.
236. Ohno Y, Hatabu H, Takenaka D, et al. Dynamic oxygen-enhanced MRI reflects diffusing capacity of the lung. *Magn Reson Med* 2002;47: 1139–1144.
237. Muller CJ, Schwaiblmair M, Scheidler J, et al. Pulmonary diffusing capacity: assessment with oxygen-enhanced lung MR imaging preliminary findings. *Radiology* 2002;222:499–506.
238. Laukemper-Ostendorf S, Scholz A, Burger K, et al. 19F-MRI of perflubron for measurement of oxygen partial pressure in porcine lungs during partial liquid ventilation. *Magn Reson Med* 2002;47:82–89.
239. Schreiber WG, Eberle B, Laukemper-Ostendorf S, et al. Dynamic (19)F-MRI of pulmonary ventilation using sulfur hexafluoride (SF(6)) gas. *Magn Reson Med* 2001;45:605–613.
240. Tajik JK, Chon D, Won C, et al. Subsecond multisection CT of regional pulmonary ventilation. *Acad Radiol* 2002;9:130–146.
241. Simon B, Marcucci C, Fung M, Lele S. Parameter estimation and confidence intervals for Xe-CT ventilation studies: a Monte Carlo approach. *J Appl Physiol* 1998;84:709–716.
242. Kreck TC, Krueger MA, Altemeier WA, et al. Determination of regional ventilation and perfusion in the lung using xenon and computed tomography. *J Appl Physiol* 2001;91:1741–1749.
243. Thiele J, Klöppel R. Computertomographische messung der lungenventilation durch inhalation von isovist 300. *Röntgenpraxis* 1995;48: 259–260.
244. Yamaguchi K, Soejima K, Koda E, Sugiyama N. Inhaling gas with different CT densities allows detection of abnormalities in the lung periphery of patients with smoking-induced COPD. *Chest* 2001;120:1907–1916.
245. Cluzel P. Respiratory mechanics: CT and MRI. In: Kauczor H-U, ed. *Functional imaging of the chest.* Berlin: Springer, 2004:201–210.
246. Suga K, Tsukuda T, Awaya H, et al. Impaired respiratory mechanics in pulmonary emphysema: evaluation with dynamic breathing. *J Magn Reson Imaging* 1999;10:510–520.
247. Suga K, Tsukuda T, Awaya H, et al. Interactions of regional respiratory mechanics and pulmonary ventilatory impairment in pulmonary emphysema: assessment with dynamic MRI and xenon-133 single-photon emission CT. *Chest* 2000;117:1646–1655.
248. Chen Q, Mai VM, Bankier AA, et al. Ultrafast MR grid-tagging sequence for assessment of local mechanical properties of the lungs. *Magn Reson Med* 2001;45:24–28.
249. Napadow VJ, Mai V, Bankler A, et al. Determination of regional pulmonary parenchymal strain during normal respiration using spin inversion tagged magnetization MRI. *J Magn Reson Imaging* 2001;13:467–474.
250. Gee J, Sundaram T, Hasegawa I, et al. Characterization of regional pulmonary mechanics from serial magnetic resonance imaging data. *Acad Radiol* 2003;10:1147–1152.
251. Dougherty L, Asmuth JC, Gefter WB. Alignment of CT lung volumes with an optical flow method. *Acad Radiol* 2003;10:249–254.
252. Kitaoka H, Johkoh T, Koyama S, et al. A novel ventilation imaging by a voxel-based registration technique between inspiratory and expiratory 3D-CT images. Abstract 1393. Radiological Society of North America, Scientific Assembly and Annual Meeting Program, 2003:665.
253. Gefter WB. Functional CT imaging of the lungs: the pulmonary function test of the new millennium? [Guest Editorial]. *Acad Radiol* 2002;9:127–129.
254. Gefter WB, Hatabu H. Functional lung imaging: emerging methods to visualize regional pulmonary physiology. [Guest Editorial]. *Acad Radiol* 2003;10:1085–1089.

Index